D1567695

Fractures and Injuries of the Distal Radius and Carpus

Fractures and Injuries of the Distal Radius and Carpus: The Cutting Edge

David J. Slutsky, MD, FRCS

Assistant Professor,
UCLA David Geffen School of Medicine, Los Angeles;
Chief of Reconstruction Hand Surgery,
Harbor-UCLA Medical Center,
Hand and Wrist Institute
Torrance, California

A. Lee Osterman, MD

Professor, Orthopaedic and Hand Surgery
President, The Philadelphia Hand Center, P.C.,
and Hand Surgery Fellowship Program
Chairman, Division of Hand Surgery,
Department of Orthopaedic Surgery
Thomas Jefferson Medical College
Philadelphia, Pennsylvania

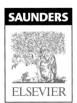

SAUNDERS

ELSEVIER

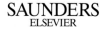

1600 John F. Kennedy Boulevard
Suite 1800
Philadelphia, Pennsylvania 19103-2899

FRACTURES AND INJURIES OF THE DISTAL RADIUS AND CARPUS: ISBN: 978-1-4160-4083-5
THE CUTTING EDGE
Copyright © 2009 by Saunders, an imprint of Elsevier Inc.

Library of Congress Cataloging-in-Publication Data
Slutsky, David J.
    Fractures and injuries of the distal radius and carpus : the cutting edge / David J. Slutsky, A. Lee Osterman.—1st ed.
        p. ; cm.
    Includes bibliographical references.
    ISBN 978-1-4160-4083-5
    1. Wrist—Wounds and injuries.   2. Wrist—Surgery.   3. Radius (Anatomy)—Fractures.   4. Radius (Anatomy)—Surgery.   I. Osterman, A. Lee.   II. Title.
    [DNLM: 1. Colles' Fracture—surgery.   2. Carpal Bones—injuries. WE 820 S634f 2009]
    RD559.S58 2009
    617.5′74044—dc22   2008020024

Acquisitions Editor: Daniel Pepper
Developmental Editor: Lucia Gunzel
Publishing Services Manager: Tina Rebane
Project Manager: Norm Stellander
Design Direction: Louis Forgione

Printed in China

Last digit is the print number: 9   8   7   6   5   4   3   2   1

Dedication

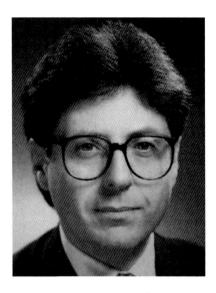

To my brother Samuel Slutsky, LLB, QC, whose work ethic and dedication to excellence inspired a sense of admiration that started me down this path.

DJS

To all the hand fellows who have taught and continue to teach me about the mysteries of life around the wrist.

ALO

Contributors

Joshua M. Abzug, MD

Chief Resident,
Department of Orthopaedic Surgery,
Drexel University,
Philadelphia, Pennsylvania
18. *Use of the T-Pin in the Treatment of Extra-articular Distal Radius Fractures*

Kimberly Z. Accardi, MD, CPT, MC, USAR

Department of Orthopaedic Surgery and Sports Medicine,
Drexel University Hahnemann Hospital,
Philadelphia, Pennsylvania
18. *Use of the T-Pin in the Treatment of Extra-articular Distal Radius Fractures*

Brian Adams, MD

Professor of Orthopaedic Surgery and Biomedical Engineering,
University of Iowa,
Iowa City, Iowa
29. *Ligament Reconstruction/Sigmoid Notch Plasty for DRUJ Instability*

B. A. Babb

Kleinert, Kutz and Associates Hand Center,
Louisville, Kentucky
37. *Distal Radioulnar Joint Prosthesis*

Alejandro Badia, MD

Chief of Hand Surgery,
Baptist Hospital,
Miami, Florida
13. *Volar Plate Fixation*

Gregory Bain, MBBS, FRCSC

Senior Lecturer, University of Adelaide;
Visiting Orthopaedic Surgeon,
Royal Adelaide Hospital;
South Australia Modbury Hospital,
Adelaide, South Australia, Australia
52. *Arthroscopic Release of Wrist Contracture*

Mark E. Baratz, MD

Professor of Orthopaedic Surgery,
Vice Chairman, Department of Orthopaedics,
Allegheny General Hospital,
Pittsburgh, Pennsylvania
34. *Sauvé-Kapandji Procedure after Distal Radius Fractures*

Ferdinando Battistella, MD

Chief Surgeon,
Center for Reconstructive Arthoscopic Shoulder Surgery,
Istituto Ortopaedico Galeazzi,
Milan, Italy
W7. *Arthroscopic Thermal Shrinkage for Scapholunate Ligament Injuries*

John M. Bednar, MD

Clinical Associate Professor of Orthopaedic Surgery,
Thomas Jefferson Medical College,
Philadelphia, Pennsylvania;
The South Jersey Hand Center,
Cherry Hill, New Jersey
26. *Arthroscopic Treatment of Triangular Fibrocartilage Complex Injuries*

Leon S. Benson, MD

Professor of Clinical Orthopaedic Surgery,
Northwestern University Feinberg School of Medicine,
Chicago;
Chief, Division of Hand and Upper Extremity Surgery,
Evanston Northwestern Healthcare,
Evanston, Illinois
12. *Fragment-Specific Fixation of Distal Radius Fractures*

Joseph Bergman, MD, FRCSC

Consulting Orthopaedic Surgeon,
Universitiy of Alberta Hospital,
Edmonton, Alberta, Canada
52. *Arthroscopic Release of Wrist Contracture*

Andrea Bialocerkowski, PhD

Senior Lecturer,
School of Physiotherapy,
The University of Melbourne,
Melbourne, Australia
W2. *A Patient-Focused Wrist Outcome Instrument—the Adelaide Questionnaire*

Adrian L. Butler, MD

Staff, Lancaster General Hospital;
Orthopaedic Associates of Lancaster,
Lancaster, Pennsylvania
33. *Arthroscopic Wafer Resection*

Douglas A. Campbell, ChM, FRCS(Ed), FRCS(Orth), FFSEM(UK)

Honorary Senior Lecturer,
University of Leeds;
Consultant, Hand and Wrist Surgery,
Leeds General Infirmary,
Leeds, United Kingdom
28. Ulnar Head and Styloid Fractures

Ronaldo S. Carneiro, MD

Head of the Hand Surgery Department,
Medical-Surgical Specialists,
Naples, Florida
10. Dorsal Plate Fixation

George D. Chloros, MD

Fellow,
Department of Orthopaedic Surgery,
Wake Forest University School of Medicine,
Winston-Salem, North Carolina
24. Complex Regional Pain Syndrome after Distal Radius Fractures

Mark S. Cohen, MD

Professor,
Department of Orthopaedic Surgery;
Director, Hand and Elbow Section;
Director, Orthopaedic Education,
Rush Universitiy Medical Center,
Chicago, Illinois
46. Open Scapholunate Ligament Repair

Randall W. Culp, MD

Professor of Orthopaedics, Hand and Microsurgery,
Thomas Jefferson University;
Attending, Thomas Jefferson University Hospital,
Methodist Hospital, Philadelphia;
Courtesy Staff, Delaware County Memorial Hospital,
Drexel Hill;
The Philadelphia Hand Center P.C.,
King of Prussia, Pennsylvania
33. Arthroscopic Wafer Resection

Phani K. Dantuluri, MD

Assistant Clinical Professor,
Department of Orthopaedics,
Thomas Jefferson Medical College;
Thomas Jefferson University Hospital;
Philadelphia Hand Center,
Philadelphia, Pennsylvania
W4. Intramedullary Fixation of Distal Radius Fractures

Lauren M. DeTullio, MS, OTR/L

Philadelphia Hand Center,
Philadelphia, Pennsylvania
W8. Rehabilitation after Carpal Ligament Injury

Joseph J. Dias, MD, MBBS, FRCS(Edin), FRCS(Eng)

Professor of Hand and Orthopaedic Surgery,
University of Leicester School of Medicine;
Department of Health Sciences,
Division of Orthopaedic Surgery,
Glenfield Hospital, Leicester, England
2. Nonoperative Treatment of Distal Radius Fractures

Dean Federman, MBBS

Department of Radiology,
The Alfred Hospital,
Melbourne, Victoria, Australia
W1. Role of Advanced Imaging in Distal Radius Fractures

Diego L. Fernandez, MD

Professor of Orthopaedic Surgery,
University of Berne;
Staff Member,
Department of Orthopaedic Surgery,
Lindenhof Hospital,
Berne, Switzerland
56. Arthroscopic-Assisted Osteotomy for Intra-articular Malunion of the Distal Radius

Alan E. Freeland, MD

Professor Emeritus,
University of Mississippi School of Medicine;
Professor Emeritus and Research Consultant,
University of Mississippi Health Care,
Jackson, Mississippi
W3. Biomechanics and Biology of Plate Fixation of Distal Radius Fractures

Marc Garcia-Elias, MD, PhD

Hand Surgeon Specialist,
Institut Kaplan,
Barcelona, Spain
53. Management of Lost Pronosupination

Steven H. Goldberg, MD

Attending Orthopaedic Surgeon and
Hand Surgeon, Hand Surgery, Ltd,
Milwaukee, Wisconsin
47. Arthroscopic Treatment of Scapholunate Ligament Tears

Renato Gonçalves, MD

Chief, Hand and Reconstructive Microsurgery,
Department of Orthopaedics,
Canta Casa de Misericordia,
Salvador, Bahia, Brazil
10. Dorsal Plate Fixation

Ruby Grewal, MD, MSc, FRCSC

Assistant Professor,
Department of Surgery,
University of Western Ontario;
Orthopaedic Surgeon,
Hand and Upper Limb Clinic,
London, Ontario, Canada
17. Kapandji Pinning of Distal Radius Fractures

Douglas P. Hanel, MD

Professor, Hand and Microsurgery,
Department of Orthopaedics and Sports Medicine,
Universitiy of Washington;
Harborview Medical Center,
Seattle, Washington
*4. Distal Radius Study Group: Purpose, Method, Results, and
  Implications for Reporting Outcomes*
19. Bridge Plating of Distal Radius Fractures

Brian J. Hartigan, MD

Assistant Professor of Clinical Orthopaedic Surgery,
Northwestern University Feinberg School of Medicine,
Chicago, Illinois
*23. Use of Bone Graft Substitutes and Bioactive Materials in
  Treatment of Distal Radius Fractures*

Michael R. Hausman, MD

Robert K. Lippmann Professor of Orthopaedic Surgery,
Mount Sinai School of Medicine;
Chief, Hand and Elbow Surgery,
Vice-Chairman, Department of Orthopaedic Surgery,
Mount Sinai Medical Center,
New York, New York
9. Surgical Approaches from an Angiosomal Perspective

Carlos Heras-Palou, MD, FRCS (Trau & Orth)

Consultant Hand Surgeon,
Pulvertaft Hand Center,
Derbyshire Royal Infirmary,
Derby, United Kingdom
42. Midcarpal Instability

Mojca Herman, MA, OTR/L, CHT

Part-time Faculty,
University of Southern California,
Los Angeles, California
W5. Rehabilitation after Distal Radius Fractures

Heather Hopkins, MA, OTR/L

Lead Occupational Therapist,
Orthopaedic Surgery and Sports Medicine,
Stamford, Connectcut
W5. Rehabilitation after Distal Radius Fractures

Asif M. Ilyas, MD

Assistant Professor, Orthopaedic Surgery,
Temple University School of Medicine;
Director, Temple Hand Center,
Temple University Hospital,
Philadelphia, Pennsylvania
14. Volar Rim and Barton's Fracture

Meghan Imrie, MD

Chief Resident,
Department of Orthopaedic Surgery,
Stanford University Medical Center,
Palo Alto, California
1. Distal Radius Fractures: A Historical Perspective

Sidney M. Jacoby, MD

Hand Fellow,
The Philadelphia Hand Center;
Thomas Jefferson University Hospital,
Philadelphia, Pennsylvania
20. Arthroscopic-Assisted Treatment of Distal Radius Fractures

Tijmen de Jong, MD

Resident, Department of Plastic and Hand Surgery,
Medical Center Leeuwarden,
Leeuwarden, The Netherlands
30. Dorsal Capsuloplasty in Volar Subluxation of the Distal Radius

Jesse B. Jupiter, MD

Hansjorg WYSS/AO Professor of Orthopaedic Surgery,
Harvard Medical School;
Director, Hand and Upper Extremity Service,
Boston, Massachusetts
14. Volar Rim and Barton's Fracture

Lana Kang, MD

Clinical Instructor of Orthopaedic Surgery,
Weill Medical College of Cornell University;
Assistant Attending Orthopaedic Surgeon,
Hospital for Special Surgery,
New York, New York
6. Bridging External Fixation with Pin Augmentation

**Eoin C. Kavanagh, MB, BCh, BAO, MRCPI, FFR, RCSI,
  MSc**

Senior Lecturer, Radiological Science,
University of Dublin School of Medicine and Medical Sciences;
Consultant Radiologist,
Mater Misericordiae Hospital,
Dublin, Ireland
W1. Role of Advanced Imaging in Distal Radius Fractures

Prakash Khanchandani, MD

Hand Fellow,
Miami Hand Center,
Miami, Florida
13. Volar Plate Fixation

Graham J. W. King, MD, MSc, FRCSC

Professor, Department of Surgery,
University of Western Ontario;
Chief, Division of Orthopaedic Surgery,
St. Joseph's Health Center,
London, Ontario, Canada
17. Kapandji Pinning of Distal Radius Fractures

William B. Kleinman, MD

Clinical Professor of Orthopaedic Surgery,
Indiana University School of Medicine;
President and Attending Surgeon,
Indiana Hand Center,
Indianapolis, Indiana
25. Stability of the Distal Radioulnar Joint

A. Richard Koch, MD

Head and Participant Teacher,
Dutch Hand Fellow Program,
Haga Hand and Wrist Center, The Hague,
Amsterdam, The Netherlands
30. Dorsal Capsuloplasty in Volar Subluxation of the Distal Radius

L. Andrew Koman, MD

Professor and Chair,
Department of Orthopaedic Surgery,
Wake Forest University School of Medicine,
Winston-Salem, North Carolina
24. Complex Regional Pain Syndrome after Distal Radius Fractures

George Koulouris, MBBS, FRANZCR, MMed, GradCertSpMed

Department of Radiology,
The Alfred Hospital,
Melbourne, Victoria, Australia
W1. Role of Advanced Imaging in Distal Radius Fractures

Kenneth J. Koval, MD

Orthopaedic Surgeon,
Dartmouth-Hitchcock Medical Center,
Lebanon, New Hampshire
4. Distal Radius Study Group: Purpose, Method, Results, and Implications for Reporting Outcomes

Scott H. Kozin, MD

Associate Professor,
Department of Orthopaedic Surgery,
Temple University School of Medicine;
Director, Upper Extremity Center of Excellence,
Shriners Hospital for Children,
Philadelphia, Pennsylvania
15. Pediatric Distal Radius Fractures

Anthony J. Lauder, MD, BS

Assistant Professor,
University of Nebraska College of Medicine;
University of Nebraska Medical Center;
Veterans Affairs Medical Center,
Omaha, Nebraska
32. The Ulnar-Shortening Osteotomy

Zhongyu Li, MD

Assistant Professor,
Department of Orthopaedic Surgery,
Wake Forest University School of Medicine,
Winston-Salem, North Carolina
24. Complex Regional Pain Syndrome after Distal Radius Fractures

Tommy Lindau, MD, PhD

Assistant Professor,
University of Derby;
Consultant Hand Surgeon,
Pulvertaft Hand Center,
Derbyshire Royal Infirmary,
Derby, United Kingdom
45. Arthroscopic Diagnosis of Carpal Ligament Injuries with Distal Radius Fractures

Kurre T. Luber, MD

Resident Physician,
Department of Orthopaedic Surgery and Rehabilitation,
University of Mississippi Medical Center,
Jackson, Mississippi
W3. Biomechanics and Biology of Plate Fixation of Distal Radius Fractures

Richard L. Makowiec, MD

Assistant Professor of Clinical Orthopaedic Surgery,
Northwestern University Feinberg School of Medicine,
Chicago, Illinois
23. Use of Bone Graft Substitutes and Bioactive Materials in Treatment of Distal Radius Fractures

K. J. Malone, MD

Fellow in Hand Surgery,
Department of Orthopaedics and Sports Medicine,
University of Washington,
Seattle, Washington
19. Bridge Plating of Distal Radius Fractures

P. A. Martineau, MD, FRCSC

Fellow in Hand Surgery,
Department of Orthopaedics and Sports Medicine,
University of Washington,
Seattle, Washington
19. Bridge Plating of Distal Radius Fractures

Christophe Mathoulin, MD

Associate Professor,
Institut de la Main,
Paris, France
44. The Role of Arthroscopy in Scaphoid Fractures

Michael K. Matthew, MD

Assistant Professor of Plastic Surgery,
Yale University, Yale New Haven Hospital,
New Haven, Connecticut
9. Surgical Approaches from an Angiosomal Perspective

Robert J. Medoff, MD

Assistant Clinical Professor of Orthopaedic Surgery,
John A. Burns School of Medicine,
University of Hawaii;
Castle Medical Center,
Kailua, Hawaii
3. Radiographic Evaluation and Classification of Distal Radius Fractures; 12. Fragment-Specific Fixation of Distal Radius Fractures

Greg A. Merrell, MD

Clinical Assistant Professor of Orthopaedic Surgery,
Indiana University School of Medicine,
Hand Surgeon, Indiana Hand Center,
Indianapolis, Indiana
21. Simultaneous Fractures of the Scaphoid and Distal Radius;
50. Bone-Ligament-Bone Reconstruction

Ather Mirza, MD

Chief of Hand and Microsurgery,
St. Catherine of Siena Medical Center,
Director, North Shore Surgi-Center, Smithtown;
Assistant Clinical Professor,
Stony Brook University,
Stony Brook, New York
7. Distal Radius Fractures Treated with the CPX System

Steven L. Moran, MD

Associate Professor of Plastic and Orthopaedic Surgery,
Mayo Clinic,
Rochester, Minnesota
49. Modified Brunelli Tenodesis for the Treatment of
  Scapholunate Instability

William B. Morrison, MD

Associate Professor,
Department of Radiology,
Jefferson Medical College,
Thomas Jefferson University,
Philadelphia, Pennsylvania
W1. Role of Advanced Imaging in Distal Radius Fractures

Chaitanya S. Mudgal, MD, MS(Orth), MCh(Orth)

Instructor in Orthopaedic Surgery,
Harvard Medical School;
Orthopaedic Hand Service,
Massachusetts General Hospital,
Boston, Massachusetts
14. Volar Rim and Barton's Fracture

Daniel J. Nagle, MD

Professor of Clinical Orthopaedics,
Northwestern Feinberg School of Medicine,
Chicago, Illinois
W6. Capsular Shrinkage in the Treatment of Wrist Instability

David Nelson, MD, BS Electronic Engineering,
  MA Physiology

Webmaster, *www.eRadius.com,*
San Francisco, California
16. Complications of Locked Volar Plates

A. Lee Osterman, MD

Professor, Orthopaedic and Hand Surgery,
Chairman, Division of Hand Surgery,
Department of Orthopaedic Surgery,
President, The Philadelphia Hand Center,
P.C. and Hand Surgery Fellowship Program,
Thomas Jefferson Medical College,
Philadelphia, Pennsylvania
20. Arthroscopic-Assisted Treatment of Distal Radius Fractures;
26. Arthroscopic Treatment of Triangular Fibrocartilage
  Complex Injuries

Anastasios Papadonikolakis, MD

Resident,
Department of Orthopaedic Surgery,
Wake Forest University School of Medicine,
Winston-Salem, North Carolina
24. Complex Regional Pain Syndrome after Distal
  Radius Fractures

Rita M. Patterson, PhD

Department of Osteopathic Manipulative Medicine,
University of North Texas Health Science Center,
Fort Worth, Texas
41. The Dorsal Ligaments of the Wrist

Soheil Payvandi, DO

Shoulder and Elbow Fellow,
Cleveland Orthopaedic and Spine Hospital at
  Lutheran Hospital,
Cleveland, Ohio
55. Scaphoid Hemiresection and Arthrodesis of the
  Radiocarpal Joint

Francisco del Piñal, MD

Chief, Unit of Hand-Wrist and Plastic Surgery,
Hospital Mutua Montañesa,
Director, Instituto de Cirugía Plástica y de la Mano,
Santander, Spain
57. Role of Advanced Imaging in Distal Radius Fractures;
W9. Reconstruction of the Distal Radius Facet by a Free
  Vascularized Osteochondral Graft

Matthew D. Putnam, MD

Professor,
Department of Orthopaedic Surgery,
Universitiy of Minnesota,
Minneapolis, Minnesota
4. Distal Radius Study Group: Purpose, Method, Results, and
  Implications for Reporting Outcomes

Cynthia Radi-Peters, OTR, CHT

Hand Therapist,
Physicians Regional Medical Center,
Naples, Florida
10. Dorsal Plate Fixation

Gregory H. Rafijah, MD

Assistant Professor,
UCLA School of Medicine, Los Angeles;
Chief of Hand Surgery,
Harbor UCLA Medical Center,
Torrance, California
43. Perilunate Injuries of the Wrist

Keith B. Raskin, MD

Clinical Associate Professor,
Department of Orthopaedic Surgery,
New York University Hospital for Joint Diseases,
New York, New York
22. Galeazzi Fracture-Dislocations

Hamid R. Redjal, MD

Resident Physician,
Harbor UCLA Medical Center,
Torrance, California
43. Perilunate Injuries of the Wrist

Mary Kate Reinhart, MS, CNP

Nurse Practitioner,
Smithtown, New York
7. Distal Radius Fractures Treated with the CPX System

Michael E. Rettig, MD

Assistant Professor,
Department of Orthopaedic Surgery,
New York University Hospital for Joint Diseases,
New York, New York
22. Galeazzi Fracture-Dislocations

Kongkhet Riansuwan, MD

Assistant Professor of Orthopaedic Surgery,
Orthopaedic Trauma Service,
Department of Orthopaedic Surgery,
Mahidol University;
Faculty of Medicine, Siriraj Hospital,
Bangkok, Thailand
47. Arthroscopic Treatment of Scapholunate Ligament Tears

Daniel A. Rikli, MD, PD

Associate Professor,
University of Basel,
Basel, Switzerland
11. Dorsal Double Plating and Combined Palmar and Dorsal Plating for Distal Radius Fractures

David C. Ring, MD, PhD

Assistant Professor of Orthopaedic Surgery,
Harvard Medical School;
Medical Director and Director of Research,
Orthopaedic Hand and Upper Extremity Service,
Massachusetts General Hospital,
Boston, Massachusetts
54. Treatment of Ununited Fractures of the Distal Radius

Marco J. P. F. Ritt, MD, PhD

Professor of Hand Surgery,
Department of Plastic Surgery,
VU University;
Head, Department of Plastic, Reconstructive and Hand Surgery,
VU University Medical Center,
Amsterdam, The Netherlands
40. Kinematics of the Lunotriquetral Joint

Melvin P. Rosenwasser, MD

Robert E. Carroll Professor of Orthopaedic Surgery,
Columbia University College of Physicians and Surgeons;
Director of the Orthopaedic Hand and Trauma Service,
Department of Orthopaedic Surgery,
New York Orthopaedic Hospital,
Columbia University Medical Center,
New York, New York
4. Distal Radius Study Group: Purpose, Method, Results, and Implications for Reporting Outcomes;
47. Arthroscopic Treatment of Scapholunate Ligament Tears

David E. Ruchelsman, MD

Department of Orthopaedic Surgery,
New York University Hospital for Joint Diseases,
New York, New York
22. Galeazzi Fracture-Dislocations

Vera Sallen, MD

Fellow, Institut de la Main,
Paris, France
44. The Role of Arthroscopy in Scaphoid Fractures

Michael Sauerbier, MD, PhD

Associate Professor,
University of Heidelberg;
Professor and Chairman,
Department for Plastic, Hand, and Reconstruction Surgery,
Main-Taunus-Hospitals, GmbH,
Academic Hospital of Frankfurt, Germany
27. Anatomy and Biomechanics of Forearm Rotation

Luis R. Scheker, MD

Assistant Consulting Professor of Surgery,
Duke University Medical Center,
Durham, North Carolina;
Associate Clinical Professor of Surgery, Plastic and Reconstructive,
University of Louisville School of Medicine;
Kleinert, Kutz and Associates Hand Center,
Louisville, Kentucky
37. Distal Radioulnar Joint Prosthesis

Jöerg van Schoonhoven, MD, PhD

Consultant Hand Surgeon,
Clinic for Surgery of the Hand,
Bad Neustadt, Germany
36. Ulnar Head Implants: Unconstrained

William H. Seitz Jr., MD

Clinical Professor of Surgery,
Cleveland Clinic Lerner College of Medicine of Case Western
 Reserve University;
Executive Director,
Cleveland Orthopaedic and Spine Hospital at
 Lutheran Hospital,
Cleveland, Ohio
*55. Scaphoid Hemiresection and Arthrodesis of the
 Radiocarpal Joint*

Alexander Y. Shin, MD

Professor,
Department of Orthopaedic Surgery,
Mayo College of Medicine,
Rochester, Minnesota
38. Carpal Anatomy

Heidi C. Shors, MD

University of Washington Hand Center,
Department of Orthopaedics and Sports Medicine,
University of Washington Medical Center,
Seattle, Washington
34. Sauvé-Kapandji Procedure after Distal Radius Fractures

Terri M. Skirven, OTR/L, CHT

Director, Hand Rehabilitation Foundation;
Director of Therapy, The Philadelphia Hand
 Center, P.C.;
Philadelphia, Pennsylvania
W8. Rehabilitation after Carpal Ligament Injury

Joseph F. Slade III, MD

Department of Orthopaedics and Rehabilitation,
Yale University School of Medicine,
New Haven, Connecticut
21. Simultaneous Fractures of the Scaphoid and Distal Radius

David J. Slutsky, MD

Assistant Professor,
UCLA David Geffen School of Medicine, Los Angeles;
Chief of Reconstruction Hand Surgery,
Harbor-UCLA Medical Center,
South Bay Hand Surgery Center,
Torrance, California
5. Factors Infuencing the Outcome of Distal Radius Fractures;
8. External Fixation of Distal Radius Fractures;
51. Dorsal Radiocarpal Ligament Tears;
W5. Rehabilitation after Distal Radius Fractures

Beth P. Smith, MD, PhD

Associate Professor,
Department of Orthopaedic Surgery,
Wake Forest University School of Medicine,
Winston-Salem, North Carolina
*24. Complex Regional Pain Syndrome after Distal
 Radius Fractures*

Kathryne J. Stabile, MD, MS

Resident in Orthopaedic Surgery,
Wake Forest University,
Winston-Salem, North Carolina
31. Essex-Lopresti Fractures

John K. Stanley, MB, ChB, MCh(Orth), FRCS(Ed), FRCS

Professor of Hand Surgery,
University of Manchester;
Chief of Staff,
Center for Hand and Upper Limb Surgery,
 Wrightington Hospital,
Appley Bridge, Lancashire, United Kingdom
39. Chronic Volar-Flexed Intercalated Segment Instability

Robert M. Szabo, MD, MPH

Professor of Orthopaedics and Plastic Surgery,
University of California, Davis School of Medicine;
Chief of Hand and Upper Extremity Surgery,
University of California, Davis Health System,
Sacramento, California
48. Dorsal Capsulodesis

Julio Taleisnik, MD

Clinical Professor,
Department of Surgery (Orthopaedics),
University of California, Irvine,
Irvine, California
Foreword

John S. Taras, MD

Associate Professor,
Department of Orthopaedic Surgery,
Thomas Jefferson Medical College;
Associate Professor and Chief,
Division of Hand Surgery,
Drexel University,
Philadelphia, Pennsylvania
*18. Use of the T-Pin in the Treatment of Extra-articular Distal
 Radius Fractures*

Matthew M. Tomaino, MD, MBA

Founder, Tomaino Orthopaedic Care for Shoulder, Hand,
 and Elbow, LLC.,
Rochester, New York
31. Essex-Lopresti Fractures

Thomas E. Trumble, MD, BS

Professor and Chief,
Division of Hand and Microvascular Surgery,
Department of Orthopaedic Surgery,
University of Washington School of Medicine;
Harborview Medical Center;
Children's Regional Medical Center,
Seattle, Washington
32. The Ulnar-Shortening Osteotomy

Frank Unglaub, MD

Resident, Department of Plastic and Hand Surgery,
University of Erlangen, Germany
27. *Anatomy and Biomechanics of Forearm Rotation*

Steven F. Viegas, MD

Professor and Chief,
Division of Hand Surgery,
Department of Orthopaedics and Rehabilitation,
Professor, Department of Anatomy and Neurosciences,
Professor, Department of Preventive Medicine and
  Community Health,
University of Texas Medical Branch,
Galveston, Texas
41. *The Dorsal Ligaments of the Wrist*

Arnold-Peter C. Weiss, MD

Professor of Orthopaedics,
Assistant Dean of Medicine (Admissions),
Warren Alpert Medical School of Brown University,
Providence, Rhode Island
50. *Bone-Ligament-Bone Reconstruction*

Lisa A. Whitty, MD

Fellow in Plastic Surgery,
Mayo School of Medicine,
Rochester, Minnesota
49. *Modified Brunelli Tenodesis for the Treatment of
  Scapholunate Instability*

Ethan R. Wiesler, MD

Associate Professor,
Department of Orthopaedic Surgery,
Wake Forest University School of Medicine,
Winston-Salem, North Carolina
24. *Complex Regional Pain Syndrome after Distal
  Radius Fractures*

Jennifer Moriatis Wolf, MD

Assistant Professor,
Department of Orthopaedic Surgery,
University of Colorado Health Sciences Center,
Denver, Colorado
38. *Carpal Anatomy*

Scott Wolfe, MD

Professor of Orthopaedic Surgery,
Weill Medical College of Cornell University;
Chief, Hand and Upper Extremity Surgery,
Hospital for Special Surgery,
New York, New York
6. *Bridging External Fixation with Pin Augmentation*

Jeffrey Yao, MD

Assistant Professor,
Robert A. Chase Hand and Upper Limb Center,
Department of Orthopaedic Surgery,
Stanford University Medical Center,
Palo Alto, California
1. *Distal Radius Fractures: A Historical Perspective*

Naoya Yazaki, MD

Chief Surgeon,
Department of Orthopaedic Surgery,
Nagoya Ekisaikai Hospital,
Nagoya, Aichi, Japan
41. *The Dorsal Ligaments of the Wrist*

David S. Zelouf, MD

Clinical Instructor,
Department of Orthopaedic Surgery,
Thomas Jefferson University Hospital,
Philadelphia, Pennsylvania
35. *Hemi-resection Interposition Arthroplasty*

Foreword

Why another textbook about the wrist and its injuries? Because this is a field that is constantly innovating.

After Etienne Destot's treatise "Traumatismes du Poignet et Rayon X" was published in 1923, there were several notable contributions to the literature on wrist anatomy, function, and injury, particularly from European investigators. It was not until the last few decades of the 20th century, however, that textbooks dedicated exclusively to the wrist saw the light of day. Simultaneously, there was an exponential growth of papers dedicated to the wrist, making each new textbook outdated almost as soon as it was published. These papers, however, were scattered through the many journals dedicated to orthopaedics and hand surgery. The practitioner in search of guidance from the peer-reviewed medical literature frequently encountered conflicting, confusing, or inconclusive answers, if answers were found. This book should correct this deficiency.

Doctors David Slutsky and Lee Osterman have undertaken a truly monumental task, both in its scope and in the selection of an incredible list of international contributors. I am convinced that I, and all readers regardless of their experience and expertise, will find much to learn. I am also convinced that this will become a "must-have" textbook for all those interested in the treatment of injuries to the distal radius and carpus. Doctors Slutsky and Osterman have assembled a distinguished panel of experts. Unlike similar endeavors in the past, with contributors generally from a single country or region, the experts for this text include a worldwide selection of innovative physicians and investigators.

I did not find a single subject that was not covered, and I expect that there will be an answer to any questions that practitioners may have when faced with the treatment of injuries to the wrist. The inclusion of video imaging on the accompaning website to further illustrate wrist kinematics, carpal instability patterns, and surgical techniques is an exciting addition to this very ambitious undertaking. I am honored to have been asked to write a foreword to this book, and I am eager to own the published work.

Julio Taleisnik, MD

Preface

There has been an explosion in the number of internal fixation devices available for the treatment of complex intra-articular distal radius fractures. Locking volar plate designs have continued to evolve along with innovative techniques for reduction of the articular fragments. Limited internal fixation of individual fragments has become a mainstay of treatment, but intramedullary fixation is also a viable option. Joint bridging external fixation is typically used to unload the joint surface, but newer external fixators allow early wrist motion in both extra-articular and intra-articular fractures. Pain on the ulnar side of the wrist has become the proverbial black box of wrist surgery and is underrepresented in most textbooks. This book includes 13 chapters devoted entirely to the diagnosis and treatment of ulnar-sided wrist pain and instability of the distal radioulnar joint as well as a thorough coverage of the latest advancements in ulnar head replacement. The treatment of carpal ligament injuries has also undergone a renaissance with many new arthroscopic and open procedures that hold promise for the future. No book would be complete without a discussion of the complications, outcome assessments, and salvage procedures.

This book is intended to serve as a user's manual for both the entry-level wrist surgeon as well as the experienced operator. The methodology and the practical aspects of each procedure are stressed along with myriad pearls and tips, oftentimes from the originators of the technique. The videos on the accompanying website illustrate the techniques and provide a glimpse into the surgical anatomy in real time.

We are indebted to our contributors, without whom this book would not exist. We appreciate the time, effort, and personal sacrifice they have put forth to educate their peers. We are also indebted to Kim Murphy, Senior Publishing Director of Global Medicine at Elsevier, for allowing us to move forward with this project, as well as the associate editors who contributed their time and energy to this project, including the tireless Lucia Gunzel, Emily Christie, and Norman Stellander. Once again Bruce Robison and his audiovisual crew did a fantastic job on the accompanying website. It was a real joy working with many of the pioneers and innovators in wrist and hand surgery and we hope the reader experiences the same.

David J. Slutsky, MD, FRCS(C)
A. Lee Osterman, MD

Contents

Web Only Chapters

Web Only Videos

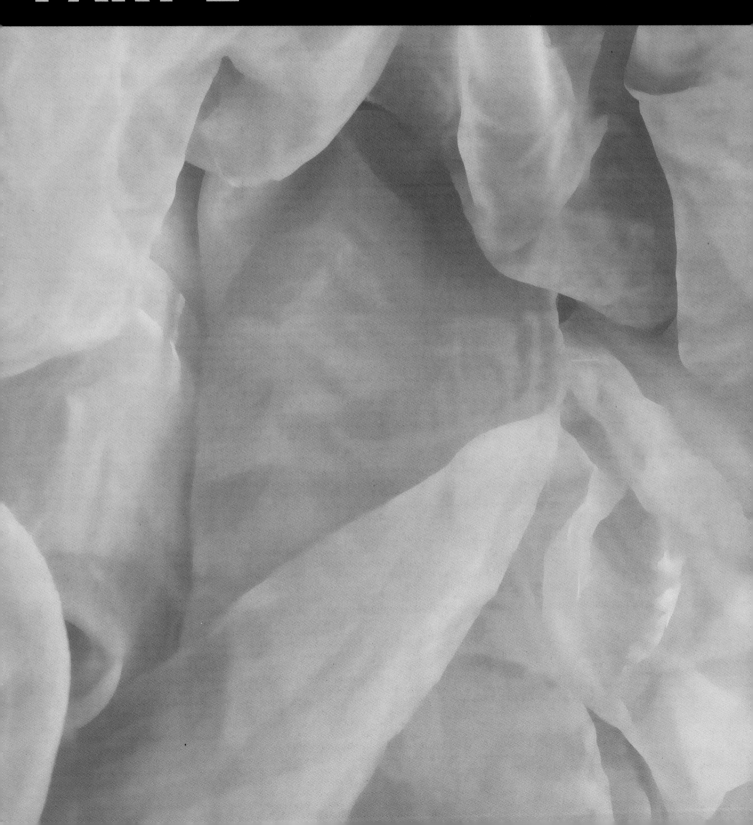

PART 1 INTRODUCTION

Distal Radius Fractures: A Historical Perspective

Meghan Imrie, MD and Jeffrey Yao, MD

Most discussions of distal radius fractures start with Colles' description published in 1814 under the title "On the Fracture of the Carpal Extremity of the Radius" and its now well-known proclamation that

"One consolation only remains, that the limb at some remote period again enjoy perfect freedom in all its motions, and be completely exempt from pain."[1]

Needless to say, the medical world has changed since the days of the eponymous Colles, and so have the etiology, diagnosis, classification, and treatment of distal radius fractures. It is an exciting time in the 21st century with many new technical advances in the treatment of this ageless injury. These advances are thoroughly discussed throughout this textbook. Before we move forward, however, it is worthwhile to look back to where we started. This chapter provides an overview of the history of the diagnosis and treatment of distal radius fractures, from the time before Colles to the present.

Fracture Description

In the Beginning

Distal radius fractures were historically thought of as dislocations of the wrist, from Hippocrates' time until the 18th century, when Petit first posed the possibility that they may be fractures.[2] The memoir of Pouteau, chief surgeon of L'Hotel Dieu in Lyon, published in 1783, described distal radius fractures as such, and recognized that there were several types.[3] This memoir predates Colles' article by 30 years, and in France, distal radius fractures are still often referred to as Pouteau-Colles fractures.[4]

Abraham Colles (**Fig. 1-1**) was born in 1773, near Kilkerny, Ireland; he presumably became interested in medicine after receiving an anatomy book in gratitude from the town surgeon after a flood swept away all of the surgeon's possessions. Colles trained in Dublin and Edinburgh, obtained his medical degree in 1797, and was elected president of the Royal College of Surgeons of Ireland in 1802 at age 29. His landmark work on distal radius fractures was published in 1814,[1] preceded by an article on surgical anatomy in 1811, and followed by an article on clubfoot (1818) and a text on venereal disease and the use of mercury (1837). His contribution to orthopaedics does not include an illustration or any description of the dissection of the injury, which is surprising given his reputation as an anatomist. His work is an explanation for his logic as to why the injury is likely a fracture rather than a dislocation. Colles made this assumption based on the presence of crepitus typical to well-described fractures at the time. He discussed the tendency of the wrist to revert to its deformity at

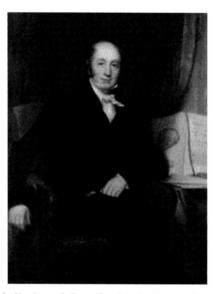

FIGURE 1-1 Abraham Colles. *(Reprinted with permission from the Colles-Graves foundation, New York.)*

the time of injury in the absence of appropriate immobilization, and the importance of guarding "against the carpal end of the radius being drawn backwards," recognizing the deleterious effect of loss of palmar tilt.

Colles concluded his work with the following remarks:

"I cannot conclude these observations without remarking that were my opinion to be drawn from those cases only which have occurred to me, I should consider this as by far the most common injury to which the wrist or carpal extremities are exposed. During the last three years I have not met a single instance of Desault's dislocation of the inferior end of the radius while I have had opportunities of seeing a vast number of the fracture of the lower end of this bone."[1]

This statement suggests that fractures of the distal radius were likely just as common in 1814 as they are today.

Colles' article was published in a narrowly distributed medical journal, the *Edinburgh Medical Surgical Journal*, and received little attention until Dupuytren brought the distal radius fracture to the attention of his students and to the surgical world at large via published lectures:

"One would have thought that the observations of these writers [Petit, Pouteau, and Desault] would have raised some doubts in

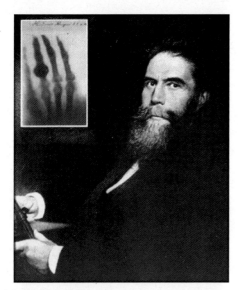

FIGURE 1-2 Wilhelm Conrad Röntgen. *(Reprinted with permission from Bill DeHope.)*

TABLE 1-1   Gartland and Werley System of Classification

Group	Description
1	Simple Colles' fracture with no involvement of the radial articular surface
2	Comminuted Colles' fracture with involvement of the radial articular surface
3	Comminuted Colles' fracture with involvement of the radial articular surface with displacement of the fragments
4	Extra-articular, nondisplaced (added by Solgaard in 1985)

Adapted from Gartland JJ, Werley CW: Evaluation of healed Colles' fractures. J Bone Joint Surg Am 1951; 33:895–907.

the minds of modern surgeons on this obscure point of doctrine: but not so; for we find Richerand, Boyer, Delpech, Leveille, Monteggia and Samuel Cooper adhering to old errors; and they have unanimously admitted four dislocations at the wrist."[5]

Goyrand in the 1830s noted that most cases of distal radius fractures had dorsal displacement, but also described occasional cases of palmar displacement and illustrated both.[6,7] Nelaton contributed to the anatomical study of these injuries and to the study of the mechanism of injury using cadavers with his paper in 1844.[8] In 1838, Barton of the United States described a fracture-dislocation of the radiocarpal joint, saying, as many authors (including Colles) prior had, that these injuries are often mistaken for sprains or dislocations of the wrist. Barton distinguished the injury under discussion, however, by describing a subluxation of the wrist resulting from a fracture through the distal radial articular surface, not to be mistaken for fractures "of the radius, or of the radius and ulna, just above, and not involving the joint."[9] Smith published a chapter, "Fractures of the Bones of the Forearm, in the Vicinity of the Wrist-Joint," in 1847 describing the anatomy of Colles' fracture and a palmarly displaced distal radius fracture, although he did not have the benefit of an anatomical specimen as Goyrand did a decade earlier.[10]

And Then There Was Röntgen

The discovery and development of roentgenography in late 1895 was a significant advance in the nature of fracture evaluation and treatment. Wilhelm Conrad Röntgen (**Fig. 1-2**) was born in Prussia and emigrated to Holland with his family as political refugees. He became Professor of Physics at Wurzburg in 1888 and developed a practical use for roentgenography in the early winter of 1895. He submitted his first paper on the topic to the local scientific community on December 28, 1895. The idea took hold quickly, and within months larger hospitals obtained and used the technology. His wife recalled:

"When Willi told me in November that his work was going well, we had no idea of the consequences it would bring. But scarcely had he published the results of his research than our peace of mind was at an end. . . . It is no small matter to become a great man."[9]

Röntgen received the Nobel Prize in 1901 for his work.

Beck and Cotton were two of the first to use roentgenograms for further investigation of distal radius fractures, publishing their findings independently from 1898 through 1900.[11-14] Cotton focused not only on the radiographic characteristics of this injury, but also on the experimental and anatomical correlations with roentgenograms on 140 patients with distal radius fractures. Several other authors studied the radiographic characteristics of these fractures, including Morton,[15] Pilcher,[16] and Destot.[17]

Classification Systems

With the advent of widespread use of radiographs, surgeons no longer relied solely on clinical examination or postmortem evaluation of distal radius fractures. They could now comment on the direction and degree of displacement and the presence or absence of articular injury, leading to the development of various classification systems.

Numerous classification systems have been published over the years, and orthopaedic surgeons have employed them, trying to realize Burstein's ideal description of a successful classification system[18]: one that is functional (with high interobserver and intraobserver reliability) and useful (one that helps determine treatment and predict outcomes of that treatment). Today, no one classification system seems to fit that description perfectly, and orthopaedists draw on a multitude of classifications to help describe and treat distal radius fractures.

In 1939, the classification system of Nissen-Lie[19] was published; this system was based on the presence or absence of intra-articular involvement, metaphyseal comminution, or singular deformity, similar to the system proposed by Gartland and Werley[20] in 1951 in the *Journal of Bone and Joint Surgery* (**Table 1-1**). This was followed by Lidstrom's system,[21] published in 1959, which expanded the evaluation criteria to describe better the direction of displacement and involvement of the joint surface.

Older and colleagues[22] published their classification of extra-articular distal radius fractures in 1965. This classification divides

TABLE 1-2 Older Classification

Type	Description
I	Nondisplaced 1. Loss of some volar angulation and ≤5 degrees of dorsal angulation 2. No significant shortening: ≥2 mm above the distal radius
II	Displaced with minimal comminution 1. Loss of volar angulation 2. Shortening: usually not below the distal ulna, but occasionally ≤3 mm below it 3. Minimal comminution of the dorsal radius
III	Displaced with comminution of the distal radius 1. Comminution of the distal radius 2. Shortening: usually below the distal ulna 3. Comminution of the distal radius fragment: usually not marked and often characterized by large pieces
IV	Displaced with severe comminution of the radial head 1. Comminution of the dorsal radius: marked 2. Comminution of the distal radius fragment: shattered 3. Shortening: usually 2-8 mm below the distal ulna 4. Poor volar cortex in some cases

fractures into four types, each with two to four subtypes, based on extent of displacement, dorsal angulation, shortening of the distal fragment of the radius, and presence and extent of comminution of the dorsal metaphyseal cortex. This system has subsequently been tested for consistency and has been evaluated prospectively. Prospective studies from the late 1980s and early 1990s showed that presence of initial dorsal comminution and the extent of the initial deformity are the best indicators for later loss of reduction (**Table 1-2**).[23-27]

The Frykman classification was introduced in 1967. This classification system differed in that it addressed the radiocarpal joint and the radioulnar joint and presence or absence of an ulnar styloid fracture (**Fig. 1-3**).[28]

Melone[29] in 1984 described distal radius fractures based on the following four components: shaft, radial styloid, dorsal medial facet, and volar medial facet. This classification system is used widely for defining indications and determining surgical approach, but its accuracy and reproducibility based on standard radiographs have not been determined (**Fig. 1-4**).

The AO/ASIF classification, used by Muller and associates[30] to describe distal radius fractures, was published in 1987. Although there are 27 subtypes of distal radius fractures within this system, it has been shown to have the highest reliability when simplified into three categories—extra-articular, partial articular, and complete articular (**Fig. 1-5**).

In 1993, Cooney and colleagues[31] from Mayo published their classification system, which was described as treatment based. It

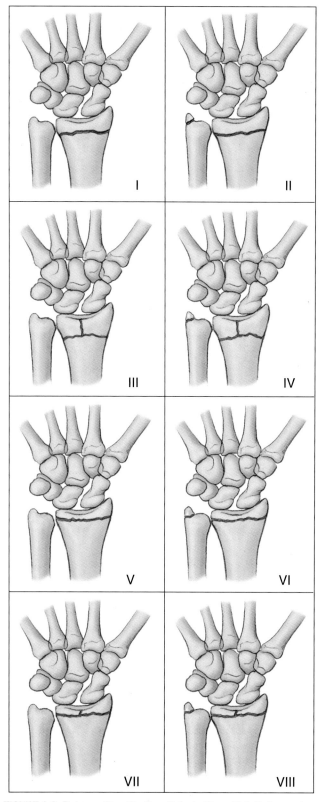

FIGURE 1-3 Frykman Classification. *(Adapted from Metz S: Comparison of different radiography systems in an experimental study for detection of forearm fractures and evaluation of the Muller-AO and Frykman classification for distal radius fractures. Invest Radiol 2006; 41:9.)*

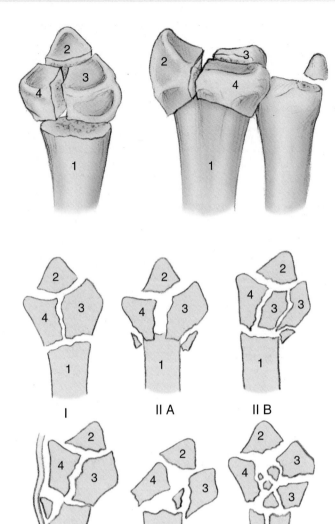

FIGURE 1-4 **Melone Classification.** *(Adapted from Melone CP Jr: Distal radius fractures: patterns of articular fragmentation. Orthop Clin North Am 1993; 24:221.)*

TABLE 1-3 Mayo Classification

Type	Description
I	Intra-articular fracture of the radiocarpal joint
II	Displaced intra-articular fracture of the radioscaphoid joint involving a significant portion of the articular surface of the distal radius (more than a radial styloid fracture)
III	Displaced intra-articular fracture of the radiolunate joint that often manifests as a "die-punch" fracture of the lunate fossa; a displaced fracture component into the distal radioulnar joint is common
IV	Displaced intra-articular fracture involving both radioscaphoid joint surfaces and usually involving the sigmoid fossa of the distal radioulnar joint; this fracture is usually comminuted

". . . while assistants hold the limb in a middle state between prona- tion and supination, let a thick and firm compress be applied transversely on the anterior surface of the limb, at the seat of the fracture, taking care that it shall not press on the ulna; let this be bound on firmly with a roller and then let a tin splint, formed to the shape of the arm, be applied to both its anterior and posterior surfaces."[9]

Wheat glues, wax, and resins were used for many centuries to make bandages set hard; egg whites also were used, up until the 18th century in England. Gypsum (plaster of Paris) was being used for casting in Arabia, and was described by the British Consul in Bassora, Eton, in 1798. The use of plaster in splinting bandages seemed to increase in popularity in Europe in the 1850s after Mathijsen described them in a medical book that was pro- moted by a friend.[9] Mathijsen used plaster bandages extensively during the Crimean War and applied them in a circumferential manner; however, he recommended splitting the cast while it was still wet to be able to loosen the cast without breaking it. He attributed to his plaster bandages the following characteristics: simplicity, easy application, quick application, instant setting, complete fixation, removability, exact retention, porosity, resil- ience ("neither urine, nor pus nor water harm its firmness or strength in any way"), and affordability.[9] Around the same time, Pirogoff, in Russia, independently advocated casting fractures in plaster bandages; St. John, an American, strongly supported the use of plaster bandages, but also introduced the concept of cast padding. Although the word of plaster casting spread out of the Crimean War, it was not until World War I that the use of plaster casts really became popular.[9]

Surgical Treatment

The factors leading to the emergence of safe, successful surgery for the treatment of fractures of the distal radius are multifacto- rial, and their respective influence is interrelated and complicated. In its simplest terms, the development of anesthesia and asepsis were the major strides leading to safe surgical techniques. Priest- ley discovered nitrous oxide in 1772. Ether was used in a demon- stration at Massachusetts General Hospital in 1846, and its use

consists of four types, based on the degree and location of dis- placement (**Table 1-3**).[32]

Ultimately, also in 1993, Fernandez[33] published a modification of the AO/ASIF system, but based his classification on the mech- anism of injury. According to the authors, this classification was developed to be practical, to suggest stable versus unstable frac- ture patterns, to include associated injuries, to identify pediatric fracture equivalents, and to suggest general recommendations for treatment (**Fig. 1-6**).

Evolution of Treatment
Splinting and Casting

Rudimentary splinting, using a variety of materials, has been used since the time of Hippocrates, who described it in 400 BC. Colles, in his 1814 paper, described treatment as closed reduction, fol- lowed by splinting and casting:

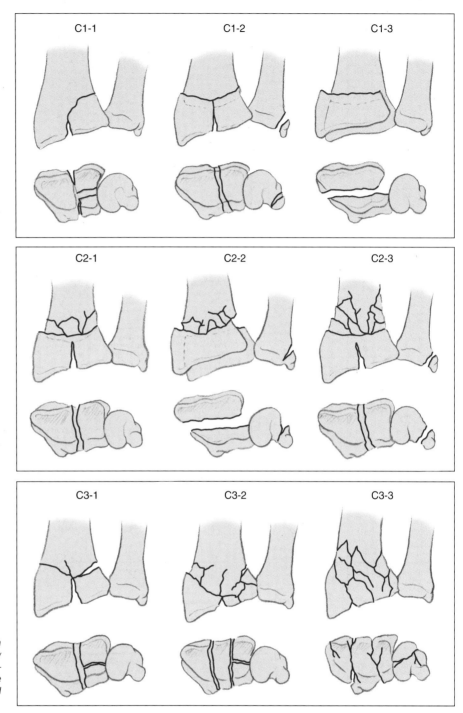

FIGURE 1-5 **AO Classification.** (Adapted from Metz S: Comparison of different radiography systems in an experimental study for detection of forearm fractures and evaluation of the Muller-AO and Frykman classification for distal radius fractures. Invest Radiol 2006; 41:9.)

became popularized in America and Europe. Lister championed antiseptic principles and published results in 1867. Until the invention of boilers by Neuber (1885) and steam sterilizers, however, Lister's principles were not widely accepted, and surgery remained a dangerous endeavor, with a high rate of morbidity and mortality.[9]

Treatments other than casting or splinting for distal radius fractures were initially described around 1930.[34] Anderson and O'Neil[35] in 1944 used a simple external fixator to treat distal radius fractures. Pins were placed proximally in the radius and distally in the second metacarpal and attached by a simple

bar. Advances in this technique led to many other designs of external fixators over the decades, and external fixation remains a viable treatment option in severely comminuted or open distal radius fractures. Such advances include fixators that are radiolucent and have adjustable bars. Nonbridging external fixation affords the benefit of not spanning the radiocarpal joint, minimizing the sequelae of external fixation on overall wrist motion.

Percutaneous pinning was introduced early in the timeline of surgical treatment of distal radius fractures and has endured in various forms to the present day. Lambotte described the

Fracture types (adults) based on the mechanism of injury	Children fracture equivalent	Stability/ instability: high risk of secondary displacement after initial adequate reduction	Displacement pattern	Number of fragments	Associated lesions carpal ligament, fractures, median, ulnar nerve, tendons, ipsilateral, fracture upper extremity, compartment syndrome	Recommended treatment
Type I Bending fracture of the metaphysis 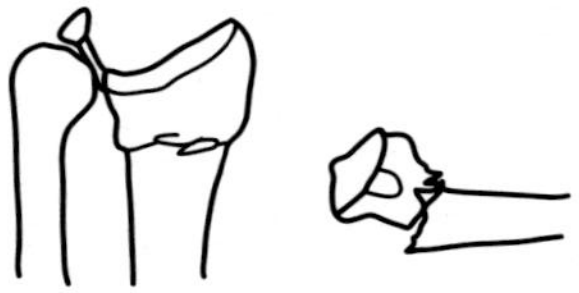	Distal forearm fracture Salter II	Stable Unstable	Nondisplaced dorsally (Colles-Pouteau) Volarly (Smith) Proximal Combined	Always 2 main fragments + Varying degree of metaphyseal comminution (instability)	Uncommon	Conservative (stable fractures) Percutaneous pinning (extra- or intrafocal) External fixation (exceptionally bone graft)
Type II Shearing fracture of the joint surface 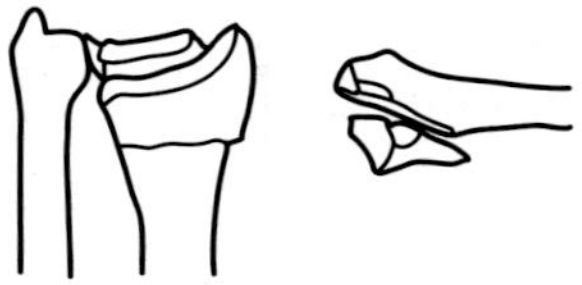	Salter IV	Unstable	Dorsal Radial Volar Proximal Combined	Two-part Three-part Comminuted	Less uncommon	Open reduction Screw-plate fixation
Type III Compression fracture of the joint surface 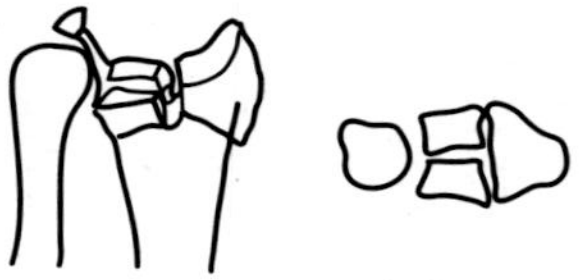	Salter III, IV, V	Stable Unstable	Nondisplaced Dorsal Radial Volar Proximal Combined	Two-part Three-part Four-part Comminuted	Common	Conservative closed, limited, arthroscopic assisted, or extensile open reduction Percutaneous pins combined with external and internal fixation Bone graft
Type IV Avulsion fractures Radiocarpal fracture Dislocation 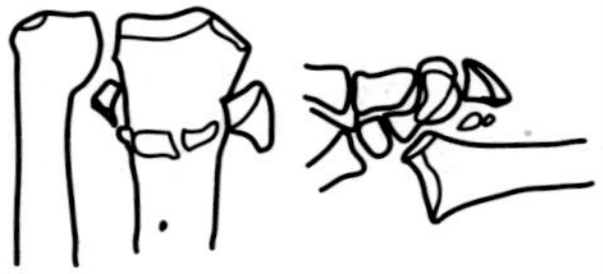	Very rare	Unstable	Dorsal Radial Volar Proximal Combined	Two-part (radial styloid, ulnar styloid) Three-part (volar, dorsal margin) Comminuted	Frequent	Closed or open reduction Pin or screw fixation Tension wiring
Type V Combined fractures (I-II-III-IV) High-velocity injury 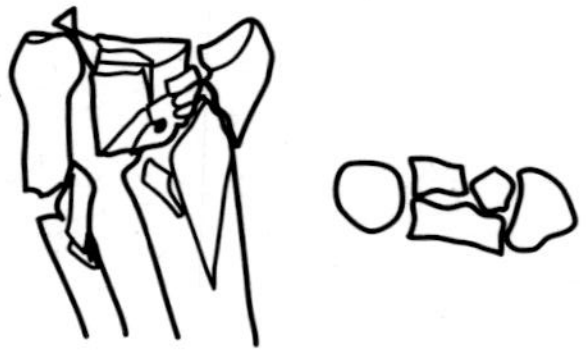	Very rare	Unstable	Dorsal Radial Volar Proximal Combined	Comminuted and/or bone loss (frequently intra-articular, open, seldom extra-articular)	Always present	Combined method

FIGURE 1-6 Fernandez Classification. *(Adapted from Jupiter JB: Comparative classification for fractures of the distal end of the radius. J Hand Surg 1997; 23A:4.)*

placement of a single pin into the radial styloid to stabilize a displaced distal radius fracture in 1908. This technique was modified by Stein and Katz in 1975 with the addition of a pin through a dorsal-ulnar radial fragment, from proximal to distal; Uhl, Lortat-Jacob, and Mortier all described in 1976 radial styloid pinning plus fixation of the posteromedial fragment with an ulnar-radial pin. Most notably, Kapandji introduced the concept of intrafocal pinning in 1976. Two pins, 0.078 inch in size, are placed directly into the fracture site and then driven proximally into the radial diaphysis, buttressing the fracture site. Kapandji later modified his description of this technique to include a third pin. This intrafocal pinning has been extensively studied and is arguably the most published percutaneous technique. It is still used extensively, especially in Europe.[36]

Open reduction and internal fixation of distal radius fractures was described well after the first description of percutaneous pinning or external fixation. Ellis[37] described the use of a volar buttress plate for Barton's fractures in 1965, but it was not until the 1980s and 1990s that the role of internal fixation in the surgical armamentarium of distal radius fractures began to grow. Concurrently, increased focus on outcome studies better defined which fracture patterns did not do as well with prior treatment methods. Similarly, outcome studies and biomechanical studies showed the importance of restoration of radial length, radial inclination, articular congruity, and palmar tilt.

More recently, advances have been made in implant technology and surgical techniques that continue to advance the treatment of distal radius fractures. Specifically, these advances have improved our ability to address severely comminuted, intra-articular fractures that would previously have been less optimally treated.[38,39]

The realization that the balance between achieving anatomical reduction with stable fixation and allowing early mobilization with rehabilitation was important has encouraged the popularity of open reduction and internal fixation with fragment-specific fixation type devices. This concept was popularized by Medoff and Kopylov[40] and has permeated throughout the development of new technology. Additionally, the use of arthroscopy (credited to Takagi, Watanabe, and Jackson in the knee) in the wrist for arthroscopically assisted management of distal radius fractures is a more recently introduced idea, useful especially in cases of complex intra-articular fractures.[41,42]

Past, Present and Future

Distal radius fractures have remained one of the most common fractures seen by physicians since the time of Hippocrates. Much has changed since that time, however. Not only has the nature of the injury changed with the increasing frequency of higher energy trauma, but also patients, their expectations, and the tools available for treatment and evaluation of success of that treatment all have undergone significant metamorphoses. At the time Colles published his article, the life expectancy for a laborer was a mere 23 years, there was no electricity, and surgery was thought to expose a patient to "more chances of death than the English soldier on the field of Waterloo."[9] Clearly, things have changed, and continue to evolve. Rang[9] described five stages of knowledge: .

1. Description
2. Ineffectual treatment
3. Effectual treatment
4. Prevention
5. Decline of disease importance

Rang used polio as an example in *The Story of Orthopaedics*.[9] In the context of distal radius fractures, we currently exist between the third and fourth stage. The coming decades will undoubtedly bring more effective treatments and a focus on prevention, including targeting osteoporosis and insufficiency fractures and high-energy accidents and injuries. The history of distal radius fractures has brought us to where we are in their diagnosis and treatment today, and we will certainly see improvements continue to evolve as we move forward.

REFERENCES

1. Colles A: On the fracture of the carpal extremity of the radius. Edinburgh Med Surg J 1814; 10:182.
2. Petit JL: L'Art de guerir les maladies des os. Paris: L. d'Houry, 1705.
3. Pouteau C: Oeuveres posthumes de M. Pouteau: memoire, contenant quelques reflexions sur quelques fractures de l'avant-bras, sur les luxations incompletes du poignet et sur le diastasis. Paris: PhD Pierres, 1783.
4. Peltier LF: Fractures of the distal end of the radius: an historical account. Clin Orthop 1984; 187:18-21.
5. Dupuytren G: On the injuries and diseases of bones, being selections from the collected edition of the clinical lectures of Baron Dupuytren. Clark F. LeGros (trans. and ed.). London: Syndenham Society, 1847.
6. Goyrand G: Memoirs sur les fractures de l'extremite inferieure de radius, qui simulent les luxations du poignet. Gazette de Medicine 1832; 3:664.
7. Goyrand G: De la fracture par contre-coup de l'extremite inferieure du radius. Journal Hebdomadaire 1836; 1:161.
8. Nelaton A: Elements de pathologie chirurgicale. Paris: Germer Bailliere, 1844.
9. Rang M: The Story of Orthopaedics. Philadelphia: WB Saunders, 1966.
10. Smith RW: A treatise on fractures in the vicinity of joints and on certain forms of accidental and congenital dislocations. Dublin: Hodges & Smith, 1847.
11. Beck C: Colles' fracture and the Roentgen-rays. Med News 1898; 72:230.
12. Cotton FJ: Experimental Colles' fracture. J Boston Soc Med Sci 1897-1898; 2:171.
13. Cotton FJ: A study of the x-ray plates of one hundred and forty cases of fracture of the lower end of the radius. Boston Med Surg J 1900; 143:305.
14. Cotton FJ: The pathology of fracture of the lower extremity of the radius. Ann Surg 1900; 32:194-218, 388-415.
15. Morton R: A radiographic survey of 170 cases clinically diagnosed as "Colles' fracture." Lancet 1907; 1:731.
16. Pilcher LS: Fractures of the lower extremity or base of the radius. Ann Surg 1917; 65:1.
17. Destot E: Injuries of the Wrist, a Radiological Study. New York: Paul B. Hoeber, 1926.
18. Burstein AH: Fracture classification systems: do they work and are they useful? J Bone Joint Surg 1993;75:1743-1744.
19. Nissen-Lie HS: Fracture radii "typical." Nord Med 1939; 1:293-303.
20. Gartland JJ, Werley CW: Evaluation of healed Colles' fractures. J Bone Joint Surg Am 1951; 33:895-907.

21. Lidstrom A: Fractures of the distal end of the radius: a clinical and statistical study of end results. Acta Orthop Scand 1959; 30:1-118.

22. Older TM, Stabler GV, Cassebaum WH: Colles' fracture: evaluation and selection of therapy. J Trauma 1965; 5:469-474.

23. Axelrod T, Paley D, Green J, et al: Limited open reduction of the lunate facet in comminuted intra-articular fractures of the distal radius. J Hand Surg [Am] 1988; 13:372-377.

24. Bartosh RA, Saldana MJ: Intra-articular fractures of the distal radius: a cadaveric study to determine if ligamentotaxis restores radiopalmar tilt. J Hand Surg [Am] 1990; 15:18-21.

25. Bradway JK, Amadio PC, Cooney WP: Open reduction and internal fixation of displaced, comminuted intra-articular fractures of the distal end of the radius. J Bone Joint Surg Am 1989; 71:839-847.

26. Putnam MD, Seitz WH: Fractures of the distal radius. In Rockwood and Green's Fractures in Adults. 5th ed. Philadelphia: Lippincott Williams & Wilkins, 2002.

27. Rikli DA, Regazzoni P: Fractures of the distal end of the radius treated by internal fixation and early function: a preliminary report of 20 cases. J Bone Joint Surg Br 1996; 78:588-592.

28. Frykman G: Fractures of the distal radius, including sequelae—shoulder- and finger-syndrome, disturbance in the distal radioulnar joint and impairment of nerve function: a clinical and experimental study. Acta Orthop Scand Suppl 1967; 108:1-153.

29. Melone CP Jr: Articular fractures of the distal radius. Orthop Clin North Am 1984; 15:217-236.

30. Muller ME, Nazarian S, Koch P, et al: The Comprehensive Classification of Long Bones. New York: Springer-Verlag, 1990, pp 54-63.

31. Cooney WP: Fractures of the distal radius: a modern treatment-based classification. Orthop Clin North Am 1993; 24:211-216.

32. Jupiter JB, Fernandez FL: Comparative classification for fractures of the distal end of the radius. J Hand Surg [Am] 1997; 22:563-571.

33. Fernandez DL: Fractures of the distal radius: operative treatment. Instr Course Lect 1993; 42:73-88.

34. Bohler L: Treatment of Fractures. 4th ed. Baltimore: William Wood, 1929.

35. Anderson R, O'Neil G: Comminuted fractures of the distal end of the radius. Surg Gynecol Obstet 1944; 78:434-440.

36. Rayhack JM: The history and evolution of percutaneous pinning of displaced distal radius fractures. Orthop Clin North Am 1993; 24:287-300.

37. Ellis J: Smith's and Barton's fractures: a method of treatment. J Bone Joint Surg Br 1965; 47:724-727.

38. Nana AD, Joshi A, Lichtman DM: Plating of the distal radius. J Am Acad Orthop Surg 2005; 13:159-171.

39. Smith DW, Henry MH: Volar fixed-angle plating of the distal radius. J Am Acad Orthop Surg 2005; 13:28-36.

40. Medoff RJ, Kopylov P: Open reduction and immediate motion of intraarticular distal radius fractures with a fragment specific system. Arch Am Acad Orthop Surg 1999; 2:53.

41. Benson LS, Minihane KP, Stern LD, et al: The outcome of intra-articular distal radius fractures treated with fragment-specific fixation. J Hand Surg [Am] 2006; 31:1333-1339.

42. Wiesler ER, Chloros GD, Mahirogullari M, et al: Arthroscopic management of distal radius fractures. J Hand Surg [Am] 2006; 31:1516-1526.

Nonoperative Treatment of Distal Radius Fractures

2

Joseph J. Dias, MD, FRCS, FRCS (Edin), MBBS

Indications

The fractures of the distal radius best suited for nonoperative treatment are (1) undisplaced and minimally displaced stable fractures, (2) bending fractures in good bone, and (3) intra-articular fractures where there is almost no step between the intra-articular fragments.

Radiographic Criteria for Nonoperative Treatment

On the assumption that the wrist was normal prior to the fracture of the distal radius my colleagues and I recommend the following radiographic criteria for nonoperative treatment after reduction if required: dorsal tilt of the distal radius articular surface of less than 10 degrees, intra-articular step of less than 1 mm, and 3 mm of ulnar variance. In very osteoporotic individuals or those who are unwell or physiologically elderly, however, we may accept up to 20 degrees of dorsal tilt, an intra-articular step of 2 mm, and 5 mm of ulnar-positive variance.

Undisplaced and Minimally Displaced Fractures

It is usual to treat undisplaced or minimally displaced stable fractures of the distal radius in a below-elbow plaster of Paris cast for 4 to 6 weeks. The wrist is usually immobilized in slight extension so as to allow some activities of daily living. Even in undisplaced fractures, the cast is applied with some molding to reduce the risk of loss of position of the fracture during bone healing.

The cast is made up of an 8-inch plaster of Paris slab extending from the distal palmar crease around the radial aspect of the wrist and proximally up to the proximal third of the forearm. A hole is cut out for the thumb. The pronated forearm is held by two assistants, one holding the arm just above the elbow and the other holding the extended fingers. These assistants must give slight traction along the line of the forearm (**Fig. 2-1**). The hand and forearm are covered firmly with synthetic wool, and the plaster slab is applied to extend around the radial side of the forearm and wrist and ulnarward both dorsally and on the palmar side. This slab is then firmly bandaged in place with a crepe bandage. As the plaster sets it is molded with three points of compression to counter the dorsal bending deformity of the distal radius fracture. The palmar point of compression overlies the site of the fracture and forms the fulcrum over which the dorsal two compression points stretch the broken bone, thereby countering the dorsal bending tendency of such a fracture (**Figs. 2-2** and **2-3**).

The cast is a radially based gutter slab encompassing four fifths of the circumference of the forearm. This leaves the ulnar side of the forearm free to accommodate for any immediate swelling. The bandaging can be tightened in the first 2 weeks as the swelling reduces. Alternatively the cast can be reapplied. The distal extent of the plaster of Paris slab extends to the distal palmar crease on the ulnar side and the proximal palmar crease on the radial side to allow full flexion of the metacarpophalangeal joints over the distal palmar edge of the cast.

In the initial day or two after reduction, patients are advised to clench and unclench the hand on the affected side and to elevate the hand on pillows when at home. Attention must be paid not to flex the elbow above a right angle to avoid circulatory compromise and stretching of the ulnar nerve. The patients are encouraged to use the hand for light activities of daily living and are told how to avoid getting the plaster wet when bathing. They are encouraged to return to the clinic if they experience any problems or if the plaster of Paris slab breaks or becomes soft. Patients are also provided with written instructions on care of the plastered extremity.

Do Undisplaced Fractures Need Immobilization?

Undisplaced or minimally displaced fractures can be safely treated in a plaster of Paris slab. Stable fractures can also be safely treated without immobilization. In a prospective randomized study of 97 fractures, Dias and associates[1] demonstrated that the treatment of such fractures without a cast did not result in greater displacement or more discomfort than those treated in a cast. Moreover, more patients treated without immobilization recovered grip and movement within 8 weeks compared to those immobilized in a cast.

Displaced Fractures
Extra-articular Fractures

Extra-articular displaced fractures need to be carefully manipulated back into place. The technique described by Charnley[2] needs to be followed to disimpact the fracture by giving traction. Traction may be easily given using manual distraction or alternatively may be provided by finger traps and weights as described by Earnshaw and coworkers.[3] Once the fracture has been disimpacted, the wrist can be manipulated in pronation to counter the tendency of the distal fragment to supinate. Although flexion of the wrist has been suggested to counter the dorsal angulation of the distal radius, the fracture can be gently manipulated to correct the dorsal tilt by molding. The physician stands facing the patient's head, on the thumb side of the pronated forearm. The physician's hand nearest the patient supports the palmar side

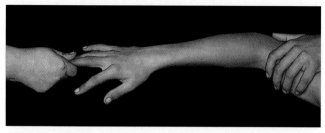

FIGURE 2-1 **Traction of the Hand.** The patient is supine with the shoulder abducted, the elbow flexed to a right angle, and the forearm pronated. One assistant holds the arm and provides countertraction as the other pulls on the index and middle fingers.

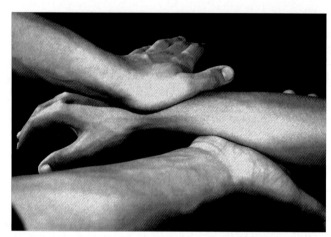

FIGURE 2-2 The precise position of the physician's hands in order to mold the fracture into its proper alignment is demonstrated. The physician is positioned facing the patient's head. The physician's hand near the patient is used to provide the fulcrum for the molding and lies close to the fracture but proximal to it. The physician's hand away from the patient is used to mold the fracture by pressing the thenar eminence over the distal fragment of the fracture. This should stretch the probably intact dorsal periosteum and reduce the fracture, provided that the palmar cortex at the site of the fracture is not comminuted.

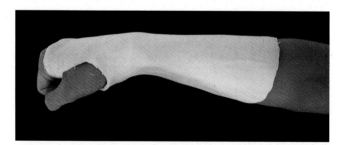

FIGURE 2-3 The below-elbow plaster of Paris slab is demonstrated with the smooth molds apparent.

of the radius just proximal to the fracture. The physician's hand away from the patient is used to push down on the dorsum of the distal fragment (see Fig. 2-2). The fracture is then assessed under fluoroscopy. If the position is satisfactory, especially with the traction released, a plaster slab is applied as described above.

Intra-articular Fractures

When there is an intra-articular nondisplaced fracture line, the fracture is treated exactly as an extra-articular fracture but care is exercised to ensure that the intra-articular fracture does not dis-

place during reduction. This is done by depending more on traction to realign the fracture.

If there is displacement of the intra-articular fracture, the position is checked after traction. A cast may be applied if the fracture and other factors indicate it or the physician decides to try nonoperative treatment in the first instance. Monitoring, discussed below, needs to be meticulous, however, and the physician must be prepared to change the method of management if the fracture displaces.

Severely displaced or comminuted fractures cannot be treated satisfactorily using a cast. Casting can only be considered in these cases if the physiologic state of the patient does not permit surgical intervention. The physician must anticipate a high rate of loss of position, with remanipulation not offering much hope of improved position.[4]

Aftercare

Nonoperative treatment in a plaster of Paris gutter slab demands regular and meticulous monitoring of the fracture and the injured limb. In our unit it is usual to review the patient, the fracture, and the injured extremity in the second week after injury. This is used to (1) confirm that the position of the fracture is maintained by obtaining radiographs of the injured limb in the cast; (2) check that the cast is still snug as the swelling of the wrist and hand settles; (3) ensure that the cast is comfortable and there is no localized discomfort to suggest excess pressure; (4) ensure that the patient is moving and exercising the hand using the six-pack of hand exercises; and (5) establish that all tendons, particularly the extensor pollicis longus tendon, and all nerves, particularly the median nerve, are functioning normally.

The plaster slab is retained until the next appointment, which occurs in the sixth week after injury. At this clinic visit the plaster slab is removed and the following are done: (1) Radiographs of the wrist are taken to confirm whether the position of the fracture obtained immediately after injury and confirmed in the second week is maintained. (2) The state of the tendons is confirmed. The extensor pollicis longus tendon is assessed by asking the patient to actively extend the thumb interphalangeal joint and noting that the interphalangeal joint extends and that the patient does not experience any soreness near Lister's tubercle to suggest an impending rupture. (3) Nerve function, especially that of the median nerve, is assessed. (4) Attention is then turned to the wrist and the following documented:

+ The persistence of swelling and the appearance of the hand and whether it is deviated radially to suggest a radial inclination malunion of the distal radius
+ The prominence of the head of the ulna and the direction of this prominence, whether palmar or dorsal
+ The range of wrist movement is measured with a goniometer to document the extension, flexion, and radial and ulnar inclination.
+ Forearm rotation is measured.
+ Any pain and its severity on movement, particularly on the ulnar side of the wrist, is noted.
+ Grip strength is recorded.

Based on these observations, the patient is taught wrist exercises, concentrating on wrist circumduction and forearm rotation. Formal physiotherapy may need to be organized if the wrist and forearm range is less than half of the opposite, uninjured side. The patient is advised to resume activity but to avoid heavy work and any activity or sport where there is a real risk of falling. This is because bone healing is still progressing.

If the assessment and function of the wrist and hand are satisfactory, the patient may be discharged with advice and instructions to return if there are any concerns. Patients with significant stiffness need to be monitored over the subsequent 6 weeks. Any concerns about tendons, nerves, or algodystrophy demand immediate appropriate investigation and frequent visits until such concerns are resolved or the appropriate treatment instituted.

Advantages, Disadvantages, and Limitations of Nonoperative Treatment

Advantages

The advantage of nonoperative treatment of a distal radius fracture is that it does not interfere with the intricate sequence of healing events at the fracture site, the patient is not exposed to the risks of surgery, and hand function recovery can begin immediately. After the early period, patients are encouraged to return to work if able.

Disadvantages

The disadvantage of nonoperative management is that it requires the wrist to be immobilized for 4 to 6 weeks. The cast imposes restrictions, particularly in bathing and driving. Patients cannot return to some occupations with a cast. For example, surgeons could not operate and those dealing with the preparation of food could not safely perform their duties when the wrist is incarcerated in a cast.

Limitations of Cast Immobilization

It must be clearly recognized that a cast cannot counter shortening at the fracture site either due to compaction of osteoporotic trabeculae or to comminution of a significant circumference of the metaphysis of the distal radius. Fractures with these attributes will lead to healing of the distal radius in a shortened position. A formal decision is required from the outset that such shortening of bone is acceptable for that particular patient. If it is not acceptable, alternative techniques to counter shortening of the distal radius need to be considered.

A plaster of Paris cast also may not maintain the reduction of a significant intra-articular step. If a cast is used for such a fracture, it needs to be monitored closely during the initial 2 weeks and any redisplacement of the fracture needs to be addressed.

For bending or minimally displaced fractures, the degree of swelling of the injured limb will help predict the risk of loss of a close fit of the plaster of Paris slab, with the consequent loss of fracture position. Patients with much swelling need to be watched carefully during the first 2 weeks, and the threshold for a change of plaster with a remanipulation should be low.

The shape and size of the forearm and wrist determine the security of immobilization in a plaster of Paris cast. In obese individuals with short forearms, the girth of the forearm is such that it is difficult to apply a plaster and mold it sufficiently to counter the dorsal bending force at the fracture site. The security of immobilization of the fracture in an obese person with a short forearm is less than that in a slender patient with a long forearm. The clinician needs to monitor the former type of patient carefully, as these patients are at greater risk of having their reduced fracture of the distal radius displace in the cast and heal in a misplaced position.

The physician must be prepared to change the method of immobilization if the fracture is showing signs of unacceptable displacement. The best person to decide on nonoperative treatment of the distal radius fracture is someone who is competent and proficient in all methods of intervention including nonoperative treatment.

Advice to Patients

Nonoperative treatment of distal radius fractures is an established method of management, and most fractures of the distal radius are treated in this manner internationally. It is, however, important to give good advice to patients so that they know what to expect from such management.

Loss of Position and Malunion

The biggest risk with nonoperative treatment of distal radius fractures is loss of position. Mackenney and colleagues[5] carefully investigated factors that could help predict loss of position after manipulation and established that the patient's age, initial metaphyseal comminution, and shortening promoted such a loss. The rate of malunion, defined as shortening of 3 mm and a dorsal tilt of 10 degrees, has been calculated as 27% for minimally displaced fractures and 60% for initially displaced fractures. This rate has also been established by other studies. Dias and associates[6] demonstrated that osteoporosis caused greater impaction at injury, a greater early loss of position, and a greater progression of deformity during the subsequent healing phase after the cast was removed because osteoporotic bone was less able to resist the deformation of bone caused by the loads borne by the wrist during everyday activity.

Recovery of Movement

It is usual to recover almost a full range of wrist and forearm rotation after distal radius fractures treated nonoperatively within 1 year.[6-8]

The outcome in the long term also remains satisfactory, with no patient treated nonoperatively changing occupation over a lifetime.[9]

Osteoarthritis After Nonoperative Treatment

Gartland and Werley[10] reviewed 60 distal radius fractures around 18 months after injury and found no arthritis if the fracture was undisplaced and mild arthritis in 11% of 27 undisplaced intra-articular fractures and 40% of 26 displaced intra-articular fractures.

Smaill[8] reported on the results of 41 fractures 5 years after injury and found that 10 (24%) had some narrowing of joint space, but only 3 had minor aching symptoms. This rate of between 21% and 33% is unchanged for minimally displaced fractures over the long term of between 32 and 38 years.[9,11]

Knirk and Jupiter[12] related the presence of radiologic arthritis to the step in the intra-articular fracture and reported an 11% arthritis rate if the joint was congruous but a 95% arthritis rate if the joint was not congruous. Their data, however, had 21 cases of intra-articular fractures treated nonoperatively and 8 (38%) had slight decrease of joint space at 6.7 years after injury. This is similar to the 40.5% slight decrease in joint space reported by Kopylov and coworkers[9] in 47 intra-articular fractures seen 32 years after injury. Ford and associates[11] reported that 24 of 40 (60%) intra-articular fractured wrists had radiologic arthritis at least one grade worse than the other wrist 38 years after injury. They calculated that the odds of developing arthritis in the fractured wrist doubled (2.4 times) with 2-mm shortening and tripled (3.2 times) in intra-articular fractures.

The possibility of remodeling of the step also needs to be borne in mind. This has been demonstrated by Ford and colleagues[11] in a prospective study following patients with fractures over 9 years. Arthritis may not be completely avoided if there is significant damage to the articular cartilage at the time of injury.

The observation that a step of greater than 2 mm results in osteoarthritis may be less true for nonoperatively treated fractures because the step may decrease with loading of the hand as the carpus pushes the articular step displacement into better alignment. This may explain why the rate of osteoarthritis is greater in fractures that are partly fixed with wires and other metal[12] where one column is better fixed than the other, resulting in inadequate correction or loss of correction during healing. This promotes the formation of a step within the articular surface, which may result in early onset of arthritis. The fixation device prevents the leveling of the intra-articular displacement and, by maintaining the step, promotes degenerative change.

All alternative methods of intervention must be able to, at the very least, deliver the rate and severity of osteoarthritis following nonoperative treatment or improve on it. The information available at present does not suggest that internal fixation methods have delivered an improved rate,[12,13] even if one were to discount the occasional serious and irreversible complications of fixation, such as screws cutting out into the radiocarpal joint and destroying it.

Tendon Rupture

The extensor pollicis tendon can rupture even after nonoperative treatment of distal radius fractures. The rate of rupture is very low, between 0.3% (14 of 4000),[14] 1.2% (7 of 565),[15] and 2% (4 of 207).[16] Up to 50% of ruptures of this tendon are due to a distal radius fracture.[17] It usually occurs soon after the cast is removed, at between 4 and 12 weeks after injury, and is often seen after minimally displaced fractures.

The tendon may fray over a sharp edge at the fracture site or as it is contained in an osseoligamentous third extensor compartment pulley. Its circulation could be compromised, causing an ischemic rupture. Heidemann and associates[18] were able to demonstrate encroachment of the third extensor compartment by the edge of the fracture at Lister's tubercle using CT scans.

The usual treatment, if needed, is a transfer of the extensor indicis proprius tendon to the extensor pollicis distal tendon with satisfactory but incomplete restoration of thumb extension.[17] Although rare, isolated cases of rupture of flexor tendons have been reported, and there are also a very few cases of rupture of more than one tendon.

Nerve Problems

Nerve symptoms occur in between 6% and 17% of patients.[7,15,16] Ulnar nerve and radial nerve symptoms are less common.

Stewart and coworkers[7] recorded that symptoms of median nerve dysfunction after nonoperatively treated distal radius fracture, with altered feeling in the thumb, index, middle, and ring fingers, occurred in 17% of 209 patients with distal radius fractures, and if treated nonoperatively, resolution of symptoms occurred in 55%.

Increasing symptoms may indicate the need for a carpal tunnel release. The prognosis must be guarded, however, as the consequences of a significant nerve injury will not be reversed by surgical release of the flexor retinaculum. It is our approach to identify nerve symptoms at the initial presentation and monitor for the first day or two if there is no other reason to operate. Usually these symptoms improve. If the symptoms do not improve and especially if the nerve symptoms worsen, we recommend an immediate flexor retinaculum release.

Algodystrophy

Algodystrophy needs early identification and rigorous management to control pain, decrease swelling, and maintain and improve movement if the devastating and essentially permanent dysfunction of the wrist and hand is to be avoided. Up to 25% of patients with distal radius fracture will have some features of algodystrophy,[19] which can be identified early and are usually exacerbated by tight circumferential casts. If inadequately treated, the consequences are lasting.

Conclusion

Patients being counseled for nonoperative treatment of their distal radius fracture need to be made aware of the probability of loss of position of the fracture of 27% for minimally displaced fractures and 60% for displaced fractures. Between 6% and 17% will have nerve symptoms, but fewer than half of these symptoms will persist. Fewer than 1% of patients will develop a tendon rupture. Algodystrophy can occur in 25% of cases, but the rate of significant algodystrophy with permanent severe disability is difficult to ascertain from the literature. Radiologic osteoarthritis will develop in 25% of minimally displaced fractures and 60% of intra-articular fractures. However, most patients in both of these groups will not develop significant symptoms. It is very unlikely that patients will need to change their occupation if their distal radius fracture is treated nonoperatively.

Any other method of treating these common fractures must clearly improve on these outcomes and not introduce other devastating risks.

Nonoperative treatment is the most common method of treatment of distal radius fractures, delivering reasonable short- and long-term outcomes. Patients need to be advised of this option. All clinicians must be competent in nonoperative treatment of distal radius fractures and be able to advise patients on the pros and cons of this method of treatment.

REFERENCES

1. Dias JJ, Wray CC, Jones JM, Gregg PJ: The value of early mobilisation in the treatment of Colles' fractures. J Bone Joint Surg [Br] 1987; 69:463-467.

2. Charnley J: The Colles Fracture. In The Closed Treatment of Common Fractures. 3rd ed. Edinburgh, E and S Livingstone, 1961, pp 128-142.

3. Earnshaw SA, Aladin A, Surendran S, Moran CG: Closed reduction of Colles fractures: comparison of manual manipulation and finger-trap traction. A prospective, randomised study. J Bone Joint Surg [Br] 2002; 84(3):354-358.

4. McQueen MM, Hajducka C, Court-Brown CM: Redisplaced unstable fractures of the distal radius: a prospective randomised comparison of four methods of treatment. J Bone Joint Surg [Br] 1996; 78(3):404-409.

5. Mackenney PJ, McQueen MM, Elton R: Prediction of instability in distal radial fractures. J Bone Joint Surg [Am] 2006; 88(9):1944-1951.

6. Dias JJ, Wray CC, Jones JM: Osteoporosis and Colles' fractures in the elderly. J Hand Surg [Br] 1987; 12(1):57-59.

7. Stewart HD, Innes AR, Burke FD: Functional cast-bracing for Colles' fractures. A comparison between cast-bracing and conventional plaster casts. J Bone Joint Surg [Br] 1984; 66(5):749-753.

8. Smaill GB: Long-term follow-up of Colles' fracture. J Bone Joint Surg [Br] 1965; 47:80-85.

9. Kopylov P, Johnell O, Redlund-Johnell I, Bengner U: Fractures of the distal end of the radius in young adults: a 30-year follow-up. J Hand Surg [Br] 1993; 18(1):45-49.

10. Gartland JJ Jr, Werley CW: Evaluation of healed Colles' fractures. J Bone Joint Surg [Am] 1951; 33(4):895-907.

11. Ford DR, Sithole J, Davis TRC: The 38-year outcome of distal radial fractures in young adults. J Hand Surg [Br] 2006; 31(Suppl 1):6-7.

12. Knirk JL, Jupiter JB: Intra-articular fractures of the distal end of the radius in young adults. J Bone Joint Surg [Am] 1986; 68(5):647-659.

13. Catalano LW 3rd, Cole RJ, Gelberman RH, et al Displaced intra-articular fractures of the distal aspect of the radius. Long-term results in young adults after open reduction and internal fixation. J Bone Joint Surg [Am] 1997; 79:1290-1302.

14. Hove LM: Delayed rupture of the thumb extensor tendon. A 5-year study of 18 consecutive cases. Acta Orthop Scand 1994; 65(2):199-203.

15. Cooney WP 3rd, Dobyns JH, Linscheid RL: Complications of Colles' fractures. J Bone Joint Surg [Am] 1980; 62:613-619.

16. McKay SD, MacDermid JC, Roth JH, Richards RS: Assessment of complications of distal radius fractures and development of a complication checklist. J Hand Surg [Am] 2001; 26(5):916-922.

17. Loos A, Kalb K, Van Schoonhoven J, et al Rekonstruktion der Extensor pollicis longus-Sehne mittels Extensor indicis-Transposition. Handchir Mikrochir Plast Chir 2003; 35(6):368-372.

18. Heidemann J, Gausepohl T, Pennig D: Einengung des dritten Strecksehnenfaches bei gering dislozierter distaler Radiusfraktur mit Gefahr einer Extensor pollicis longus-Sehnenruptur. Handchir Mikrochir Plast Chir 2002; 35(5):324-327.

19. Atkins RM, Duckworth T, Kanis JA: Algodystrophy following Colles' fracture. J Hand Surg [Br] 1989; 14(2):161-164.

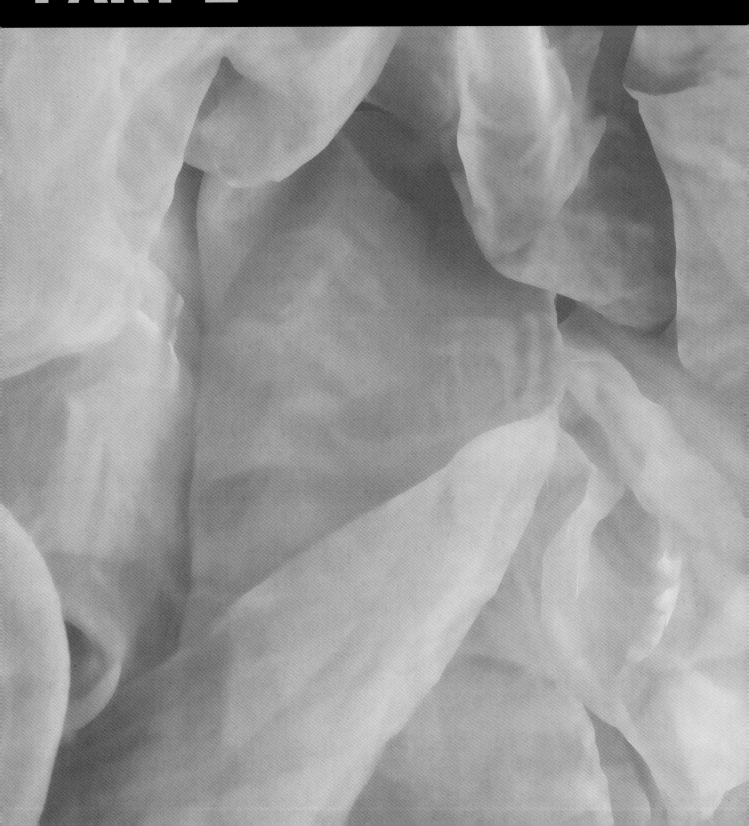

PART 2 ANATOMY, IMAGING, AND OUTCOMES

Radiographic Evaluation and Classification of Distal Radius Fractures

3

Robert J. Medoff, MD

X-rays are essential to the treatment of distal radius fractures. When combined with the age and baseline level of activity of the patient, the interpretation of a patient's x-rays significantly influences the type of treatment selected. Radiographs form the basis for nearly every system of classification of distal radius fractures. Radiographs also are used during procedures to judge residual fragment displacements and to determine whether hardware has been placed appropriately. Ultimately, x-rays are the means used to assess the quality of the final reduction and treatment.[1] By improving the interpretation of standard x-rays, a better understanding of the pattern of injury emerges, which improves algorithms for treatment and ultimately results in better clinical outcomes.

Radiographic Landmarks
Posteroanterior View

An x-ray image is a two-dimensional representation of a three-dimensional structure. Orthogonal views, such as posteroanterior (PA) and lateral views, show the outline of the cortical profile in two projections perpendicular to one another and reveal fracture lines traversing the cortical profile tangential to the beam. Oblique films may provide additional information by rotating other sections of the cortical outline into profile. Because the distal radius is not a simple rectangular solid, however, a more sophisticated analysis of the radiographic images is usually needed to create a clear mental image of the components of a particular injury.

The actual x-ray technique directly affects the quality and characteristics of the visual information that is presented on the radiographic image. It is not unusual to receive injury films that have been poorly positioned or were taken with poor radiographic technique from emergency staff members who were unwilling to move an injured arm for fear of causing additional pain or injury to the patient. X-rays of an unreduced, highly displaced fracture compound the difficulties of interpretation because of the distortion from abnormal displacement and rotation of fracture components. In some cases, determining the nature of a complex injury is no more complicated than simply obtaining a second set of films after a closed reduction with proper positioning and technique. Finally, articular visualization on the PA view may be improved by angling the x-ray beam 10 degrees proximally.[2]

The rotational position of the forearm also can change the appearance of the radiographic image (**Fig. 3-1**).[3] On a standard PA view of the wrist with the forearm in neutral position, the cortical bone along the ulnar border of the ulnar styloid connects smoothly with the cortical bone along the ulnar border of the shaft. In addition, the cortical outline of the ulnar head does not extend behind the ulnar styloid, and the lateral border of the

distal ulnar shaft has a concave outline on its radial side. Subtle changes occur if this view is taken with the forearm in full supination (typically done as an anteroposterior [AP] view). In this situation, the position of the ulnar styloid shifts radially to align more toward the central longitudinal axis of the ulnar shaft. In addition, the ulnar shaft shows a more linear appearance along its radial border, and the subchondral bone of the ulnar head can be seen superimposed over the ulnar styloid.

With the forearm in a position of full pronation, the radius crosses over the ulna resulting in an obligate but physiological shortening of the radius in relation to the ulna. In this position of forearm rotation, a normal loss of about 0.5 mm of radial length is common. In addition, the radial and ulnar shafts appear to converge proximally, and the cortical outline of the ulnar head can be identified behind the base of the ulnar styloid. With pronation of the forearm, measured values of radial inclination, volar tilt, and radial height decrease; with supination of the forearm, these values increase.[4]

The radial column is a pillar of bone that forms the lateral border of the distal radius. The radial column is an important structure that maintains carpal length and cradles and guides the kinematics of the carpus during wrist motion from a position of radial deviation and extension to ulnar deviation and flexion. Distally, the radial column forms the scaphoid facet; dorsally, it extends to the base of Lister's tubercle. Along the volar surface, the radial column merges with the distal radial ridge that forms the distal insertion of the pronator quadratus. Radiographically, the outline of this anatomical structure can be easily recognized on the standard PA view. Oblique x-rays are sometimes used to project the outline of a more volar portion of the radial border into greater profile.

The ulnar border of the radius flares distally to form the sigmoid notch and has been referred to as the intermediate column. Normally, there is a uniform joint interval present between the ulnar head and the subchondral bone of the sigmoid notch; typically, this interval measures about 1 mm. Separation of the distal radioulnar joint (DRUJ) and joint interval to more than 2 mm implies that a ligamentous injury to this joint has occurred. Distally, the margins of the sigmoid notch end in a dorsal and volar corner. If the forearm is positioned in significant pronation or supination, the appearance of the DRUJ and joint interval is altered. Finally, if the wrist is in neutral position in terms of radial and ulnar deviation, the lunate is normally positioned between the ulnar border of Lister's tubercle and the radial one third of the ulnar head.

The carpal facet horizon is a radiodense line that appears on a normal PA view near the distal articular surface and extends from the ulnar side of the radius across most of the width of the

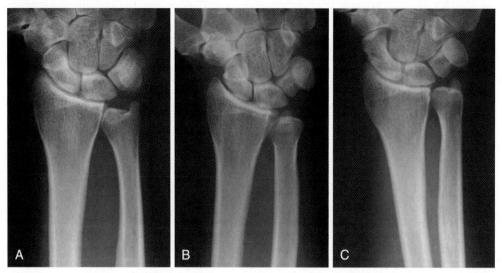

FIGURE 3-1 Change in Appearance of Posteroanterior View with Different Forearm Rotation. A, With the forearm in neutral, the ulnar border of the ulnar styloid is contiguous with the ulnar border of the ulnar shaft, the lateral side of the ulnar shaft has a concave appearance, and no subchondral bone is seen superimposed over the ulnar styloid. **B,** With the forearm in supination, the outline of the ulnar styloid is aligned with the central axis of the ulnar shaft, the lateral side of the ulnar shaft is more linear in appearance, and the subchondral bone of the ulnar head can be seen behind the ulnar styloid. **C,** With forearm pronation, the subchondral bone of the ulnar head can be seen behind the ulnar styloid, the radius undergoes a relative but obligate shortening in relation to the ulna, and the radius and ulna converge proximally.

bone (**Fig. 3-2**). In a normal wrist, the carpal facet horizon is inclined at an angle of about 10 degrees to a perpendicular of a line extended from the longitudinal axis of the radius. The carpal facet horizon is a radiographic landmark that is produced by the x-ray beam as it crosses a portion of the curved arc of dense subchondral bone that is tangential to the axis of the beam. Because a normal distal radius has a volar tilt of 5 to 8 degrees, under normal circumstances, the volar portion of the subchondral plate is the part of the articular surface that is parallel to the x-ray beam. As a result, in a PA view of a normal wrist, the carpal facet horizon identifies the volar rim of the lunate facet and extends ulnar to the volar corner of the sigmoid notch.

In addition, close inspection of a PA view of a normal wrist often reveals the dorsal rim and dorsal corner more distally, overlying the proximal articular surface of the scaphoid and the lunate. In contrast, if a fracture has caused the distal fragment to rotate dorsally, the curved arc of the subchondral plate displaces into dorsal tilt. In this situation, the dorsal portion of the curved subchondral plate becomes aligned tangential to the longitudinal axis of the x-ray beam, and the carpal facet horizon instead identifies the dorsal rim. In this case, this landmark is congruent with the dorsal rim and dorsal corner of the sigmoid notch, and close inspection often reveals the volar rim extending more distally over the proximal edge of the carpus.

Identification of the carpal facet horizon has several clinical applications. Discontinuity of this landmark suggests the presence of a separate intra-articular fracture component. Isolated volar shear fractures with proximal and volar displacement of a free volar rim fragment can show an obvious step-off in the carpal facet horizon on the PA projection and imply the presence of an articular fragment (**Fig. 3-3**). The carpal facet horizon also is used to identify whether a particular fragment on the PA view involves the dorsal rim or volar rim. In fractures that are volarly displaced

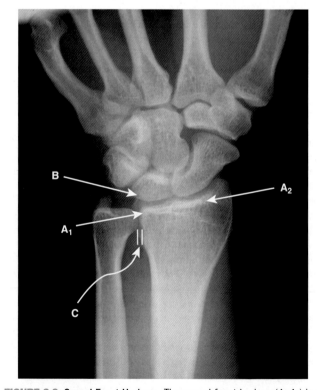

FIGURE 3-2 Carpal Facet Horizon. The carpal facet horizon (A_1-A_2) is a radiodense line that is produced by the portion of the curved subchondral bone that is positioned tangential to the radiographic beam. In a normal wrist that has some volar tilt of the articular surface, the carpal facet horizon represents the volar rim of the lunate facet. In this instance, this finding can be used to distinguish the volar rim (A_1) from the dorsal rim (*B*). Also note the distal radioulnar joint interval (*C*).

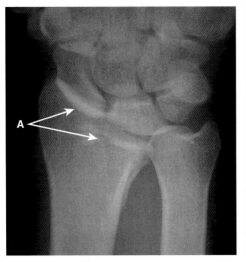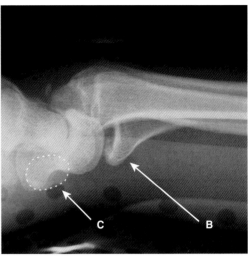

FIGURE 3-3 **Step-off in the Carpal Facet Horizon.** *Left,* The step-off in the carpal facet horizon is caused by an articular fracture component (*A*). Note the overlap of the proximal carpal row over the intact portion of the carpal facet horizon. *Right,* The lateral view shows the displaced volar rim fragment (*B*) with volar subluxation of the carpus into the palmar soft tissues. The position of the pisiform over the distal pole of the scaphoid (*C*) confirms that this view is a true lateral x-ray.

in which there is volar tilt of the articular surface on the lateral x-ray, the carpal facet horizon identifies the volar rim of the lunate facet. In fractures that are dorsally displaced in which there is dorsal tilt of the articular surface on the lateral x-ray, the carpal facet horizon identifies the dorsal rim of the lunate facet. Determining whether a particular articular fragment is located dorsally or volarly on the PA view can be crucial in assessing the pattern of instability and in considering surgical approaches (**Fig. 3-4**).

Lateral View

The lateral x-ray is normally taken with the forearm in neutral rotation. The accuracy of obtaining a true lateral film can be checked by noting the position of the pisiform in relation to the distal pole of the scaphoid on the lateral view. On a true lateral x-ray, the pisiform is located directly over the distal pole of the scaphoid (see Fig. 3-3). If the pisiform lies dorsal to the distal pole of the scaphoid, the forearm is rotated into pronation, and the x-ray is more oblique. Although this type of oblique view can put the volar portion of the radial column in profile, it also results in suboptimal visualization of the volar rim.

In addition to a standard lateral view, the 10-degree lateral view provides a sharper image of the articular surface. The 10-degree lateral view is so named because the ulnar two thirds of the articular surface is normally at an inclination of about 10 degrees to a perpendicular of a line extended along the longitudinal axis of the radius. In some patients, this angle may be greater to correspond to variations in the tilt of the ulnar two thirds of the articular surface.[5,6] The technique for taking the 10-degree lateral view is simple. The forearm is initially positioned horizontally on the plate as if to take a standard lateral x-ray and then elevated 10 degrees off the horizontal plane. If done properly, the articular outline of the ulnar two thirds of the radiocarpal joint is placed into sharp relief (**Fig. 3-5**). This view positions the outline of the radial styloid more proximally than is normally seen on the standard lateral view and may affect the appearance of hardware placed on or into the radial styloid.

Although the radius and ulna overlie one another on the lateral projection, in most cases it is not difficult to follow the cortical outline of each forearm bone to distinguish one from the other. If the film has been properly exposed, the superimposed outline

of the radial styloid over the scaphoid can be identified. On the lateral view, the volar surface of the radial column can be seen to project volar to the outline of the part of the cortical shaft proximal to the lunate facet. As a result, the volar portion of the radial column can be distinguished from the volar cortex of the radial shaft on the lateral view.

The teardrop is a dense, U-shaped outline seen at the distal end of the radius on the lateral view; it is formed from the confluent outlines of the distal shaft and distal radial ridge, and terminates in the volar rim of the lunate facet (**Fig. 3-6**). The thickness of the cortical bone that forms the base of the teardrop is noted to be significantly greater than the thickness of the dorsal cortical bone and reflects the greater loading forces that normally occur along the volar surface of the radius. In addition, a line that extends from the volar cortex of the radial shaft nearly bisects the curve of the articular surface (typically passing just volar to the center of the articular surface on the lateral view), suggesting that the carpal load is nearly balanced along the volar cortex.

The distal articular surface of the radius on a normal wrist has an arc of curvature that matches the arc of curve of the proximal pole of the lunate; this uniform joint interval is more clearly seen on the 10-degree lateral x-ray. Fractures that result in a joint interval that is nonuniform from the dorsal to volar margin or show incongruent arcs of curvature between the articular surface of the distal radius and the proximal pole of the lunate imply discontinuity between the volar and dorsal joint surfaces with independent articular fracture components (**Fig. 3-7**).

Carpal alignment also is an important feature to observe on the lateral x-ray. With a wrist in neutral to slight dorsiflexion, a line extended from the volar cortex of the radial shaft should be nearly collinear with the center axis of rotation of the proximal pole of the capitate (see Fig. 3-6). Fractures with dorsal angulation or displacement cause translation of the carpus dorsally, resulting in dorsal migration of the proximal pole of the capitate relative to the volar cortex of the radial shaft (**Fig. 3-8**). Fractures that displace to the volar side result in volar migration of the capitate from its normal alignment with the radial shaft and are highly unstable. Significant displacement of the carpus in either direction changes the functional moment arm of tendons that cross the wrist and may contribute to adverse affects on grip strength.

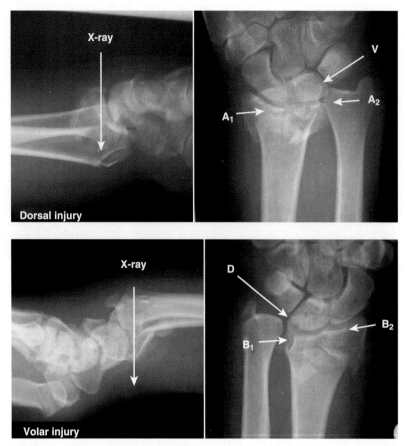

FIGURE 3-4 Clinical Application of the Carpal Facet Horizon. *Top panel,* In the dorsal injury, the distal fragment has rotated dorsally causing the dorsal portion of the subchondral bone to align with the axis of the x-ray beam. In this case, the carpal facet horizon (A_1-A_2) identifies the dorsal rim of the lunate facet. Note the position of the dorsal ulnar corner (A_2) and the volar corner of the sigmoid notch (*V*). Discontinuity of the carpal facet horizon indicates an additional free articular fragment. *Bottom panel,* In the volar injury, the distal fragment has rotated volarly. As a result, the volar rim of the lunate facet is aligned with the x-ray beam, and the carpal facet horizon (B_1-B_2) identifies the volar rim. Note the position of the volar corner (B_1) and dorsal corner (*D*) of the sigmoid notch. Also note the irregularity of the carpal facet horizon indicating a separate volar rim and radial column fragment.

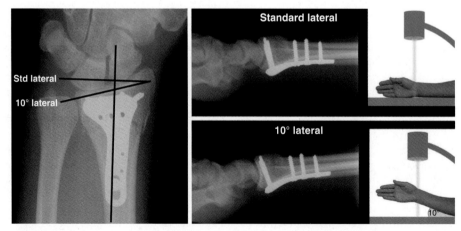

FIGURE 3-5 10-Degree Lateral X-ray. A standard lateral x-ray is taken with the forearm in the horizontal plane and crosses the articular surface obliquely. As a result, incongruity and displacements of the articular surface are obscured, and assessments of fracture reduction or hardware placement are less accurate. With the 10-degree lateral x-ray, the forearm is elevated off the horizontal plane to place the ulnar two thirds of the articular surface into profile, resulting in a more accurate image of the subchondral bone.

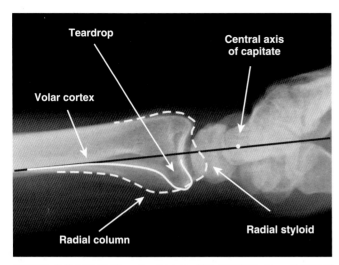

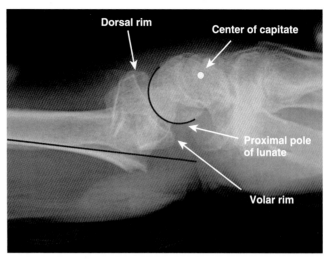

FIGURE 3-6 Lateral View Landmarks. The teardrop is a U-shaped outline caused by the confluence of the volar shaft, the distal radial ridge, and the volar rim of the lunate facet. Note the outline of the radial styloid superimposed over the carpus, and the volar border of the radial column that normally extends more volar than the volar cortex of the shaft. A line extended from the volar cortex of the radial shaft normally nearly bisects the articular surface of the distal radius and passes through the central axis of rotation of the base of the capitate with the wrist in neutral position. Also note the uniform joint interval from dorsal to volar between the lunate and the distal articular surface of the radius.

FIGURE 3-7 Nonuniform Joint Interval. This intra-articular fracture with dorsal displacement clearly shows a nonuniform joint interval between the proximal articular surface of the lunate and the distal articular surface of the radius. A nonuniform joint interval implies discontinuity across the articular surface of the distal radius from separate dorsal and volar fragments. On this x-ray, also note the significant depression of the teardrop angle and the dorsal translation of the center of rotation of the base of the capitate away from its normal alignment with the volar cortex of the shaft.

FIGURE 3-8 Abnormal Carpal Alignment. *Left,* Intraoperative image shows a depressed tear-drop angle (32 degrees) and dorsal translation of the central axis of rotation of the base of the capitate during application of a volar plate. Also note the incongruity of the joint interval and the widened anteroposterior distance. *Right,* Intraoperative image taken after the surgical approach was modified shows correction of the tear-drop angle using a Volar Buttress Pin (TriMed, Valencia, CA) and restoration of a normal joint interval and carpal alignment.

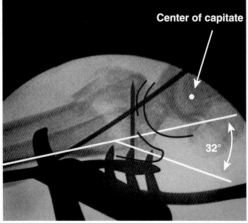

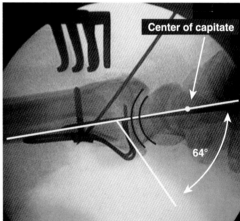

Radiographic Parameters
Anteroposterior View

Radiographic parameters are measured values used to quantify the amount of displacement or amount of angulation that has occurred with a distal radius fracture. Although recommendations are often made to define indications for operative treatment based on threshold values of individual parameters, in nearly all fractures abnormalities of multiple parameters are often present and may act synergistically in terms of the functional impairment caused by the total deformity. Generally, abnormalities of a single parameter should not be considered in isolation, but rather in the context of the entire fracture pattern before committing to a particular approach for treatment. Understanding of which combinations of abnormal parameters have the greatest clinical significance

continues to evolve. In addition, because there is a certain amount of normal variation of most parameters within a typical population, it can be quite helpful to take x-rays of the normal contralateral wrist to establish baseline values.

Radial inclination and ulnar variance are two parameters measured on the PA view that often are defined using the most distal corner of the ulnar border of the distal radius as a point of reference. As discussed previously, this radiographic landmark does not correspond to a single anatomical structure, but may vary, representing either the dorsal corner of the sigmoid notch or the volar corner of the sigmoid notch depending on whether the distal articular surface has a volar or dorsal tilt. Because these measurements should ideally remain independent of the tilt of the articular surface on the lateral view, a central reference point (CRP) should be used for the measurement of radial inclination and

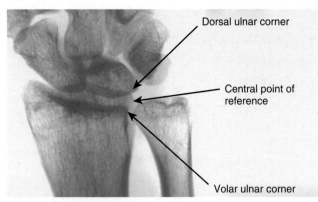

FIGURE 3-9 **Central Reference Point.** Because the most distal point on the ulnar side of the radius may be on the volar or dorsal side of the radius depending on the tilt of the articular surface, this landmark is not a reliable point of reference for parameters such as ulnar variance. The central reference point is a more reliable reference point for measurement of radial inclination and ulnar variance and is found by bisecting a line drawn between the dorsal and volar corners of the sigmoid notch. Because the central reference point sits near the coronal center of the sigmoid notch, it is not as dependent on the amount of volar or dorsal tilt.

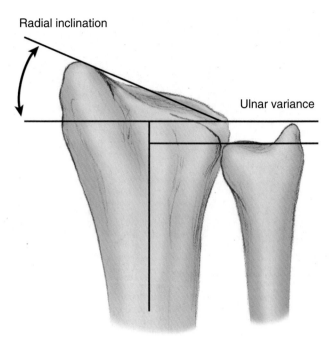

FIGURE 3-10 **Radial Inclination and Ulnar Variance.** Radial inclination is measured as the angle between a line drawn from the tip of the radial styloid to the central reference point and a line that is perpendicular to the long axis of the radial shaft (normal value 24 degrees). Ulnar variance is defined as the separation between two lines that are perpendicular to the long axis of the radial shaft, where one line intersects the central reference point, and the other line intersects the distal edge of the ulnar head (normal value −0.6 mm).

ulnar variance. The CRP can be identified by determining the center of a line that is drawn between the volar and dorsal corners on the AP view (**Fig. 3-9**). Because the CRP coincides with the coronal center of the distal edge of the sigmoid notch, it is relatively independent of changes in the volar tilt of the articular surface. Using the CRP is particularly important for assessing ulnar variance because this measurement can be significantly affected by changes in volar tilt.

Radial inclination is a parameter that is defined as the angle between a line drawn from the tip of the radial styloid to the CRP and a line perpendicular to the long axis of the radius (**Fig. 3-10**). In normal wrists, radial inclination measures about 24 degrees.[7] Generally, displaced fractures of the distal radius reduce radial inclination; radial inclination less than 15 degrees is a relative indication for operative treatment.

Ulnar variance is a parameter used in the context of distal radius fractures to help quantify the loss of radial length. Ulnar variance is determined by measuring the distance between two lines drawn perpendicular to a reference line extended along the axis of the radial shaft where one perpendicular intersects the distal edge of the ulnar head, and the second perpendicular intersects the CRP (see Fig. 3-10). Negative values indicate that the radius extends beyond the ulna; positive values indicate that the ulna extends beyond the radius. Ulnar variance is normally −0.6 mm with a standard deviation of 1 mm. Shortening of more than 5 mm is a relative indication for operative treatment.

Radial height is another parameter that can be used to assess the loss of radial length. This measurement is made by measuring the distance between two lines drawn perpendicular to a reference line extended along the axis of the radial shaft where one perpendicular intersects the tip of the radial styloid, and the second perpendicular intersects the CRP. The normal value for radial height is 11.6 mm. Radial height is related to the loss of radial inclination and the width of the bone.

Articular step-off is a parameter used with intra-articular fractures to measure discontinuity in height between two adjacent articular fragments.[8] Generally, articular step-off of greater than 1 to 2 mm is considered a relative indication for operative treatment. Residual articular step-offs greater than these values have been associated with a high incidence of osteoarthritis in young patients. In addition, if significant depression between the scaphoid and lunate facet is seen on the PA view, the clinician should have a high index of suspicion for scapholunate injury.

The radiocarpal interval is the distance that separates the base of the scaphoid from the base of the scaphoid facet. Normally, this interval measures 2 mm. This parameter can be particularly useful in the context of a spanning external fixator to judge the relative degree of distraction across the joint. A radiocarpal interval greater than 3 mm suggests excessive distraction across the wrist joint.

Lateral View

On the lateral view, volar tilt is used to measure the angular change of the articular surface. Volar tilt is defined as the angle between a line perpendicular to the central axis of the radial shaft and a line that connects the corner of the dorsal rim and the corner of the volar rim on the lateral view (**Fig. 3-11**). Normal wrists have about 10 degrees of volar tilt; dorsally angulated fractures with greater than 10 degrees of dorsal tilt are a relative indication for reduction. Fractures displaced to the volar side often show an increase in volar tilt. These fractures tend to be highly unstable and require some form of stabilization.

The AP distance is the point-to-point distance between the corner of the dorsal rim and the corner of the volar rim on the lateral view (**Fig. 3-12**). Normal AP distance measures 20 mm in men and 18 mm in women. Elevation of the AP distance more than 21 mm in men and 19 mm in women suggests discontinuity across the lunate facet with a separate dorsal and volar fragment.

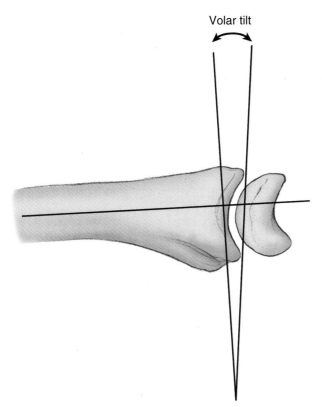

FIGURE 3-11 **Measurement of Volar Tilt.** Volar tilt is measured as the angle between a line that connects the dorsal rim and volar rim of the articular surface of the radius on the lateral view with a line perpendicular to the long axis of the radial shaft.

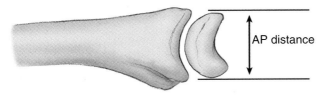

FIGURE 3-12 **Measurement of Anteroposterior (AP) Distance.** AP distance is measured as the distance between the dorsal and volar rims of the articular surface on the lateral view. Increased AP distance is sometimes the only sign of coronal fracture lines that split the lunate facet into independent volar and dorsal fragments.

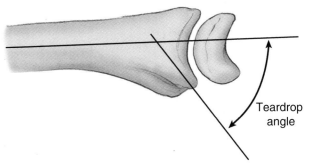

FIGURE 3-13 **Measurement of Teardrop Angle.** The teardrop angle is measured as the angle between a line drawn down the longitudinal axis of the radial shaft with a line drawn down the center of the teardrop (parallel to the subchondral bone along the volar rim). Generally, articular fractures of the volar rim with depression of the teardrop below 45 degrees indicate a dorsiflexed volar rim fragment. Dorsal translation of carpal alignment is routinely present with significant depression of the teardrop angle.

Marked widening of the AP interval may be the only evidence of sigmoid notch involvement that would be otherwise difficult to visualize on standard x-rays.[9] It is usually better to measure the AP distance on the 10-degree lateral projection.

The teardrop angle is used to measure the angular position of the teardrop, or volar rim of the lunate facet, on the lateral view. In extra-articular fractures with dorsal angulation, the depression of the teardrop angle is directly proportional to the change in volar tilt and does not add any new information. In contrast, in intra-articular fractures with axial compression, impaction of the lunate into the lunate facet can generate a free volar rim fragment that is driven by the carpus into significant dorsiflexion. As a result, significant depression of the teardrop angle can occur, which is often independent and greater than the loss of volar tilt. If correction of the teardrop angle is not addressed in the context of a dorsiflexed volar rim fragment, significant residual intra-articular incongruity and dorsal subluxation of the carpus may go unnoticed. For instance, simple buttress plate application on a dorsiflexed volar rim may aggravate an existing depression of the teardrop angle.

The teardrop angle is determined by measuring the angle between a line extended along the longitudinal axis of the radial shaft and a line that is drawn down the center of the teardrop; if the complete cortical outline of the teardrop is difficult to determine, a line drawn parallel to the subchondral bone of the volar rim can be used instead (**Fig. 3-13**). Depression of the teardrop angle below 45 degrees indicates significant dorsiflexion deformity of the volar rim of the lunate facet and should be corrected.

Fragmentation Patterns

Over the past 5 decades, many different classifications of distal radius fractures have been proposed, both as a suggestion for guidelines to treatment and as a predictor of the natural history of different patterns of injury. Traditional classifications of distal radius fractures were based on early descriptions of simple extra-articular fractures by Colles, Barton, and Smith.[10] These initial observations described angulation of the distal fragment in a volar or dorsal direction. Further iterations of these descriptions incorporated the presence of comminution, involvement of the radial articular surface, displacement, direction of displacement and degree of articular surface involvement, length of the radial styloid, presence of dorsal angulation, and extent of metaphyseal comminution.[11] Frykman[12] identified the presence of radiocarpal joint, radioulnar joint, and ulnar styloid involvement. Later classification systems, such as the Melone[13] and Mayo[14] classifications, have underscored the importance of basic fragmentation patterns of the articular surface.

More recently, the AO[15] and Fernandez/Jupiter[16] classifications have proposed grouping patterns by the mechanism of injury. The AO system broadly divides fractures into bending, shear, and axial loading categories, with the Fernandez/Jupiter system adding carpal avulsions and high-energy trauma as additional categories. Although the AO classification divides patterns further into 27 subcategories, there is poor interobserver and intraobserver correlation beyond the three basic types.[17-19]

The fragment-specific classification system is based on the observation that fracture lines in distal radius fractures generally

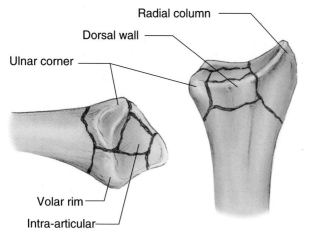

Radial column

Dorsal wall

Ulnar corner

Volar rim

Intra-articular

FIGURE 3-14 Fragment-Specific Classification. Articular fractures of the distal radius tend to propagate along recurrent pathways, resulting in generation of five basic fracture components: radial column, ulnar corner, dorsal wall, free intra-articular, and volar rim. In addition to these distal radius fracture elements, impaction of the metaphyseal bone, distal radioulnar joint and distal ulna injuries, and intracarpal pathology may affect the natural history of a particular fracture pattern.

TABLE 3-1   Distal Radius Fracture Personalities

Mechanism	Personality
Shear	Dorsal shear
	Volar shear
Bending	Dorsal bending
	Volar bending
Bending + axial	Three-part articular
Axial	Comminuted articular
	Comminuted articular with volar rim dorsiflexion
	Comminuted articular with DRUJ instability

DRUJ, distal radioulnar joint.

propagate along recurrent pathways, resulting in five basic fracture components: the radial column, ulnar corner, dorsal wall, volar rim, and free intra-articular fragments (**Fig. 3-14**). The radial column fragment is often a major fragment along the radial border of the wrist and is important to maintain radial length and provide support to the carpus across the radioscaphoid joint. The ulnar corner fragment involves the dorsal side of the lunate facet and the dorsal portion of the sigmoid notch, and typically migrates dorsally and proximally; significant displacement of this fragment can adversely affect movement and function of the DRUJ. Dorsal wall fragmentation is often a contributing factor in dorsal instability. The volar rim fragment is formed by the distal radial ridge and the volar portion of the lunate facet and is often a major element of fracture instability. This fragment can either displace volarly into the palmar soft tissue or impact axially, rotating into dorsiflexion with depression of the teardrop angle and dorsal subluxation of the carpus. Finally, free intra-articular fragments may displace and rotate into the metaphyseal cavity creating articular step-offs and joint incongruity.

Fractures of the distal ulna are usually classified based on the position of the fracture.[20] Simple avulsions of the tip of the styloid are rarely clinically important, although they may be associated with more significant tears of the triangular fibrocartilaginous complex. Fractures through the base of the ulnar styloid may be associated with instability of the DRUJ, particularly if widely displaced with the carpus in a radial direction. Ulnar head fractures may involve the congruency of the articular surface of the DRUJ and cause dysfunction or late arthritis if left unreduced. Fractures through the neck or shaft of the ulna can compromise rotational stability of the forearm.

One contemporary approach to distal radius fractures is to combine the fragment-specific classification system with a characterization of fracture "personality," which is based on mechanism, magnitude, and direction of injury.[1] Because forces on the volar side of the radius are typically much higher than forces along the dorsal side, the direction of displacement of the distal fragment can significantly affect the characteristics and natural history of a particular fracture pattern. For this reason, extra-articular

fractures with dorsal displacement from a dorsal bending mechanism are considered different from extra-articular fractures with volar displacement from a volar bending mechanism. Similarly, dorsal shear fractures have different characteristics in terms of prognosis and treatment from volar shear fractures. Finally, axial loading injuries may result in several different patterns based on the magnitude and direction of applied force (**Table 3-1**).

Dorsal bending injuries occur from a dorsal bending moment and result in compressive failure on the dorsal side and simple tensile failure on the volar cortex (**Fig. 3-15**). Characteristically, they manifest as a large single distal fragment that includes the articular surface of the radiocarpal joint and fragmentation of the dorsal wall along with compression of the metaphyseal cavity. In many cases, apposition of the volar cortex at a single fracture line between the proximal and distal fragment provides a stable fulcrum on which to hinge the reduction. In this situation, the amount of dorsal comminution and metaphyseal impaction is the primary determinant of the degree of dorsal instability. Although ligamentous damage to the DRUJ also may be present, often DRUJ stability is restored simply by reduction of the distal fragment.

Although supination of the distal fragment relative to the proximal fragment is typically present, this deformity is difficult to assess radiographically. In dorsal bending injuries, the x-ray evaluation should be directed at determining the degree of dorsal wall fragmentation and metaphyseal involvement and the extent of DRUJ involvement. Loss of length and radial inclination are characteristic features. In addition, dorsal subluxation of the center of rotation of the base of the capitate is usually observed. Although depression of the teardrop angle is a typical characteristic of the x-ray findings in dorsal bending injuries, in this situation it simply reflects and is proportional to the loss of volar tilt.

In contrast to dorsal bending injuries, displaced volar bending injuries are nearly always unstable and are subject to an entirely different environment of deforming forces (**Fig. 3-16**). In this fracture personality, the distal fragment and carpus displace into the palmar soft tissues, and stable reduction across the volar cortex is often impossible with closed methods of management. Rotational deformities are difficult to assess radiographically. In contrast to dorsal bending injuries, in which the volar cortex can often be used as a fulcrum for balancing the dorsal instability pattern against the strong pull of the flexor tendons, the deform-

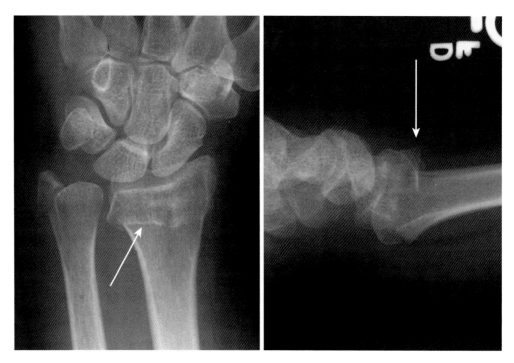

FIGURE 3-15 **Dorsal Bending Personality.** This dorsally angulated extra-articular fracture shows loss of radial inclination, dorsal tilt of the articular surface, and ulnar-positive variance from loss of length. Note the dorsal wall fragment has rotated to align with the x-ray beam and is seen as a horizontal radiodense line on the posteroanterior view and in a vertical attitude on the lateral view (*arrows*).

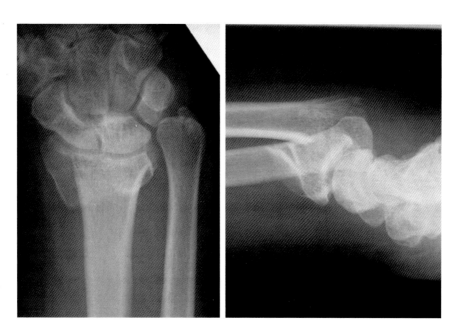

FIGURE 3-16 **Volar Bending Injury.** Note the significant volar subluxation of the carpus with the distal fragment, the loss of length, and volar wall comminution in this highly unstable volar bending pattern.

ing pull of the flexor tendons in volar bending injuries results in palmar and proximal migration of the carpus and distal fragment. Volar bending injuries are characterized by volar subluxation of the rotational center of the base of the capitate in relation to the volar cortex of the shaft. In some cases, additional fragmentation of the volar wall also may be observed. In addition, displaced volar bending injuries show proximal carpal migration with loss of overall length and radial inclination. Volar tilt may be increased, and disruption of the DRUJ is commonly observed. Typically, these injuries require some type of operative intervention to achieve a stable reduction.

In volar shear fractures, the carpus is driven into the volar rim of the lunate facet, resulting in volar and proximal translation of this fragment (see Fig. 3-3). The carpus is carried by the volar rim

fragment and dislocates off the remaining intact dorsal rim of the lunate facet. Volar and proximal migration of the teardrop occurs, and overlap of the dorsal rim and the carpus is seen on the PA view. As noted previously, discontinuity of the carpal facet horizon also may be noted on the PA view. On the lateral view, displacement of the carpus and volar rim is usually obvious, and increased AP distance is frequently noted. Particular focus should be on examination of the volar rim component for additional secondary fracture lines within the volar rim. Fragmentation into the radial column also may be present. In addition to injury views, postreduction x-rays should confirm that the center of rotation of the base of the capitate is restored to its normal relationship to a line extended from the volar cortex of the shaft, indicating that complete correction of volar subluxation of the carpus has been obtained. X-rays also should confirm that reduction has brought the volar rim back out to length, resulting in complete correction of the carpal facet horizon to its normal spatial alignment on the PA view.

A pure dorsal shear fracture is a more uncommon pattern of injury. In this pattern, the impact of the carpus against the dorsal rim of the lunate facet results in a shear failure with varying degrees of dorsal subluxation and proximal migration of the carpus (**Fig. 3-17**). In dorsal shear fractures, significant articular step-offs are present in the sagittal plane, producing a sharp edge that can grind against the proximal pole of the lunate during flexion movements of the wrist. In volar shear fractures, the predominant clinical concern is correction of the significant volar instability of the carpus caused from the strong pull of the flexor tendons. In contrast, in dorsal shear fractures, the predominant clinical concern is the restoration of a smooth and congruous articular surface, eliminating deep articular offsets dorsally that may result in accelerated wear of the lunate during flexion movements of the wrist.

On the PA view, dorsal shear fractures may show a reduction in the radiocarpal interval as the carpus shifts proximally from the dorsal subluxation. On the lateral view, dorsal subluxation of the carpus is easily noted with an increase in the AP distance. The DRUJ interval may or may not be affected. Dorsal wall fragments and an ulnar corner fragment are typically present; free intra-articular fragments also may be impacted within the metaphysis. Articular offset is often observed on the lateral view.

Simple three-part distal radius fractures consist of a proximal shaft fragment, an ulnar corner fragment, and a large distal articular fragment that contains the radial column and the volar rim (**Fig. 3-18**). Although this injury pattern is often described as the result of axial loading, it is probably the result of a combination of axial loading and simple bending mechanisms. The ulnar corner fragment often involves the dorsal portion of the sigmoid notch and usually includes the insertion of the dorsal ligament of the DRUJ. Three-part fractures usually show some loss of radial

length and radial inclination on the PA view. On the lateral view, dorsal angulation of the distal fragment is frequently observed. Dorsal and sometimes proximal displacement of the ulnar corner fragment may occur. In addition, fragmentation of the dorsal wall is often seen.

Complex articular fractures tend to occur in two patterns, based on the direction and instability of the volar rim of the lunate facet. These complex axial load injuries can generate any or all of the five basic fracture components, resulting in significant step-offs or separations within the articular surface. In one pattern of injury, the impact of the carpus causes the articular surface to explode peripherally, resulting in displacement of the volar rim fragment volarly and proximally. In this pattern, volar or proximal migration of the carpus is observed. An independent radial column fragment is almost always present. In addition, free intra-articular fragments may be impacted into the metaphysis, and ulnar corner and dorsal wall fragments are commonly present (**Fig. 3-19**). Depressed radial inclination, widened AP interval, and incongruity of the articular surface are frequent radiographic findings with this injury. An inconsistent joint interval between the distal radius and proximal pole of the lunate on the lateral view can indicate articular disruption across the lunate facet. Dorsal or excessive volar tilt also may be present and depends on the principal direction of injury.

In a second comminuted articular pattern, the carpus impacts axially into the articular surface, resulting in dorsiflexion of the volar rim of the lunate facet and dorsal subluxation of the carpus. In addition to the radiographic abnormalities discussed previously, these injuries manifest with depression of the teardrop angle and dorsal subluxation of the carpus. Widening of the AP distance also is a consistent feature of this pattern. Correction of the dorsiflexion deformity of the volar rim of the lunate facet should be an integral part of a complete reduction of the articular surface.

Comminuted articular fractures of the distal radius also may affect the ulna or DRUJ or both, which may complicate the injury

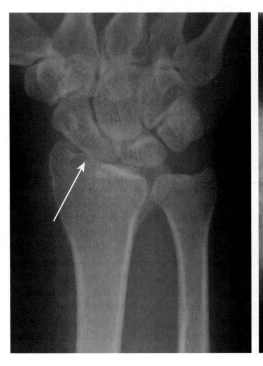
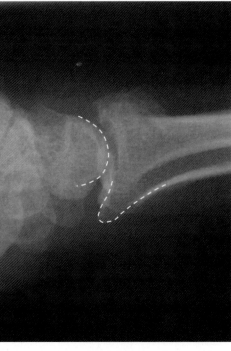

FIGURE 3-17 Dorsal Shear Fracture. *Left,* On the posterior view, the radiocarpal interval appears reduced because of the proximal migration of the carpus into the dorsal defect (*arrow*). *Right,* Note on the lateral view how the proximal articular surface of the lunate has slipped off the volar rim of the lunate facet into the dorsal defect.

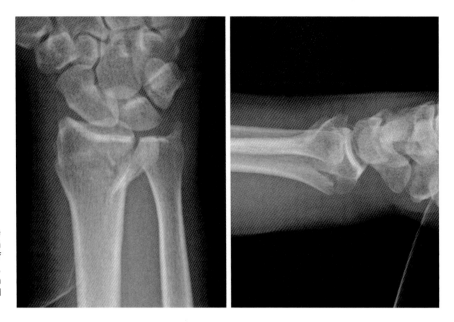

FIGURE 3-18 Three-Part Articular Fracture. The three-part articular fracture is a low injury pattern that is probably the result of a combination of dorsal bending and axial loading mechanisms. Note the ulnar corner fragment dorsally, which involves the dorsal portion of the sigmoid notch.

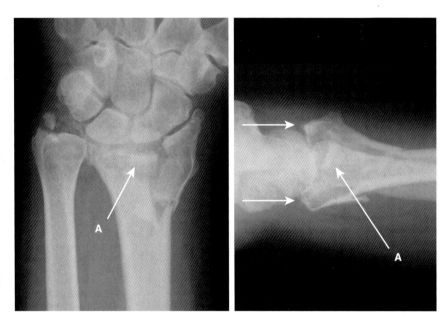

FIGURE 3-19 Comminuted Articular Fracture. This injury is the result of an axial loading mechanism and shows a depressed, free intra-articular fragment (A) and an increased anteroposterior distance (horizontal arrows, right panel). The lunate has collapsed within the central articular defect into the metaphysis. Note the incidental signs of degenerative arthritis with spurring of the tip of the radial styloid and chondrocalcinosis of the radiocarpal joint medially.

pattern further (Fig. 3-20). Significant disruption of the DRUJ may occur with volar or dorsal subluxation of the distal ulna in relation to the distal radius. In some cases, excessive widening of the DRUJ may be noted. These fractures are usually associated with extreme comminution of the articular surface and malalignment of the carpus on the lateral view. Widening of the AP distance and a nonuniform joint interval on the lateral view are often features of this pattern. In addition to reconstruction of the articular surface, restoration of stability of the DRUJ is required and may include soft tissue reconstruction of the ligamentous structures.

Radial shear fractures are an unusual form of distal radius fractures. In radial shear fractures, translation of the carpus results in a shear fracture across the tip of the radial styloid, rather than the radial column type of injury seen with other fracture patterns. Radial translation of the carpus may be observed along with ulnar styloid injuries that have displaced toward the radius. In these

fractures, the extent of articular surface damage is often underestimated by the radiographic findings, and supplemental arthroscopic evaluation may be required to assess fully the degree of joint damage. Marked widening of the DRUJ or bones of the forearm may implicate syndesmotic disruption; these injuries are particularly unstable in terms of DRUJ function (Fig. 3-21). In addition, particular attention should be directed toward assessing these injury patterns for additional intracarpal ligament pathology.

Carpal avulsions and high-energy trauma also have been included as forms of distal radius fractures, although these injuries have their own distinct features. Carpal avulsions are primarily ligamentous injuries to the carpus in which osseous fragments are avulsed from the radius. High-energy trauma injuries are associated with highly comminuted fractures of the distal articular surface of the radius along with extension well up into the shaft of the radius or ulna or both. Although these injuries may have

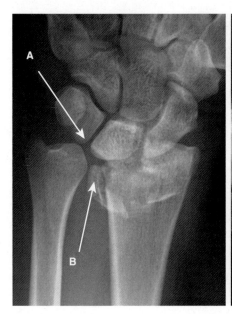

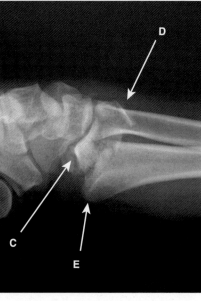

FIGURE 3-20 Comminuted Articular Fracture with Dorsiflexion of the Volar Rim and Disruption of the Distal Radioulnar Joint. In this injury, note the significant widening of the distal radioulnar joint interval indicating severe ligamentous disruption (*A*). An ulnar corner fragment is noted dorsally (*B*). The volar rim of the lunate facet has rotated into dorsiflexion (*C*), allowing the carpus to displace dorsally. A free dorsal wall fragment also is present (*D*). Note the sharp edge of the volar metaphysis (*E*) that puts the median nerve at risk of injury.

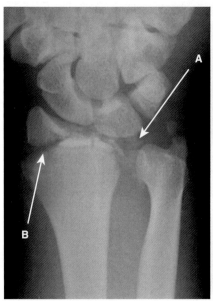

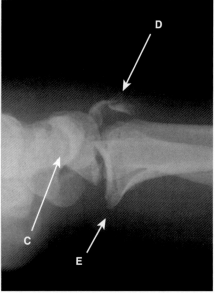

FIGURE 3-21 Radial Shear Fracture. *Left,* A transverse fracture of the radial styloid (*A*) has a different appearance from the more common radial column fragment. Significant widening of the distal radioulnar joint is noted (*B*), and may suggest syndesmotic rupture in addition to disruption of the dorsal and volar ligaments. Note the marked irregularity of the articular surface on the posteroanterior view, which often underscores the extent of articular damage. *Right,* On the lateral view, dorsal subluxation of the carpus (*C*) and dorsal fragmentation (*D*) are seen. Note the dorsal displacement of the lunate out of its normal position adjacent to the teardrop (*E*).

an extensive osseous component, it is not unusual to have a substantial soft tissue component completely overshadow the clinical treatment of these fracture patterns.

Conclusion

In many respects, the treatment of distal radius fractures really begins with the x-ray examination. A wealth of information is present on standard views that can significantly influence the decision and type of treatment that is ultimately selected. Although radial inclination and volar tilt are well-known parameters used to assess the angulation of the distal fragment in the coronal and sagittal planes, several other landmarks and parameters should be routinely evaluated as part of every injury assessment. On the PA view, the carpal facet horizon can help distinguish whether a fragment on the ulnar border of the radius is actually the volar or dorsal corner. Radial translation of the carpus or excessive widening of the DRUJ can imply instability along the

ulnar column. Significant offset of the articular surface, particularly between the scaphoid and lunate facet, may increase the possibility of an intercarpal ligament disruption. On the lateral view, a nonuniform joint interval or increased AP distance suggests disruption and discontinuity across the lunate facet. Depression of the teardrop angle and subluxation of the central rotational axis of the capitate may alter the approach to treatment.

In addition to an awareness of the essential radiographic landmarks and parameters, radiographic evaluation of distal radius fractures requires an understanding of the basic patterns of injuries to appreciate the anatomy of the injury and the mechanical basis of instability. Recognizing which fracture elements are present allows a mental picture of the injury to be developed. Categorizing the mechanism, direction, and magnitude of injury as one of several fracture personalities provides clinically useful information that relates to the source of instability and the possible modes of failure. With improved understanding of the structural anatomy and biomechanical basis of the injury, better treatment and clinical outcomes are likely to follow.

ACKNOWLEDGMENTS

The author would like to thank James Chen, MD, for the research and assistance he provided in the preparation of this chapter.

REFERENCES

1. Medoff R: Essential radiographic evaluation for distal radius fractures. Hand Clin 2005; 21:279-288.

2. Boyer M, Korcek K, et al: Anatomic tilt x-rays of the distal radius: an ex vivo analysis of surgical fixation. J Hand Surg [Am] 2004; 29:116-122.

3. Pennock A, Phillips C, et al: The effects of forearm rotation on three wrist measurements: radial inclination, radial height and palmar tilt. Hand Surg 2005; 10:17-22.

4. Yeh G, Beredjiklian P, et al: Effects of forearm rotation on the clinical evaluation of ulnar variance. J Hand Surg [Am] 2001; 26:1042-1046.

5. Lundy D, Quisling S, et al: Tilted lateral radiographs in the evaluation of intra-articular distal radius fractures. J Hand Surg [Am] 1999; 24:249-256.

6. Mekhail A, Ebraheim N, et al: Anatomic and x-ray film studies of the distal articular surface of the radius. J Hand Surg [Am] 1996; 21:567-573.

7. Szabo R, Weber S: Comminuted intraarticular fractures of the distal radius. Clin Orthop 1988; 230:39-48.

8. McCallister W, Smith J, et al: A cadaver model to evaluate the accuracy and reproducibility of plain radiograph step and gap measurements for intra-articular fracture of the distal radius. J Hand Surg [Am] 2004; 29:841-847.

9. Rozental T, Bozentka D, et al: Evaluation of the sigmoid notch with computed tomography following intra-articular distal radius fracture. J Hand Surg [Am] 2001; 26: 244-251.

10. Peltier L: Fractures of the distal end of the radius. Clin Orthop 1984; 187:18-22.

11. Gartland J, Werley C: Evaluation of healed Colles' fractures. J Bone Joint Surg Am 1951; 33:895-907.

12. Frykman G: Fractures of the distal radius, including sequelae—shoulder and finger syndrome, disturbance in the distal radioulnar joint and impairment of nerve function: a clinical and experimental study. Acta Orthop Scand Suppl 1967; 108:1-153.

13. Melone CJ: Distal radius fractures: patterns of articular fragmentation. Orthop Clin North Am 1993; 24:239-253.

14. Cooney W: Fractures of the distal radius: a modern treatment-based classification. Orthop Clin North Am 1993; 24:211-216.

15. Muller M, Nazarian S, et al: The Comprehensive Classification of Fractures of Long Bones. Berlin: Springer-Verlag, 1990.

16. Jupiter J, Fernandez D: Comparative classification for fractures of the distal end of the radius. J Hand Surg [Am] 1997; 22:563-571.

17. Andersen DJ, Blair WF, et al: Classification of distal radius fractures: an analysis of interobserver reliability and intraobserver reproducibility. J Hand Surg [Am] 1996; 21:574-582.

18. Flinkkilä T, Nikkola-Sihto A, et al: Poor interobserver reliability of AO classification of fractures of the distal radius. J Bone Joint Surg Br 1998; 80:670-672.

19. Kreder H, Hanel D, et al: Consistency of AO fracture classification for the distal radius. J Bone Joint Surg Br 1996; 78:726-731.

20. Biyani A, Simison A, et al: Fractures of the distal radius and ulna. J Hand Surg [Br] 1995; 20:357-364.

Distal Radius Study Group: Purpose, Method, Results, and Implications for Reporting Outcomes

4

Matthew D. Putnam, MD, Melvin P. Rosenwasser, MD, Kenneth Koval, MD, and Douglas P. Hanel, MD

Distal radius fracture care has undergone substantial changes in tools and methods since the first commercial introduction of dorsal and volar fixed angle subchondral fixation plates in 1996.[1] Are these changes good? Is plating "good" in general and specifically?

What is "quality care" as related to distal radius fractures? In *Zen and The Art of Motorcycle Maintenance*, Pirzig[2] examines the concept of Quality. His argument cannot be restated within the context of this chapter; however, his premise of Quality as a unification of all values implies that the true "Quality" of distal radius fracture care can be found only in understanding the whole problem. There are participants (insurers, hospital administrators, equipment manufacturers) in the care process that measure and assign value to only a segment or segments of the "results pie." For the purpose of this chapter, we contend that the physician is the participant with sufficiently broad and specific training to enable "asking the big question": that is, does the addition of new technology matter to the patient, and where should the technology be delivered? We posit that "asking this big question" is the physician's obligation, and that doing so requires ongoing comparative examination of outcome.

In assessing the utility of a new method or technology as it relates to care of a diagnosed condition, we hypothesize the following:

1. A new method or technology does not alter the primary outcome of care of distal radius fractures.
2. The location or physician name associated with distal radius care does not affect the outcome (primary or secondary outcomes).

The above-listed hypotheses assume the reader is familiar with basic concepts of outcomes medicine and some concepts related to manufacturing. Specifically, the reader should be aware that a primary outcome can be selected from three broad categories: (1) general health, (2) condition-specific health, and (3) satisfaction.[3] It also is assumed that the reader accepts the validity of structured patient questionnaires to measure outcomes within the three broad categories. As related to manufacturing, the second hypothesis examines the generalized utility of the method/technology; this is crucial when a tool requires a manipulation/skill-set. Physicians are generally familiar with the need to include patient compliance as a factor to consider when testing medication effec-

tiveness. In physician-administered, "tool-based" medicine, it is essential to examine the ability of physicians to "comply" with a method/device requirement to achieve a desired outcome, and not to assume that success can be generalized outward from a motivated cohort (the surgeon designer's experience). The need to prove treatment efficacy by providers can be assumed to vary directly in relationship to the potential variation in skill and treatment risk. Although large outcome differences cannot be categorically stated to occur in all of medicine, it is known that significant differences in treatment response to specific musculoskeletal diagnoses do occur throughout the United States, and so it seems likely that physician/region specific differences in outcomes already exist.[4]

Traditionally, the best medical experiments manipulate a single variable with the experiment's designer separated from the introduction of the variable and the data collection process. This type of randomized clinical trial (RCT) has many qualities to recommend its use whenever possible. Clinical work makes such studies expensive, however, at a level that practically cannot be sustained as a means to reconfirm and monitor surgeon/system efficacy. Also, randomization requires patient enrollment that is predicated on the physician's belief that selected treatments are equivalent. Often, it is impossible to find providers without treatment prejudice. Prejudiced physicians could not follow the principles of clinical equipoise (a state of genuine uncertainty on the part of the clinical investigator regarding the comparative therapeutic merits of each arm in a trial).[5] Taken together, cost and the need for clinical equipoise argue for an alternative method of prospective enrollment and clinical data acquisition.

"Practical clinical trials" (PCT) is a phrase coined by Tunis and colleagues.[6] By the authors' definition, such trials (1) select relevant information/interventions to compare, (2) include a diverse population of study participants (providers), (3) include patients from a heterogeneous mix of practice settings, and (4) collect a broad range of health outcomes.

For the purpose of studying the effects of distal radius fracture treatment, these instructions are particularly useful. Using this set of instructions enables the study participants to choose the treatment that they believe, based on their skill and experience, would best meet a specific patient's needs. Also, a "high" percentage of eligible patients can be expected to enroll because the relative risk to their health is clinically unchanged compared with not enrolling. Most important in the context of understanding the results of clinical care, such a study can still yield meaningful future treatment guidance assuming that data input is structured and standardized, and assuming that treatment selection bias is low.

Conclusions reached from observational studies have been shown to resemble RCTs when available treatments carry similar indications and risk.[7] RCTs are valuable, but, assuming that the patients who "fall" by their choice or physician's recommendation into specific treatment groups in the PCT are similar (equivalent propensity after analyses), the PCT is able to provide equal or better guidance regarding treatment efficacy (real-world applicability) compared with the effectiveness guidance gained from the RCT (result in an expert world within a specified set of patients willing to be randomly assigned).[8]

The final point just mentioned leads to the issues of privacy and scalability. That is, the size of the observational trial matters as well as its longevity. A meaningful analogy might be as follows: Imagine that we know the number of small planes that took off and landed (without crashing) in Florida in the spring of 2007. What can this tell us about the spring of 2008 in Florida and in the United States? The obvious answer is "not much." We need more data. To acquire these greater data on an ongoing basis within the budget allowed for many studies would be impossible. Hence, the concept of registries has evolved from processes concerned mostly with larger public health issues to registries that "are now vital to quality-improvement programs that assess the safety of new drugs and procedures, identify best clinical practice and compare healthcare systems."[9]

The problem discussed by Williamson and colleagues[9] concerns the clear need for a tracking mechanism across systems that while being respectful of privacy also addresses the need to "see" the patient specifically across systems and across time. In conjunction with the foregoing, the need for such a system to use an open and scalable means of data display, acquisition, and storage is obvious. That such a system must be deployed via the Internet to be affordable and universally available should go without saying.

Methods

The Distal Radius Study Group (DRSG) was formed in 2003. Original group membership included four academic centers, one single-specialty group practice with academic affiliation, and one single-specialty group with no academic experience. The Primary Investigator (PI) acted in an oversight capacity and did not enroll patients.

The group was formed with the intent to examine the possibility of an Internet-based data set as a means of detecting differences in distal radius care. The data to be collected had been agreed on by group members at the outset and were presented from the fixed data set via the Internet to document enrollment, baseline data, treatment data, and follow-up data at specified intervals. The data set was kept constant throughout the study interval (December 2003 to February 2007). Two of the six sites never entered patients (the site housing the oversight PI and the single-specialty group with no academic experience). In 2006, a seventh site (fifth active) joined the DRSG and has successfully enrolled patients using the complete functionality of the collection system (real-time use with direct data transfer into an electronic medical record).

The study was designed in the manner of a PCT. As such, the inclusion and exclusion criteria were kept as broad as possible. The primary exclusion criteria were (1) open epiphysis, (2) open fracture, (3) history of inflammatory arthritic process, (4) fractures with associated nerve or tendon injuries requiring surgical repair, and (5) inability to read or write English. For the DRSG, institutional review board approval has been obtained and maintained at all sites.

The purpose of our choosing an observational model for the study was threefold:

- Inability to choose what should be randomized without bias: Factors that could or should be reasonably randomized are not agreed on. Also, substantial variance in treatment exists without apparent rationale. Before beginning a more discriminating study (randomized), it seemed reasonable to gather structured data regarding this disease/treatment process and outcome so that hypotheses could be formulated.

- Desire to enroll as many patients as possible without an expensive process: The PCT reduced patients' resistance to having their outcome observed without risk that an unknown treatment would be applied was attractive.

- Testing of a method that could support a registry of specific problems and, in this case, distal radius fractures: Of all study models, an observational Internet-based standardized data-element model may come closest to enabling an affordable, easily shared and distributed data set that facilitates subsequent data analyses.

Previously reported variables were used as a guideline to create structured data sets for demographics, baseline, operative (pathology, equipment, complications), outcomes, and adverse events. The Disabilities of the Arm, Shoulder, and Hand (DASH) score was selected as the patient-reported instrument and designated as primary outcome for comparison. Fracture type as designated by the Orthopaedic Trauma Association classification system for distal radius fractures was selected as the primary means of fracture/disease classification.[10] A conceptual model for treatment of distal radius fractures was designed (**Fig. 4-1**). The model depicts the basic treatment/measurement process and identifies the primary outcome and independent variables.

A study booklet was created for each site that summarized the data entry process and was used to familiarize the users with structure of the "screen" that would be seen during the process of data entry. This included a view of all patients enrolled and their follow-up schedule (divided into five postoperative intervals: 2 weeks, 6 weeks, 13 weeks, 26 weeks, and 52 weeks [±20%]) (**Fig. 4-2**). The type of data element to be collected was seen by the user and enforced by the system (range with specific end point using slider bars, single possible choice of data element from a list, multiple possible choice data element or elements from a list, and open text entry) (**Fig. 4-3**).

To enable individual treatment site data entry, an Internet-based data entry method was designed. BoundaryMedical Incorporated (www.boundarymedical.com) developed, deployed, and hosted the method as employed. No software applications or databases were installed at any remote site computers. A monitor, Internet connection, and browser (any) were the only required products at the remote site. The methods met Health Insurance Portability and Accountability Act (HIPAA) compliance and data integrity and security standards.

Each site monitored completion of individual patient follow-up data of enrolled patients using a site-specific follow-up screen that was continuously updated and available via the Internet. In some cases, outstanding DASH scores were obtained via an Internet-based patient portal from home or elsewhere. Data were

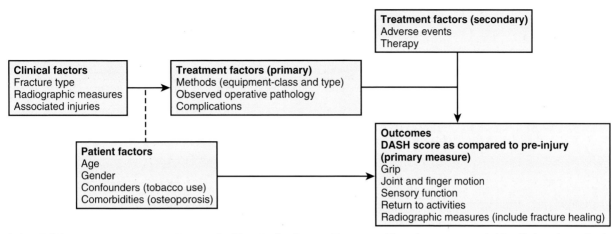

FIGURE 4-1 Outcome Study Design Diagram for Distal Radius Fracture Treatment. The primary outcome is identified as the patient's DASH score. Independent variables (fracture type, physician, treatment site, treatment type [device and technique], and patient) also are shown.

STUDY GROUP PATIENT LIST

Patients in study

Patient	Site/hospital	Baseline	Surgery	0–17 days	18–34 days	35–50 days	51–101 days
Mary Smith 00002SL	Mercy Hospital	7/7/04	7/7/04 Signed	7/7/04 7/24/04 No record	7/24/04 8/10/04 8/5/04 DASH	8/10/04 8/26/04 No record	8/26/04 10/16/04 10/12/04 DASH
Beverly White 00001UU	Southwest Surgery Center	12/30/05	12/30/05 Signed	12/30/05 1/16/06 No record	1/16/06 2/2/06 2/1/06 DASH	2/2/06 2/18/06 2/18/06 DASH	2/18/06 4/9/06 No record DASH 3/3/06
John Sanford 000045W	University Hospital	3/8/05	3/8/05 Signed	3/8/05 3/25/05 No record	3/25/05 4/11/05 3/30/05 DASH	4/11/05 4/27/05 4/27/05 DASH	4/27/05 6/17/05 6/7/05 DASH

FIGURE 4-2 Screen Shot Showing Follow-up Schedule.

obtained for analyses using a secure download method into a specifically formatted Access database that was used to create relational comparisons that were statistically analyzed using SAAS.

Results

Since inception, 280 patients have been identified as meeting the enrollment criteria for study inclusion. Of these, 220 met all inclusion and exclusion criteria and chose to enroll. The primary author (M.D.P.) enrolled one third of all patients treated (**Fig. 4-4**). Enrollment was offered to qualified patients at the time of treatment initiation. **Figure 4-5** depicts the distribution of patient ages, gender, and season at time of fracture. These and other patient factors (e.g., osteoporosis) appear similar across sites.

Sites were instructed to offer enrollment to all patients seen regardless of planned treatment. Treatment numbers suggest that this offer was not made. The frequency of closed cast management varied substantially among sites (**Table 4-1**). Because the distributions of intervention by season, gender, and age are otherwise

similar per site, however, it may be true that the enrollment instruction was observed for surgical treatments at each site during the time period of study participation. Also, the enrollment and rejection rates were similar among sites, providing additional evidence that each site attempted to enroll eligible patients.

Patients' medical characteristics and behavior seem to be similar among sites. Comorbidities revealed an 8% incidence of patients receiving medical treatment for osteoporosis before fracture. This incidence was not significantly different among sites. All patients included in this report completed follow-up examinations. Interval 2 (6 weeks) participation was 72%, but participation decreased to 40% by 1 year (interval 5). The follow-up participation percentage was not statistically different among sites.

The combined average primary outcome measure (DASH score) was similar at all but one site. The dissimilar site seemed to restore function over a longer time interval. This finding was significant and could not be explained by average age or gender bias.

Observation date (mandatory!): Month: [Select... ▲▼] Day: [Select... ▲▼] Year: [2007 ▲▼]

Group	Description
813.42 OTHER CLOSED FRACTURES OF DISTAL END OF RADIUS (ALONE) forearm and wrist	
RIGHT grip KG (average of 3 trials using a Jaymar at position #2. In KG).	Range 0 to 100 KG (5 KG increments) ☐ ◇———°—°—°— 0
LEFT grip KG (average of 3 trials using a Jaymar at position #2. In KG).	Range 0 to 100 KG (5 KG increments) ☐ ◇———°—°—°— 0
RIGHT lateral key pinch KG (average of 3 trials. In KG).	Range 0 to 20 KG (2 KG increments) ☐ ◇—°—°—°—°— 0
LEFT lateral key pinch KG (average of 3 trials. In KG).	Range 0 to 20 KG (2 KG increments) ☐ ◇—°—°—°—°— 0
Supination RIGHT	Greatest degree of active motion (10 degree increments) ☐ ——°—◇—°—°— 0
Supination LEFT	Greatest degree of active motion (10 degree increments) ☐ ——°—◇—°—°— 0
Pronation RIGHT	Greatest degree of active motion (10 degree increments) ☐ ——°—◇—°—°— 0

FIGURE 4-3 Screen Shot Showing Data-Entry Screen as Seen via the Internet.

Inclusion criteria	Closed distal radius fracture (any type) (any treatment) with or without other fractures (ICD-9 = 813.41 Colles' fracture closed, 813.42 fracture distal radius OT closed, 813.44 fracture low radius W ULNA closed) (CPT = 20690, 25600, 25605, 25611, 25620, 29847)
Exclusion criteria	1. Open epiphysis 2. Open fracture 3. Inflammatory arthritic process 4. Nerve, tendon, or vessel injury requiring surgical repair 5. Unable to read English

Patients in study	Potential patients	Enrolled patients
Matthew D. Putnam, MD	97	75
All MDs	280	220

FIGURE 4-4 Enrollment Screen Showing Enrollment Criteria and Case Count.

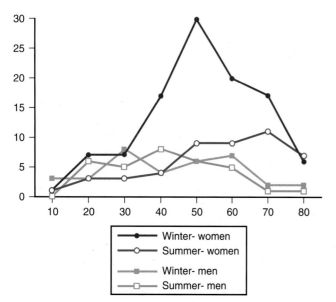

FIGURE 4-5 Demographics Summary Sorted into Gender, Age, and Season at Injury.

Primary outcome measure (DASH score) recovery was similar for A (extra-articular) fractures compared with C (intra-articular) fractures. Primary outcome measure (DASH score) recovery was faster for men compared with women. This trend was true at all intervals and approaches significance (**Fig. 4-6**).

Excluding bilateral injuries, grip strength recovery (compared with percentage of unaffected side), digital motion recovery (total active motion of affected hand fingers [measure the worst finger]), visual analog scale pain scores (0 to 10), and work status (coded in an ordinal manner as to ability to perform "original" work tasks) are the best clinical (physician-collected) values as correlated to DASH recovery ($P < .001$). Wrist motion does not correlate to DASH recovery. Forearm motion is important, but not to the same degree as grip strength recovery and digital motion preservation (**Table 4-2**).

Radiographic measurements were not generally predictive of DASH recovery. Only lateral tilt (volar or dorsal tilt captured in 5-degree increments on the true lateral view) moved significantly with DASH and only at interval 2.

Fixation differences by site and fracture type are listed in **Table 4-3**. Excluding patients with bilateral injuries, weak evidence

TABLE 4-1 **Treatments Used According to Fracture and Site**

Device	Manufacturer	Site 1		Site 2		Site 3		Site 4		All	
		A	C	A	C	A	C	A	C	A	C
Cast only	—	2	1					4	5	6	6
DBP	Avanta/SBI		1							0	1
DFAP	Avanta/SBI		3							0	3
DFAP	EBI						1			0	1
DFAP	Stryker/Howmedica						1			0	1
Ext Fix Br	EBI			1	1					1	1
Ext Fix Br	OrthoFix		1							0	1
Ext Fix Br	Stryker/Howmedica		1			4	4			4	5
Ext Fix Br	Synthes								1	0	1
Ext Fix Br	Other					2	1			2	1
Ext Fix Non Br	Stryker/Howmedica			1						1	0
Ext Fix Non Br	Synthes			2						2	0
IM Rod	Wright	9	7							9	7
K Wires	Stryker/Howmedica					3	4			3	4
K Wires	Tri-med					1				1	0
K Wires	Generic	1								1	0
K Wires	Other						1		1	0	2
RBP	EBI						1			0	1
RBP	Stryker/Howmedica						1			0	1
RBP	Other						1			0	1
RFAP	EBI					2	5			2	5
VBP	Synthes					1				1	0
VBP	Other						1			0	1
VFAP	Avanta/SBI	11	10			1		11	4	23	14
VFAP	EBI					2	7			2	7
VFAP	Hand Innovations								10	0	10
VFAP	Stryker/Howmedica			4	11					4	11
VFAP	Other	1						1	1	2	1
Totals		24	24	8	12	16	28	16	22	64	86

DBP, dorsal buttress plate; DFAP, dorsal fixed angle plate; Ext Fix Br, bridging external fixation; Ext Fix Non Br, non-bridging external fixation; IM Rod, intramedullary rod with fixed angle support; K wires, Kirschner wires; RBP, radial buttress plate; RFAP, radial fixed angle plate; VBP, volar buttress plate; VFAP, volar fixed angle plate.

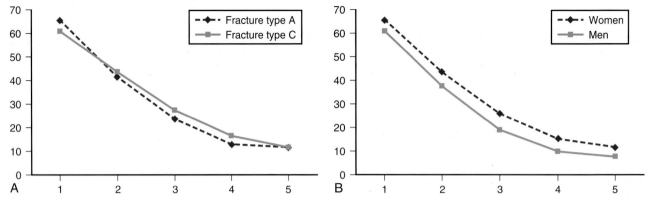

FIGURE 4-6 **Median DASH Scores.** **A,** Median DASH score by fracture type at follow-up intervals 1-5. **B,** Median DASH score by gender at follow-up intervals 1-5.

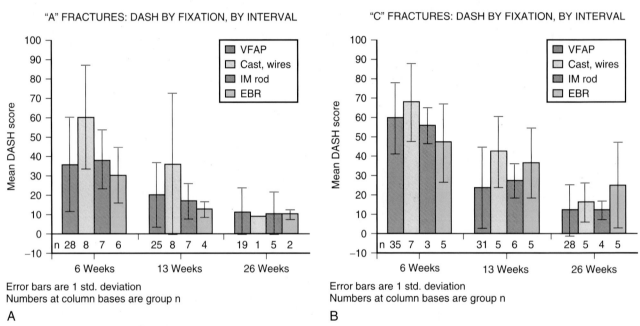

FIGURE 4-7 **DASH Score Recovery (Median).** DASH score recovery (median) by interval (**A**) and sorted by treatment device (**B**).

suggests external fixation bridging is best early (interval 2 [6 weeks]) compared with volar fixed-angle plating (VFAP). At later (interval 3 [13 weeks] and beyond) follow-up, VFAP (no difference between manufacturers observed) is different (lower DASH) from external fixation bridging. As previously noted, cast care and primary "pin" fixation recover most slowly (**Fig. 4-7**).

Adverse events were recorded. Conversion from original intended treatment to a second type at a later date was considered an adverse event. Two scenarios were seen: (1) conversion from cast immobilization to internal fixation after loss of reduction (several cases) and (2) failure of original fixation to achieve reduction (one case). The adverse events in this series were sufficiently different and infrequent to prevent analyses.

Data were entered to the database from all sites via the Internet. In some instances, the data were entered contemporaneously with the episode of care (including operative documentation). Some of these data were directly incorporated into the electronic medical record present at the site of care using a VPN connection and HL-7 protocol. Most (70%) data were collected by investigators using patient-specific treatment, paper-based

booklets, and entered into the database at some point after the visit.

One case is used to illustrate the data capture process in this study. A patient presented with a new closed fracture. The patient was an otherwise healthy English-speaking woman with no prior injury or chronic medical concerns. No nerve or tendon injuries were present. An unstable fracture with a dorsal-ulnar corner fragment and associated laxity of the distal radioulnar joint was diagnosed. Fixation maintained reduction of this intra-articular fracture and early active-assisted range of motion was initiated. DASH score recovery was progressive and nearly complete. The patient presented nearly 10 months after fixation with dorsal tenderness over a fixation bolt (adverse event) that resolved after removal of the screw only and no change in the DASH score (**Figs. 4-8** to **4-10**).

Discussion

One goal of this study was to employ this Internet-based method of data collection to examine our first hypothesis:

TABLE 4-2 Relatedness of Physician-Measured Data to the DASH Score at All Five Intervals

DASH versus 2-Sample Tests (t or Rank-Sum)	Value	Interval 1		Interval 2		Interval 3		Interval 4		Interval 5	
		Mean [N]	P	Mean [N]	P	Mean [N]	P	Mean [N]	P	Mean [N]	P
Ulnar styloid fracture	N	61.6 [64]	.31	40.8 [86]	.33	23.2 [62]	.45	15.2 [49]	.76	10.1 [47]	.97
	Y	65.1 [70]		44.2 [75]		26 [68]		14.3 [47]		10.2	
Adverse event in interval	N	63.9 [136]	.86	42.4 [164]	.82	24.1 [131]	.46	[98]		[88]	
	Y	64.5 [4]		39.4 [3]		35.4 [4]		[0]		[1]	
Adverse event ever	N	64.1 [130]	.72	42.5 [156]	.71	23.2 [124]	.0419*	14 [87]	.18	10.6 [84]	.62
	Y	61.7		40 [11]		39.1 [11]		20.9 [11]		11.9 [5]	
Spearman Rank Correlations		Rs [N]	P	Rs [N]	P	Rs [N]	P	Rs [N]	P	Rs [N]	P
Grip Pct		−0.262 [38]	.11	−0.409 [105]	<.0001**	−0.453 [96]	<.0001**	−0.389 [51]	.0048**	−0.659 [30]	.0001**
Pronation Pct		0.144 [37]	.4	−0.085 [100]	.40	0.107 [101]	.29	0.034 [54]	.81	−0.109 [32]	.55
Range of motion loss (coded 1-5)		0.260 [76]	.0235*	0.333 [104]	.0006**	0.349 [84]	.0005**	0.175 [48]	.24	0.196 [33]	.27
Supination Pct		−0.043 [54]	.76	−0.270 [111]	.0042**	−0.102 [100]	.31	−0.181 [56]	.18	−0.150 [33]	.41
Visual analog scale		0.356 [77]	.0015**	0.189 [110]	.0478*	0.456 [86]	<.0001**	0.502 [51]	.0002**	0.524 [30]	.0030**
Work status (coded 1-3)		0.218 [106]	.0246*	0.423 [148]	<.0001**	0.523 [107]	<.0001**	0.462 [54]	.0004**	0.205 [34]	.25
Wrist extension		−0.085 [59]	.52	−0.155 [113]	.10	−0.219 [102]	.0269*	0.092 [58]	.49	−0.171 [33]	.34
Wrist flexion		−0.427 [59]	.0008**	−0.165 [113]	.0809 TR	−0.276 [102]	.0049**	−0.091 [58]	.50	−0.143 [33]	.43
X-ray lateral inclination		−0.155 [86]	.16	−0.273 [127]	.0019**	−0.130 [78]	.26	−0.070 [46]	.64	−0.150 [26]	.46
X-ray radial-ulnar length		0.048 [85]	.66	0.075 [121]	.41	−0.016 [79]	.89	0.213 [46]	.16	0.231 [24]	.28

TR trend, $P < .10$
*Significant, $P < .05$
**Strongly significant, $P < .01$.
Rs, Spearman rank; [N], number of instances; P, percentage of opposite.

TABLE 4-3   Relatedness of Device to the DASH Score at All Five Intervals

Fixation	Manufacturer	Fracture	2 Weeks		6 Weeks		13 Weeks		26 Weeks		52 Weeks	
			N	DASH	N	DASH	N	DASH	N	DASH	N	DASH
Cast only		A	3	88.3	4	76.9	4	60				
		C	2	61.8	4	47.9	1	21.6	3	19.1	2	6.7
DBP	Avanta/SBI	C			1	62.1	1	5				
DFAP	Avanta/SBI	C	1	60.7	2	64.6	2	36.7	2	17.9	2	14
	EBI	C			1	21.7	1	32.5	1	12.5		
	Stryker/Howmedica	C	1	47.5	1	49.2					1	11.7
Ext Fix Br	EBI	A			1	39.3	1	17.2	1	8.6	1	8.6
		C	1	42.9	1	48.3	1	21.7	1	10	1	8.6
	OrthoFix	C			1	59.2	1	35.8	1	33.3	1	9.2
	Stryker/Howmedica	A	2	57.4	3	36.9	2	10.4	1	12.5	1	14.2
		C	3	42.1	5	42.3	2	29.6	2	12.1	2	22.1
	Synthes	C	1	68.8	1	50	1	67	1	58		
	Other	A	1	39.2	2	17.9	1	14.2				
Ex Fix Non Br	Stryker/Howmedica	A	1	81.7	1	68.3						
	Synthes	A	2	35	2	19.2	2	2.9	2		2	1.7
IM Rod	Wright	A	9	66.1	7	38.4	7	17.7	5	10.5	2	12
		C	3	56	6	48.7	6	27.5	4	11.9	2	17.9
K Wires	Generic	A	1	97.5	1	53.3	1	11.6	1	9.3		
	Stryker/Howmedica	A	3	68.9	2	31.7	2	7.5			1	12.9
		C	3	71.4	4	60	3	49.3	1	0.8		
	Tri-med	A			1	62.5	1	21.7				
	Other	C	2	70	2	70.8	1	43.1	1	22.5	1	25
RBP	Stryker/Howmedica	C	1	89.2			1	50.8	1	48.3		
	Other	C			1	53.3						
RFAP	EBI	A	2	90.4	1	60.8	1	24.2			1	16.7
		C	4	66	3	34.2	5	24.7	5	18.2	2	15
VBP	Synthes	A			1	68.3	1	75.8	1	43.3	1	34.2
	Other	C					1	55				
VFAP	Avanta/SBI	A	19	63.3	20	35	17	20.6	14	11.2	13	9
		C	9	55	13	39.5	8	21.7	9	10		
	EBI	A	2	72.9	2	40.8	2	20.8			2	12.1
		C	4	68.1	5	54	3	34.1	2	16.3	2	25.4
	Hand Innovations	C	7	67.7	8	30.4	6	19.6	9	13.9	5	4.7
	Stryker/Howmedica	A	4	49.4	4	31.3	4	13.1	4	7.6	4	5.8
		C	11	53.3	11	34.6	10	26.9	7	16.3	6	10.7
	Other	A	2	76.3	2	57.1	2	36.7	1	31		
		C	1	44.8	1	12.5	1	11.7	1	4.2	1	10

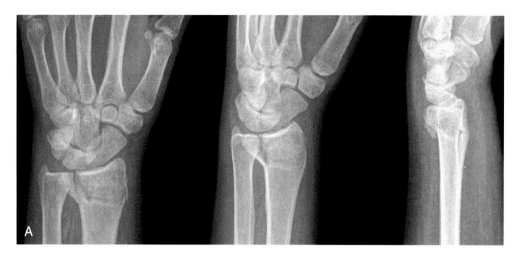

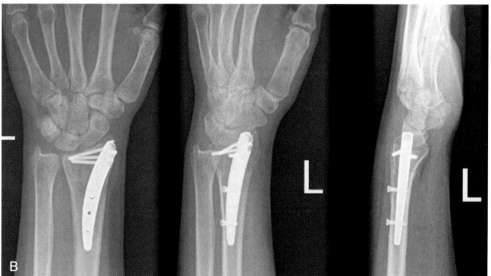

FIGURE 4-8 **Three X-ray Views of an Unstable Distal Radius Fracture. A**, Before treatment. **B**, After treatment using an IM nail.

1. A new method or technology does not alter the primary outcome of care of distal radius fractures.

As such, differences in primary outcome related to equipment factors are observed in this study, but are not large and seem to vary with time of analysis. Also, power analysis confirms that the number of patients required to detect meaningful and predictive difference between fixation types by manufacturer within specific groups (e.g., VFAP) cannot be estimated, with this data set, owing to the similarity of results by fixation manufacturer within fixation groups. Assuming that a difference might exist, our estimate suggests that each group would need to number in the thousands of patients to find any clinical difference between VFAPs. It would seem that a range of VFAPs are clinically identical.

External fixation (bridging) is different (trend) and better early during recovery. We believe this observation warrants special emphasis in the face of the number of plating products with strong messages being communicated to physicians via advertising and data reported to support VFAP published by Chung and associates.[11] Earlier work published by Kreder and coworkers[12] found no difference between fixation with plating versus external fixation for unstable fractures of the radius when the patients

were randomly assigned to one of the two groups.[12] This article cannot be compared directly with the current work in that the plating techniques chosen for open fixation did not share the same characteristics as the techniques now presented to the market and represented within Chung's work.

Proof that fixed-angle fixation of the radius would improve fixation rigidity using an in vitro extra-articular distal radius fracture fixation model was first shown by Gesensway and colleagues[13] and later compared with fixation forces needed to allow early rehabilitation vis-à-vis a low load gripping (finger motion) model by Putnam and colleagues.[14] Given generally understood knowledge of joint and ligament function, it is probably impossible to argue logically against restoration of function of all joints as early as possible. To be useful in the context of a utility/disutility analysis, however, at the outset of introducing alternative fixation methods into the matrix of fracture care, the instant and widely applicable benefits should be known. A specific analysis of distal radius fractures regarding utility/disutility has not been done. Inferring from the work of Gandjour and Lauterbach,[15] one issue to be understood is the expected and observed volume of "greater benefit" for all distal radius patients who receive the best care compared with alternative (and, for argument's sake, less expensive) care. In this example, "dollars available for health care" can be

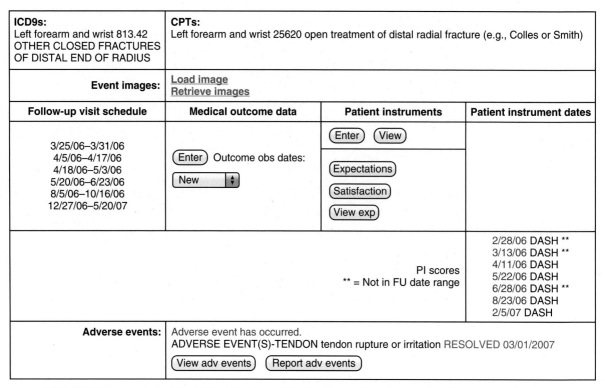

ICD9s: Left forearm and wrist 813.42 OTHER CLOSED FRACTURES OF DISTAL END OF RADIUS	CPTs: Left forearm and wrist 25620 open treatment of distal radial fracture (e.g., Colles or Smith)		
Event images:	Load image Retrieve images		
Follow-up visit schedule	**Medical outcome data**	**Patient instruments**	**Patient instrument dates**
3/25/06–3/31/06 4/5/06–4/17/06 4/18/06–5/3/06 5/20/06–6/23/06 8/5/06–10/16/06 12/27/06–5/20/07	(Enter) Outcome obs dates: New ▼	(Enter) (View) (Expectations) (Satisfaction) (View exp)	
		PI scores ** = Not in FU date range	2/28/06 DASH ** 3/13/06 DASH ** 4/11/06 DASH 5/22/06 DASH 6/28/06 DASH ** 8/23/06 DASH 2/5/07 DASH
Adverse events:	Adverse event has occurred. ADVERSE EVENT(S)-TENDON tendon rupture or irritation RESOLVED 03/01/2007 (View adv events) (Report adv events)		

FIGURE 4-9 Screen Shot of the "Patient Dashboard" Used to Manage Data Entry during Treatment and Follow-up.

PATIENT INSTRUMENT SCORES, DASH

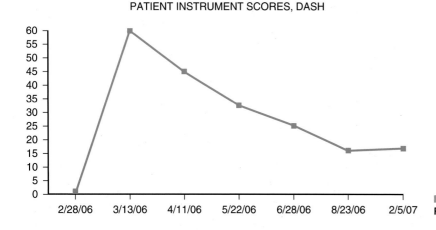

FIGURE 4-10 Plot of Specific Patient's DASH Score Recovery after Treatment.

assumed to equal energy and are subject to the laws of thermodynamics, wherein they can neither be created nor be destroyed. To achieve utility, any increase in energy spent on radius fracture care should ideally result in greater societal health compared with spending these same dollars elsewhere.

Based on the lack of consistent differences in recovery speed seen in this study when comparing fixed-angle plates (any side or manufacturer), intramedullary rod fixation, and external fixation, and the lack of any formal comparative utility/cost analysis, we recommend that the surgeon should choose the fixation type to be employed based on factors other than device design.

A second goal of this study was to assess if:

2. The location or physician name associated with distal radius care does not affect the outcome (primary or secondary outcomes).

Separating DASH averages by site was reassuring and surprising. As seen in **Figure 4-11**, the sites are more similar than different when the DASH alone is examined. One site does trend to recover more slowly, however. Ultimately the true test of such a display would be the ability to detect a best (or worst) process. Ideally, such a method could confirm a competent result (single event) and competent method (many events by many physicians). The concept of measuring and displaying surgical competence is gaining acceptance as a goal. The CUSUM (CUmulative SUM) method of presenting surgical success/competence data may prove reliable and acceptable to the users.[16,17]

Figure 4-12 shows examples of how physician-derived data and patient instrument might be combined to represent distal radius fracture recovery at specific intervals. To create this graph, the physician values that most closely correlated with DASH score (grip, finger range of motion, visual analog scale, and work

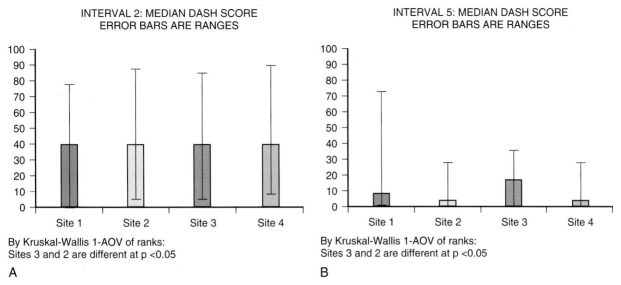

FIGURE 4-11 **DASH Score Median. A,** DASH score median with ranges at interval 2 showing site difference. **B,** DASH score median with ranges at interval 5 showing site difference.

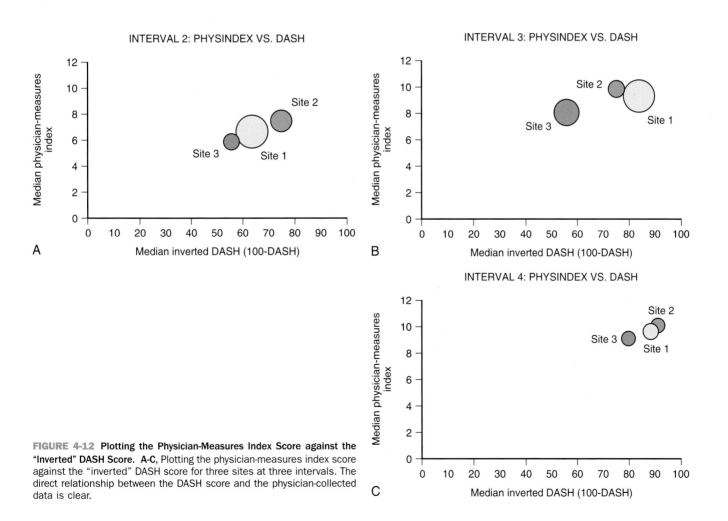

FIGURE 4-12 **Plotting the Physician-Measures Index Score against the "Inverted" DASH Score. A-C,** Plotting the physician-measures index score against the "inverted" DASH score for three sites at three intervals. The direct relationship between the DASH score and the physician-collected data is clear.

status) were assigned values to create a physician index. This index score can be seen to move in the same direction and approximate proportion compared with the DASH instrument. The importance of this fact can be surmised from the difference in number of sites represented in Figures 4-11 and 4-12. Specifically, site 4 was not successful at collecting values for physician-derived data. Although site 4 did collect patient instrument data that could be analyzed to create Figure 4-11, the frequency and completeness of data collection were insufficient to enable inclusion of site 4 in Figure 4-12.

The importance of the DASH score accurately reflecting the movement/improvement in physician-derived data (physician-measures index) seems obvious. Assuming that stakeholders could agree on a desired standard percent of DASH score recovery without adverse event occurrence, a binary process could be constructed to represent expected recovery parameters. These data could enable the building of a CUSUM representation of care success without substantial change in the regular medical work process (i.e., limited physician data gathering requirement and patient data gathering via novel and inexpensive means [Internet]).

In this observational study, we intended to enroll "all comers" as related to distal radius fracture patients who met the inclusion/exclusion criteria. Strictly speaking, all patients presenting with a specific diagnosis should be enrolled. Enrollment numbers suggest, however, that patients receiving cast care as treatment were not enrolled as frequently as patients undergoing surgical intervention. Notwithstanding this limitation of the current study, for purposes of formulating some conclusions from the collected data set, the distribution of patient characteristics is encouraging in that it compares favorably with an earlier demographic study by Falch.[18]

Differences in primary outcome related to clinical factors were observed in this study. Some of these are significant. Taken together, it seems that using radiographs as a means of assessing fracture recovery is less meaningfully related to the primary outcome (DASH recovery) than comparative grip strength and finger motion. Forearm motion may be important in DASH score recovery, whereas pure wrist motion is not. That collecting the aforementioned data is less expensive and without x-radiation risk compared with routinely obtained radiographs is potentially important. If we assume that current practice is to obtain postsurgical radiographs at 2, 6, and 12 weeks; that each radiographic series costs $100 to the institution; that 300,000 distal radius events are treated in the United States per year; and that the 6-week and 12-week radiographs could be eliminated 90% of the time, the direct cost savings to the health care providers and institutions would be $[(100 + 100) \times 270,000 = US\$54,000,000]$. Although such a number is only three ten-thousandths of the U.S. health care budget, the value of identifying such opportunities is obvious.

Considering the need to conserve resources in medicine and the inability of orthopaedic equipment to possess sufficient embedded knowledge so as to make the physician's decision making and physical skills of minimal importance, it seems obvious that true and ongoing tests of widespread efficiency (ability of each user to employ a tool effectively [desired outcome]) are needed with continuous comparison with an existing standard when new and differently priced tools are introduced to the market.[19]

Incomplete capture of late follow-up data occurred secondary to patients failing to return for later examination. The current data set has not been examined using an "intention to treat"

method.[20] Presumably, this method would enable a better explanation of trends, although it may "downgrade" seemingly good results. In the absence of completing this analysis, the trend differences between sites and some equipment must be viewed with caution. The clinical correlations between DASH and grip and finger motion are so significant and largely dependent on earlier, more complete data that we expect these correlations to remain positive regardless of any new data points gained vis-à-vis our planned intention-to-treat analysis.

The database as used shows the Internet's greatest strength: the ability to deploy and gather data with greatest efficiency and enforced accuracy. Widespread deployment would not be simple, however. Not everyone is ready and willing to understand individual effectiveness. Patients, who arguably have the most to gain, have almost no voice. Third parties (operating sites, payers, manufacturers) have variable and conflicting opinions ranging from "I am already doing it" (payers) to "I cannot do it" (operating sites). Physician leadership is stating that measurement is a necessity, but must deal with "push back" from many physicians who see quality measurement as an unfunded mandate or a "hidden agenda" or both.

In this study, we identified an ability to use a primary outcome instrument to observe individual and group recovery of function over time using a validated outcomes instrument (DASH) as the primary outcome measure. Separation of treated fractures into comparative groups is not likely to have occurred in a uniformly agreeable manner. Dahlen and colleagues[21] describes the "under" classification of extra-articular fractures by plain radiographs. Because of this, these authors suggested classification following routine computed tomography scan after original radiographs. If operative treatment expense is an issue, however, imagine the utility, or disutility, of obtaining a computed tomography scan in all patients presenting with a distal radius fracture. That intraobserver and interobserver reliability of fracture classification is poor for any but the simplest classification scheme is also known.[22] One clear opportunity, if the power of a clinical database distributed via the Internet is to have maximal benefit for clinical studies, occurs at the moment a disease or image is classified. Whether the physician is simply given enough information to become more consistent or, ideally, a machine algorithm is used to validate any crucial classification, the value to a clinical data collection and sorting process is evident.

Summary

As related to the primary outcome of distal radius fracture treatment, we have shown that:

1. New treatment methods do not alter the primary outcome to a significant and consistent degree.
2. The location or physician name associated with care seems to have the most significant impact on the primary outcome.

This message moves against the differentiation sought by the medical equipment industry and the uniformity of payment for service enjoyed by insurers as it relates to professional service payments.

Pirzig[2] relates the story of a South Indian monkey whose hand is caught in a coconut with rice inside. The monkey cannot remove its hand when holding onto rice because his hand closed around the rice is larger than the hole he reached through with his open flat hand. There are hunters coming. So, the monkey must choose to forego his hunger or be caught. Maintaining his frame of reference, the monkey will lose his freedom, or worse.

Medicine's situation is more problematic. The "hunters" may not be here tomorrow and so, depending on the variable ages and needs of physicians, the need to remove one's "hand" from the "food" would be viewed differently. The trick becomes to see the need from the "eyes of the future." From this vantage point, it might be possible to place the greatest value on the overall quality achieved and, in this context, the need for patient-validated measurement of equipment, physicians, and sites is apparent. The database method presented fills the need to compare variables in a manner that enables an ongoing understanding of real-world efficiency and simultaneously provides individual understanding of effectiveness.

ACKNOWLEDGMENTS

The authors acknowledge N. J. Meyer, MD, R. Strauch, MD, and C. Jennings, MD, for working to refine the data set and allowing their cases to be included, and J. Agel and P. Lender for working to analyze the data set and providing monitoring and maintenance of the institutional review board status.

Dr. Putnam has an ownership interest in the Database method (BoundaryMedical) employed by this study with oversight supplied by the University of Minnesota. Dr. Putnam has a royalty interest in distal radius fracture fixation products sold by SBI and Wright Medical Technology.

REFERENCES

1. Putnam MD, Gesensway D: Method and apparatus for fixation of distal radius fractures. US Patent 5586985 issued December 24th, 1996.
2. Pirzig RM: Zen and the Art of Motorcycle Maintenance. William Morrow & Company, 1974.
3. Kane R, ed. Understanding Health Care Outcomes Research. Gaithersburg, MD: Aspen Publications, 1997.
4. Wennberg JE, Fisher ES, Skinner JS: Geography and the debate over Medicare reform. J Health Affairs, February 13, 2002. Available at: http://content.healthaffairs.org/cgi/content/abstract/hlthaff.w2.96v1.
5. Freedman B: Equipoise and the ethics of clinical research. N Engl J Med 1987; 317:141-145.
6. Tunis SR, Stryer DB, Clancy CM: Practical clinical trials. JAMA 2003; 290:1624-1632.
7. Stukel T, Fisher ES, Wennber DE, et al: Analysis of observational studies in the presence of treatment selection bias. JAMA 2007; 297:278-285.
8. D'Agostino RB Jr, D'Agostino RB Sr: Estimating treatment effects using observational data. JAMA 2007; 297:314-316.
9. Williamson O, Cameron P, McNeil J: Medical registry governance and patient privacy. Med J Aust 2004; 181:125-126.
10. Orthopaedic Trauma Association/Committee for Coding and Classification: OTA fracture classification. J Orthop Trauma 1996; 10(Suppl 1):27-30.
11. Chung KC, Watt AJ, Kotsis SV, et al: Treatment of unstable distal radial fractures with the volar locking plating system. J Bone Joint Surg Am 2006; 88:2687-2694.
12. Kreder HJ, Hanel DP, Agel J, et al: Indirect reduction and percutaneous fixation versus open reduction and internal fixation for displaced fractures of the distal radius: a randomized, controlled trial. J Bone Joint Surg Br 2005; 87:829-836.
13. Gesensway D, Putnam MD, Mente PL, et al: Design and biomechanics of a plate for the distal radius. J Hand Surg [Am] 1995; 20:1021-1027.
14. Putnam MD, Meyer NJ, Nelson EW, et al: Distal radial metaphyseal forces in an extrinsic grip model: implications for postfracture rehabilitation. J Hand Surg [Am] 2000; 25:469-475.
15. Gandjour A, Lauterbach KW: Utilitarian theories reconsidered: common misconceptions, more recent developments, and health policy implications. Health Care Anal 2003; 11:229-244.
16. Lim TO, Soraya A, Ding LM, et al: Assessing doctors' competence: application of CUSUM technique in monitoring doctors' performance. Int J Qual Health Care 2002; 14:251-258.
17. Yap C-H, Colson ME, Watters DA: Cumulative sum techniques for surgeons: a brief review. Aust N Z J Surg 2007; 77:583-586.
18. Falch JA: Epidemiology of fractures of the distal forearm in Oslo, Norway. Acta Orthop Scand 1983; 54:291-295.
19. Madhavan R, Grover R: From embedded knowledge to embodied knowledge: new product development as knowledge management. Journal of Marketing 1998; 62:1-12.
20. Hollis S, Campbell F: What is meant by intention to treat analysis? Survey of published randomized controlled trials. BMJ 1999; 319:670-674.
21. Dahlen HC, Franck WM, Saburi G, et al: Incorrect classification of extra-articular distal radius fractures by conventional x-rays: comparison between biplanar radiographic diagnostics and CT assessment of fracture morphology. Unfallchirurg 2004; 107:491-498.
22. De Oliveira Filho OM, Belangero WD, Teles JB: Distal radius fractures: consistency of the classifications. Rev Assoc Med Bras 2004; 50:55-61.

Factors Influencing the Outcome of Distal Radius Fractures

5

David J. Slutsky, MD

The anatomical results of fracture treatment have no meaning unless they are considered in light of the functional outcome.[1] Myriad factors affect the clinical result after a distal radius fracture. Most of these predictions are based on the radiographic findings, although the surrounding soft tissue envelope and the intracarpal ligaments have a marked influence. It is useful to identify the variables that have some predictive value regarding the ultimate result to maximize the chances of a favorable outcome.

Anatomical Predictors of Fracture Instability

Fracture instability may be defined as an inability to resist displacement after an anatomical reduction. The standard radiographic parameters of the distal radius include a radial inclination of 23 degrees (range 13 to 30 degrees), a radial length of 12 mm (range 8 to 18 mm), and an average volar tilt of 12 degrees (1 to 21 degrees).[2-5] There are difficulties in reliably predicting fracture instability based on radiographs alone. Algorithms have been developed to gauge the risk of redisplacement of a fracture after reduction, but to no avail. Two separate scoring systems have been devised to calculate this risk based on the initial injury films. In a prospective study of 80 patients, both scoring systems were found to underestimate the degree of fracture instability and to have a poor correlation with the predicted and the actual instability.[6]

In a now classic article, Lafontaine and colleagues[7] identified numerous risk factors that were associated with redisplacement of a distal radius fracture despite an initial satisfactory reduction. These included the presence of dorsal tilt greater than 20 degrees, comminution, intra-articular involvement, an associated fracture of the ulna, and age older than 60 years. If three or more of these factors were present, there was a high likelihood of fracture collapse. Altissimi and coworkers[8] noted that the severity of the initial radial shortening alone seemed to be a reliable indicator of late instability.

Advanced age influences fracture instability because of the associated osteopenia. In patients older than 60 years, Leone and coworkers[9] found that the degree of radial shortening, volar tilt, the amount of dorsal comminution, and advanced age were predictive of early or late failure. An unexpected finding was that one third of undisplaced fractures occurred in patients older than 65 years. Abbaszadegan and colleagues[10] determined that age was the only statistically significant predictor of secondary displacement. After obtaining an acceptable initial closed reduction, patients who were older than 60 years had four times the risk for 4-week failure over patients younger than 60 years. The risk for displacement increased as age increased.

One can surmise from these observations that there is a higher likelihood of secondary fracture collapse in elderly patients even with less initial displacement. In this age group, Dicpinigaitis and associates[11] found that fracture site settling may occur for up to 6 months. Because of the risk of late collapse, adjuvant internal fixation with locking plates should be considered in elderly and osteopenic patients.

Greater force is necessary to fracture the radius in younger patients because of their higher bone density, which can result in more comminution and a higher risk of subsequent fracture collapse.[12] In young patients, lesser degrees of fracture site displacement can be tolerated, so adjuvant external or internal fixation should be considered. Trumble and coworkers[13,14] recommend internal fixation if there is more than 2 mm of radial shortening and more than 15 degrees of dorsal tilt after a closed reduction, if there is comminution of more than two cortices, or if there is a displaced intra-articular component.

Anatomical Predictors of Osteoarthritis

Articular congruity is paramount in the development of post-traumatic osteoarthritis. In a classic article, Knirk and Jupiter[15] retrospectively reviewed 43 intra-articular fractures in 40 young adults (mean age 27.6 years) that were treated at Massachusetts General Hospital, with a mean follow-up of 6.7 years. Because most of the fractures (38 of 43) were treated with older, nonrigid fixation methods that were popular at that time, including cast or pins and plaster, there was a high incidence of residual intra-articular incongruity. Knirk and Jupiter[15] noted that radiographic evidence of arthritis was present in 8 of 8 of the fractures in which articular incongruity was 2 mm or more, in contrast to only 2 of 19 of the fractures that healed with a congruous joint. Osteoarthritis was found in 22 of 24 of the patients who had any step-off whatsoever.[15]

In their study of 59 patients, Altissimi and coworkers[16] found a 31% incidence of osteoarthritis when there was 2 mm or more of articular step-off at the 3.5-year follow-up. Catalano and colleagues[17] studied 21 patients younger than 45 years old who had undergone internal fixation of displaced intra-articular fractures. At an average of 7.1 years, osteoarthrosis of the radiocarpal joint was radiographically apparent in 16 wrists (76%). A strong association was found between the development of osteoarthrosis of the radiocarpal joint and residual displacement of articular fragments at the time of bony union ($P < .01$). The authors revisited 16 of these patients at 15 years. Arthrosis was present in 13 of 16 of the wrists, and there was an additional 67% reduction of the joint space.[18] Even 1 mm of intra-articular

47

congruence has been associated with the development of arthrosis.[19]

The predictive value of these studies is that articular incongruity after a distal radius fracture is the most significant factor in the development of radiocarpal osteoarthritis. Articular displacement that is identified on the initial injury films warrants a more aggressive surgical approach.

Predictors of Residual Impairment
Radiographic Predictors

The landmark article by Gartland and Werley[20] was instrumental in establishing the link between the anatomical restoration of a distal radius fracture and the functional outcome. This finding has been corroborated by many studies since then. Aro and Koivunen[21] looked at the outcomes in 92 patients older than 55 years. They noted that even minor axial shortening of the radius after a Colles' fracture affected the outcome. The functional end result was unsatisfactory in 4% of the patients with an acceptable anatomical result, in 25% of the patients with radial shortening of 3 to 5 mm, and in 31% of the patients with shortening of more than 5 mm. Fujii and associates[22] also determined that radial shortening of 6 mm or more was associated with a poor functional outcome. Combined deformities also are significant. Axial compression of more than 2 mm and dorsal angulation of more than 15 degrees adversely affect the end results.[13] Radiographic evidence of carpal instability also has been shown to correlate with poor functional results.[23]

Intracarpal Lesions

Arthroscopic evaluation of extra-articular and intra-articular distal radius fractures has revealed that triangular fibrocartilage and interosseous ligament tears are much more common than previously suspected. Several authors have examined the incidence of intracarpal soft tissue injuries associated with distal radius fractures. Geissler and colleagues[24] studied 60 patients and found a triangular fibrocartilage complex injury in 26 (43%). In the series by Lindau and associates[25] of 51 patients, 43 (84%) had a triangular fibrocartilage complex injury: 24 had a peripheral tear, 10 had a central perforation, and 9 had a combined central and peripheral tear. In the series by Richards and colleagues[26] of 118 patients, triangular fibrocartilage complex injury occurred in 35% of the intra-articular fractures and 53% of the extra-articular fractures. They noted, however, that the preoperative radiographs had no predictive value for assessing interosseous ligament injury. Unrecognized chondral and ligamentous lesions may explain poor outcomes after seemingly well-healed fractures in young adults.[25]

Post-traumatic Osteoarthritis

Experimental work on displaced intra-articular distal radius fractures has measured significant changes in mean contact stresses with step-offs of only 1 mm.[27] Pain has been significantly related to the size of the intra-articular step.[28] These findings have prompted some authors to recommend surgical treatment for residual articular incongruity of more than 1 mm.[13,29]

Ulnar Wrist Pain

One study of 109 Colles' fractures treated with closed reduction and casting determined that the most important factor for predicting ulnar wrist pain was incongruity of the distal radioulnar joint as a result of residual dorsal angulation of the radius.[30] Other studies have found that an increase in the ulnar variance was the most important radiological parameter affecting outcome.[31] Ulnocarpal impingement and distal radioulnar joint incongruency are related to the amount of radial shortening and are a common cause of ulnar-sided wrist pain.[32] In young patients, distal radioulnar joint instability is another cause for residual pain after a distal radius fracture. Lindau and coworkers[33] could not correlate this instability with any specific radiographic parameter, however.

Grip Strength Loss

More than 10 degrees of dorsal tilt leads to a dorsal carpal shift with compressive forces, which causes pain and insecurity with gripping. This condition has been associated with increased difficulty with everyday activities and work.[34] Dorsal angulation of more than 20 degrees and a reduction of the radial angle to less than 10 degrees can result in a reduction in grip strength.[35]

Work-Related Injury

Injury compensation is a predictive factor with regard to patient-reported pain and disability. In a prospective study of 120 patients sustaining a distal radius fracture, the most influential predictor of pain and disability at 6 months was injury compensation. Wrist impairment was moderately correlated with patient-reported pain and disability.[36] Fernandez and colleagues[19] found that patients with work-related injuries were more than four times less likely to return to work than patients injured outside of work.

The message gleaned from these data is that aggressive efforts should be made to achieve a congruent joint reduction and to circumvent an excessive loss of radial length or abnormal tilt of the articular surface to prevent residual impairment and pain. Intracarpal pathology should be suspected in patients with persistent wrist pain despite an acceptable anatomical result. Patients with work-related injuries are apt to have poorer outcomes regardless of the anatomical result.

Predictors of Loss of Wrist Motion

Experimentally, dorsal tilt of up to 30 degrees and radial translation of up to 10 mm leads to no significant restriction in forearm pronation or supination. Radial shortening of 10 mm reduces forearm pronation by 47% and supination by 29%. Five millimeters of ulnar translation deformity results in a mean 23% loss of pronation.[37] Clinical experience has shown that axial compression of more than 2 mm and dorsal angulation exceeding 15 degrees were directly related to diminished range of motion.[38]

Comminution and intra-articular involvement also predispose toward a loss of movement.[35] In a study of 169 distal radius fractures in adults younger than 50 years, fracture union with a step in the radiocarpal articular surface was associated with loss of wrist mobility and difficulty with fine dexterous tasks.[34] The predictive value of this evidence is that if a loss of motion is due to bony malalignment, prolonged therapy would be of no benefit.

Predictors of Patient Satisfaction
Wrist Pain and Grip Strength

A total of 53 items were evaluated by a group of 55 patients recovering from a fracture of the distal radius, which established the prevalence, mean severity score, and overall severity score (or impact) of each item as it related to physical function and social and emotional impact. The amount of residual wrist pain influenced patient satisfaction more than motion. Hand dominance also was a significant factor.[39]

Trumble and colleagues[14] devised a combined injury score rating system that included grip strength, range of motion, and pain relief to score the results after internal fixation of displaced intra-articular distal radius fractures. In this retrospective study, 43 patients were evaluated at a mean of 38 months. Patient satisfaction seemed to correlate best with pain relief and grip strength, rather than the postoperative loss of palmar tilt or radial tilt. Preoperative step-off and gap and radial shortening were equated with worse outcomes.[14]

In other clinical trials, Fujii and associates[22] noted that the grip power was the most significant factor related to subjective evaluation. A prospective study of 31 patients recovering from unstable fractures of the distal radius investigated the association between objective variables and the level of post-traumatic disability of the wrist as measured by the patient-rated wrist evaluation (PRWE) score. Grip strength was shown to be a significant predictor of the PRWE score and seemed to be a sensitive indicator of return of wrist function.[40]

Osteoporosis

A study of the bone mineral densitometry in women older than 40 years who sustained a distal radius fracture showed that the clinical results correlated better with bone mineral density than with the radiological parameters.[41] The gist of this observation is that although surgeons continue to strive for perfection, some degree of malalignment seems to be well tolerated. Patient satisfaction often hinges on pain relief and return of grip strength over anatomical restoration. This observation was affirmed by one prospective study of 85 patients who were randomly assigned to either bridging external fixation or plaster immobilization for treatment of a Colles' type distal radius fracture. Despite a high level of radiographic malunion (50%), overall function, range of movement, and activities of daily living were not limited.[42] Involvement of the dominant hand and osteopenia may compromise the end result.

Factors That Are Not Invariably Predictive
Acceptable Reduction

The relationship between form and function is not invariable. Acceptable radiographic reduction of dorsal/volar tilt criteria was not associated with better self-reported functional outcomes or increased satisfaction at 6 months in elderly patients with conservatively treated distal radius fractures.[43] A retrospective study of Colles' fractures in patients 60 years or older revealed an 82% incidence (11 patients) of a good to excellent outcome in undisplaced fractures compared with a 68% incidence (25 patients) in redisplaced fractures.[44]

Malunion

In the evaluation of the outcomes using the Short-Form 36 survey, a study of 50 patients (mean age 49.6 years) found no correlation with residual radial height, radial tilt, or palmar tilt after internal or external fixation of distal radius fractures. Intra-articular incongruence of 1 mm or greater did correlate with a lower score, however.[19]

Gliatis and colleagues[34] assessed the outcome of 169 fractures of the distal radius in adults younger than 50 years at a mean follow-up of 4.9 years. No measure of either intra-articular or extra-articular malunion influenced the severity or frequency of persistent wrist pain.

Dayican and coworkers[45] investigated the results of 108 patients older than 70 years with intra-articular distal radial fractures who would not consent to an operation. At a mean follow-up of 39.5 months, 88.9% were considered to have good and excellent functional results even though 25.9% of the patients had fair and poor anatomical scores.[45]

In another study, 85 patients with displaced Colles' fractures were reviewed 10 years after the injury. Initial and 10-year radial shortening and early finger stiffness significantly correlated with final outcome. Dorsal angulation influenced early, but not 10-year, function. Sixty-two percent of patients with an unsatisfactory result had objective features of reflex sympathetic dystrophy compared with only 6% of patients with a satisfactory result.[46]

A more recent article clarifies this point further. Grewal and MacDermid[47] prospectively followed 216 patients with extra-articular distal radius fractures for 1 year and assessed the patient-reported outcomes using the Disabilities of the Arm, Shoulder, and Hand (DASH) score and PRWE. The overall alignment of the distal radius fracture was designated as "unacceptable" if the dorsal angulation was greater than 10 degrees, if the radial inclination was less than 15 degrees, or if there was 3 mm or more of ulnar-positive variance. Patients younger than 65 years showed a very strong link between poor outcomes and the presence of malalignment of the distal radius. Patients 65 years and older showed no significant relationship between malalignment of the distal radius and patient reports of pain and disability. Based on relative risk, malalignment increased the risk of having a poor outcome (DASH > 20 or PRWE > 20) in all age groups. Using the DASH score, patients older than 65 years experience one bad outcome for every eight patients who present with unacceptable alignment. This finding contrasts with younger patients, in whom one in two (based on the DASH) or one in three (based on the PRWE) experience a poor outcome if left with a malaligned distal radius fracture.[47]

Osteoarthritis

The radiographic presence of osteoarthritis does not always adversely affect the functional outcome.[42] In a series of 21 patients with surgically treated intra-articular fractures, osteoarthrosis of the radiocarpal joint was radiographically apparent in 16 (76%) of the wrists at an average follow-up of 7.1 years. The functional status did not correlate, however, with the magnitude of the residual step and gap displacement at the time of fracture healing. All patients had a good or excellent functional outcome regardless of radiographic evidence of osteoarthrosis of the radiocarpal or distal radioulnar joint.[17]

Wrist Motion

Forearm rotation and flexion and extension of the wrist were not significantly associated with the PRWE score.[40] Absolute wrist motions have been found to be subjectively less relevant than grip strengths and residual wrist pain.[39]

Summary

Myriad factors determine the outcome after a distal radius fracture, including anatomical alignment, age, motion, pain, and hand dominance. Elderly patients may tolerate greater degrees of residual deformity because of lower functional demands. Unrecognized intracarpal pathology may account for poor functional results despite acceptable radiographic alignment. By exerting control over the factors that can be altered by treatment, the surgeon is better prepared to shepherd the patient on a course toward a functional and pain-free wrist.

REFERENCES

1. Carrozzella J, Stern PJ: Treatment of comminuted distal radius fractures with pins and plaster. Hand Clin 1988; 4:391-397.

2. Feipel V, Rinnen D, Rooze M: Postero-anterior radiography of the wrist: normal database of carpal measurements. Surg Radiol Anat 1998; 20:221-226.

3. Friberg S, Lundstrom B: Radiographic measurements of the radio-carpal joint in normal adults. Acta Radiol Diagn (Stockh) 1976; 17:249-256.

4. Mann FA, Wilson AJ, Gilula LA: Radiographic evaluation of the wrist: what does the hand surgeon want to know? Radiology 1992; 184:15-24.

5. Solgaard S: Angle of inclination of the articular surface of the distal radius. Radiologe 1984; 24:346-348.

6. Jeong GK, Kaplan FT, Liporace F, et al: An evaluation of two scoring systems to predict instability in fractures of the distal radius. J Trauma 2004; 57:1043-1047.

7. Lafontaine M, Delince P, Hardy D, et al: Instability of fractures of the lower end of the radius: apropos of a series of 167 cases. Acta Orthop Belg 1989; 55:203-216.

8. Altissimi M, Mancini GB, Azzara A, et al: Early and late displacement of fractures of the distal radius: the prediction of instability. Int Orthop 1994; 18:61-65.

9. Leone J, Bhandari M, Adili A, et al: Predictors of early and late instability following conservative treatment of extra-articular distal radius fractures. Arch Orthop Trauma Surg 2004; 124:38-41.

10. Abbaszadegan H, Jonsson U, von Sivers K: Prediction of instability of Colles' fractures. Acta Orthop Scand 1989; 60:646-650.

11. Dicpinigaitis P, Wolinsky P, Hiebert R, et al: Can external fixation maintain reduction after distal radius fractures? J Trauma 2004; 57:845-850.

12. Weber ER: A rational approach for the recognition and treatment of Colles' fracture. Hand Clin 1987; 3:13-21.

13. Trumble TE, Schmitt SR, Vedder NB: Factors affecting functional outcome of displaced intra-articular distal radius fractures. J Hand Surg [Am] 1994; 19:325-340.

14. Trumble TE, Wagner W, Hanel DP, et al: Intrafocal (Kapandji) pinning of distal radius fractures with and without external fixation. J Hand Surg [Am] 1998; 23:381-394.

15. Knirk JL, Jupiter JB: Intra-articular fractures of the distal end of the radius in young adults. J Bone Joint Surg Am 1986; 68:647-659.

16. Altissimi M, Mancini GB, Ciaffoloni E, et al: Comminuted articular fractures of the distal radius: results of conservative treatment. Ital J Orthop Traumatol 1991; 17:117-123.

17. Catalano LW, Cole RJ, Gelberman RH, et al: Displaced intra-articular fractures of the distal aspect of the radius: long-term results in young adults after open reduction and internal fixation. J Bone Joint Surg Am 1997; 79:1290-1302.

18. Goldfarb CA, Rudzki JR, Catalano LW, et al: Fifteen-year outcome of displaced intra-articular fractures of the distal radius. J Hand Surg [Am] 2006; 31:633-639.

19. Fernandez JJ, Gruen GS, Herndon JH: Outcome of distal radius fractures using the short form 36 health survey. Clin Orthop 1997; 341:36-41.

20. Gartland JJ Jr, Werley CW: Evaluation of healed Colles' fractures. J Bone Joint Surg Am 1951; 33:895-907.

21. Aro HT, Koivunen T: Minor axial shortening of the radius affects outcome of Colles' fracture treatment. J Hand Surg [Am] 1991; 16:392-398.

22. Fujii K, Henmi T, Kanematsu Y, et al: Fractures of the distal end of radius in elderly patients: a comparative study of anatomical and functional results. J Orthop Surg (Hong Kong) 2002; 10:9-15.

23. Batra S, Gupta A: The effect of fracture-related factors on the functional outcome at 1 year in distal radius fractures. Injury 2002; 33:499-502.

24. Geissler WB, Freeland AE, Savoie FH, et al: Intracarpal soft-tissue lesions associated with an intra-articular fracture of the distal end of the radius. J Bone Joint Surg Am 1996; 78:357-365.

25. Lindau T, Arner M, Hagberg L: Intraarticular lesions in distal fractures of the radius in young adults: a descriptive arthroscopic study in 50 patients. J Hand Surg [Br] 1997; 22:638-643.

26. Richards RS, Bennett JD, Roth JH, et al: Arthroscopic diagnosis of intra-articular soft tissue injuries associated with distal radial fractures. J Hand Surg [Am] 1997; 22:772-776.

27. Baratz ME, Des Jardins J, Anderson DD, et al: Displaced intra-articular fractures of the distal radius: the effect of fracture displacement on contact stresses in a cadaver model. J Hand Surg [Am] 1996; 21:183-188.

28. Mehta JA, Bain GI, Heptinstall RJ: Anatomical reduction of intra-articular fractures of the distal radius: an arthroscopically-assisted approach. J Bone Joint Surg Br 2000; 82:79-86.

29. Fernandez DL, Geissler WB: Treatment of displaced articular fractures of the radius. J Hand Surg [Am] 1991; 16:375-384.

30. Tsukazaki T, Iwasaki K: Ulnar wrist pain after Colles' fracture: 109 fractures followed for 4 years. Acta Orthop Scand 64:462-464, 1993.

31. Hollevoet N, Verdonk R: The functional importance of malunion in distal radius fractures. Acta Orthop Belg 69:239-245, 2003.

32. Geissler WB, Fernandez DL, Lamey DM: Distal radioulnar joint injuries associated with fractures of the distal radius. Clin Orthop 1996; 327:135-146.

33. Lindau T, Hagberg L, Adlercreutz C, et al: Distal radioulnar instability is an independent worsening factor in distal radial fractures. Clin Orthop 2000; 376:229-235.

34. Gliatis JD, Plessas SJ, Davis TR: Outcome of distal radial fractures in young adults. J Hand Surg [Br] 2000; 25:535-543.

35. Porter M, Stockley I: Fractures of the distal radius: intermediate and end results in relation to radiologic parameters. Clin Orthop 1987; 220:241-252.

36. MacDermid JC, Donner A, Richards RS, et al: Patient versus injury factors as predictors of pain and disability six months after a distal radius fracture. J Clin Epidemiol 2002; 55:849-854.

37. Bronstein AJ, Trumble TE, Tencer AF: The effects of distal radius fracture malalignment on forearm rotation: a cadaveric study. J Hand Surg [Am] 1997; 22:258-262.

38. Leung F, Ozkan M, Chow SP: Conservative treatment of intra-articular fractures of the distal radius—factors affecting functional outcome. Hand Surg 2000; 5:145-153.

39. Beaule PE, Dervin GF, Giachino AA, et al: Self-reported disability following distal radius fractures: the influence of hand dominance. J Hand Surg [Am] 2000; 25:476-482.

40. Karnezis IA, Fragkiadakis EG: Association between objective clinical variables and patient-rated disability of the wrist. J Bone Joint Surg Br 2002; 84:967-970.

41. Hollevoet N, Verdonk R: Outcome of distal radius fractures in relation to bone mineral density. Acta Orthop Belg 2003; 69:510-514.

42. Young CF, Nanu AM, Checketts RG: Seven-year outcome following Colles' type distal radial fracture: a comparison of two treatment methods. J Hand Surg [Br] 2003; 28:422-426.

43. Anzarut A, Johnson JA, Rowe BH, et al: Radiologic and patient-reported functional outcomes in an elderly cohort with conservatively treated distal radius fractures. J Hand Surg [Am] 2004; 29:1121-1127.

44. Chang HC, Tay SC, Chan BK, et al: Conservative treatment of redisplaced Colles' fractures in elderly patients older than 60 years old—anatomical and functional outcome. Hand Surg 2001; 6:137-144.

45. Dayican A, Unal VS, Ozkurt B, et al: Conservative treatment in intra-articular fractures of the distal radius: a study on the functional and anatomic outcome in elderly patients. Yonsei Med J 2003; 44:836-840.

46. Warwick D, Field J, Prothero D, et al: Function ten years after Colles' fracture. Clin Orthop 1993; 295:270-274.

47. Grewal R, MacDermid JC: The risk of adverse outcomes in extra-articular distal radius fractures is increased with malalignment in patients of all ages but mitigated in older patients. J Hand Surg [Am] 2007; 32:962-970.

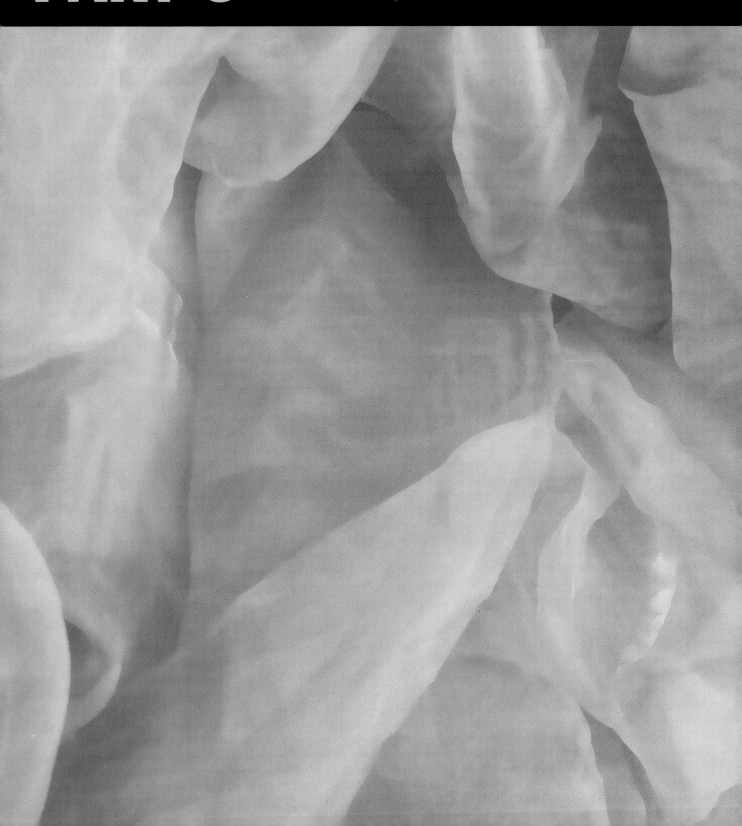

PART 3 EXTERNAL FIXATION

Bridging External Fixation with Pin Augmentation

6

Scott Wolfe, MD and Lana Kang, MD

External fixation is fundamental to the principles of orthopaedic trauma. It provides a rapid, simple, and effective surgical treatment for osseous, articular, and soft tissue injuries. Patients with fractures and injuries of the distal radius have and continue to achieve good results after immediate and definitive treatment with external fixation.[1-4]

The term "bridging" refers to the design of the frame in which the radiocarpal joint is spanned, and fracture stability is achieved via distraction and ligamentotaxis, which refers to the support provided by soft tissue tension to align and hold the reduction.[5] Additional fixation is supplemented by Kirschner wire (K-wire) pins, which are percutaneously or internally placed into the distal radius. This is the concept referred to collectively as "bridging external fixation with pin fixation" or "augmented external fixation."[6] "Nonbridging external fixation" refers to a frame design that fixes the metaphyseal/articular fragments to the proximal diaphysis without spanning the wrist joint, sparing the capsule and the ligaments from the potentially damaging effects of traction.[7-11]

Although the specific roles of external and internal methods of fixation in the treatment of distal radius fractures continue to evolve, restoration of articular congruity, radial length, radial height, and dorsal tilt remains a common tenet to all modes of treatment.[12] After Vidal and colleagues[5] introduced the concept of ligamentotaxis as a means to align bony fragments using soft tissue tension, the use of the external fixator soared. A decade later after widespread adoption of the technique internationally, an increased awareness of its limitations and attendant complications, such as loss of reduction, digital and wrist stiffness, and complex regional pain syndrome, unfolded.[13,14]

As we have developed an improved and more sophisticated understanding of fracture healing and wrist biomechanics, we have been better able to refine the application of external fixation for distal radius fractures. Its combined use with limited internal,[15] arthroscopic,[16-20] and percutaneous fracture reduction techniques,[21] and supplemental bone graft or bone graft substitutes has enhanced the stability of the fixation construct,[22-30] and simultaneously minimized the dependency on traction for maintenance of reduction.

Despite its effectiveness, and similar to other forms of treatment, external fixation has its problems and concerns. These include poor patient tolerance or acceptance, pin tract infection, iatrogenic injury to the small branches of the superficial radial nerve, loss of fixation, settling, radioulnar joint dysfunction, radiocarpal arthrofibrosis, and, as stated previously, hand and digital stiffness.[13,31-34] In addition, external fixation without supplementation inherently lacks the capacity to fix rigidly impacted or comminuted articular "die-punch" fragments and, by itself, has been

associated with loss of articular reduction and articular incongruency.[35] In the last few years, the ease of application and increased fixation strength of volar locking plates have led to an unprecedented increase in the popularity of internal fixation and a concomitant shift away from external fixation of distal radius fractures.

Although correct principles of application of augmented external fixation are in danger of becoming a lost art among orthopaedic surgical training programs, the technique continues to be the only viable treatment option in certain situations. In addition, more recent randomized clinical studies attest not only to its clinical utility, but also to improved functional and satisfaction outcomes compared with internal fixation.[1-3] It is imperative that hand and upper extremity surgeons who routinely provide care for fractures and injuries of the distal radius be well versed in techniques of external fixation and prepared to use this form of treatment when applicable.

Basic Science

The basic biomechanical principles of external fixation apply to the distal radius. Strength and stability are indirect, and reduction is attained by distraction and ligamentotaxis. Stability of the fixation construct is improved with the following:

- Direct contact of the fracture ends
- Larger diameter pins
- Decreased rod-bone distance
- Increased spacing of pins relative to the fracture (near-near and far-far)
- Pins in different planes
- Increased number of bars (stacking)[36]

In contrast to nonbridging applications of external fixation to long bones, such as the tibia, femur, or humerus, peculiar to the distal radius is the need to span the neighboring radiocarpal and intercarpal joints, and the associated deleterious effect of distraction on the intrinsic and extrinsic carpal ligaments. Although it is important to *gain* reduction of fracture fragments, it is crucial that the principle of ligamentotaxis not compromise soft tissue viability or tendon gliding by prolonged maintenance of traction. Lengthy or excessive traction predictably results in digital stiffness and joint contractures,[37] and the resultant dysfunction of the hand and wrist negates any of the goals of fracture healing with external fixation.

Principles of Augmented External Fixation

Augmentation with percutaneous or open pin fixation or bone graft or both is needed to provide increased stability to the external fixator construct and reduce the need for applied distraction.[27,38] Although application of an external fixator can acutely restore radial height and correct angular rotation alignment, there is a tendency for the fracture fragments to settle over time because of the stress-relaxation of the surrounding collagenous soft tissue envelope.[38] This settling of fracture fragments especially occurs when there is metaphyseal comminution and bone loss, which precludes firm bony contact, diminishing construct stability. In addition, traction alone does not restore articular congruency when there is impaction and displacement of intra-articular fragments, in which case a limited open incision is required to attain reduction.[27,29]

Biomechanical studies have shown that supplemental pin fixation decreases the dependency on ligamentotaxis for maintenance of reduction by minimizing the extremes of positioning and need for distraction.[33] A pin placed through the radial styloid neutralizes the deforming force of the brachioradialis[38] and the powerful wrist radial deviators of the first dorsal compartment. A single pin placed dorsally (dorsal transfixation wire [DTW]) provides a statistically significant increase in resistance to deformation, by gaining purchase on the stout volar metaphyseal cortex and directly opposing the strong dorsally deforming forces of the wrist and digital extensors. The increased stability gained by the augmentation pins more than offsets the biomechanical differences in the material strength of different external fixation models[39]; consequently, a fixator should be chosen because of ease of application and use, rather than because of its size or material properties.

Bone Grafting with Augmentation of External Fixation

Several studies have shown that the addition of bone graft or bone graft substitutes supports the articular surface and effectively prevents fragment settling.[22,28,40] Leung and colleagues[22-24] showed that bone graft application into the metaphyseal void that is created after reduction of dorsally displaced and articular impaction injuries enables earlier removal of the external fixator by expediting healing and providing firm support for the reduced articular surface. Subsequent studies have shown that bone graft substitutes are equally effective in provision of articular support and minimization of fracture fragment settling.[25,30]

Indications

The indications for external fixation with pin augmentation depend on an array of factors that should be tailored to the individual case. These include patient factors (age, dominance, occupation, comorbidities, other injuries, compliance), the personality of the fracture pattern, availability of equipment, and surgeon skill level and preference.

The patient should be apprised of the different options and expected outcomes and be involved in the decision-making process. The patient may accept the additional risk of open reduction and internal fixation to allow for a shorter period of cast immobilization. The patient should understand that an initial attempt at minimally invasive percutaneous reduction before open reduction is an acceptable treatment algorithm that is well supported by clinical studies.[1-3] Kreder and colleagues[3] showed that if an optimal and stable reduction is achieved with percutaneous fixation, open reduction is unnecessary, and function is superior.

The ideal candidate for external fixation with pin augmentation is a patient who has an unstable intra-articular fracture of the distal radius (**Fig. 6-1**). Specific indications for operative management include articular depression (1 mm) after attempted closed reduction, or loss of reduction, defined as a dorsal tilt exceeding 10 degrees, loss of radial length exceeding 5 mm, or articular depression exceeding 1 mm.[12,28] The technique of augmented external fixation is useful for a variety of fracture patterns, however, which may include intra-articular and extra-articular

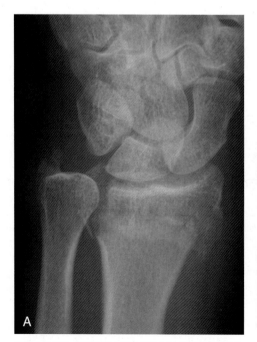
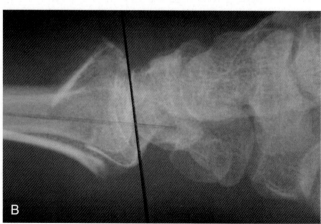

FIGURE 6-1 Anteroposterior (**A**) and lateral (**B**) plain radiographs of an unstable intra-articular fracture of the distal radius that is amenable to treatment with external fixation with pin augmentation.

fractures that are displaced and unstable. Other indications for external fixation include injuries with soft tissue compromise, grossly contaminated open fractures, and unstable multitrauma patients who are brought to the operating room for other life-threatening injuries. These emergent situations potentially apply to patients of all age groups. Percutaneous techniques for fracture fixation should not be delayed longer than 10 to 14 days because of the early callus and soft tissue scarring that would preclude closed fracture manipulation and the effects of ligamentotaxis.

Contraindications

There are very few contraindications to augmental external fixation. Absolute contraindications include medical comorbidities that disallow the safety of the manipulation or the required degree of anesthesia, ongoing systemic infection, and local infection at the planned site of external fixator and K-wire pin placement. Relative contraindications include gross comminution that would preclude augmented pin fixation, volar lip fracture patterns that are not amenable to percutaneous fixation, and severely osteoporotic bone that would hold fixation pins poorly and may be more amenable to simple closed reduction or locked plate internal fixation.

Surgical Technique

The patient is positioned supine on the operating room table. Anesthesia can be either regional or general, the choice of which is based on the preference and skill level of the anesthesiologist and the medical conditions of the patient. Complete muscle relaxation of the patient should be achieved. Antibiotic prophylaxis is provided. A tourniquet is placed above the elbow of the involved extremity, which is sterilely prepared over a radiolucent hand board attachment. Intraoperative fluoroscopic imaging is mandatory.

The external fixator generally can be placed without the need for a tourniquet, diminishing reactive postoperative edema, and allowing more time later if a complicated open reduction and grafting is required. A preliminary reduction is performed to align the fracture fragments grossly and ensure that the frame would be appropriately aligned with the fracture. The guiding philosophy is that the fixator is applied exclusively to neutralize muscle forces and maintain overall fracture alignment, and should not be thought of as a tool to gain reduction through application of force, excessive traction, or extremes of positioning.

A 2.5-cm longitudinal incision is made at the level of the mid radial shaft about 10 cm proximal to the radial styloid and a minimum of 3 cm from the most proximal fracture line. We prefer this mini-incision approach over percutaneous placement of the external fixator pins because of the unpredictable proximity of the superficial branch of the radial nerve (SBRN) and the lateral antebrachial cutaneous nerve.[29] The preferred interval is between the extensor common radialis brevis and longus muscles,[41] such that the fixator lies in an oblique plane midway between the coronal and sagittal planes of the forearm. A deep muscular interval between the brachioradialis and extensor radialis longus[38] also is acceptable, although there is an increased risk of neurapraxic injury or irritation of the radial sensory nerve (**Fig. 6-2**). Soft tissue is reflected sharply off the bone without stripping periosteum to allow for secure positioning of the pin guide.

Two 4-mm-diameter pins are drilled across two cortices of the shaft. Whether the pins are placed in parallel or convergent depends on the particular fixator design, and there is some suggestion that the obliquity of convergent pin placement increases bone purchase. Although various pin sizes are available, 4-mm pins have been shown to have the best pullout strength and resistance to bending without increasing risk of pin site fracture.[42] Pin placement is confirmed with fluoroscopy.

A 2-cm longitudinal incision is made in the oblique plane over the index metacarpal distal to the flare of the metacarpal base. The extensor tendon and first dorsal interosseous muscle are sharply reflected to allow exposure to the bone (see Fig. 6-2). Care is taken to avoid injury to the small branches of the SBRN. With the index metacarpophalangeal joint flexed to tension the intrinsics properly, two 3-mm pins are drilled across two cortices in a similar fashion as was done for the radius. Bicortical purchase is again confirmed with fluoroscopy.

The surgical wounds are irrigated, and small bleeding points are coagulated. Skin closure is done with 4-0 or 5-0 nylon sutures, before application of the fixator frame. We have found that closure of the skin at this stage of the procedure is much easier than at the end of the case because of the difficulty of suturing around the fixator frame after it has already been secured and tightened.

The external fixator frame is applied (**Fig. 6-3**). Most systems comprise a single radiolucent bar that is secured with metal clamps to the stainless steel pins. Subtle variations exist, and technical guidelines should be studied and learned before use.

The frame is first loosely applied to the pins, and the final reduction is guided by intraoperative fluoroscopy. A surgical assistant is helpful during the manipulation to provide a gentle countertraction force on the proximal forearm; the assistant also may

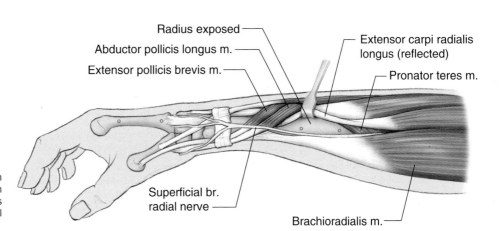

FIGURE 6-2 Diagrammatic illustration of the deep muscular interval between the brachioradialis and extensor radialis longus for placement of the proximal external fixator pins.

Radius exposed

Abductor pollicis longus m.

Extensor pollicis brevis m.

Extensor carpi radialis longus (reflected)

Pronator teres m.

Superficial br. radial nerve

Brachioradialis m.

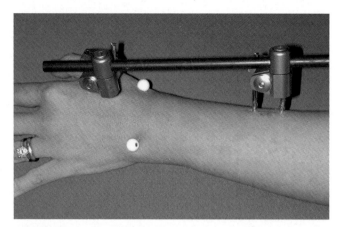

FIGURE 6-3 Clinical photograph of the external fixator frame after application.

be asked to secure and tighten the bar to the distal pins while the fracture reduction is held. An alternative method that may be useful when an assistant is unavailable is to suspend the hand with sterile finger traps and apply 5 to 10 lb of countertraction.[21]

Fracture reduction is achieved by a combination of longitudinal traction, ulnar deviation, and dorsal or volar translation of the carpus relative to the shaft of the radius.[43,44] Manual pressure placed directly on the tip of the radial styloid by the surgeon's thumb helps to restore radial length and inclination. When the fracture is displaced dorsally, a palmarly directed translation force on the carpus is helpful at this time to optimize reduction. When the fracture is displaced volarly, a dorsally directed translation force combined with slight wrist extension and supination is performed. The external fixator is then provisionally locked in position.

A closed reduction alone is usually attainable with fractures that have a simple intra-articular component.[29] Additional reduction maneuvers are then required, however, to fix individual fracture fragments directly and obviate the need for maintenance of distraction or extremes of positioning. K-wire placement into the major fracture fragments can be used as joysticks to help guide reduction.

Because of the indirect nature of the external fixator, the frame alone is insufficient to reduce impacted articular fragments. After the larger fragments are aligned or provisionally fixed with K-wires, we perform percutaneous, limited open reduction as described by Fernandez and Geissler.[21,45] Reduction of these fragments is achieved with a 2- to 3-cm longitudinal dorsal mini-incision that is based slightly ulnar to Lister's tubercle. The interval between the third and fourth dorsal compartments is dissected, and the extensor pollicus longus tendon is transposed radially. The fracture lines in the metaphysis are identified and exposed, and lifting a single large dorsal cortical fragment (trapdoor) exposes the entire metaphysis and the impacted articular pieces. A Freer elevator or dental pick is used to elevate the impacted articular fragments (**Fig. 6-4**). The displaced fragment is reduced against the lunate; it is important at this phase of the procedure that traction is reduced to allow the lunate and scaphoid to act as a guide to a congruent reduction.

Bone graft or bone graft substitute is packed behind the reconstituted subchondral bone (**Fig. 6-5**). The articular surface is supported with a subchondral 0.045- or 0.062-cm K-wire placed transversely from the radial styloid directed toward the dorsal radial cortex of the sigmoid notch, taking care not to penetrate the radioulnar joint.[21,45] Restoration of radiocarpal articular con-

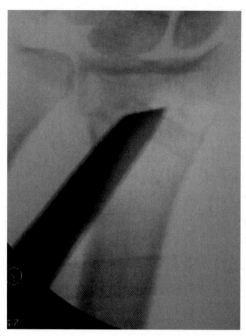

FIGURE 6-4 Intraoperative fluoroscopic image showing use of a Freer elevator to elevate the impacted articular fragments.

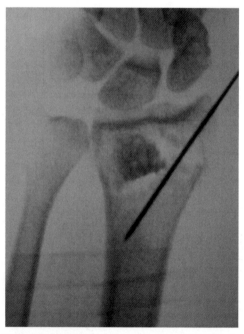

FIGURE 6-5 Intraoperative fluoroscopic image after application of bone graft or bone graft substitute.

gruency is guided and confirmed with fluoroscopy. In addition, congruency of the distal radioulnar joint should be ensured at this stage.

One (or two) additional K-wires are inserted through the tip of the radial styloid just dorsal to the crossing of the first dorsal compartment and positioned at a relatively acute angle to the radial shaft to cross the fracture and gain purchase in the strong diaphyseal ulnar cortex of the radial shaft. A 14-gauge or 16-gauge angiocatheter is important as a drill guide to prevent injury to the nearby branches of the radial sensory nerve. (If using more than one wire through the styloid, we prefer a parallel configuration.) A DTW is placed in a 45-degree angle to the sagittal plane of the radial shaft through the dorsal rim of the distal radius between the fourth and fifth dorsal compartments. This wire is positioned to cross the fracture site and capture the stout volar cortex of the radial shaft. The placement of this DTW in combination with the pin placed through the radial styloid (**Fig. 6-6**) has been shown to provide maximal stability to the external fixation construct.[38]

Lastly, the distal radioulnar joint should be assessed for stability after radiocarpal fixation. If grossly unstable, numerous techniques can be used to effect stability. Casting in the position of maximal stability (usually partial or complete supination) for 3 to 4 weeks is effective for restoration of stability.[26,46,47] Alternatively, an ulnar styloid pin or two cross pins can be placed through radial and ulnar cortical shafts approximately 5 to 6 cm proximal to the joint and left proud to facilitate removal in the event of fatigue failure. Large basi-styloid fragments can be fixed with K-wires, tension bands, or a small cannulated screw as needed to reattach the disrupted dorsal and volar radioulnar ligaments, which insert at its fovea.

At this point, distraction of the carpus and radiocarpal joint should be checked, and traction is diminished to ensure that the carpus is not overdistracted. Fluoroscopic imaging in the anteroposterior plane should show no more than 1 mm of distraction of the radiocarpal joint beyond that of the midcarpal joint. In addition, passive digital motion should be supple with metacarpophalangeal flexion to 90 degrees.

The skin around the external fixator and K-wire pins is assessed to ensure that there is no undue tension with the final frame configuration. Relaxing incisions should be made as deemed necessary. All pin sites are covered with povidone-iodine (Betadine)–soaked or xeroform dressings. The K-wire pins are either left out of the skin and cut short or cut just below skin level and buried. The patient is immobilized in a sugar tong cast in full supination

for the initial few days postoperatively because pain may otherwise initiate a protective posture of wrist flexion and forearm pronation that may be difficult to reverse later.

Technical Pearls and Pitfalls

1. Be familiar with the specific nuances of the chosen external fixator system.
2. Use a mini-incision to avoid iatrogenic injury to the radial nerve, the lateral antebrachial cutaneous nerve, or the SBRN.
3. Use power drilling and saline cooling to avoid thermal necrosis of the bone and to prevent eccentric pin placement, which increase the risk of fracture.
4. Use the DTW and radial styloid K-wires to augment strength of fixation.
5. Freely use intraoperative fluoroscopy to guide pin placement and to ensure optimal fracture reduction.
6. Check and avoid overdistraction by assessing digital motion and distance of the radiocarpal interval compared with the midcarpal interval after frame application has been secured.
7. Avoid skin tension on the K-wire and external fixation pin sites to minimize pin tract infections; place relaxing T-incisions around the pins if needed.
8. Prevent postoperative stiffness and complex regional pain syndrome that is associated with prolonged immobilization and overdistraction; use bone graft to accelerate fracture healing, prevent collapse, and allow a decreased period of immobilization.

Postoperative Course and Rehabilitation

The wrist and hand should be elevated for the first 48 to 72 hours. Digital motion exercises are begun immediately after surgery. The

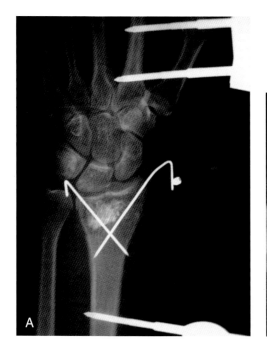
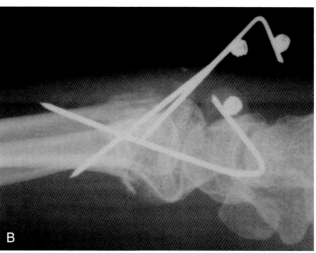

FIGURE 6-6 Anteroposterior (**A**) and lateral (**B**) plain radiographs after placement of the dorsal transfixation wire and radial styloid pins.

skin sutures and postoperative dressing are maintained for 10 to 14 days, and then twice daily pin site care is begun with diluted hydrogen peroxide. If the distal radioulnar joint is determined to be stable at surgery, forearm supination and pronation exercises are begun at the first postoperative visit. Patients are encouraged to use their hand for light activities, such as eating, writing, dressing, and light typing. Lifting, squeezing, and gripping are prohibited until all hardware has been removed. Patients may shower with the frame in place, provided that all wounds are healed and dry, but should avoid immersion in standing water. Fracture healing and maintenance of fracture reduction are checked with plain radiographs every 2 to 3 weeks. Hand therapy is generally instituted early in the postoperative course, especially if stiffness or edema develops. Peroxide pin tract care is supplemented by a short course of oral antibiotics if pin erythema develops; frank pin tract infection requiring premature removal is rare.

The external fixator frame is removed in the office after 4 to 6 weeks, and the K-wire pins are generally removed 2 to 3 weeks later. The exact timing may vary depending on pin site integrity, pin purchase or loosening, bone graft incorporation, degree of articular and metaphyseal comminution, and radiographic evidence of healing. The pin sites are cleaned and covered with a dry sterile dressing. A volar wrist splint is applied, and hand therapy is continued immediately on removal of the external fixator.

Complications

As stated previously, complications include pin tract irritation or infection, injury to the SBRN, radiocarpal arthrofibrosis, and digital stiffness. Injury to the SBRN is more difficult to treat and is best avoided by meticulous open pin placement. Radiocarpal or digital stiffness is treated by intense and early hand therapy. Complex regional pain syndrome must be recognized early and treated with a multifaceted approach involving therapy, pain management, and frequent office visits. This syndrome is almost always associated with nerve injury, excessive or prolonged traction, or both, and these causes must be ruled out and treated

before irreparable injury ensues. Patients should be reassured that motion gains continue to be made in radiocarpal and radioulnar joints for the first year after surgery, as is the case with patients after open reduction and internal fixation.

Results

Although biomechanical studies suggest superior fixation strength with internal fixation compared with augmented external fixation,[38,48] clinical studies show little significant difference in functional outcome between dorsal plating, augmented external fixation, or closed reduction and casting.[1,4,49] With augmental external fixation, we have achieved excellent radiographic healing (**Fig. 6-7**) and restoration of functional wrist motion (**Fig. 6-8**). In a retrospective cohort of 21 patients consecutively treated with augmented external fixation and bone graft, wrist motion averaged 90% of the uninjured wrist, and grip strength measured 75% of the uninjured side. Of cases, 94% had good or excellent radiographic results by the modified Lidstrom radiographic scoring system and were rated as good or excellent by the criteria of Gartland and Werley. The average DASH functional/symptom score was 90.3 (maximum 100). Radiographic parameters were restored to an average of 12 mm radial length, 4 degrees volar tilt, 23 degrees radial inclination, and 0.6 mm ulnar-positive variance. Articular reduction was maintained in all patients.[28]

There are few level I studies that effectively compare internal fixation and external fixation; the studies that exist support percutaneous fixation over the added surgical dissection and risk of internal fixation, provided that articular congruence and stability can be achieved.[1,3] Although a few more recent studies suggest superiority of locked volar plate fixation,[50,51] no randomized trials have been reported to date. More data are needed to compare sufficiently various fixation techniques that are stratified to patient demographics and specific fracture patterns. Under many circumstances, external fixation with pin augmentation continues to be an ideal method of treatment, supported by decades of clinical and basic research. With proper planning and surgical technique,

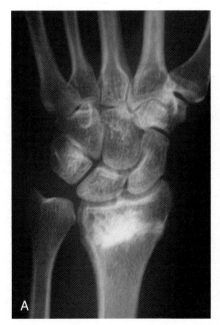 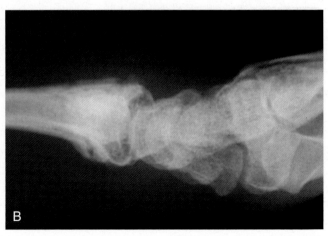

FIGURE 6-7 Anteroposterior (**A**) and lateral (**B**) plain radiographs confirming fracture healing after external fixation with pin augmentation.

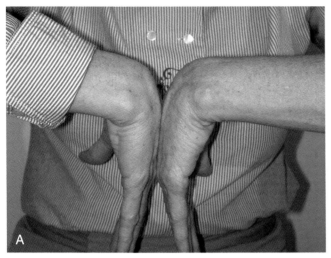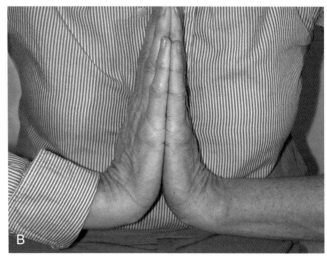

FIGURE 6-8 Clinical photographs of bilateral wrist flexion (**A**) and extension (**B**) showing restoration of functional motion after external fixation with pin augmentation.

excellent results can be achieved in a wide variety of fracture patterns.

REFERENCES

1. Grewel R, Perey B, Wilmink M, et al: A randomized trial on the treatment of intra-articular distal radius fractures: open reduction internal fixation with dorsal plating versus mini open reduction, percutaneous pinning and external fixation. J Hand Surg [Am] 2005; 30:764-772.

2. Kapoor H, Agarwal A, Dhaon BK: Displaced intra-articular fractures of distal radius: a comparative evaluation of results following closed reduction, external fixation and open reduction with internal fixation. Injury 2000; 31:75-79.

3. Kreder HJ, Hanel DP, Agel J, et al: Indirect reduction and percutaneous fixation versus open reduction and internal fixation for displaced intra-articular fractures of the distal radius. J Bone Joint Surg Br 2005; 87:829-836.

4. Margaliot Z, Haase SC, Kotsis SV, et al: A meta-analysis of outcomes of external fixation versus plate osteosynthesis for unstable distal radius fractures. J Hand Surg [Am] 2005; 30:1185-1199.

5. Vidal J, Buscayret C, Fischbach C, et al: New method of treatment of comminuted fractures of the lower end of the radius: "ligamentary taxis." Acta Orthop Belg 1977; 43:781-789.

6. Seitz WH Jr, Froimson AI, Leb R, et al: Augmented external fixation of unstable distal radius fractures. J Hand Surg [Am] 1991; 16:1010-1016.

7. McQueen MM: Non-spanning external fixation of the distal radius. Hand Clin 2005; 21:375-380.

8. McQueen MM: Metaphyseal external fixation of the distal radius. Bull Hosp Jt Dis 1999; 58:9-14.

9. McQueen MM: Redisplaced unstable fractures of the distal radius: a randomised, prospective study of bridging versus non-bridging external fixation. J Bone Joint Surg Br 1998; 80:665-669.

10. Slutsky DJ: Nonbridging external fixation of intra-articular distal radius fractures. Hand Clin 2005; 21:381-394.

11. Gradl G, Jupiter JB, Gierer P, et al: Fractures of the distal radius treated with a nonbridging external fixation technique using multiplanar K-wires. J Hand Surg [Am] 2005; 30:960-968.

12. Lafontaine M, Hardy D, Delince P: Stability assessment of distal radius fractures. Injury 1989; 20:208-210.

13. Cooney WP III, Dobyns JH, Linscheid RL: Complications of Colles' fractures. J Bone Joint Surg 1980; 62:613-619.

14. Sanders RA, Keppel FL, Waldrop JI: External fixation of distal radial fractures: results and complications. J Hand Surg [Am] 1991; 16:385-391.

15. Cooney WP, Berger RA: Treatment of complex fractures of the distal radius: combined use of internal and external fixation and arthroscopic reduction. Hand Clin 1993; 9:603-612.

16. Wolfe SW, Easterling KE, Yoo H: Arthroscopic-assisted reduction of distal radius fractures. J Arthr Rel Surg 1995; 11:706-714.

17. Freeland AE, Geissler WB: The arthroscopic management of intra-articular distal radius fractures. Hand Surg 2000; 5:93-102.

18. Geissler WB: Arthroscopically assisted reduction of intra-articular fractures of the distal radius. Hand Clin 1995; 11:19-29.

19. Geissler WB, Freeland AE: Arthroscopic management of intra-articular distal radius fractures. Hand Clin 1999; 15:455-465, viii.

20. Geissler WB, Freeland AE: Arthroscopically-assisted reduction of intraarticular distal radial fractures. Clin Orthop 1996; 327:125-134.

21. Geissler WB, Fernandez DL: Percutaneous and limited open reduction of the articular surface of the distal radius. J Orthop Trauma 1991; 5:255-264.

22. Leung KS, Shen WY, Leung PC, et al: Ligamentotaxis and bone grafting for comminuted fractures of the distal radius. J Bone Joint Surg Br 1989; 71:838-842.

23. Leung KS, Shen WY, Tsang HK, et al: An effective treatment of comminuted fractures of the distal radius. J Hand Surg [Am] 1990; 15:11-17.

24. Leung KS, So WS, Chiu VD, et al: Ligamentotaxis for comminuted distal radial fractures modified by primary cancellous grafting and functional bracing: long-term results. J Orthop Trauma 1991; 5:265-271.

25. Pike LM, Wolfe SW: Alternatives to bone graft in the treatment of distal radius fractures. Atlas Hand Clin 1997; 2:125-150.

26. Ruch DS, Weiland AJ, Wolfe SW, et al: Current concepts in the treatment of distal radial fractures. Instr Course Lect 2004; 53:389-401.

27. Swigart CR, Wolfe SW: Limited incision open techniques for distal radius fracture management. Orthop Clin North Am 2001; 32:317-327, ix.

28. Wolfe SW, Pike L, Slade JF III, et al: Augmentation of distal radius fracture fixation with coralline hydroxyapatite bone graft substitute. J Hand Surg [Am] 1999; 24:816-827.

29. Seitz WH Jr, Putnam MD, Dick HM: Limited open surgical approach for external fixation of distal radius fractures. J Hand Surg [Am] 1990; 15:288-293.

30. Herrera M, Chapman CB, Roh M, et al: Treatment of unstable distal radius fractures with cancellous allograft and external fixation. J Hand Surg [Am] 1999; 24:1269-1278.

31. Sanders RA, Keppel FL, Waldrop JI: External fixation of distal radial fractures: results and complications. J Hand Surg [Am] 1991; 16:385-391.

32. Seitz WH Jr: Complications and problems in the management of distal radius fractures. Hand Clin 1994; 10:117-122.

33. Seitz WH Jr, Froimson AI, Leb RB: Reduction of treatment-related complications in the external fixation of complex distal radius fractures. Orthop Rev 1991; 20:169-177.

34. Weber SC, Szabo RM: Severely comminuted distal radial fracture as an unsolved problem: complications associated with external fixation and pins and plaster techniques. J Hand Surg [Am] 1986; 11:157-165.

35. Catalano LW, Cole RJ, Gelberman RH, et al: Displaced intra-articular fractures of the distal aspect of the radius. J Bone Joint Surg [Am] 1997; 79:1290-1302.

36. Pollak AN, Ziran BH: Principles of external fixation. In Browner B, Jesse B, Jupiter JB, et al, eds: Skeletal Trauma. 3rd ed. Philadelphia: WB Saunders, 2003.

37. Kaempffe FA, Wheeler DR, Peimer CA, et al: Severe fractures of the distal radius: effect of amount and duration of external fixator distraction on outcome. J Hand Surg [Am] 1993; 18:33-41.

38. Wolfe SW, Swigart CR, Grauer BS, et al: Augmented external fixation of distal radius fractures: a biomechanical analysis. J Hand Surg [Am] 1998; 23:127-134.

39. Wolfe SW, Austin G, Lorenze MD, et al: Comparative stability of external fixation: a biomechanical study. J Hand Surg [Am] 1999; 24:516-524.

40. Ladd AL, Pliam NB: The role of bone graft and alternatives in unstable distal radius fracture treatment. Orthop Clin North Am 2001; 30:337-351.

41. Raskin KB, Rettig ME: Distal radius fractures: external fixation and supplemental K-wires. Atlas Hand Clin 2006; 11:187-196.

42. Seitz WH Jr, Froimson AI, Brooks DB, et al: Biomechanical analysis of pin placement and pin size for external fixation of distal radius fractures. Clin Orthop 1990; 251:207-212.

43. Agee JM, Szabo RM, Chidgey LK, et al: Treatment of comminuted distal radius fractures: an approach based on pathomechanics. Orthopedics 1994; 17:1115-1122.

44. Agee JM: Distal radius fractures: multiplanar ligamentotaxis. Hand Clin 1993; 9:577-585.

45. Fernandez DL, Geissler WB: Treatment of displaced articular fractures of the radius. J Hand Surg [Am] 1991; 16:375-384.

46. Cole DW, Elsaidi GA, Kuzma KR, et al: Distal radioulnar joint instability in distal radius fractures: the role of sigmoid notch and triangular fibrocartilage complex revisited. Injury 2006; 37:252-258.

47. Ruch DS, Lumsden BC, Papadonikolakis A: Distal radius fractures: a comparison of tension band wiring versus ulnar outrigger external fixation for the management of distal radioulnar instability. J Hand Surg [Am] 2005; 30:969-977.

48. Dodds SD, Cornelissen S, Jossan S, et al: A biomechanical comparison of fragment-specific fixation and augmented external fixation for intra-articular distal radius fractures. J Hand Surg [Am] 2002; 27:953-964.

49. Harley BJ, Scharfenberger A, Beaupre LA, et al: Augmented external fixation versus percutaneous pinning and casting for unstable fractures of the distal radius—a prospective randomized trial. J Hand Surg [Am] 2004; 29:815-824.

50. Orbay JL, Fernandez DL: Volar fixed-angle plate fixation for unstable distal radius fractures in the elderly patient. J Hand Surg [Am] 2004; 29:96-102.

51. Wright TW, Horodyski M, Smith DW: Functional outcome of unstable distal radius fractures: ORIF with a volar fixed-angle tine plate versus external fixation. J Hand Surg [Am] 2005; 30:289-299.

Distal Radius Fractures Treated with the CPX System

7

Ather Mirza, MD and Mary Kate Reinhart, CNP

There are many ways to treat distal radius fractures. Over the years, many techniques and instruments have evolved in this frequently changing landscape. The basic principles of fracture treatment, however—fracture reduction, restoration of joint congruency, maintenance of reduction throughout healing, early mobilization, and the resumption of activities of daily living—remain the same.[1]

This ubiquitous fracture has become very important to our aging population. Life expectancy has increased dramatically, and people are more active as they age.[2,3] A cavalier attitude in treating these fractures can lead to unhappy patients who are unwilling to accept either the deformity or the functional compromise of such injuries despite their age.

Deforming angular, compressive, and torsional forces affect fractures of the distal radius.[4,5] Such forces are generated by musculotendinous units, gravity, and patient activity, and can lead to collapse of the fracture, especially in elderly patients with osteoporotic bone.[2,3] This collapse occurs in four radiological dimensions—radial height, radial inclination, palmar tilt, and ulnar variance—resulting in deformity and functional loss to the patient.[5-8]

To counteract these deforming forces, many forms of immobilization are used. The traditional method of cast immobilization still has a place in the treatment of distal radius fractures.[6-10] In unstable intra-articular fractures, the treatment becomes challenging. Casting alone or in combination with the application of percutaneous Kirschner wires (K-wires), pins in plaster, or external fixators has not solved the problems associated with these fractures.[7,11-13] Although dorsal plating and, more recently, volar plating techniques provide stable fixation, they require extensive soft tissue dissection.[14-19]

Biomechanical Concepts of Internal Fixation

A review of the literature provides an understanding of the basic biomechanical principles of internal fixation applied to distal radius fractures. A single wire (pin) through a fracture fragment allows rotation and translation along the axis of the wire.[4,20,21] A second wire through the fragment provides stability between the two fragments as long as the second wire is not parallel to the first.[4,21,22] If the second wire is parallel to the first, the fragment can still translate along the pin axis; complete stability is not insured.[4] In an experimental cadaver model, Graham and Louis found that as the number of pins was increased from one to four, the construct became more stable.[20] In this model, the pins that crossed each other at different angles through the ulnar shaft provided the greatest stability.

Rogge and colleagues,[4] in a three-dimensional finite element model, showed that two pins traversing the fracture, as in cross-pinning, are more stable than two parallel pins. Naidu and coworkers[23] reported similar findings. Crossed K-wires capture the larger fragments and buttress the smaller fragments, preventing gross articular collapse. In the wrist, where loads of 100 to 180 lb are anticipated in the postoperative phase, it is beneficial to distribute the load over multiple crossed K-wires in the Kapandji fashion.[24,25] This configuration also allows the surgeon to decrease the diameter of the pins significantly, from 3.5 to 1.6 mm.

Cross pin fixation has been in use for a long time.[26] Cross pin fixation alone does not hold an unstable distal radius fracture, however, unless another means of further support is provided, either by a cast or an external fixator.[26,27] The application of a cast or a bridging external fixator carries specific inherent problems that are well known within the orthopaedic community.[28-34] The CPX system was conceived as a hybrid of cross pin fixation and a nonbridging external fixator. The nonbridging external fixator provides stability to the cross pin construct, holding reduction of the distal radius fracture without compromising wrist mobilization.

The CPX system is a minimally invasive technique using closed reduction and internal fixation with percutaneous cross pin fixation and a nonbridging external fixator. The CPX device consists of an adjustable two-part aluminum sliding bar (11.5 to 14.5 cm) (**Fig. 7-1**). Two screws adjust the length of the bar, and at each end of the bar there is a head with three adjustable K-wire fixators. Each K-wire fixator has a guide hole, allowing freedom to angle the K-wire 10 degrees from center, and two screws, one to control the angle of the K-wire insertion and the other to lock the K-wire to the fixator (**Fig. 7-2**). The CPX system is indicated for treatment of displaced reducible extra-articular and nondisplaced and displaced reducible intra-articular distal radius fractures.

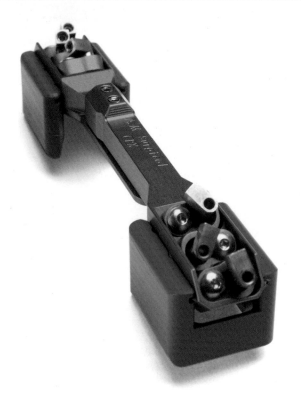

FIGURE 7-1 **CPX Device with Spacers.** *(Courtesy of AM Surgical.)*

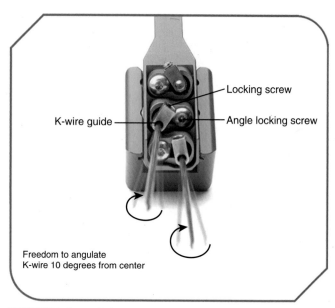

FIGURE 7-2 **Head of CPX Device with Adjustable K-wire Fixators.** *(Courtesy of AM Surgical.)*

CPX System
Biomechanics of CPX System

To achieve successful outcomes, it is important to understand how this system works biomechanically and how it differs from other systems available today. It has been shown that the stability of the fixation with K-wires is greatly enhanced by increasing the number of K-wires.[20] As noted, ensuring that these wires are not parallel to each other provides three-dimensional stability.[21] To minimize motion of the fragments and prevent articular step-off or deformity, it is important to achieve multiplanar (three-dimensional) stability of all major fragments (**Fig. 7-3**).[7] The CPX system, with a minimum of four wires (two distally and two proximally) crossing each other at different angles, greatly enhances the stability of the construct.

In traditional bridging and nonbridging external fixators, the pins are perpendicular to the long axis of the bone. This configuration unloads the fracture.[5] Comparatively, the pins of the CPX system are more longitudinally oriented and do not unload the fracture (**Fig. 7-4**). Wires with small diameters (1.6 mm), which flex when the construct is loaded and allow load sharing across the fracture fragments, facilitate callus formation[27] and reduce the risk of nonunion because of stress shielding. Also, the cross positioning of K-wires fixes the larger fracture fragments while buttressing the smaller fragments, helping to maintain joint congruency (see Figs. 7-3 and 4).

The cross pin configuration works similar to reinforced concrete (i.e., the pin is similar to steel, and the bone is similar to cement), and the external device acts like a pillar giving rigidity to the whole system (resisting compressive, torsional, and angular forces) (see Fig. 7-4). Among external fixators, bilateral and three-dimensional frames give more stability because of their multiplanar configuration compared with unilateral frames.[34,35] Conversely,

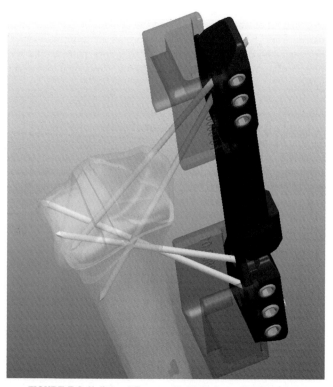

FIGURE 7-3 **Unilateral Frame with Multiplanar Configuration.**

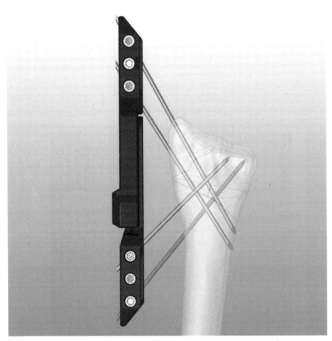

FIGURE 7-4 Biomechanical Concept of the CPX System. The cross pin fixation stabilizes the major fragments while buttressing the smaller fragments as in Kapandji fashion. This system allows for loading the fracture. The external bar gives rigidity to the system and resists angular and torsional forces.

the CPX system is lightweight (41 g, with the pins), and despite its unilateral frame, achieves three-dimensional stability because of its multiplanar K-wire configuration (see Fig. 7-3).

Indications and Contraindications

Using AO classification, the CPX system is indicated for extra-articular A2 and A3 fractures; simple articular B1 fractures; non-displaced or reducible and minimally displaced three-part fractures; and C1 and comminuted C2.1, C2.2, and C3.1 fractures. Although, I have successfully treated dorsal shear B2.2 and volar shear B3.3 fractures (see Illustrated Cases later), further investigation and clinical studies are needed to recommend these fractures and C2.3, C3.2, and C3.3 fractures further as indications for the CPX system. Osteoporosis and an unstable distal radioulnar joint are not contraindications. A small distal fragment (<1 cm) is not an absolute contraindication, as long as it is reducible and stable. This system is not recommended for patients with massive swelling, an unstable soft tissue envelope, open fractures, dementia, or advanced Parkinson's disease, or for patients who are not willing to commit to the postoperative protocol.

Surgical Technique

The surgery can be performed at an ambulatory surgical center under axillary block, regional intravenous (Bier) block, or general anesthesia. In some cases, a forearm tourniquet is used with a Bier block. In patients with shorter forearms, difficulty may arise inserting the proximal pins. In such cases, an upper arm Bier block may be used.

The fracture is reduced by using the classic maneuver, palmar flexion and ulnar deviation.[36] If this maneuver fails, finger trap traction can be used. Finger traps are applied to the thumb and index finger and sometimes to the middle finger, with 10 lb of

traction or more, if needed. If greater radial inclination is desired, only the thumb is placed in a finger trap. The only drawback to longitudinal traction is that palmar tilt is not restored.[37] This problem can be overcome by applying dorsal pressure to the distal fragment, pushing in the volar direction to maintain palmar tilt until the first K-wire is in place.

After reduction, it is important to FluoroScan and assess the fracture in the anteroposterior, lateral, and oblique planes for restoration of radial inclination, radial height, palmar tilt, ulnar variance, and articular joint congruency. The tissue protector is placed against the radial styloid between the first and second dorsal compartment, and FluoroScan is done to determine placement of the first K-wire (**Fig. 7-5A**). The tissue protector is removed, and a small stab wound is made in its place (**Fig. 7-5B**). Through the stab wound, a clamp is introduced, and the soft tissues are spread through to the bone (**Fig. 7-5C**).

Some surgeons might elect to make a small incision and identify and protect the radial sensory nerve. Early in the development of this technique, I (AM) began this way. I subsequently switched to making a stab wound and using a tissue protector. The tissue protector has a sharp end that can be anchored directly against the bone while driving the K-wire, protecting the radial sensory nerve and minimizing any potential for damage.

A 1.6-mm K-wire is driven freehand at a 40- to 45-degree angle through the tissue protector into the bone (**Fig. 7-6A**). The aim is to cross the fracture site and come out on the opposite side proximally in the mid lateral plane, penetrating the ulnar cortex (**Fig. 7-6B**). This can be very easily assessed under FluoroScan by imaging a lateral view and making sure that the K-wire is not too dorsal or too volar; otherwise, the K-wire may snag either the extensor or the flexor tendon (**Fig. 7-6C**). After satisfactorily driving the first pin, the fracture is stable enough so that one does not have to continue the dorsal pressure on the distal fragment to maintain the palmar tilt. The radial inclination and radial height continue to be maintained by the traction.

Before applying the CPX device, it is important to loosen all of the screws. The device is provided with two blue plastic spacers; these are used to ensure that the device is a certain distance away from the skin, allowing for mobilization of the wrist (see Fig. 7-1). With the spacers attached to the device, one slides the device over the K-wire through the distalmost guide hole. The length of the fixator can be adjusted to accommodate for the insertion of the proximal K-wire.

I find it helpful at this point to take a K-wire and place it on the dorsal aspect of the skin, and FluoroScan in the anteroposterior plane showing that the K-wire is aimed at the lunate fossa. I draw a line along the K-wire with a marking pen (**Fig. 7-7**). Using this line as a guide, make the proximal stab wound in the mid lateral plane on the radial side approximately 1 to 2 cm distal to the line drawn, introduce the clamp and spread the tissue down to the bone. Subsequently, slide the proximal head of the CPX fixator to the desired length, slide the tissue protector through the proximal-most K-wire guide hole, into the stab wound, ensuring that there are no intervening soft tissues.

Next, a 1.6-mm K-wire is passed through the tissue protector and driven into the bone at an angle that aims at the lunate fossa (**Fig. 7-8A**). One verifies that the wire is aiming toward the lunate fossa by checking the anteroposterior view on the fluoroscan; one proceeds only if satisfied with its position. Otherwise, the K-wire is removed, the angle of the tissue protector is changed, and the K-wire is reinserted until one satisfactorily aims the wire at the lunate fossa (**Fig. 7-8B**). One of the most important things to

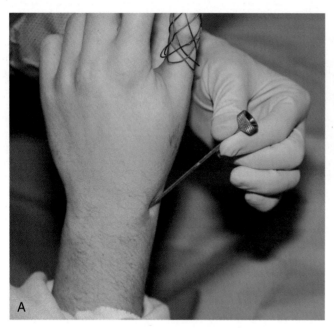

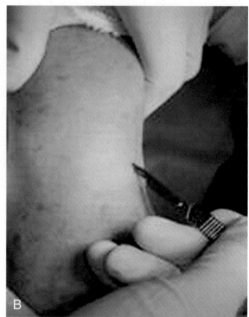

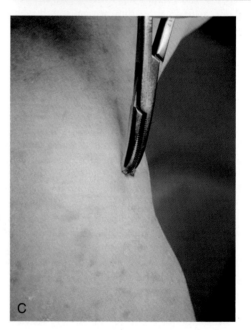

FIGURE 7-5 **A,** Placement of the tissue protector against the radial styloid to determine with FluoroScan placement of the first K-wire. **B,** Stab wound. **C,** Insertion of clamp into stab wound.

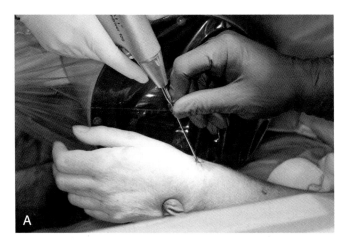

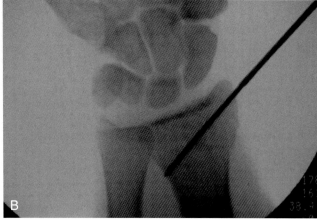

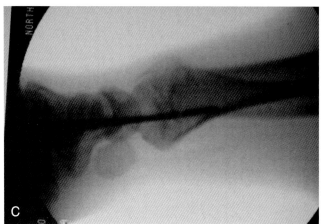

FIGURE 7-6 **Insertion of First K-wire. A,** Freehand insertion of the K-wire through the tissue protector. **B,** FluoroScan—anteroposterior view. **C,** FluoroScan—lateral view.

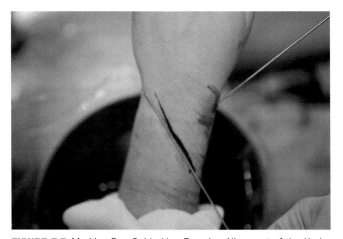

FIGURE 7-7 Marking Pen Guide Line Ensuring Alignment of the K-wire to the Lunate Fossa with Fluoroscan.

remember is that the cortical bone is difficult to penetrate proximally; take your time and continue driving the K-wire until it penetrates the cortex.

After driving the second K-wire almost to the subchondral bone, tighten the screws, that adjust the length of the CPX device. Then tighten the screws that affix the K-wires to the device and remove the blue spacers.

An alternative technique for the insertion of the second K-wire would be to take the fixator apart by completely loosening the screws on the bar and driving the proximal K-wire freehand through the tissue protector precisely in the mid lateral border of the forearm. Then one slides the proximal and distal component of the CPX device on the K-wires. One attaches the pieces of the CPX bar together, slides it to the desired length, and tightens the screws.

Next, working from a proximal to distal direction, one makes another stab wound and, using the tissue protector to limit soft tissue damage, drives the third K-wire toward the lunate fossa. After this is accomplished, one drives the fourth K-wire from distal to proximal, again using a tissue protector so as not to damage the radial nerve. I prefer two pins proximally and two pins distally, which should suffice in most cases (**Fig. 7-9**). One might consider using a third K-wire proximally or distally. FluoroScan x-rays should be taken in the anteroposterior and lateral planes to ensure the pin alignment. One tightens the screws to affix the additional K-wires to the device, then checks each screw one by one and tightens if indicated.

The pins are cut at a convenient level, and pin caps are placed on the cut ends for protection. The traction is then removed, and FluoroScan views are taken to ascertain that there is no loss of reduction. Bupivacaine (Marcaine) with epinephrine is injected around the pins proximally and distally and into the fracture hematoma. This medication makes the patient comfortable postoperatively. Xeroform dressings are applied around the pins followed by a soft dressing and a wrist/forearm volar splint (**Fig. 7-10**). The patient is sent home with instructions to move the

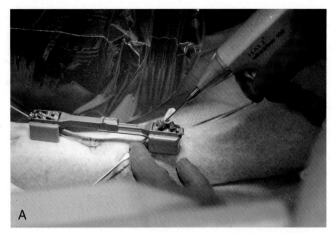

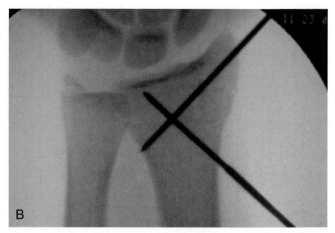

FIGURE 7-8 **Insertion of the Second K-wire. A,** Through the tissue protector, the second pin is driven proximal to distal to the lunate fossa. **B,** FluoroScan of K-wire position.

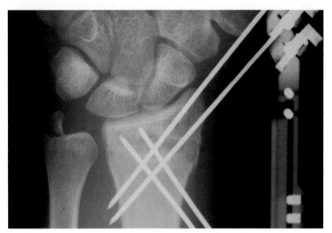

FIGURE 7-9 FluoroScan of Anteroposterior View Showing Four K-wires.

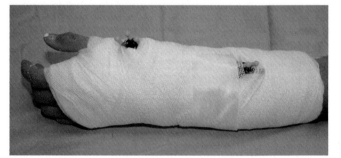

FIGURE 7-10 **Postoperative Dressing with Volar Splint.**

fingers through their entire range of motion and to keep the arm elevated.

Caveats

It is most important to remember that the fracture assessment is of paramount importance. In a displaced multifragment fracture, it is difficult to understand the various components of the fracture and to decide whether the fracture is reducible or not. X-rays routinely understate and computed tomography (CT) scans tend to overstate these fracture fragment configurations. After reduction of the fracture, the surgeon has a much better understanding of which form of fixation to use.

In our experience, the best thing to do is to reduce the fracture and assess by FluoroScan in the anteroposterior, lateral, and oblique planes, confirming proper restoration of fracture alignment and joint congruency. The dictum here is: *no reduction, no decision*. If the fracture is reducible and stable, one can proceed using the CPX system; otherwise, one should plan on open reduction and internal fixation.

Postoperative Study Protocol

The patient is seen in the office 3 to 5 days postoperatively for evaluation and referral to an occupational therapist. During this visit, a custom removable orthosis is applied (**Fig. 7-11**), and the

patient is instructed to begin a formal home exercise program for the wrist and fingers.

Occupational therapy three times per week begins 5 to 7 days post surgery, for further active finger, wrist, and forearm range of motion, and resumption of usual activities. The patient is instructed to remove the splint six times each day to perform the home exercise program. Additionally, at 4 weeks post surgery, patients are encouraged to remove the splint for general light activities, such as mealtime, personal care, folding laundry, and computer use. Goniometric measurements in flexion, extension, radial and ulnar deviation, supination and pronation, and grip and pinch strengths are recorded by the occupational therapist at designated intervals.

Postoperative x-rays are taken at 2, 4, 6, 8, and 12 weeks and again at 6 months to evaluate radial height, palmar tilt, radial inclination, and ulnar variance. Pin care is rendered during office visits by applying Hibiclens-soaked gauze to the pin sites. Patient completion of the patient-rated wrist and hand evaluation (PRWHE) and the Disabilities of the Arm, Shoulder, and Hand (DASH) score assisted us in assessing pain, return to activities, and upper extremity functional disability and symptoms. The CPX device and K-wires are removed when trabecular bridging and obliteration of distinct fracture lines are verified radiologically, 6 to 8 weeks post reduction.

Author's Experience

Cross pin fixation with a plaster bar strut, an experimental precursor to the CPX system, was used to treat 14 distal radius

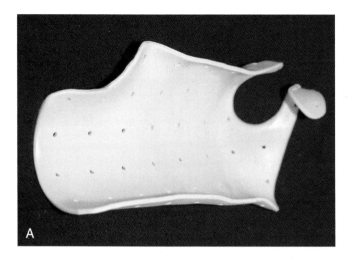

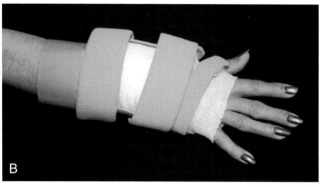

FIGURE 7-11 A and B, Removable Custom Splint.

fractures between September 2001 and February 2004. Between September 2004 and July 2007, 45 patients, 29 women and 15 men, with 48 distal radius fractures, were treated with the CPX system. The average age was 55 years (range 17 to 87 years).

Three patients were excluded. One patient was excluded because of noncompliance in the early postoperative period, and two patients with severe osteoporosis, bone loss, and irreducibility refused open reduction; the CPX system was used with a synthetic bone graft. Additionally, one patient at 12 weeks post surgery fell and refractured the wrist, requiring reapplication of the CPX system.

Results

Radiographic parameters of radial height, palmar tilt, radial inclination, and ulnar variance were fully restored in all but three fractures. One had a persistent 3-degree dorsal tilt, and all three had radial height and ulnar variance out of range. When the CPX system was applied, these three fractures held without angular or longitudinal collapse. Overall, fracture reduction was maintained in all but two, which had a loss in ulnar variance of 1 mm and 2 mm, without loss of radial inclination or palmar tilt. On final evaluation, one patient had a persistent 1-mm step-off in the lunate fossa. There was no loss of fracture reduction or nonunion. The CPX device was removed an average of 47 days (range 39 to 61 days) post application.

Initial occupational therapy evaluation (6 to 10 days post surgery) revealed that the patients' mean wrist range of motion of the operative wrist was as follows: dorsiflexion 22 degrees (range −20 to 52 degrees), volar flexion 23 degrees (range 9 to 50 degrees), pronation 64 degrees (range −14 to 86 degrees), and supination 25 degrees (range −3 to 87 degrees). Range of motion continued to progress throughout recovery. **Figure 7-12** shows assisted range of motion relative to the uninjured hand/wrist at 1 year.

The PRWHE revealed improved functional ability with decreasing pain and resumption of usual and specific activities throughout recovery. Total mean scores were 68 (range 34 to 97.5) at baseline, 29 (range 0 to 81.5) at 12 weeks, and 14 (range 0.5 to 51) at 1 year. Similarly, DASH scores revealed a clinically significant improvement in physical function. The mean DASH baseline score was 64 (range 16 to 100), improving to 45 (range

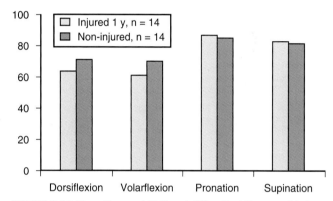

FIGURE 7-12 Mean Range of Motion at 1-Year Post Surgery with Comparison to Noninjured Wrist.

10 to 69) at 4 weeks, 26 (range 0 to 78) at 12 weeks, and 14 (range 0 to 68) at 1 year.

Two patients developed superficial radial nerve sensitivity, which resolved to mild transient sensitivity without functional compromise when treated with gabapentin and desensitization. One patient, who sustained multiple injuries in addition to a distal radius fracture, had a protracted recovery and was diagnosed with type 1 complex regional pain syndrome, which resolved, requiring no formal treatment. One other patient with a protracted recovery had a significant improvement after the 1-year follow-up, status post endoscopic carpal tunnel release and manipulation of the wrist. There were no pin tract infections or tendon ruptures.

Illustrated Cases

Three cases are illustrated with preoperative, postoperative, and healed anteroposterior and lateral radiographic views in addition to range of motion, DASH, and PRWHE scores from the patient's most recent follow-up visit. **Figure 7-13** shows a 17-year-old boy with a left nondominant C2.2 fracture. At 8 weeks post surgery, dorsiflexion was 76 degrees, volar flexion was 76 degrees, pronation was 90 degrees, supination was 90 degrees, DASH score was 16.67, and PRWHE was 10. **Figure 7-14** shows a 48-year-old woman with osteoporosis and a left non-

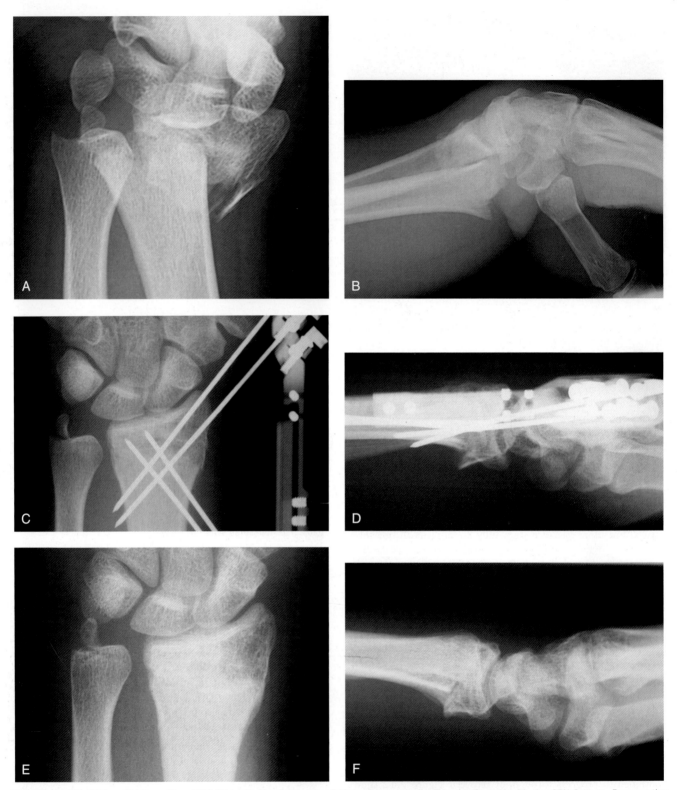

FIGURE 7-13 A 17-Year-Old Boy with a C2.2 Distal Radius Fracture and Major Extra-articular Element Treated with the CPX System. Preoperative views—posteroanterior (**A**) and lateral (**B**). Postoperative views—posteroanterior (**C**) and lateral (**D**). Views after healing—posteroanterior (**E**) and lateral (**F**).

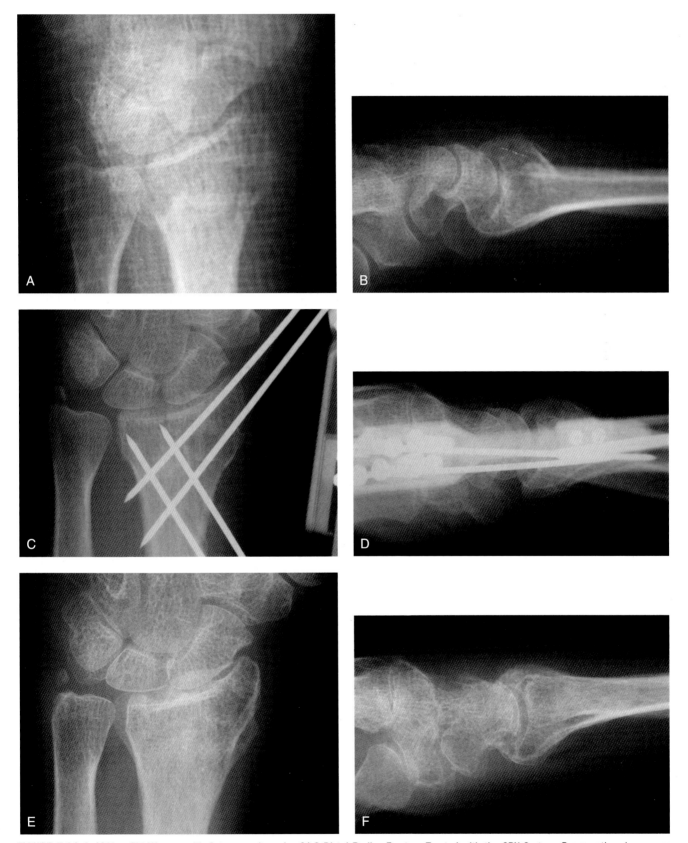

FIGURE 7-14 **A 48-Year-Old Woman with Osteoporosis and a C1.2 Distal Radius Fracture Treated with the CPX System.** Preoperative views—posteroanterior (**A**) and lateral (**B**). Postoperative views—posteroanterior (**C**) and lateral (**D**). **E** and **F**, View after healing—posteroanterior.

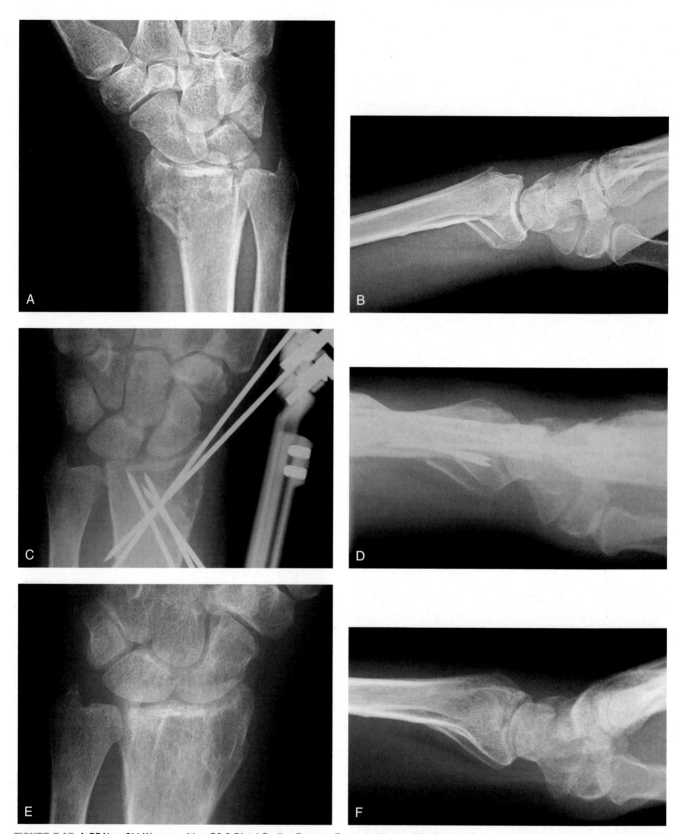

FIGURE 7-15 A 55-Year-Old Woman with a B3.3 Distal Radius Fracture Treated with the CPX System. Preoperative views—posteroanterior (**A**) and lateral (**B**). Postoperative views—posteroanterior (**C**) and lateral (**D**). Views after healing—posteroanterior (**E**) and lateral (**F**).

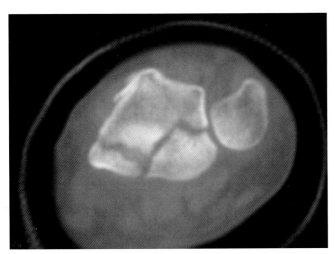

FIGURE 7-16 Computed Tomography Scan View of Figure 7-15 (B3.3 Volar Barton Fracture).

dominant C1.2 distal radius fracture. At 6 months post surgery, dorsiflexion was 76 degrees, volar flexion was 66 degrees, pronation was 88 degrees, supination was 88 degrees, DASH score was 11.66, and PRWHE was 17. **Figure 7-15** shows a 55-year-old woman with a B3.3 volar Barton distal radius fracture of the right dominant hand. At 1 year post surgery, dorsiflexion was 60 degrees, volar flexion was 50 degrees, pronation was 82 degrees, supination was 77 degrees, DASH score was 9.48, and PRWHE was 17. A CT scan view of the B3.3 volar Barton fracture is shown in **Figure 7-16**.

Summary

The CPX system is a minimally invasive technique, using a non-bridging, single-frame external fixator, which integrates internal fixation with a multiplanar pin configuration. This fixation system significantly maintains reduction, while allowing wrist rehabilitation during fracture healing. Soft tissue dissection is minimal, and the risk to anatomical structures is negligible. From a technical standpoint, the CPX device provides the surgeon flexibility when positioning the K-wire, with 10 degrees of rotation from the insertion point. Finally, the learning curve for this technique is manageable.

REFERENCES

1. Krishnan J, Chipcase S, Slavotinek J: Intraarticular fractures of the distal radius treated with metaphyseal external fixation. J Hand Surg [Br] 1998; 23:396-399.
2. Mallmin H, Ljunghall S: Distal radius fracture is an early sign of general osteoporosis: bone mass measurements in a population based study. Osteopor Int 1994; 4:357-361.
3. Gausepohl T, Worner S, Pennig D, et al: Extraarticular external fixation in distal radius fractures pin placement in osteoporotic bone. Injury 2001; 32:79-85.
4. Rogge R, Adams B, Goel VK: An analysis of bone stresses and fixation stability using a finite element model of simulated distal radius fractures. J Hand Surg [Am] 2002; 27:86-92.
5. Bindra RR: Biomechanics and biology of external fixation of distal radius fractures. Hand Clin 2005; 21:363-373.
6. Nesbitt KS, Faille JM, Les C: Assessment of instability factors in adult distal radius fractures. J Hand Surg [Am] 2004; 29:1128-1138.
7. Gradl G, Jupiter JB, Gierer P, et al: Fractures of the distal radius treated with a nonbridging external fixation technique using multiplanar K-wires. J Hand Surg [Am] 2005; 30: 960-968.
8. Slutsky DJ, Herman M: Rehabilitation of distal radius fractures: a biomechanical guide. Hand Clin 2005; 21:455-468.
9. Rogachefsky RA, Lipson SR, Applegate B, et al: Treatment of severely comminuted intra-articular fractures of the distal end of the radius by open reduction and combined internal and external fixation. J Bone Joint Surg Am 2001; 83:509-519.
10. Hanel DP, Jones MD, Trumble TE: Wrist fractures. Orthop Clin North Am 2002; 33:35-37.
11. Agee JM: Distal radius fractures: multiplanar ligamentotaxis. Hand Clin 1993; 9:577-585.
12. Kapoor H, Agarwal A, Dhaon BK: Displaced intra-articular fractures of distal radius: a comparative evaluation of results following closed reduction, external fixation. Injury 2000; 31:75-79.
13. Wolf J, Weil W, Hanel D, et al: A biomechanic comparison of an internal radiocarpal-spanning 2.4-mm locking plate and external fixation in a model of distal radius fractures. J Hand Surg [Am] 1999; 24:516-524.
14. Rozental TD, Blazar PE: Functional outcome and complications after volar plating for dorsally displaced, unstable fractures of the distal radius. J Hand Surg [Am] 2006; 31:359-365.
15. Smith DW, Henry MH: Volar fixed-angle plating of the distal radius. J Am Acad Orthop Surg 2005; 13:28-36.
16. Ruch DS, Papadonikolakis A: Volar versus dorsal plating in the management of intra-articular distal radius fractures. J Hand Surg [Am] 2006; 31:9-16.
17. Harness NG, Meals RA: The history of fracture fixation of the hand and wrist. Clin Orthop 2006; 445:19-29.
18. Ruch DS, Yang C, Patersen Smith B: Result of palmar plating of the lunate facet combined with external fixation for the treatment of high-energy compression fractures of the distal radius. J Orthop Trauma 2004; 18:28-33.
19. Rush LV: Closed medullary pinning of Colles' fracture. Clin Orthop 1954; 3:152-162.
20. Graham TJ, Louis DS: Biomechanical aspects of percutaneous pinning for distal radius fractures. In Saffar P, Cooney W, eds: Fractures of the Distal Radius. London: Martin Dunitz, 1995.
21. Heatherly RD, Adams BD, Goel VK: An evaluation of distal radius fracture pinning techniques using experimentally validated FE model. Summer Bioengineering conference, ASMEM, Big Sky, Montana, 1999.
22. Stein AH Jr, Katz SF: Stabilization of comminuted fractures of the distal inch of the radius: percutaneous pinning. Clin Orthop 1975; 108:174-181.
23. Naidu SH, Capo JT, Moulton M, et al: Percutaneous pinning of distal radius fractures: a biomechanical study. J Hand Surg [Am] 1997; 22:252-257.

24. Ruschel PH, Albertoni WM: Treatment of unstable extra-articular distal radius fractures by modified intrafocal Kapandji method. Tech Hand Up Extrem Surg 2005; 9:7-16.

25. Weil WM, Trumble TE: Treatment of distal radius fractures with intrafocal (Kapandji) pinning and supplemental skeletal stabilization. Hand Clin 2005; 21:317-328.

26. Clancey GJ: Percutaneous Kirschner-wire fixation of Colles' fractures: a prospective study of thirty cases. J Bone Joint Surg [Am] 1984; 66:1008-1014.

27. Wolfe SW, Austin G, Lorenze M, et al: A biomechanical comparison of different wrist external fixators with and without K-wire augmentation. J Hand Surg [Am] 1999; 24:516-524.

28. Gutow AP: Avoidance and treatment of complication of distal radius fractures. Hand Clin 2005; 21:295-305.

29. Anderson JT, Lucas GL, Buhr BR: Complications of treating distal radius fractures with external fixation: a community experience. Iowa Orthop J 2004; 24:53-59.

30. Weber SC, Szabo RM: Severely comminuted distal radius fractures as an unsolved problem: complications associated with external fixation and pin and plaster techniques. J Hand Surg [Am] 1986; 11:156.

31. Sanders RA, Keppel FL, Waldrop JI: External fixation of distal radial fractures: results and complications. J Hand Surg [Am] 1991; 16:385-391.

32. Moroni A, Vannini F, Mosca M, et al: State of the art review: techniques to avoid pin loosening and infection in external fixation. J Orthop Trauma 2002; 16:189-195.

33. Parameswara AD, Roberts CS, Seligson D, et al: Pin tract infection with contemporary external fixation: how much of a problem? J Orthop Trauma 2003; 17:503-507.

34. Davenport WC, Miller G, Wright TW: Wrist ligament strain during external fixation: a cadaveric study. J Hand Surg [Am] 1999; 24:102-107.

35. Lindsay CS, Richards RS, King GJ, et al: Ilizarov hybrid external fixation for fractures of the distal radius, part I: feasibility of transfixion wire placement. J Hand Surg [Am] 2001; 26:210-217.

36. Fernandez DL, Jupiter JB: Fractures of the Distal Radius: A Practical Approach to Management. 2nd ed. New York: Springer, 2003.

37. Bartosh RA, Saldana MJ: Intraarticular fractures of the distal radius: a cadaveric study to determine if ligamentotaxis restores radiopalmar tilt. J Hand Surg [Am] 1990; 15:18-21.

External Fixation of Distal Radius Fractures

8

David J. Slutsky, MD

External fixation has been used for the treatment of distal radius fractures for more than 50 years. Although the fixator configurations have undergone considerable modification over time, the type of fixator itself is not as important as the underlying principles that provide the foundation for external fixation. Although volar plate fixation is currently popular, the indications for external fixation remain largely unchanged. Newer fixator designs also have expanded the traditional usage to include nonbridging applications, which allow early wrist motion. This chapter focuses on the myriad uses for external fixation and the shortcomings and potential pitfalls.

Anatomy

There are some important anatomical points one must bear in mind when considering external fixation of the distal radius. The articular surface of the radius is triangular with the apex of the triangle at the radial styloid. It slopes in a volar and ulnar direction with a radial inclination of 23 degrees (range 13 to 30 degrees), a radial length of 12 mm (range 8 to 18 mm), and an average volar tilt of 12 degrees (range 1 to 21 degrees).[1] The dorsal surface of the distal radius is convex and irregular, and it is covered by the six dorsal extensor compartments. The dorsal cortex is thin, which often results in comminution that may lead to an abnormal dorsal tilt. Lister's tubercle acts as a fulcrum for the extensor pollicis longus (EPL) tendon, which lies in a groove on the ulnar side of the tubercle. The volar side of the distal radius, which is covered by the pronator quadratus, is flat and makes a smooth curve that is concave from proximal to distal. When inserting the dorsal pins, it is important to engage the volar ulnar lip of the distal radius where the bone density is highest, especially in osteopenic bone.[2]

The dorsum of the radius is cloaked by the arborizations of the superficial radial nerve (SRN) and the dorsal cutaneous branch of the ulnar nerve. The SRN exits from under the brachioradialis approximately 5 cm proximal to the radial styloid and bifurcates into a major volar and a major dorsal branch at a mean distance of 4.2 cm proximal to the radial styloid (**Fig. 8-1**). Either partial or complete overlap of the lateral antebrachial cutaneous nerve with the SRN occurs up to 75% of the time.[3] The dorsal cutaneous branch of the ulnar nerve arises from the ulnar nerve 6 cm proximal to the ulnar head and becomes subcutaneous 5 cm proximal to the pisiform. It crosses the ulnar snuffbox and gives off three to nine branches that supply the dorsoulnar aspect of the carpus, small finger, and ulnar ring finger. Open pin insertion allows identification and protection of these branches.

The proximal pins are placed at the junction of the proximal and middle thirds of the radius. At this level, the radius is covered by the tendons of the extensor carpi radialis longus, extensor carpi radialis brevis, and extensor digitorum communis. The proximal pins can be inserted in the standard mid lateral position by retracting the brachioradialis tendon and the SRN, in the dorsoradial position between the extensor carpi radialis longus and extensor carpi radialis brevis, or dorsally between the extensor carpi radialis brevis and extensor digitorum communis, which carries less risk of injury to the SRN.[4]

Ligamentotaxis

External fixation of distal radius fractures may be used in a bridging or nonbridging manner. Bridging external fixation of distal radius fractures typically relies on ligamentotaxis to obtain and maintain a reduction of the fracture fragments. As longitudinal traction is applied to the carpus, the tension is transmitted mostly through the radioscaphocapitate and long radiolunate ligaments to restore the radial length. In a similar vein, pronation of the carpus can indirectly correct the supination deformity of the distal fragment.

Limitations of Ligamentotaxis

Ligamentotaxis has many shortcomings when applied to the treatment of displaced intra-articular fractures of the distal radius. First, because ligaments exhibit viscoelastic behavior,[5] there is a gradual loss of the initial distraction force applied to the fracture site through stress relaxation.[6] The immediate improvements in radial height, inclination, and volar tilt are significantly decreased by the time of fixator removal (**Fig. 8-2**).[7]

Traction does not correct the dorsal tilt of the distal fracture fragment because the stout volar radiocarpal ligaments are shorter,

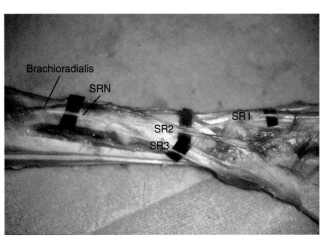

FIGURE 8-1 Proximity of the Superficial Radial Nerve (SRN) Branches (SR1, SR2, SR3) to Potential Pin Placement Sites. (© *South Bay Hand Surgery, LLC; 2007. Used by permission.*)

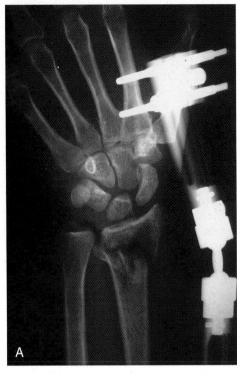

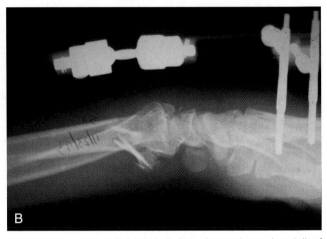

FIGURE 8-2 **Limitations of Ligamentotaxis. A,** Initial overdistraction restores radial length. **B,** Note the persistent dorsal tilt of the articular surface even with maximum distraction. *(© South Bay Hand Surgery, LLC; 2007. Used by permission.)*

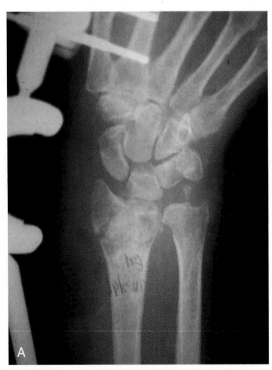

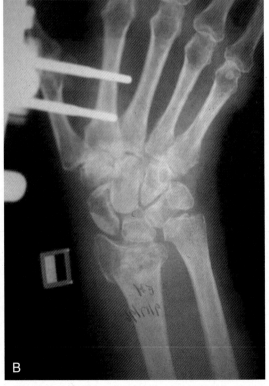

FIGURE 8-3 **Stress Relaxation. A,** Note overdistraction of the radiocarpal joint and restoration of radial length. **B,** Two weeks later, there is a loss of the radial length, and the joint space is no longer overdistracted. *(© South Bay Hand Surgery, LLC; 2007. Used by permission.)*

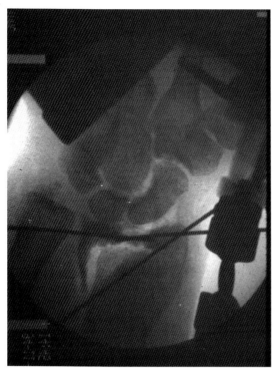

FIGURE 8-4 Unstable Distal Radioulnar Joint. The medial (sigmoid notch) fragment follows the ulnar head because of the intact radioulnar ligaments and cannot be stabilized with K-wires and bridging external fixation. *(© South Bay Hand Surgery, LLC; 2007. Used by permission.)*

and they pull out to length before the thinner dorsal radiocarpal ligaments exert any traction.[8] Excessive traction may increase the dorsal tilt (**Fig. 8-3**).[9] A dorsally directed vector is still necessary to restore the normal volar angulation. This vector is usually accomplished by applying manual thumb pressure over the dorsum of the distal fragment. With intra-articular fractures, ligamentotaxis reduces the radial styloid fragment, but for the aforementioned reasons, it does not reduce a depressed lunate fragment.[10] When there is a sagittal split of the medial fragment, traction causes the volar medial fragment to rotate, which often necessitates an open reduction. External fixation cannot control radial translation and cannot be used with an unstable distal radioulnar joint (**Fig. 8-4**).

Biomechanical Considerations for External Fixation

Fracture Site Loads

External fixation is considered flexible fixation.[11] The biomechanical requirements of external fixation for fractures of the distal radius have not been ascertained because until more recently, the magnitude and direction of the physiological loads on the distal radius were dynamic and unknown. Work by Rikli and colleagues[12] has shed new light on this point, however. Using a new capacitive pressure-sensory device, these investigators measured the in vivo dynamic intra-articular pressures under local anesthesia in the radioulnocarpal joint of a healthy volunteer. With the forearm in neutral rotation, the forces ranged from 107N with wrist flexion to 197N with wrist extension. The highest forces of 245N were seen with the wrist in radial deviation and the forearm

in supination. Presumably, any implant or external fixator would need to be strong enough to neutralize these loads to permit early active wrist motion. Rikli and colleagues[12] also identified two centers of force transmission. The first center was opposite the scaphoid pole, which would represent the radial column. The second center, which would represent the intermediate column of the wrist, took a considerable amount of the load and was opposite the lunate, extending ulnarly over the triangular fibrocartilaginous complex.

Construct Rigidity

Increasing the rigidity of the fixator does not appreciably increase the rigidity of fixation of the individual fracture fragments.[13] The stability of the construct can be augmented in many ways, however. After restoration of radial length and alignment by the external fixator, percutaneous pin fixation can lock in the radial styloid buttress and support the lunate fossa fragment.[14] A fifth radial styloid pin attached to the frame of a spanning AO external fixator (Synthes, Paoli, PA) prevents a loss of radial length through settling and leads to improved wrist range of motion compared with a four-pin external fixator.[15] The addition of a dorsal pin attached to a sidebar easily corrects the dorsal tilt found in many distal radius fractures.[16,17]

Kirschner wire (K-wire) fixation enhances the stability of external fixation. The combination of an external fixator augmented with 0.62-inch K-wires approaches the strength of a 3.5-mm dorsal AO plate (Synthes, Paoli, PA).[18] Supplemental K-wire fixation is more crucial to the fracture fixation than the mechanical rigidity of the external fixator itself.[13] Stabilizing a fracture fragment with a nontransfixing K-wire that is attached to an outrigger is just as effective as a K-wire that transfixes the fracture fragments.[19]

Bridging External Fixation

Temporary External Fixation: Indications

Web Video

8-2

Compared with conventional plate fixation, bridging external fixation may be used in a temporary manner, or it may be used for definitive management of the distal radius fracture. Bindra[20] listed the following indications for this technique:

1. Initial management of severe-grade open fractures with extensive soft tissue loss (**Fig. 8-5**)
2. Temporizing measure to resuscitate a patient with polytrauma
3. Pending transfer to a tertiary referral facility for definitive fracture management

Rikli and colleagues[21] use temporary bridging external fixation for complex fractures to aid in the provisional fracture reduction and to allow a better computed tomography (CT) evaluation of the fracture characteristics before double-plate fixation.

Definitive External Fixation: Indications

Indications for definitive external fixation include the following:

1. Unstable extra-articular distal radius fractures
2. Two-part and selected three-part intra-articular fractures without displacement
3. Combined internal and external fixation

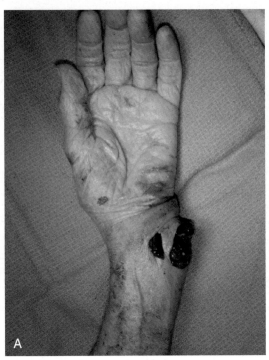 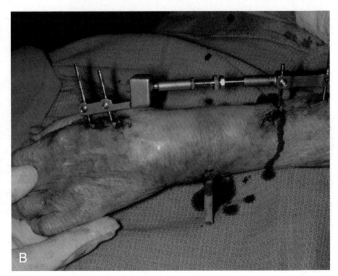

FIGURE 8-5 A, Open distal radius fracture. **B,** Temporary stabilization with a bridging external fixator. *(© South Bay Hand Surgery, LLC; 2007. Used by permission.)*

Contraindications

Bridging external fixation should not be used as the sole method of stabilization in the following situations:

1. Ulnar translocation resulting from an unstable distal radioulnar joint
2. Intra-articular volar shear fractures (Barton's, reverse Barton's)
3. Disrupted volar carpal ligaments and radiocarpal dislocations
4. Marked metaphyseal comminution

Combined index and middle finger metacarpal fractures preclude the use of this technique because of the interference with distal pin site placement.

Complications

Fixator loosening with loss of fracture position can be avoided by periodically checking and tightening the fixator connections. Fixator failure by itself is uncommon, but many commercially available fixators are approved for single use only because of the risk of unrecognized material fatigue or failure of any locking ball joints. Pin site complications include infection, loosening, and interference with extensor tendon gliding. The risk of injury to branches of the SRN mandate open pin site insertion. Bad outcomes associated with external fixation are often related to overdistraction. One biomechanical study documented the effect of distraction of the wrist on metacarpophalangeal joint motion. More than 5 mm of wrist distraction increases the load required for the flexor digitorum superficialis to generate metacarpophalangeal joint flexion for the middle, ring, and small fingers. For the index finger, however, 2 mm of wrist distraction significantly increases the load required for flexion at the metacarpophalangeal

joint.[22] Many cases of intrinsic tightness and finger stiffness that are attributed to reflex sympathetic dystrophy are a consequence of prolonged and excessive traction, which can be prevented by limiting the duration and amount of traction and instituting early dynamic metacarpophalangeal flexion splinting even while in the fixator.

The degree and duration of distraction correlate with the amount of subsequent wrist stiffness.[23] Distraction, flexion, and locked ulnar deviation of the external fixator encourage pronation contractures (**Fig. 8-6**). Distraction also increases the carpal canal pressure,[24] which may predispose to acute carpal tunnel syndrome. Metaphyseal defects should be grafted to diminish bending loads and to allow fixator removal after 6 to 7 weeks, which minimizes the fixator-related complications.

Results

Margaliot and associates[25] did a meta-analysis of 46 articles with 28 (917 patients) external fixation studies and 18 (603 patients) internal fixation studies. They did not detect a clinically or statistically significant difference in pooled grip strength, wrist range of motion, radiographic alignment, pain, or physician-rated outcomes between the two treatment arms. There were higher rates of infection, hardware failure, and neuritis with external fixation and higher rates of tendon complications and early hardware removal with internal fixation. Considerable heterogeneity was present in all of the studies, which adversely affected the precision of the meta-analysis.

Augmented External Fixation

The use of supplemental K-wire fixation can expand the indications for external fixation. As noted earlier, K-wire fixation not only enhances the reduction of the fracture fragments, but also

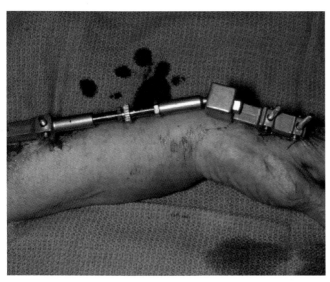

FIGURE 8-6 Fixator Frame Is Improperly Applied with Wrist in Marked Flexion. *(© South Bay Hand Surgery, LLC; 2007. Used by permission.)*

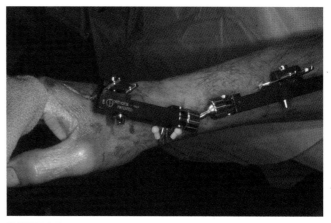

FIGURE 8-7 Fracture Reduction Is Captured with Percutaneous K-wires, then Neutralized with an External Fixator with Wrist in Slight Extension. *(© South Bay Hand Surgery, LLC; 2007. Used by permission.)*

increases the rigidity of the entire construct. Many authors have stressed the importance of using the external fixator as a neutralization device rather than a traction device. Ligamentotaxis is used to obtain a reduction of the fracture fragments, which is then captured with percutaneous K-wire fixation. The traction on the fixator can be reduced, which allows positioning of the wrist in neutral or slight extension (**Fig. 8-7**).[9] This positioning serves to reduce extensor tendon tightness and facilitates finger motion. In a study of intrafocal pinning, Weil and Trumble[26] noted that in patients older than 55 years and younger patients with comminution involving two or more surfaces of the radial metaphysis (or >50% of the metaphyseal diameter), bridging fixation was necessary in addition to percutaneous pin fixation to prevent late fracture collapse. In four-part fractures in which there is a sagittal split of the medial fragment, longitudinal traction accentuates the palmar translation and rotation of the volar medial fragment (**Fig. 8-8**). Dorsal to volar K-wire placement carries the risk of injury to the volar neurovascular bundles, especially with K-wire migration. For these reasons, any sagittal split of the articular surface typically requires open treatment[27] (**Fig. 8-9**).

Indications

1. Intra-articular radial styloid fractures
2. Three-part intra-articular fractures
3. After percutaneous reduction of a depressed lunate fragment
4. Arthroscopic-aided reduction of distal radius fractures

Contraindications

1. Marked metaphyseal comminution
2. Volar/dorsal intra-articular shear fractures

Results

Kreder and associates[28] compared the results of open reduction and internal fixation (ORIF) versus external fixation and pinning. The study randomly assigned 179 adult patients with displaced intra-articular fractures of the distal radius to receive indirect percutaneous reduction and external fixation ($n = 88$) or ORIF ($n = 91$). There was no statistically significant difference in the

radiological restoration of anatomical features or the range of movement between the groups at 2 years. The patients who underwent indirect reduction and percutaneous fixation had a more rapid return of function and a better functional outcome, however, than the patients who underwent ORIF, provided that the intra-articular step and gap deformity were minimized.

Complications

In one study of 70 cases of external fixation and percutaneous pinning, 49% of cases lost more than 5 degrees of volar tilt after reduction at the 6-month follow-up despite the use of pinning. Initial deformity, patient age, use of bone graft, and duration of external fixation were not predictors of loss of reduction. No specific predictor of loss of reduction was noted, although there was a trend toward a loss of reduction in younger patients.[29]

Nonbridging External Fixation
Extra-articular Fractures
Indications

Nonbridging external fixation is indicated in any extra-articular fracture in which there is a high risk of late collapse, or if there is redisplacement of the fracture after an acceptable closed reduction (**Fig. 8-10**). When there is significant displacement on the injury films, there is a high likelihood of collapse even if the initial reduction is satisfactory. Trumble and colleagues[30] recommend supplemental internal or external fixation in younger patients for fractures with more than 2 mm of radial shortening and more than 15 degrees of dorsal tilt after a closed reduction, especially if there is comminution of two or more cortices.

Contraindications

Nonbridging external fixation is contraindicated when the distal fragment is too small for pin placement. At least 1 cm of intact volar cortex is required for pin purchase. Dorsal comminution does not preclude a successful result. This technique is not applicable in patients with volar displaced or volar shear fractures or in children with open epiphyses.[40]

Surgical Technique

The technique is similar to bridging external fixation, with the use of a tourniquet and intraoperative fluoroscopy, but a traction tower is not required. Two dorsal 3-mm pins are inserted in

Web Video

8-4

b Video

8-3

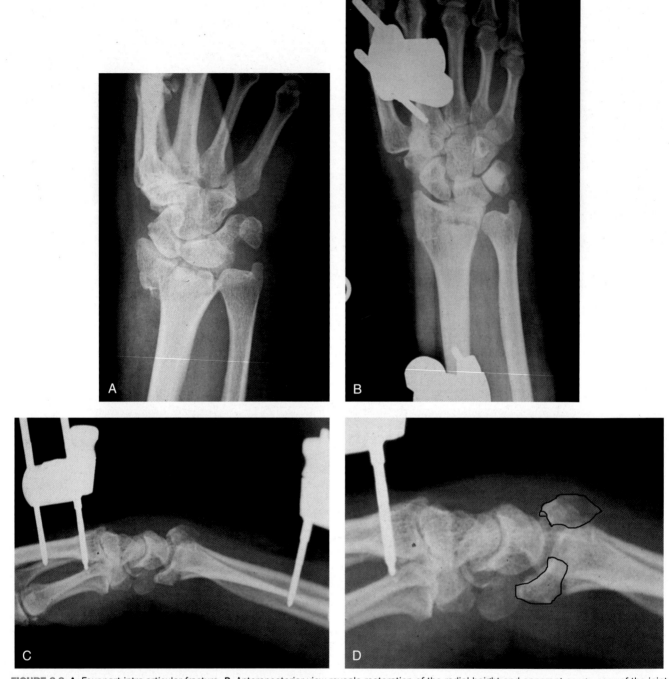

FIGURE 8-8 A, Four-part intra-articular fracture. **B,** Anteroposterior view reveals restoration of the radial height and apparent congruency of the joint surface. **C,** Lateral view reveals the sagittal split and increased rotation of the palmar medial fragment. **D,** Close-up with the volar medial and dorsal medial fragments outlined. *(© South Bay Hand Surgery, LLC; 2007. Used by permission.)*

the distal fragment through separate longitudinal incisions. The pins can be placed on either side of Lister's tubercle or the EPL tendon and between the extensor digitorum communis and the extensor digiti minimi. The starting position of the pin should be approximately halfway between the fracture and the radiocarpal joint. A temporary K-wire can be used to gauge the proper angle. The first pin is inserted through Lister's tubercle parallel to the joint surface in the lateral plane until it engages the volar cortex. The second dorsal pin is inserted in a similar manner, but on the ulnar side of the EPL

or extensor digitorum communis tendons. The dorsal tilt is corrected by levering the pins distally until the normal volar inclination has been restored. The fixator frame is applied and tightened.

Complications

Pin pullout resulting from fracture of the distal fragment can occur if the distal fragment is too small or osteopenic, or if the reduction is too vigorous. If this occurs, the fixator can be

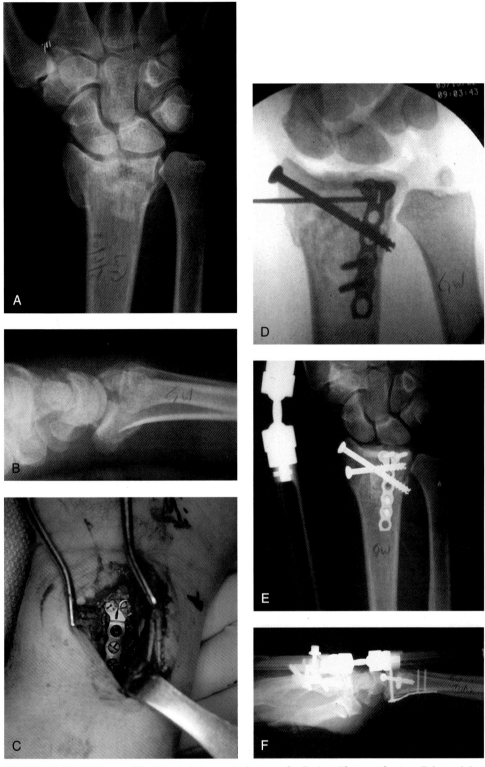

FIGURE 8-9 Limited Internal Fixation. A, Anteroposterior x-ray of a displaced four-part fracture. **B,** Lateral view shows a sagittal split of the medial fragment. **C,** Internal fixation of medial fragment through a limited volar ulnar approach. **D,** Subchondral K-wire inserted to support the joint surface. **E,** Second K-wire replaced by a percutaneous screw, which stops short of the distal radioulnar joint. **F,** Lateral view shows restoration of normal tilt and reduction of the sagittal split. *(© South Bay Hand Surgery, LLC; 2007. Used by permission.)*

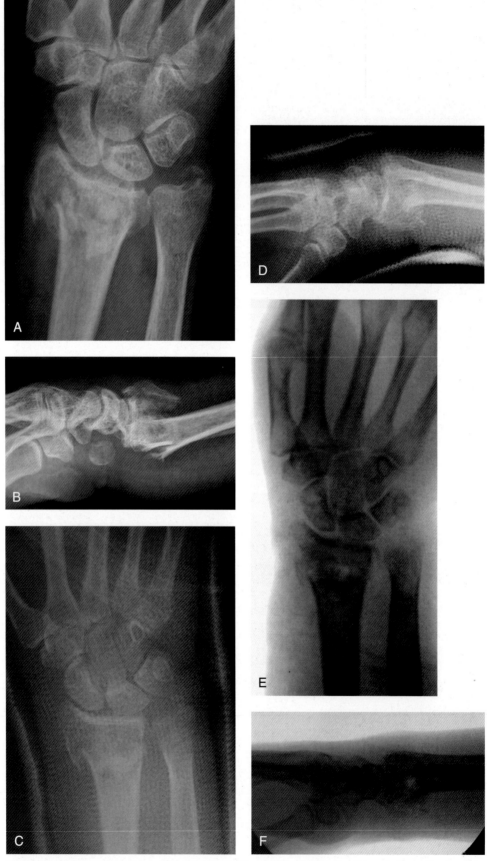

FIGURE 8-10 Nonbridging External Fixation. A, A 55-year-old woman with extra-articular radius fracture. **B,** Note the marked dorsal comminution. **C,** Redisplacement at 8 days with loss of radial height. **D,** Loss of volar tilt. **E,** Appearance after percutaneous bone grafting. **F,** Lateral view after bone grafting.

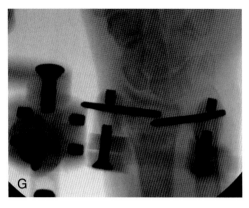
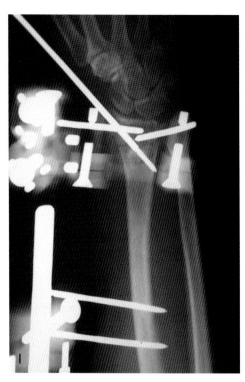
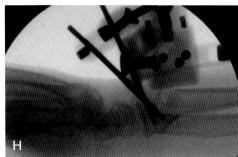

FIGURE 8-10, cont'd **G,** Insertion of dorsal fixator pins. **H,** Lateral view with nonbridging external fixator. **I,** Postoperative x-ray at 1 week with additional radial styloid pin. (© *South Bay Hand Surgery, LLC; 2007. Used by permission.*)

converted to a bridging construct. An incomplete reduction also is possible, especially with nascent malunions. Over-reduction of the fracture also can occur, especially when there is volar comminution.[31]

Results

McQueen[31] performed a prospective study of 641 patients with unstable fractures of the distal radius treated with external fixation. Of these cases, 59% were treated with nonbridging external fixation, mostly AO type A3.2 and C2.1 fractures. Patients treated with nonbridging external fixation had statistically significantly better radiological results throughout the period of review. In particular, this technique consistently restored the volar tilt and carpal alignment. Radiological improvement was mirrored by functional improvement. Most functional indices were statistically better at an early stage, whereas wrist flexion and grip strength remained significantly better at the final review. Complication rates were similar between the two groups.

Intra-articular Fractures

Early wrist motion after intra-articular fractures provides many possible benefits, including diminished stiffness, stimulation of cartilage repair,[32] and decreased osteopenia of the distal fragments.[33] To accomplish this with nonbridging external fixation, the construct must be able to withstand the forces generated during active and passive wrist motion.

Biomechanical Considerations

The author undertook a biomechanical study to examine the feasibility of nonbridging external fixation of simulated three-part and four-part intra-articular fractures.[34] All of the fractures were stabilized using a single custom nonbridging external fixator that has an integrated dorsal sidearm (Fragment Specific Fixator; South Bay Hand Surgery LLC, Torrance, CA) (see Fig. 8-10).

The study conclusion was that nonbridging external fixation with new fixator designs could be applied to the treatment of intra-articular fractures. Putnam and coworkers[35] have shown that for every 10N of grip force, 26N is transmitted through the distal radius metaphysis. They recommended that the rehabilitation grip forces should be kept at less than 140N with external fixation to prevent or minimize fixation failure. This also seems to be a safe limit because it pertains to nonbridging external fixation as well.

Similar to a fixed-angle plate, the biomechanical rationale for the Fragment Specific Fixator is to transfer load from the fixed support of the articular surface to the intact radial shaft, bypassing any metaphyseal comminution (**Fig. 8-11**). In contrast to a

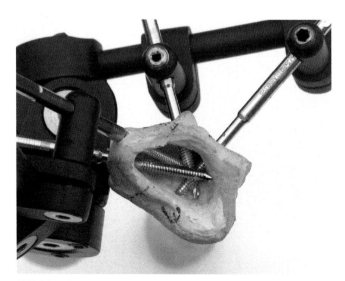

FIGURE 8-11 Cut-away View of Distal Radius Showing Stacking of Fixator Pins in Multiple Planes Similar to a Fixed-Angle Plate. (© *South Bay Hand Surgery, LLC; 2007. Used by permission.*)

fixed-angle blade plate, the fixator pin angle is freely adjustable so that it can be adapted to the fracture site plane, which may diminish fracture malalignment.

Indications

Nonbridging external fixation is ideally suited for the treatment of two-part and three-part intra-articular fractures of the distal radius, provided that there is good bone density and a stable distal radioulnar joint. Its use after an arthroscopic-aided reduction and K-wire fixation of an intra-articular fracture permits early protected wrist motion, although bridging fixation is warranted in the presence of marked articular comminution.

Contraindications

Volar and dorsal marginal fractures (Barton's and reverse Barton's) are excluded and should be treated with internal fixation. Fractures with extensive metaphyseal and diaphyseal comminution require supplemental internal fixation.

Surgical Technique Using the Fragment Specific Fixator

Radial Styloid Reduction With the aid of a traction tower, the radial styloid fragment is reduced with ligamentotaxis under fluoroscopic control. Any excessive supination or radial translation of the distal fragment is corrected before pin insertion. The styloid may be held with a provisional 0.062″ K-wire. An oblique 3-mm pin is hand drilled at approximately a 45-degree angle from the tip of the radial styloid across the fracture site to engage the ulnar cortex of the proximal fragment. The pin is fastened to a single pin clamp attached to the distal fixator arm. A more proximal pin clamp is used as a drill guide for insertion of a horizontal styloid pin to fixate and provide subchondral support for the lunate fragment. The K-wire can be removed or left in place for added support as necessary. Next, two proximal pins are inserted in the mid radius using the double-pin clamp as a drill guide.

Reduction of Dorsal Tilt The dorsal tilt can be corrected by using a Freer elevator inserted percutaneously in the fracture site after the radial styloid reduction. Alternatively, the tilt can be corrected as described for the extra-articular fractures. In this case, the radial styloid is reduced secondarily. Two dorsal 3-mm pins are inserted in the distal fragment through separate longitudinal incisions as described for the extra-articular fractures. The first 3-mm pin is inserted through Lister's tubercle parallel to the joint surface in the lateral plane until it engages the volar cortex. The dorsal sidearm is positioned parallel to the joint space. A single-pin clamp attached to the dorsal sidearm is fastened to this pin, then both are locked in place. After the two proximal pins are inserted in the mid radius, the distractor unit is used to lengthen the fixator until the volar tilt of the articular surface has been restored. An additional dorsal pin is inserted on the ulnar side of the EPL or extensor digitorum communis tendons using the second single-pin clamp on the outrigger bar as a drill guide. The radial styloid pins are inserted as described earlier (**Fig. 8-12**).

Protected wrist motion is allowed after the first week. If there is difficulty regaining supination, the patient is held in a long arm splint in supination in between wrist motion exercises. The fixator is typically removed in the office at 6 weeks.

Caveats

Nonbridging external fixation of intra-articular distal radius fractures should be reserved for manually active patients with good bone quality without evidence of prior wrist arthritis. The lunate fragment must be sufficiently large to support two 3-mm pins. A CT scan with anteroposterior, lateral, and coronal views is helpful to assess the fracture line patterns to aid pin insertion (**Fig. 8-13**).

Complications

Immediate complications consist of injury to branches of the SRN or dorsal cutaneous branches of the ulnar nerve. Loss of fixation because of poor pin placement or interference with extensor tendon gliding can be minimized by careful technique and open rather than percutaneous pin insertion. The use of many standard external fixator frames applied in a nonbridging manner

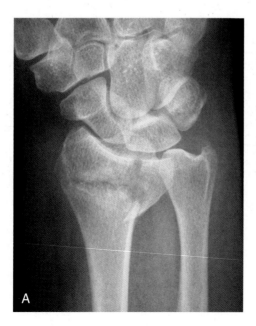
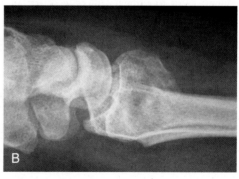

FIGURE 8-12 A, Displaced three-part distal radius fracture. **B,** Dorsal tilt of the joint surface.

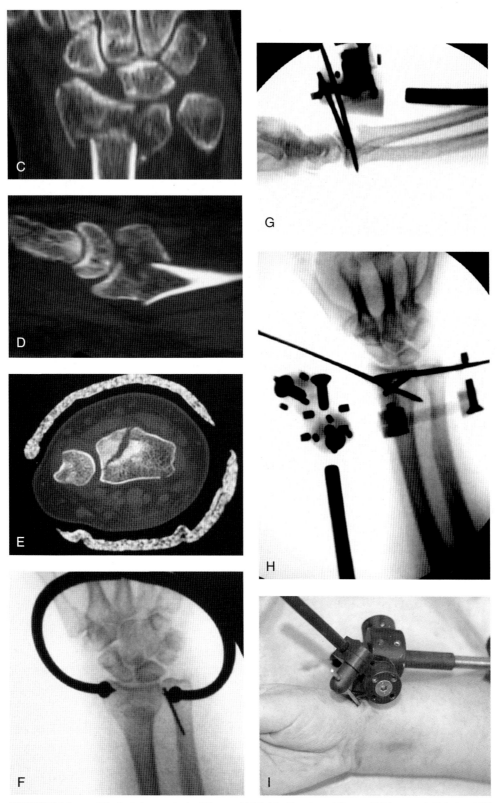

FIGURE 8-12, cont'd   C, Anteroposterior CT scan highlights the size of the medial fragment. **D,** Lateral CT scan shows the sagittal split of the medial fragment. **E,** Coronal CT scan shows disruption of the sigmoid notch. **F,** Reduction of coronal split with percutaneous bone forceps. **G,** Reduction of dorsal tilt and application of nonbridging fixator. **H,** Insertion of an oblique radial styloid pin. **I,** Palmar view of the radial styloid pin, which does not interfere with thumb motion. *(© South Bay Hand Surgery, LLC; 2007. Used by permission.)*

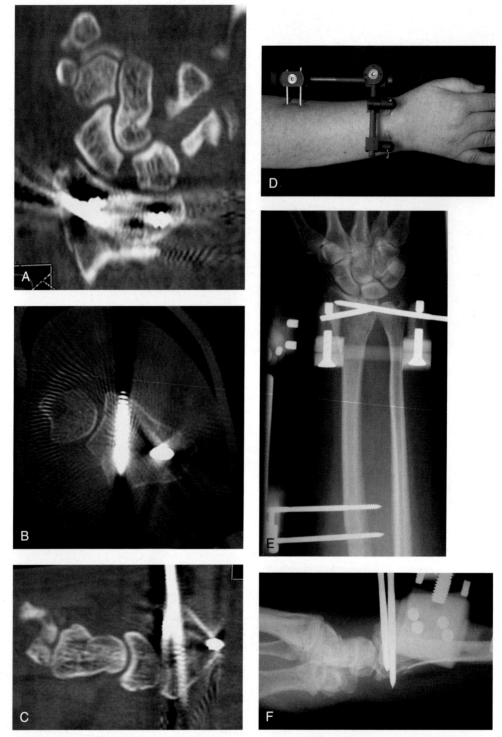

FIGURE 8-13 A, Anteroposterior CT scan shows the anatomical reconstruction of the joint space. **B,** Coronal CT scan shows fixation of the dorsomedial fragment with the fixator pin. **C,** Correction of dorsal tilt seen on lateral CT scan. **D,** Appearance at 4 weeks after removal of radial styloid pin. **E,** Anteroposterior view. **F,** Lateral view.

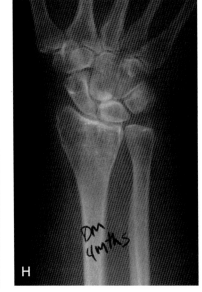
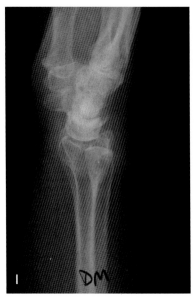

FIGURE 8-13, cont'd **G,** Wrist flexion in fixator at 4 weeks. **H,** Anteroposterior view at 4 months. **I,** Lateral view at 4 months. *(© South Bay Hand Surgery, LLC; 2007. Used by permission.)*

can result in articular incongruity. Late collapse after fixator removal can occur in osteopenic bone, which often requires subchondral support beyond the 6 weeks of fixator application. Because of the risk of late collapse, adjuvant internal fixation with locking plates is advised in elderly and osteopenic patients, as fracture site settling may occur for up to 6 months.[29]

Results

Reports of nonbridging external fixation (or radioradial external fixation) for the treatment of intra-articular fractures are sparse and mostly restricted to the European literature. Krishnan and colleagues[36] reported a clinical trial of 30 patients with Frykman type 7 and 8 fractures who were treated with the Delta frame nonbridging external fixator (Mathys Medical Ltd., Bettlach, Switzerland). Although favorable wrist motion was reported, the median intra-articular step was 2.8 mm (range 0 to 9.1 mm) with a median intra-articular gap of 1.8 mm (range 0 to 13.4 mm).[33]

Gradl and coworkers[37] examined 25 consecutive patients with fractures of the distal radius who were treated with nonbridging external fixation for 6 weeks. The stepwise surgical technique comprised a preliminary joint-bridging construction for reduction purposes, the subsequent insertion of three to four K-wires in the distal fragment, the assembling of the K-wires to a dorsal outrigger bar that was nearly parallel to the fracture line, and lastly the removal of the joint-bridging part. Clinical and radiological evaluation was performed on the first and seventh days, at 6 weeks, and 2 years after surgery. All fractures united with a palmar tilt (≥0) and articular step-off (<2 mm). A loss of radial length occurred in four patients in whom only three K-wires were inserted in the distal fragment. No radial shortening was seen in fractures with four K-wires inserted in the distal fragment. The functional results at 2 years after surgery showed an average extension of 55 degrees and flexion of 64 degrees without significant differences between extra-articular and intra-articular fractures. There were no instances of extensor tendinitis or pin

loosening in the distal fragment; however, there were three cases of proximal pin tract infections.[37]

Arthroscopic-Assisted Reduction and Nonbridging External Fixation

Indications

A typical indication for surgical treatment is more than 2 mm of articular displacement or gap. Isolated radial styloid fractures and simple three-part fractures are most suited to this technique. Four-part fractures should be tackled only after one has gained experience with simpler fracture patterns. After reduction and percutaneous pin fixation, many authors use a bridging external fixator as a neutralization device or apply a volar locking plate. In many instances, I prefer to use the Fragment Specific Fixator in a nonbridging application to allow early wrist motion.

Contraindications

Large capsular tears that carry the risk of marked fluid extravasation, active infection, neurovascular compromise, and distorted anatomy are some typical contraindications. Marked metaphyseal comminution, shear fractures, and volar rim fractures require open treatment, although the arthroscope can be inserted to check the adequacy of the joint reduction.

Surgical Technique

Web Video

8-5

Intraoperative fluoroscopy is used frequently throughout the case, with the C-arm positioned horizontal to the floor. It is preferable to wait 3 to 10 days to allow the initial intra-articular bleeding to stop. I have found it useful to perform much of the procedure without fluid irrigation using the dry technique of del Pinal and colleagues,[38] which eliminates the worry of fluid extravasation. If fluid irrigation is used, inflow is through a large-bore cannula in the 4U, 5U, or 6U portal with the outflow through the arthroscope cannula. The working portals include the volar radial (VR) and 6R portal for fracture visualization and the 3/4 portal for instrumentation, but all of the portals are used interchangeably.

Lactated Ringer's solution is preferred over saline solution, and the forearm is wrapped with Coban to limit extravasation.

The fracture hematoma and debris are lavaged, and any early granulation tissue is débrided with a resector. Mehta and colleagues[39] described a five-level algorithm for reducing the fracture fragments. This algorithm included the "London technique" for comminuted intra-articular fractures in which the K-wires were advanced through the distal ulna into the subchondral distal

radius and withdrawn from the radial aspect so that they did not encroach on the distal radioulnar joint (Fig. 8-14).

The radial styloid is reduced through ligamentotaxis while the arm is suspended in the traction tower. A Freer elevator also may be placed in the fracture site under fluoroscopic control to facilitate this step. A 1-cm incision is made over the styloid to prevent injury to the SRN, and two 0.62-inch K-wires are inserted for manipulation of the styloid fragment. The fracture site is best

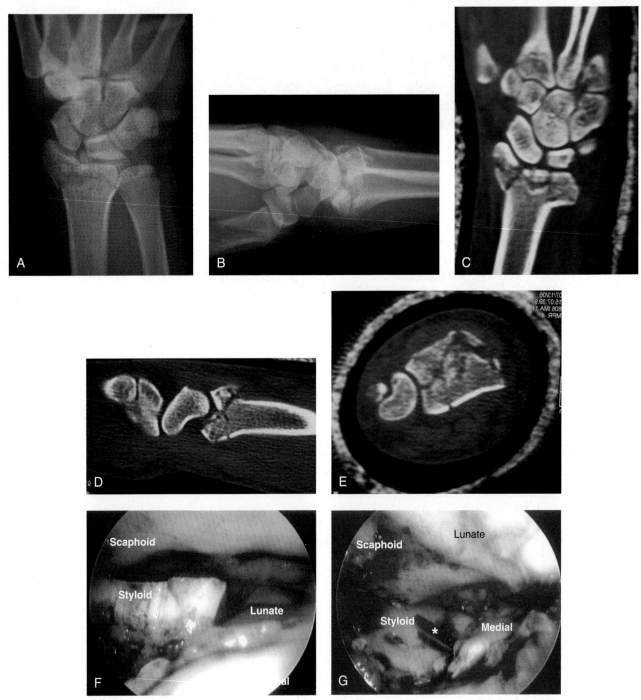

FIGURE 8-14 Arthroscopic-Guided Pinning and Nonbridging External Fixation. A, Comminuted intra-articular distal radius fracture. B, Lateral view. C, Anteroposterior CT scan reveals the extent of the intra-articular fragmentation. D, Lateral CT scan highlights the small dorsal rim fragments. E, Coronal CT scan shows the sigmoid notch disruption. F, Arthroscopic view of joint surface shows the degree of comminution. G, A percutaneous styloid is inserted through the ulna to capture and control the medial fragment.

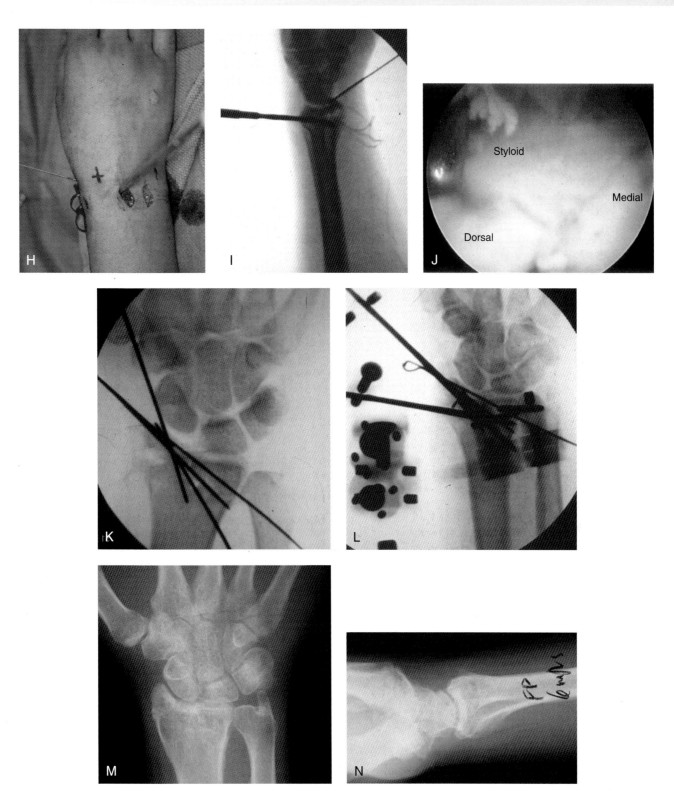

FIGURE 8-14, cont'd   H, Percutaneous reduction of dorsal tilt. **I,** Fluoroscopic appearance. **J,** Arthroscopic view after reduction and pinning. **K,** Fluoroscopic view after arthroscopic reduction. **L,** Application of nonbridging external fixator. **M,** Result at 6 months with restored radial height and tilt. **N,** Congruent joint space with neutral lateral tilt. *(© South Bay Hand Surgery, LLC; 2007. Used by permission.)*

assessed by viewing across the wrist with the scope in the 6R portal, to gauge the rotation of the styloid. The K-wires are used as joysticks to manipulate the fragment, then one K-wire is driven forward to capture the reduction. The radial styloid fragment is used as a landmark to which the depressed lunate fragment is reduced. An elevator or large pin is inserted percutaneously to elevate the lunate fragment, which is held reduced with large tenaculum forceps. Forceps with large curved jaws are preferred to prevent crushing the SRN. The tips of the forceps may be placed directly against the ulna to facilitate this step.

When the fracture fragments are anatomically reduced, horizontal subchondral K-wires are inserted, stopping short of the distal radioulnar joint. It is paramount to bone graft the metaphyseal defect through a small dorsal incision to prevent late collapse. If a dorsal die punch fragment is present, it is important that the K-wires and pins are aimed dorsally to capture this fragment. In this case, use of the volar radial portal allows superior views of this dorsal fragment. Alternatively, the K-wire can be inserted retrograde through a cannula in the VR portal and brought out dorsally.

In a four-part fracture, the lunate facet is split into a volar and dorsal fragment. The volar medial fragment usually must be reduced through an open incision because wrist traction rotates this fragment and prevents reduction by closed means. The radial styloid fragment is reduced with ligamentotaxis and temporarily held with K-wires. A standard volar approach to the distal radius through the flexor carpi radialis tendon sheath is then performed. The pronator quadratus is elevated until the volar medial fragment is seen. Alternatively, a limited volar ulnar incision can be made, with radial retraction of the flexor tendons. The volar medial fragment is reduced back to the shaft and the radial styloid fragment. A 2-mm volar locking plate is provisionally applied to hold the reduction.

The reduction is checked through the 6R and VR portals. The dorsomedial fragment is elevated back to the radial styloid and reduced to the volar medial fragment, which is used as a landmark. A small dorsal locking plate can be applied at this point, or

alternatively the distal screws of the volar plate can be used to lag the volar medial and dorsomedial fragments. In this event, one or more of the distal screws should be placed in a nonlocking fashion to help compress the fragments.

Ulnar Styloid Fractures and Distal Radioulnar Joint Instability

Ulnar styloid fractures may or may not be associated with disruption of the deep foveal insertion of the triangular fibrocartilaginous complex and secondary distal radioulnar joint instability. The deep fibers of the distal radioulnar joint can be directly assessed through a volar distal radioulnar joint portal.[40] If there is a disruption of the deep fibers of the triangular fibrocartilaginous complex, an open foveal repair can be done.[41] If the triangular fibrocartilaginous complex remains well attached to the ulnar styloid fragment, ORIF of the styloid using K-wires and tension band fixation and cannulated screws as bone anchors is performed.

Combined Fixation

Combined fixation can be performed with the fixator applied in either a bridging or a nonbridging mode. In many instances, the Fragment Specific Fixator is applied in a radial uniplanar configuration in conjunction with a combination of a volar or a dorsal plate or both (**Fig. 8-15**). In these instances, the fixator acts as a "third plate," which replaces the radial styloid plate. Alternatively, the fixator can be combined with two volar plates when there is marked periarticular dorsal comminution (**Fig. 8-16**). The fixator can be applied in a bridging fashion with dorsal outrigger support (**Fig. 8-17**). It also can be applied in a nonbridging fashion after plate fixation (**Fig. 8-18**).

Indications

Despite the plethora of volar plate designs, fixation of a small radial styloid fragment is often tenuous. The Fragment Specific Fixator can be applied in a uniplanar radial application when there is a small radial styloid fragment that cannot be adequately

Text continued on p. 95

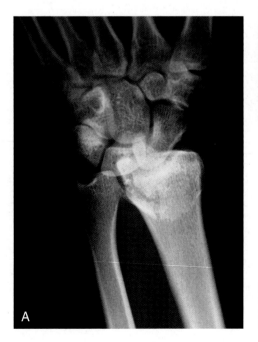

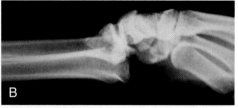

FIGURE 8-15 **A 3-Year-Old Boy with Displaced Intraarticular Fracture. A,** Anteroposterior view shows marked radial shortening. **B,** Lateral view shows a small distal fragment and marked dorsal tilt.

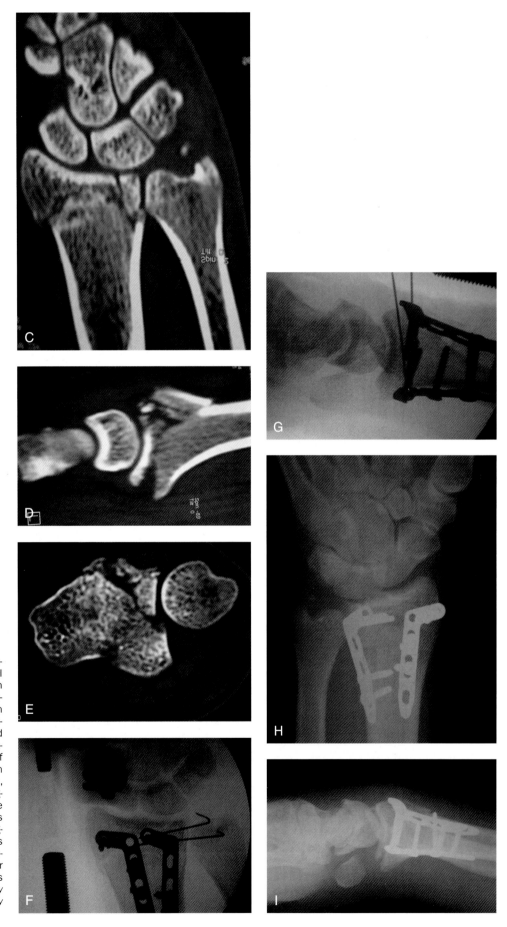

FIGURE 8-15, cont'd C, Anteroposterior CT scan reveals the small medial fragment. D, Lateral CT scan highlights the thin volar medial articular fragment. E, Coronal CT scan reveals a small, comminuted dorsomedial wall fragment with sigmoid notch disruption. F, Intraoperative x-ray shows anatomical restoration of the joint surface, but nonrigid pin fixation of the dorsal wall fragments, which necessitates temporary bridging external fixation to unload the joint space. G, Lateral view shows sandwiching of the fracture fragments with volar and dorsal plates with restored volar tilt. H, Posteroanterior view at 4 weeks after fixator removal. I, Lateral view at 4 weeks after fixator removal. (© South Bay Hand Surgery, LLC; 2007. Used by permission.)

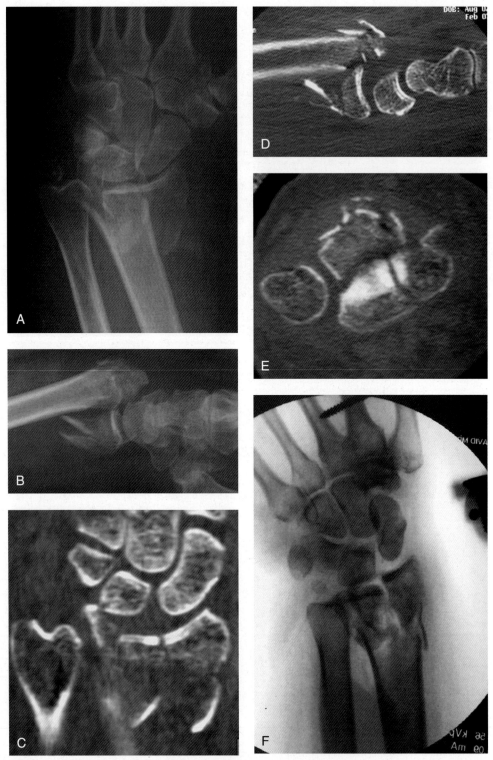

FIGURE 8-16 Volar Shear Fracture with Dorsal Comminution. A, Intra-articular fracture with marked radial shortening. **B,** Lateral x-ray shows a volar shear pattern with dorsal comminution. **C,** Anteroposterior CT scan reveals an undisplaced sagittal split of the volar articular fragment. **D,** Lateral CT scan highlights the marked periarticular dorsal comminution that precludes plate fixation. **E,** Coronal CT scan shows sigmoid notch disruption. **F,** Initial joint bridging external fixation clarifies the fracture anatomy.

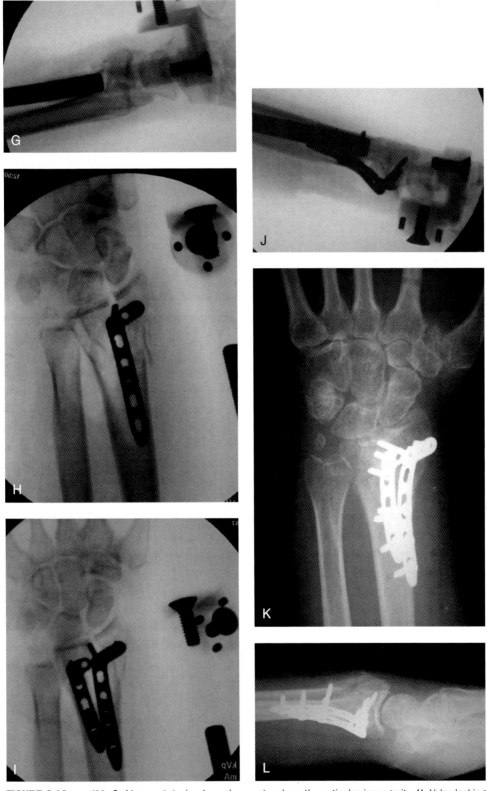

FIGURE 8-16, cont'd **G**, Ligamentotaxis alone does not reduce the articular incongruity. **H**, Volar locking plate applied to the radial column. **I**, Second volar plate applied to the intermediate column. **J**, Articular congruity is restored. **K**, Anteroposterior view at 8 weeks. **L**, Lateral view at 8 weeks. (© *South Bay Hand Surgery, LLC; 2007. Used by permission.*)

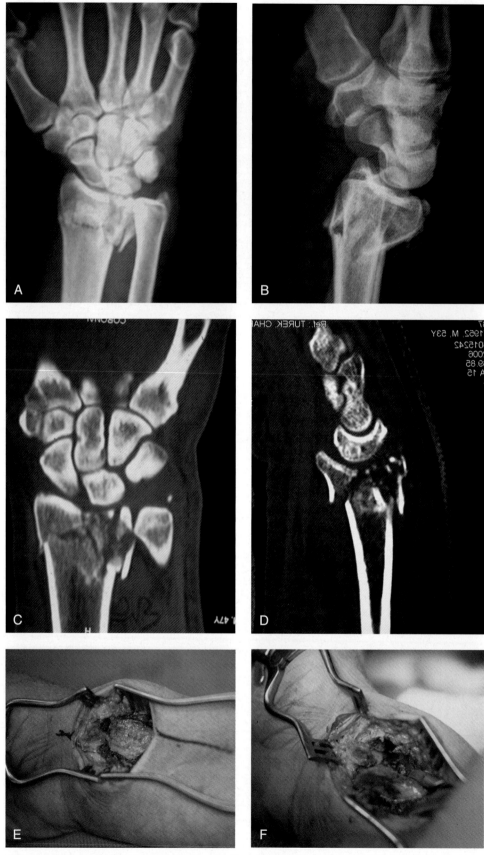

FIGURE 8-17 Joint Bridging External Fixation with Dorsal Outrigger. A, Comminuted intra-articular fracture. **B,** Marked dorsal tilt. **C,** Fragmentation of medial fragments. **D,** Sagittal split with periarticular dorsal comminution. **E,** Volar approach highlights the cortical comminution. **F,** Lunate is visible through the sagittal split.

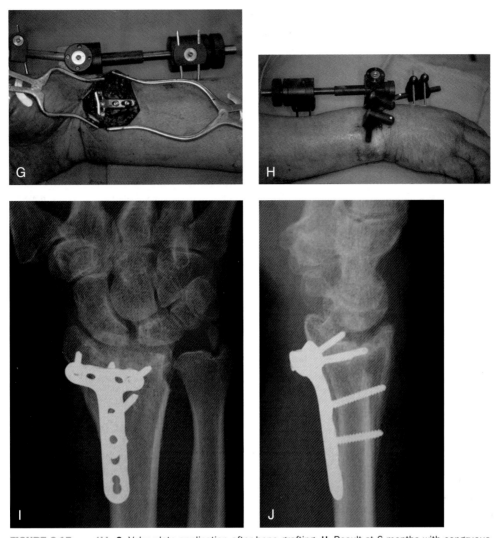

FIGURE 8-17, cont'd **G,** Volar plate application after bone grafting. **H,** Result at 6 months with congruous sigmoid notch and restored radial height. **I,** Anteroposterior view. **J,** Lateral view. Reasonable joint congruity, but some residual central depression. *(© South Bay Hand Surgery, LLC; 2007. Used by permission.)*

captured with a plate. Any sagittal split of the medial fragment that cannot be successfully reduced with percutaneous or arthroscopic methods is treated with fragment-specific implants. Joint bridging fixation is indicated when there is central comminution to help unload the articular fragments.

Contraindications

Inadequate or unstable soft tissue coverage or marked swelling would preclude the use of multiple skin incisions and implants.

Surgical Technique

Various authors have reported the use of joint bridging external fixation to facilitate fracture reduction and plate application.[21,37] A joint bridging external fixator is applied in a standard fashion as described earlier. The volar medial fragment can be approached in many ways. A 3-cm volar ulnar incision is made along the ulnar border of the flexor tendons, which are retracted radially. The interposed tendons protect the median nerve, and working through the floor of the flexor tendons gains more distance from the ulnar neurovascular bundle. The pronator quadratus is identi-

fied and elevated from its ulnar insertion and then reflected radially. Some authors use an extended carpal tunnel approach, which simplifies exposure of the volar ulnar fragment. I prefer to use the standard flexor carpi radialis approach, and then use a broad periosteal elevator to retract the flexor tendons and expose the volar ulnar corner. Alternatively, the flexor carpi radialis approach can be combined with a volar ulnar approach through the same skin incision.

My preferred technique is first to reduce the volar medial fragment to the radial shaft and to the reduced radial styloid fragment. A unicortical locking pin is placed through the distal limb of an L-shaped 2-mm plate to engage the volar ulnar fragment; this allows one to control and reduce the fragment. The traction is released, and the proximal aspect of the plate is fixed to the radial shaft. The wrist is distracted again, and a dorsal approach through the third extensor compartment is performed. The EPL tendon is removed from its compartment and retracted. The fourth extensor compartment is elevated without disrupting the extensor tendons to gain access to the dorsomedial fragment. The dorsal cortex is typically quite comminuted and

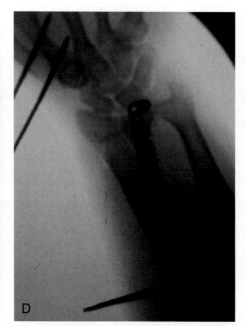

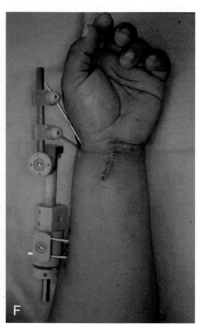

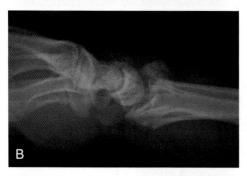

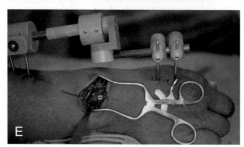

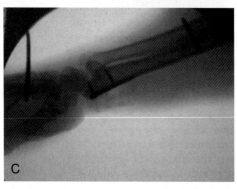

FIGURE 8-18 Volar Plating with Nonbridging External Fixation. A, Intra-articular fracture with metaphyseal extension. **B,** Depression and dorsal tilt of articular fragments. **C,** Fixation of palmar medial fragment; note distal screw does not engage the dorsal fragment yet. **D,** Restoration of sigmoid notch. **E,** Distraction with temporary joint bridging external fixation facilitates reduction of dorsal fragments. **F,** Fixator is applied in a nonbridging configuration.

often can be opened like a book to expose the articular surface. Any tilted or depressed articular fragments are elevated and supported by subchondral structural bone graft. The dorsal cortex is folded back down and held in place with a dorsal 2-mm locking plate. It is not always possible to place more than one distal screw because of the small size of the fragments. Additional bicortical locking screws can now be applied, however, through the more proximal holes to "sandwich" the volar and dorsal medial fragments.

The traction is released before attaching the plate to the proximal shaft. When using a standard joint bridging fixator, the radial column can be held with K-wires or a cannulated screw. Unless there is marked articular comminution, I insert the two radial styloid pins and apply the Fragment Specific Fixator in a nonbridging manner to allow early protected motion.

Complications

The complications are similar to those described earlier. There is a greater risk of hardware interference with tendon gliding and cutaneous nerve branches as the number of plates increases. The volar and dorsal exposure also may devascularize small fragments; this can lead to delayed healing or late collapse, which is the rationale for the use of locking plates rather than conventional mini-plates. In elderly patients with osteopenic bone, some fracture site settling cannot be avoided even after bone grafting, external fixation, and locking plates (**Fig. 8-19**).

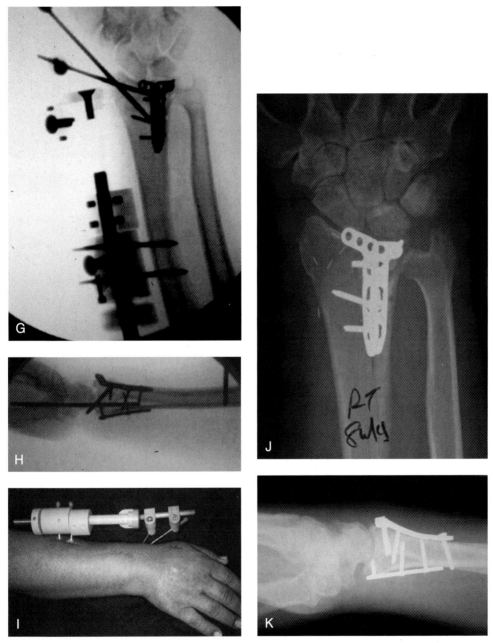

FIGURE 8-18, cont'd G, Anteroposterior view shows restoration of radial height and tilt. H, Lateral view shows reconstitution of joint surface "sandwiched" between volar and dorsal plates. I, Clinical appearance at 4 weeks. J, Anteroposterior view at 8 weeks. K, Maintenance of congruent joint after fixator removal. (© South Bay Hand Surgery, LLC; 2007. Used by permission.)

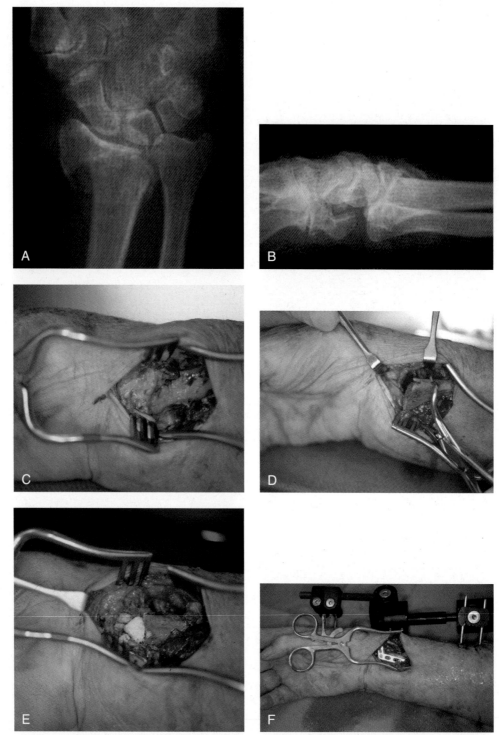

FIGURE 8-19 An 80-Year-Old Woman with Fragile Skin. A, Anteroposterior view of an unstable periarticular fracture with marked radial shortening. **B,** Lateral view highlights dorsal comminution and dorsal tilt. **C,** Volar approach to the fracture site. **D,** Pronation of the proximal radial shaft exposes the fracture. **E,** Allograft is packed into the metaphyseal defect. **F,** Neutralization plate is applied.

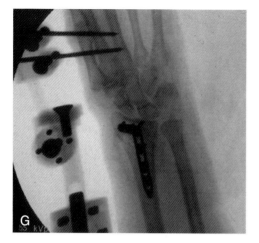

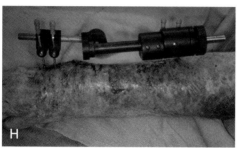

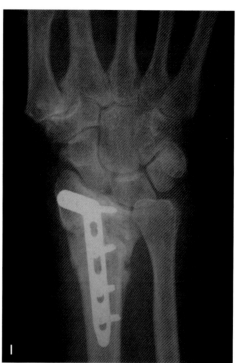

FIGURE 8-19, cont'd **G,** External fixation restores 1-mm ulnar variance. **H,** Note the fragile skin envelope, which precludes a large dorsal dissection. **I,** Result at 3 months. Note the late settling at the fracture site despite external fixation, plating, and bone grafting, resulting in a 3-mm ulnar-positive variance, but preserved radial tilt. *(© South Bay Hand Surgery, LLC; 2007. Used by permission.)*

Summary

Although currently not popular, ligamentotaxis still has its uses, especially in situations that would preclude internal plate fixation. Novel fixator designs are opening new horizons, but multicenter clinical trials are necessary to determine whether the superior results obtained with nonbridging fixation of extra-articular fractures can be duplicated with intra-articular fractures. The combination of external fixation with limited internal fixation is a useful adjunctive technique with multifragmented fractures. Gaining an understanding of the principles and limitations of external fixation allows one to be flexible and adapt the fixation to the specific fracture pattern to maximize the chances for an acceptable outcome.

REFERENCES

1. Feipel V, Rinnen D, Rooze M: Postero-anterior radiography of the wrist: normal database of carpal measurements. Surg Radiol Anat 1998; 20:221-226.

2. Gausepohl T, Worner S, Pennig D, et al: Extraarticular external fixation in distal radius fractures pin placement in osteoporotic bone. Injury 2001; 32(Suppl 4):SD79-SD85.

3. Mackinnon SE, Dellon AL: The overlap pattern of the lateral antebrachial cutaneous nerve and the superficial branch of the radial nerve. J Hand Surg [Am] 1985; 10:522-526.

4. Emami A, Mjoberg B: A safer pin position for external fixation of distal radial fractures. Injury 2000; 31:749-750.

5. Woo SL, Gomez MA, Akeson WH: The time and history-dependent viscoelastic properties of the canine medial collateral ligament. J Biomech Eng 1981; 103:293-298.

6. Winemaker MJ, Chinchalkar S, Richards RS, et al: Load relaxation and forces with activity in Hoffman external fixators: a clinical study in patients with Colles' fractures. J Hand Surg [Am] 1998; 23:926-932.

7. Sun JS, Chang CH, Wu CC, et al: Extra-articular deformity in distal radial fractures treated by external fixation. Can J Surg 2001; 44:289-294.

8. Bartosh RA, Saldana MJ: Intraarticular fractures of the distal radius: a cadaveric study to determine if ligamentotaxis restores radiopalmar tilt. J Hand Surg [Am] 1990; 15:18-21.

9. Agee JM: Distal radius fractures: multiplanar ligamentotaxis. Hand Clin 1993; 9:577-585.

10. Sanders RA, Keppel FL, Waldrop JI: External fixation of distal radial fractures: results and complications. J Hand Surg [Am] 1991; 16:385-391.

11. Juan JA, Prat J, Vera P, et al: Biomechanical consequences of callus development in Hoffmann, Wagner, Orthofix and Ilizarov external fixators. J Biomech 1992; 25:995-1006.

12. Rikli DA, Honigmann P, Babst R, et al: Intra-articular pressure measurement in the radioulnocarpal joint using a novel sensor: in vitro and in vivo results. J Hand Surg [Am] 2007; 32:67-75.

13. Wolfe SW, Austin G, Lorenze M, et al: A biomechanical comparison of different wrist external fixators with and

without K-wire augmentation. J Hand Surg [Am] 1999; 24:516-524.

14. Seitz WH Jr, Froimson AI, Leb R, et al: Augmented external fixation of unstable distal radius fractures. J Hand Surg [Am] 1991; 16:1010-1016.

15. Werber KD, Raeder F, Brauer RB, et al: External fixation of distal radial fractures: four compared with five pins: a randomized prospective study. J Bone Joint Surg Am 2003; 85:660-666.

16. Markiewitz AD, Gellman H: Five-pin external fixation and early range of motion for distal radius fractures. Orthop Clin North Am 2001; 32:329-335, ix.

17. Braun RM, Gellman H: Dorsal pin placement and external fixation for correction of dorsal tilt in fractures of the distal radius. J Hand Surg [Am] 1994; 19:653-655.

18. Dunning CE, Lindsay CS, Bicknell RT, et al: Supplemental pinning improves the stability of external fixation in distal radius fractures during simulated finger and forearm motion. J Hand Surg [Am] 1999; 24:992-1000.

19. Wolfe SW, Swigart CR, Grauer J, et al: Augmented external fixation of distal radius fractures: a biomechanical analysis. J Hand Surg [Am] 1998; 23:127-134.

20. Bindra RR: Biomechanics and biology of external fixation of distal radius fractures. Hand Clin 2005; 21:363-373.

21. Rikli DA, Businger A, Babst R: Dorsal double-plate fixation of the distal radius. Oper Orthop Traumatol 2005; 17:624-640.

22. Papadonikolakis A, Shen J, Garrett JP, et al: The effect of increasing distraction on digital motion after external fixation of the wrist. J Hand Surg [Am] 2005; 30:773-779.

23. Kaempffe FA, Wheeler DR, Peimer CA, et al: Severe fractures of the distal radius: effect of amount and duration of external fixator distraction on outcome. J Hand Surg [Am] 1993; 18:33-41.

24. Baechler MF, Means KR Jr, Parks BG, et al: Carpal canal pressure of the distracted wrist. J Hand Surg [Am] 2004; 29:858-864.

25. Margaliot Z, Haase SC, Kotsis SV, et al: A meta-analysis of outcomes of external fixation versus plate osteosynthesis for unstable distal radius fractures. J Hand Surg [Am] 2005; 30:1185-1199.

26. Weil WM, Trumble TE: Treatment of distal radius fractures with intrafocal (Kapandji) pinning and supplemental skeletal stabilization. Hand Clin 2005; 21:317-328.

27. Fernandez DL, Geissler WB: Treatment of displaced articular fractures of the radius. J Hand Surg [Am] 1991; 16:375-384.

28. Kreder HJ, Hanel DP, Agel J, et al: Indirect reduction and percutaneous fixation versus open reduction and internal fixation for displaced intra-articular fractures of the distal radius: a randomised, controlled trial. J Bone Joint Surg Br 2005; 87:829-836.

29. Dicpinigaitis P, Wolinsky P, Hiebert R, et al: Can external fixation maintain reduction after distal radius fractures? J Trauma 2004; 57:845-850.

30. Trumble TE, Schmitt SR, Vedder NB: Factors affecting functional outcome of displaced intra-articular distal radius fractures. J Hand Surg [Am] 1994; 19:325-340.

31. McQueen MM: Non-spanning external fixation of the distal radius. Hand Clin 2005; 21:375-380.

32. Salter RB, Simmonds DF, Malcolm BW, et al: The biological effect of continuous passive motion on the healing of full-thickness defects in articular cartilage: an experimental investigation in the rabbit. J Bone Joint Surg Am 1980; 62:1232-1251.

33. Mehta JA, Slavotinek JP, Krishnan J: Local osteopenia associated with management of intra-articular distal radial fractures by insertion of external fixation pins in the distal fragment: prospective study. J Orthop Surg (Hong Kong) 2002; 10:179-184.

34. Slutsky DJ, Dai QG: Fragment specific external fixation of distal radius fractures. Presented at the American Society for Surgery of the Hand, 58th Annual Meeting. Chicago, IL. 2003.

35. Putnam MD, Meyer NJ, Nelson EW, et al: Distal radial metaphyseal forces in an extrinsic grip model: implications for postfracture rehabilitation. J Hand Surg [Am] 2000; 25:469-475.

36. Krishnan J, Chipchase LS, Slavotinek J: Intraarticular fractures of the distal radius treated with metaphyseal external fixation: early clinical results. J Hand Surg [Br] 1998; 23:396-399.

37. Gradl G, Jupiter JB, Gierer P, et al: Fractures of the distal radius treated with a nonbridging external fixation technique using multiplanar K-wires. J Hand Surg [Am] 2005; 30:960-968.

38. del Pinal F, Garcia-Bernal FJ, Pisani D, et al: Dry arthroscopy of the wrist: surgical technique. J Hand Surg [Am] 2007; 32:119-123.

39. Mehta JA, Bain GI, Heptinstall RJ: Anatomical reduction of intra-articular fractures of the distal radius: an arthroscopically-assisted approach. J Bone Joint Surg Br 2000; 82:79-86.

40. Slutsky D: DRUJ arthroscopy and the volar ulnar portal. Tech Hand Up Extrem Surg 2007; 11:1-7.

41. Atzei AL, Carità E, Papini Zorli I, et al: Arthroscopically assisted foveal reinsertion of peripheral avulsions of the TFCC. J Hand Surg [Br] 2005; 30:40.

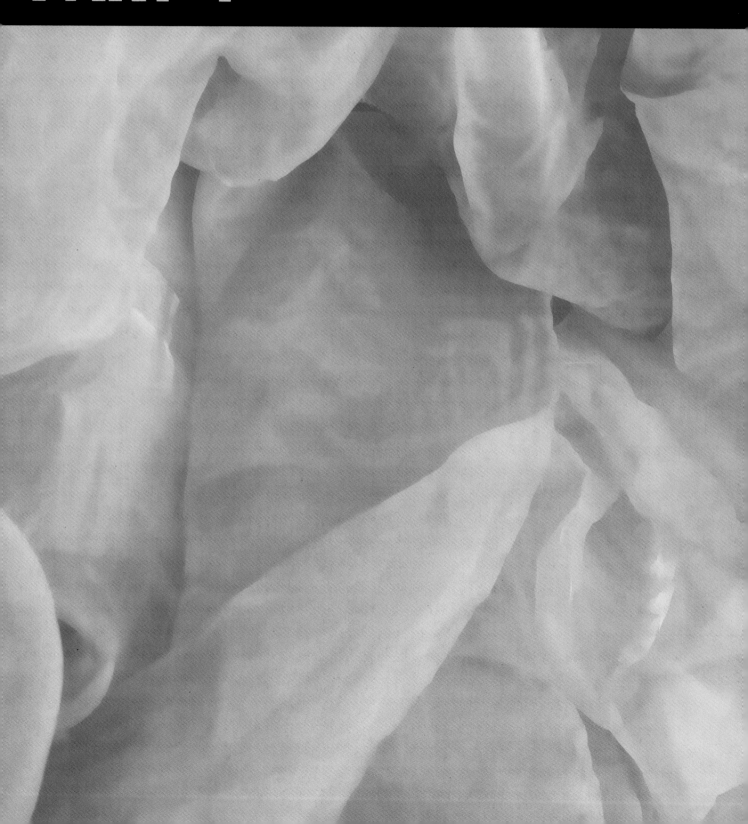

PART 4 PLATE FIXATION

Surgical Approaches from an Angiosomal Perspective

9

Michael K. Matthew, MD and Michael R. Hausman, MD

The concept of the angiosome was initially described in the cutaneous blood supply,[1] but has subsequently been shown to pertain to the underlying viscera and skeleton.[2] Devascularization of these deeper structures is less obvious than skin necrosis, but is known to occur, resulting in problems such as nonunion of fractures and avascular necrosis of bones. We seek to organize such information, using the angiosome concept, to present a cogent, comprehensible surgical approach to the three-dimensional vascular anatomy of the forearm and wrist.

Functional Microvascular Anatomy

The distal forearm, including the radius, ulna, carpal bones, and overlying soft tissues, is supplied by a network of longitudinal vessels: the radial artery, ulnar artery, anterior interosseous artery (AIA), and posterior interosseous artery (PIA). They are interconnected by dorsal and volar transverse arches (**Figs. 9-1** and **9-2**). The overlying skin is supplied by direct or septocutaneous perforators arising from these longitudinal vessels (**Fig. 9-3**), which are small arteries and veins that course along the fibrous septa that separate the muscles in the forearm.

Most of the distal radius and proximal carpal row are supplied via the radial and anterior interosseous arteries, which have a rich collateral circulation. The single exception is the pisiform, which is supplied by the ulnar artery. In contrast, the ulna is primarily supplied by the posterior interosseous and ulnar arteries. The distal carpal row is supplied from the dorsal intercarpal arch and deep palmar arch and has contributions from the radial, ulnar, and anterior interosseous arteries. The skin of the distal forearm is supplied on the radial/palmar side by the radial artery; on the ulnar/palmar side by the ulnar artery; and dorsally by the AIA, PIA, and dorsal ulnar artery. These skin territories overlap significantly secondary to the connections afforded by the subdermal and subfascial plexus.

An angiosome is a section of tissue that can remain viable based on a single feeding vessel. These angiosomes do not have absolute boundaries, or necrosis from skin incisions would be very common. There is some "built-in" redundancy from the fact that each angiosome connects with the adjacent one via small arteriole branches termed "choke vessels."[1] These vessels respond to ischemic insults within an adjacent angiosome by increasing their diameter to increase blood flow to provide adequate, collateral circulation to the adjacent, compromised angiosome.[3] This phenomenon explains the physiology behind the delay procedure commonly used to extend the margins of a flap to be transposed. This process takes 3 days in animal models. In most human clinical applications, the flaps are delayed 1 to 2 weeks before flap transposition. One angiosome may be expanded to include an adjacent angiosome, but it may not cover a more distant angiosome. Adjacent angiosomes tend to interconnect within tissue

rather than between intercompartmental fascia separations as might seem intuitive.[2] In a traumatic incident or in a surgical dissection if a specific angiosome is rendered ischemic along with its neighboring angiosomes, that angiosome becomes devitalized, predisposing to nonunion or infection.

Radial Artery Angiosome

The radial artery (**Fig. 9-4**) directly supplies bone (radius, scaphoid, and trapezium), muscle (pronator teres, extensor carpi radialis longus and brevis, brachioradialis, flexor carpi radialis [FCR], flexor digitorum sublimus [FDS], and flexor pollicis longus), and overlying volar radial skin of the forearm, including the mobile extensor wad (see Fig. 9-9).[2] The radial forearm flap based on this angiosome has been used as a pedicled septocutaneous flap for coverage of the antecubital fossa; as a pedicled reverse flow septocutaneous flap for hand coverage; and as a free flap to provide skin, muscle, and bone to distant sites.[4,5] The radial artery travels between the brachioradialis and FCR, and gives off numerous perforators along the lateral intermuscular septum that either ascend to the overlying skin or dive down to supply the underlying radius and flexor pollicis longus. The versatility of this pedicle and its associated composite flaps is well documented.[5-9]

The radial artery not only supplies the voloradial aspect of the distal radius, as might seem intuitively obvious, but also the dorsal aspect of the bone via the 1,2 supraretinacular artery (1,2 SRA), and the dorsal radiocarpal arch (DRCA). The 1,2 intercompartmental artery (ICA) originates from the radial artery approximately 5 cm proximal to the radiocarpal joint. It traverses superficial to the extensor retinaculum over the 1,2 intercompartmental septum sending branches down to the cortical and rarely cancellous bone. Sheetz and colleagues[10] described a branch from the 1,2 SRA to the second compartment floor, which penetrates into cancellous bone. This artery connects variably to the radial artery, DRCA, or dorsal intercarpal arch (DICA). The 1,2 SRA also gives off the dorsal supraretinacular arch (DSRA), which connects variably to the 2,3 supraretinacular artery (2,3 SRA), fourth intercarpal artery, fifth intercarpal artery, or ulnar artery. The DRCA, which arises from a direct branch off the radial artery, gives several small feeding vessels to the ridge of the radius at the radiocarpal joint, which descend to the cancellous bone of the metaphysis.[10]

The radial artery supplies the volar distal radius in a retrograde fashion via the palmar metaphyseal arch (PMA) and palmar radiocarpal arch (PRCA). The PMA originates from the palmar AIA within the pronator quadratus and courses through the muscle to connect with the radial artery giving off scattered perforating branches to the underlying, largely cortical bone. Sheetz and colleagues[10] pointed out that the more proximal perforating branches are more likely to penetrate into cancellous bone. This

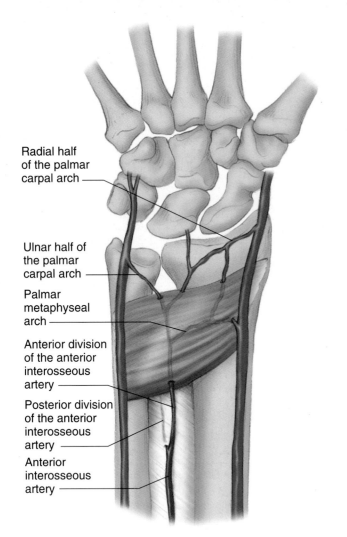

Radial half
of the palmar
carpal arch

Ulnar half of
the palmar
carpal arch

Palmar
metaphyseal
arch

Anterior division
of the anterior
interosseous
artery

Posterior division
of the anterior
interosseous
artery

Anterior
interosseous
artery

FIGURE 9-1 Palmar Vascularity. *(From Cooney WP, Linscheid RL, Dobyns JH: The Wrist: Diagnosis and Operative Treatment. St Louis: Mosby, 1998, p 108.)*

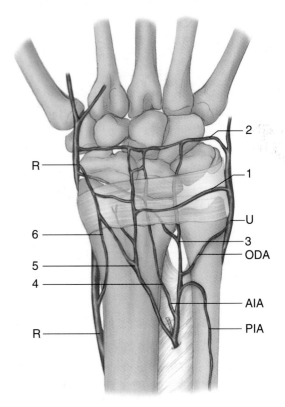

FIGURE 9-2 Dorsal Vascularity. *1,* dorsal supraretinacular arch; *2,* dorsal intercarpal arch; *3,* fifth intercompartmental artery; *4,* fourth intercompartmental artery; *5,* 2,3 intercompartmental artery; *6,* 1,2 intercompartmental artery; *U,* ulnar artery; *AIA,* anterior interosseous artery; *PIA,* posterior interosseous artery; *ODA,* oblique dorsal artery. *(From Cooney WP, Linscheid RL, Dobyns JH: The Wrist: Diagnosis and Operative Treatment. St Louis: Mosby, 1998, p 107.)*

observation was consistent for all of the penetrating vessels of the distal radius in their observations. The PMA pedicle has been used for vascularized bone grafts to the scaphoid. Some authors consider the results of this vascularized bone graft to be inconsistent, which is likely due to the variable penetrating vessels. A larger bone graft rather than a smaller one based on this pedicle is advisable to capture as many perforators as possible. Also, the more proximally the bone graft is harvested to obtain a larger arc of rotation, the more likely it is to have a perforator that penetrates into cancellous bone.

The PRCA is located just proximal to the radiocarpal joint, travels within the palmar wrist capsule, and connects with the palmar AIA and ulnar artery. The PRCA is subdivided into a radial and ulnar component by the palmar AIA forming the T-anastomosis described by Haerle and associates (see Fig. 9-1).[11] The radial PRCA gives off multiple branches to the distal radius periosteum supplying cortical and cancellous bone.[10]

The radial artery supplies the carpus from proximal to distal through (1) branches off the DRCA, (2) branches to the scaphoid tubercle and dorsal ridge, (3) a branch to the DICA, (4) a branch to the trapezium, and (5) branches off the deep palmar arch

(**Fig. 9-5**; see Figs. 9-4 and 9-14). The DRCA arises at the level of the radiocarpal joint and supplies the distal radius, lunate, and triquetrum. It continues to connect to the ulnar artery and possibly the AIA. The branches to the scaphoid arise at the level of the scaphotrapezial joint to enter the distal scaphoid. The volar scaphoid branch frequently connects to the superficial palmar arch (**Fig. 9-6**), and the dorsal branch connects to the DICA (**Fig. 9-7**). These arches serve as collateral circulation if the radial artery should become occluded proximally. The DICA originates just distal to the dorsal scaphoid branch and supplies the distal carpal row. Similar to the DRCA, the DICA traverses the wrist to connect with the AIA and ulnar arteries. The branch to the trapezium is the last branch to the carpus before continuing as the dominant vessel to the deep palmar arch. The vascular anatomy of the arches is discussed in further detail later.

Anterior Interosseous Artery Angiosome

The AIA (**Fig. 9-8**) supplies bone (central distal radius and portions of the proximal carpal row), muscles (abductor pollicis longus [APL], extensor pollicis brevis [EPB], extensor pollicis longus [EPL], pronator quadratus, and part of the flexor pollicis longus), and skin and soft tissues of the deep volar and distal dorsal forearm and hand (**Fig. 9-9**).[2] The AIA travels along the anterior surface of the interosseous membrane, then divides into a palmar and dorsal branch just before the pronator quadra-

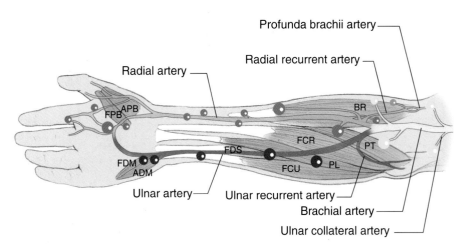

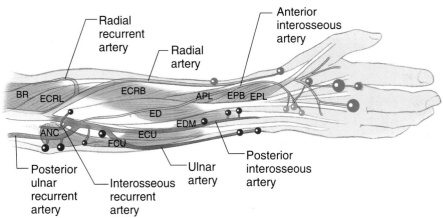

FIGURE 9-3 **Perforators of the Forearm, Wrist, and Hand.** ADM, abductor digiti minimi; ANC, anconeus muscle; APB, abductor pollicis brevis; APL, abductor pollicis longus; BR, brachioradialis; ECRB, extensor carpi radialis brevis; ECRL, extensor carpi radialis longus; ECU, extensor carpi ulnaris; ED, extensor digitorum; EDM, extensor digiti minimi; EPB, extensor pollicis brevis; EPL, extensor pollicis longus; FCR, flexor carpi radialis; FCU, flexor carpi ulnaris; FDM, flexor digiti minimi; FDS, flexor digitorum sublimus; FPB, flexor pollicis brevis; PL, palmaris longus; PT, pronator teres. *(From Inoue Y, Taylor GI: The angiosomes of the forearm: anatomic study and clinical implications. Plast Reconstr Surg 1996; 98:198.)*

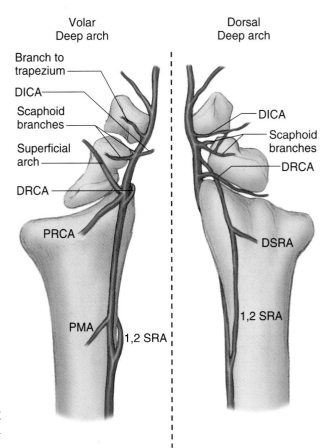

FIGURE 9-4 **Radial Artery Angiosome.** DICA, dorsal intercarpal arch; DRCA, dorsal radiocarpal arch; DSRA, dorsal supraretinacular arch; PMA, palmar metaphyseal arch; PRCA, palmar radiocarpal arch; 1,2 SRA, 1,2 supraretinacular artery.

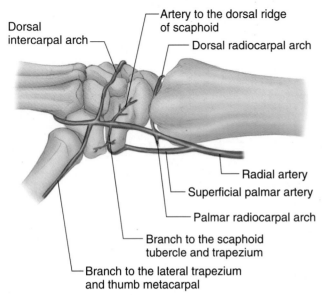

Dorsal intercarpal arch — Artery to the dorsal ridge of scaphoid — Dorsal radiocarpal arch — Radial artery — Superficial palmar artery — Palmar radiocarpal arch — Branch to the scaphoid tubercle and trapezium — Branch to the lateral trapezium and thumb metacarpal

FIGURE 9-5 **Schematic of Radial Artery Angiosome.** *(From Cooney WP, Linscheid RL, Dobyns JH: The Wrist: Diagnosis and Operative Treatment. St Louis: Mosby, 1998, p 109.)*

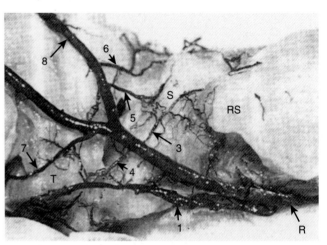

FIGURE 9-6 **Injection of Radial Artery Angiosome.** *RS,* Radial styloid; *S,* scaphoid; *T,* trapezium; *R,* radial artery; *1,* superficial palmar branch of radial artery; *3,* dorsal radiocarpal arch; *4,* branch to the tubercle of the scaphoid and trapezium; *5,* artery to dorsal ridge of scaphoid; *6,* dorsal intercarpal arch; *7,* branch of the lateral trapezium and thumb metacarpal; *8,* medial branch of radial artery (seen in 22% of the specimens) penetrating the base of the index-long web space. (Note, in this view, *2* the palmar radiocarpal arch, cannot be seen. *(From Cooney WP, Linscheid RL, Dobyns JH: The Wrist: Diagnosis and Operative Treatment. St Louis: Mosby, 1998, p 109.)*

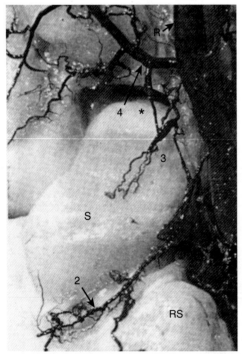

FIGURE 9-7 Injection of Scaphoid Vascularity. Close-up view of the dorsoradial aspect of the wrist, demonstrating nutrient vessels entering the dorsal ridge of the scaphoid. *RS,* Radial styloid; *S,* scaphoid; *R,* radial artery; *2,* dorsal radiocarpal arch; *3,* branch to the dorsal ridge of the scaphoid; *4,* dorsal intercarpal arch. *,* communication between DICA and dorsal branch to scaphoid. *(From Gelberman RH, Panagis JS, Taleisnik J, et al: The arterial anatomy of the human carpus, part I: the extraosseous vascularity. J Hand Surg 1983; 8A:371.)*

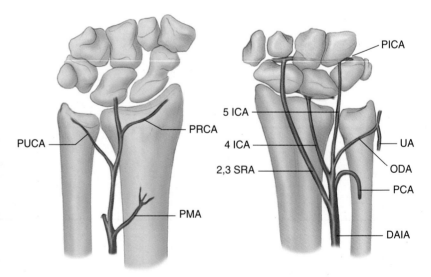

FIGURE 9-8 Anterior Interosseous Artery Angiosome. DAIA, dorsal anterior interosseous artery; 4 ICA, fourth intercompartmental artery; 5 ICA, fifth intercompartmental artery; ODA, oblique dorsal artery; PICA, palmar intercarpal arch; PMA, palmar metaphyseal arch; PRCA, palmar radiocarpal arch; PUCA, palmar ulnocarpal arch; 2,3 SRA, 2,3 supraretinacular artery; UA, ulnar artery.

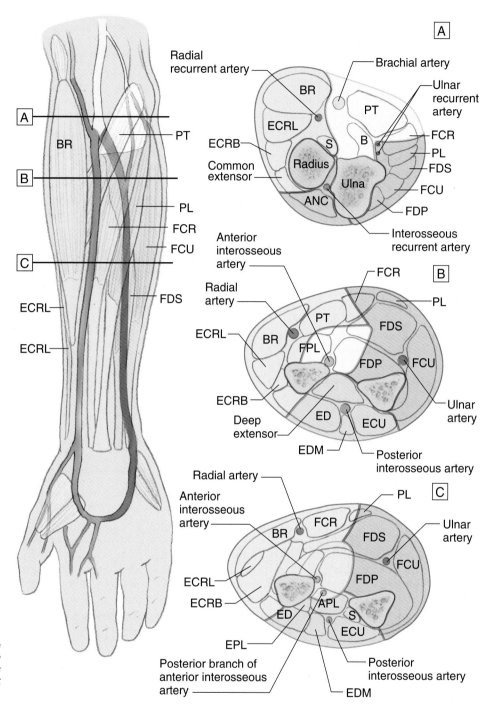

FIGURE 9-9 Angiosome of the Forearm. *(From Inoue Y, Taylor GI: The angiosomes of the forearm: anatomic study and clinical implications. Plast Reconstr Surg 1996; 98:207.)*

tus muscle. The palmar AIA gives rise to the PMA and then forms the radial PRCA and ulnar PRCA. As discussed earlier, the PRCA is subdivided into a radial and ulnar component by the palmar AIA. The radial PRCA gives off multiple branches to the distal radius, and the ulnar PRCA, originating just proximal to the radial PRCA, supplies the distal palmar ulnar head. The ulnar PRCA frequently connects to the ulnar artery or the PIA via the oblique dorsal artery to the distal ulna.

Displaced fractures of the distal radius are frequently associated with tearing and damage to the pronator quadratus; this likely damages the AIA contributions to the distal radial metaphysis and epiphysis via the PMA and PRCA. The PRCA contribu-

tions to the distal radius via flow from the adjacent radial artery angiosome become important to retain vascularity. As care is taken to avoid damage to the volar radiocarpal ligaments in the volar approach, avoiding injury to the PRCA and its connection to the radial artery also is prudent.

The dorsal branch of the AIA travels through the interosseous membrane into the posterior compartment to supply the dorsal distal radius and contributes to the dorsal arterial arches. Either the common AIA or the proximal dorsal AIA gives off a second dorsal perforating branch, which travels through the interosseous membrane and travels within a septum between the EPB and EPL that segmentally supplies the overlying skin of the distal dorsal radius. These septocutaneous branches have been used as the vascular base of a reverse flap that is able to incorporate skin, dorsal distal radius, and distal posterior interosseous nerve as a composite flap.[12,13]

The 2,3 SRA arises variably from the common AIA or dorsal branches of the AIA. It courses over the extensor retinaculum and Lister's tubercle, sending deep perforating branches that usually penetrate into cancellous bone. The 2,3 SRA then connects to the DICA. Other anastomoses between the 1,2 SRA, DRCA, and 4th ICA have been described. Similar to the 1,2 SRA, Sheetz and colleagues[10] described a branch from the 2,3 SRA to the second compartment floor.

The 4th ICA is a branch off the dorsal AIA or the 5th ICA and runs in the fourth compartment just lateral to the posterior interosseous nerve connecting with the DICA and variably the DRCA, 2,3 ICA, or 5th ICA. Along the floor of the fourth compartment, the 4th ICA gives off branches to the underlying bone that frequently enter cancellous bone.

The 5th ICA arises from the dorsal AIA and connects distally with the DICA. Sheetz and colleagues[10] found contributions to the distal radius from the 5th ICA dorsal compartment in only 39% of their specimens. In most cases, the 5th ICA does not directly supply the distal radius or carpus, but serves as a conduit between the radial artery, AIA, and ulnar artery via the DICA.

Posterior Interosseous Artery Angiosome

The PIA supplies bone (ulnar head and neck), muscles (APL, extensor digitorum communis, extensor digiti quinti, extensor carpi ulnaris, EPB, and extensor indicis proprius), and skin of the deep and proximal dorsal forearm (see Fig. 9-9).[2] Proximally in the forearm after entering the posterior compartment at the level of the distal edge of the supinator, the PIA continues on top of the APL and beneath the extensor digitorum and extensor carpi ulnaris. It then becomes more superficial in the mid forearm traveling between the extensor carpi ulnaris and extensor digiti quinti. Between the extensor carpi ulnaris and extensor digiti quinti lies a septum from which multiple cutaneous perforators arise supplying the overlying skin of the proximal and mid dorsal forearm. Pedicled flaps for elbow coverage, reverse flow pedicle flaps for distal dorsal hand coverage, and free flaps have been described using this pedicle.[14,15]

The PIA supplies the distal ulna via the oblique dorsal arteries, which arise from an arch formed by the PIA and the dorsal AIA. The oblique dorsal artery gives off branches that supply the ulnar neck and head and frequently connects to the ulnar artery. The PIA does not have any significant contribution to the radius or carpus (see Fig. 9-2).

Ulnar Artery Angiosome

The ulnar artery (**Fig. 9-10**) supplies bone (ulna, pisiform, and distal carpal row), muscle (flexor carpi ulnaris, palmaris longus, FCR, FDS, and flexor digitorum profundus), and skin of the ulnar forearm (see Fig. 9-9).[2] The ulnar artery travels on the radial side of the flexor carpi ulnaris with the ulnar nerve in the distal two thirds of the forearm. The ulnar artery gives off multiple septocutaneous branches within the medial intermuscular septum to supply the volar/ulnar skin of the entire forearm and wrist. Branches from the ulnar artery to the FDS of the ring and small finger allow for vascularized tendon transfers[16] along

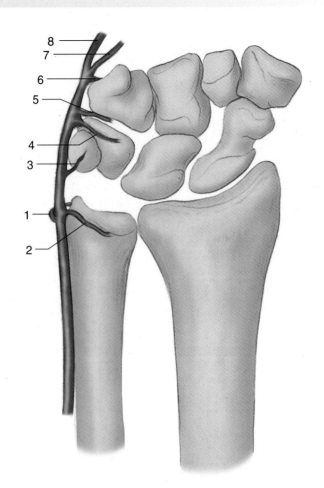

FIGURE 9-10 **Ulnar Artery Angiosome.** *1*, dorsal radiocarpal arch; *2*, palmar radiocarpal arch; *3*, branch to pisiform; *4*, palmar intercarpal arch; *5*, dorsal intercarpal arch; *6*, dorsal metacarpal arch; *7*, superficial palmar arch; *8*, deep palmar arch.

with overlying fascia and skin. The ascending branch of the dorsal ulnar artery, a branch from the ulnar artery arising 2 to 5 cm proximal to the pisiform, travels superficially and proximally to supply a large area of skin (up to 20 cm long), which may be transferred as a pedicled flap for hand soft tissue coverage.[4]

The ulnar artery gives off multiple branches to the distal ulna and carpus largely through the volar and dorsal arches. From proximal to distal, the branches are to the (1) DRCA; (2) PRCA; (3) proximal pisiform and triquetrum; (4) palmar intercarpal arch; (5) distal pisiform and medial hamate, which continues to the DICA; (6) basal metacarpal arch; and (7) superficial and deep palmar arches (**Fig. 9-11**; see Fig. 9-10). The ulnar artery directly supplies only the ulnar head, pisiform, and medial hamate.

Arches

The arches (**Fig. 9-12**) serve as bypass routes when one or more of the longitudinal vessels become disrupted and supply the central carpal bones (lunate, triquetrum, trapezoid, capitate).[17] There are five volar arches: the PMA, PRCA, palmar intercarpal arch, superficial palmar arch, and deep palmar arch. The PMA and PRCA are interconnected by the radial artery and AIA and supply the radial styloid, volar distal radius, lunate, and triquetrum. Their anatomy was detailed earlier. The palmar intercarpal arch is a diminutive vessel without significant independent contributions arising from the superficial palmar arch and connecting to the ulnar artery at the level of the proximal carpal row. The

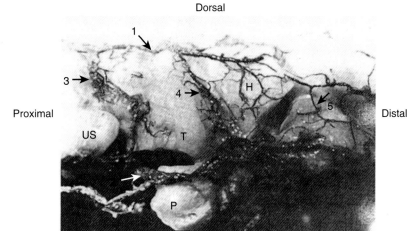

Dorsal

Proximal

Distal

FIGURE 9-11 Injection of Ulnar Artery Angiosome. *US,* Ulnar styloid; *T,* triquetrum; *P,* pisiform; *H,* hamate; *1,* dorsal branch of anterior interosseous artery; *2,* medial branch of ulnar artery; *3,* dorsal radiocarpal arch; *4,* dorsal intercarpal arch; *5,* basal metacarpal arch. *(From Gelberman RH, Panagis JS, Taleisnik J, et al: The arterial anatomy of the human carpus, part I: the extraosseous vascularity. J Hand Surg [Am] 1983; 8:372.)*

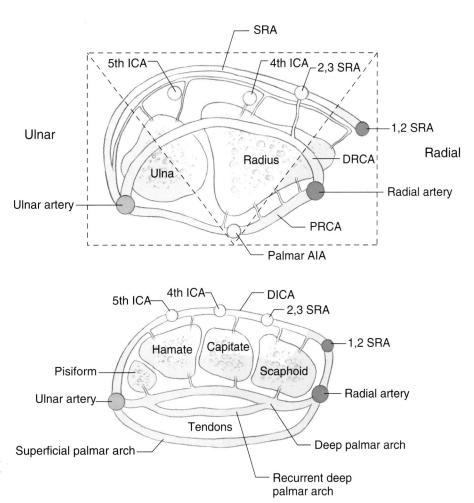

Dorsal
Anterior interosseous artery

FIGURE 9-12 Radiocarpal Arches and Anastomoses. ICA, intercarpal artery; DICA, dorsal intercarpal arch; SRA, supraretinacular artery; DRCA, dorsal radiocarpal arch; PRCA, palmar radiocarpal arch.

superficial and deep palmar arches connect the radial to the ulnar arteries. The superficial arch is the continuation of the ulnar artery and supplies the common digital branches, but it does not give any contribution to the carpal vascularity.

The deep palmar arch is the continuation of the radial artery and traverses the wrist just distal to the metacarpal bases. The deep palmar arch gives rise to the radial and ulnar recurrent branches, which combine 45% of the time[17] to form a deep recurrent arch. As a group, this deep arch arcade is the dominant supply to the palmar distal carpal row. The radial recurrent artery originates at the level of the index metacarpal and supplies the trapezium and trapezoid.[7] The ulnar recurrent branch originates between the bases of the long and ring metacarpals and continues proximally supplying the capitate and hamate, and may connect to the end of the palmar AIA.[17] The hook of the hamate is supplied via an accessory ulnar recurrent artery or from direct branches from the ulnar artery.[17]

There are four dorsal arches: the DSRA, DRCA, DICA, and dorsal metacarpal arch (**Fig. 9-13**). The supraretinacular arch connects the radial artery, 1,2 ICSRA, 2,3 ICSRA, variably the 4th ICA or 5th ICA, and the ulnar artery. It does not directly supply any underlying bone. The DRCA arises from the radial artery supplying the radius, lunate, and triquetrum, and sometimes connecting to the ulnar artery at the ulnocarpal joint. It also connects to the DICA via interconnecting branches to the lunate and triquetrum. The DICA serves as a conduit between the radial artery, ulnar artery, and dorsal AIA via the 2,3 ICSRA or 5th ICA. The DICA supplies the dorsal distal carpal row. The dorsal metacarpal arch is a series of vascular retes arising from the deep palmar arch and connecting to the DICA, providing a sagittal arch for vascularity of the distal carpal row.

The dorsal approach to the carpus divides the DSRA leaving the DRCA and the DICA as pathways of collateral flow. If the incision is carried too distally to the level of the midcarpal joint, the DICA is in jeopardy, and if the dissection is too close to the radiocarpal joint, the DRCA may be divided or its perforators stripped of the bone. The volar arches in the distal radius and proximal row mainly serve to connect the radial artery to the AIA, but they are frequently damaged in high-energy injuries. In these high-energy injuries to the distal radius or proximal carpal row, care must be taken when using the dorsal approach because this may be the only path of collateral flow.

Surgical Approaches (Box 9-1)
Dorsal Approaches

The dorsal distal radius can be approached radially between the first and second compartments, centrally between the third and fourth compartments, or ulnarly between the fifth and sixth compartments. There is little need to cross the dorsal wrist crease at

BOX 9-1 Vessels at Risk	
Dorsal radial approach	Branches to the scaphoid Distal 1,2 SRA 2,3 SRA DICA DSRA
Dorsal central approach	DSRA DRCA 2,3 SRA DICA
Dorsal ulnar approach	DSRA DRCA DICA 5th ICA
Palmar "FCR" approach	PMA PRCA Palmar AIA Superficial palmar arch
Palmar midline approach	PRCA Palmar AIA

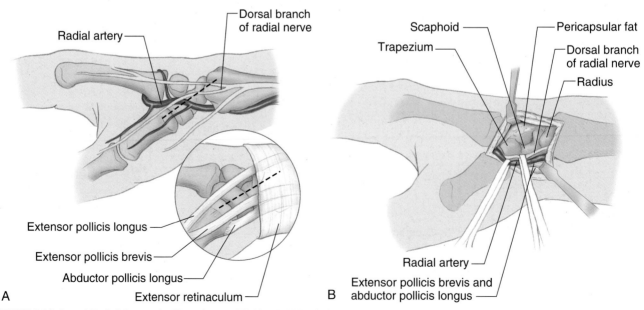

FIGURE 9-13 Dorsal Radial Approach. *(From Cooney WP, Linscheid RL, Dobyns JH: The Wrist: Diagnosis and Operative Treatment. St Louis: Mosby, 1998, p 134.)*

acute angles because extension contractures are uncommon, secondary to the stronger pull of the flexors and the mobility of the dorsal skin. The tips of triangular flaps can be prone to ischemia and wound healing complications.[18,19] When opening the extensor retinaculum, it should be incised at an oblique angle creating two peripherally based flaps that may be allowed to slide across one another making for easier closure. The decision to place a flap of retinaculum beneath the extensor tendons in cases of rheumatoid arthritis or hardware placement also should be made on opening instead of closing.

The dorsal radial approach uses a skin incision over the anatomical snuffbox extending proximally or distally depending on the underlying structures to be examined (see Fig. 9-13). Care is taken to identify and retract the radial sensory nerve, which lies just beneath the superficial vein. Perforators to the skin arise more proximally from the lateral intermuscular septum via the radial artery and from the dorsal AIA from the septum between the EPB and EPL (see Fig. 9-3). This is a common approach to the scaphoid. At the level of the scaphotrapezial joint, the volar and dorsal branches to the scaphoid, the reinsertion of the 1,2 SRA, and the origin of the DICA from the radial artery are at risk for injury (see Figs. 9-5 and 9-6). If possible, the branches to the scaphoid should be preserved by identifying and incising the capsule over the scaphocapitate joint. The dissection can be extended laterally to expose the scaphoid, protecting the dorsal ridge vessels if exposure of the entire dorsal surface of the scaphoid is required. If connections between the superficial palmar arch and the volar scaphoid branch or between the DICA and the dorsal scaphoid branch exist, it may be possible to mobilize the radial artery further without injury to the scaphoid vascular supply (see Figs. 9-6 and 9-7).

When using this approach for the radial styloid, the DRCA at the radiocarpal joint and the origin of the 1,2 ICSRA are visualized. The DRCA lies just above the radiocarpal joint capsule underneath the extensor tendons, whereas the 1,2 ICSRA originates 4 to 5 cm proximal to the joint and courses dorsally and superficial to the extensor retinaculum to supply the radial styloid. It is safe to take the origin of the 1,2 ICSRA because it receives collateral flow from the 2,3 ICSRA and the supraretinacular arch. The DRCA divided on its radial side still supplies the styloid from the dorsal AIA and ulnar artery, but any additional dorsal approaches should maintain the ulnar DRCA, 4th ICA, and DICA as pathways of collateral flow to the dorsoradial radius. When the vasculature has been identified, mobilized, and retracted palmarly, the joint capsule can be opened exposing the radius through the trapezium.

To approach the radial styloid with access to the voloradial radius, the incision can be placed over the first dorsal compartment. The first dorsal compartment then is partially released, leaving the distal end intact to avoid bowstringing. The base of the first dorsal compartment is incised, and the dissection is continued volarly releasing the brachioradialis. Only the voloulnar corner is not adequately visualized. One should take caution to maintain the vascularity of the dorsoradial radius if additional approaches are used for the voloulnar corner.

The central or standard dorsal approach to the wrist uses a linear skin incision starting at the base of the second metacarpal and extending proximally and obliquely crossing just ulnar to Lister's tubercle.[20] Alternatively, one may begin at the base of the third metacarpal and extend proximally (**Fig. 9-14**). By necessity, the supraretinacular arch is divided. The extensor retinaculum is divided obliquely just ulnar to Lister's tubercle, and the EPL is

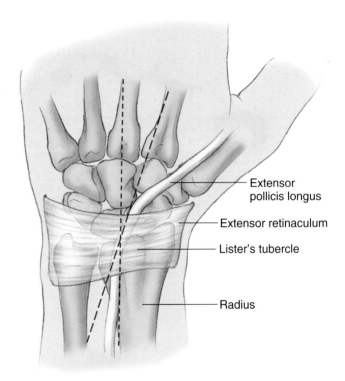

FIGURE 9-14 **Dorsal Approach.** *(From Cooney WP, Linscheid RL, Dobyns JH: The Wrist: Diagnosis and Operative Treatment. St Louis: Mosby, 1998, p 127.)*

— Extensor pollicis longus
— Extensor retinaculum
— Lister's tubercle
— Radius

released from its compartment. The subperiosteal plane is entered at the base of the third compartment, and the remaining compartments are elevated off the radius, being mindful to attempt to leave the perforators from the 1,2 ICSRA at the base of the second compartment along with the origin of the dorsal radiocarpal ligament radially, and the dorsal radioulnar ligament and dorsal AIA branches ulnarly.

If the dorsal radiocarpal joint capsule is opened, and the DRCA is divided, collateral flow is sustained by the DICA. The joint capsule can be opened many ways, including a linear, triangular flap sparing the dorsal radiocarpal and dorsal intercarpal ligaments or extending this triangular flap with a back cut along the radiocarpal joint (**Fig. 9-15**).

The ulnar dorsal approach uses a variable skin incision from the triquetral tuberosity and extending proximally down the shaft of the ulna (**Fig. 9-16**). Care is taken not to injure the ulnar sensory nerve traveling dorsally 1 to 2 cm distal to the ulnar head. The DSRA is cauterized, and the extensor retinaculum is entered between the fifth and sixth compartments. Bowers[21] uses a radially based flap of extensor retinaculum, taking care not to enter the fourth compartment and the 4th ICA. The 5th ICA is likely to need to be cauterized, but, as mentioned previously, the 5th ICA rarely nourishes the underlying radius serving as a conduit between the dorsal AIA and the DICA. At this point, the radioulnar joint capsule or the dorsal ulnar wrist capsule may be opened, exposing the distal radioulnar joint or ulnocarpal joint. The DRCA is divided in exposing the distal radioulnar joint, but the dorsal vascularity to the triangular fibrocartilage complex is kept largely intact if the 4th ICA is not entered. As the dissection is extended proximally, the oblique dorsal artery from the ulnar artery is likely to be divided, but this is of little significance to the distal vascularity.

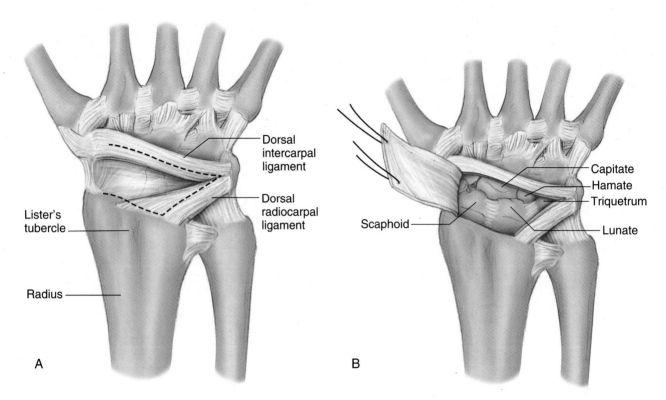

FIGURE 9-15 **Capsular Incision.** *(From Cooney WP, Linscheid RL, Dobyns JH: The Wrist: Diagnosis and Operative Treatment. St Louis: Mosby, 1998, p 130.)*

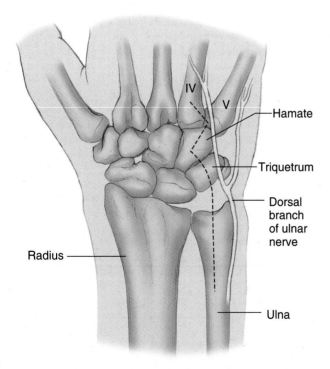

FIGURE 9-16 **Dorsal Ulnar Approach.** *(From Cooney WP, Linscheid RL, Dobyns JH: The Wrist: Diagnosis and Operative Treatment. St Louis: Mosby, 1998, p 137.)*

Palmar Approaches

The two basic palmar approaches are the FCR and midline approach. The FCR approach uses a skin incision over the FCR tendon. The dissection is carried down through the FCR sheath. The FCR may be retracted ulnarly to expose the radial border or radially to access the palmar surface of the radius. The palmar cutaneous branch of the median nerve classically lies between the FCR and the palmaris longus, but caution is prudent to avoid injury. The branches from the radial artery to the pronator quadratus are divided, and a transverse incision is made at the end of the pronator quadratus muscle proximal to the origin of the radiocarpal ligaments. The pronator quadratus is incised on its radial border leaving a small cuff to facilitate closure. The pronator quadratus can now be elevated off the distal radius in the subperiosteal plane, taking care not to cross the ulnar border of the radius and injure the palmar AIA.

As the dissection is performed near the radiocarpal joint, especially on the medial column of the radius, the volar RCA is likely to be encountered if the dissection plane is above the periosteum as the radial volar RCA arises from the palmar AIA coursing obliquely and distally toward the radial artery. The superficial arch as it arises from the radial artery also may need to be divided if the incision is carried distal in an oblique fashion toward the scaphoid tubercle across the volar wrist crease, as in Russe's approach[22] to the scaphoid. If the radiocarpal joint needs to be exposed, the floor of the FCR sheath is opened, the FCR is retracted, and the volar RCA is visualized and controlled. Caution should be exercised not to injure the volar RCA at its origin at the volar AIA and at the radial artery, or there would be a segment of devascularized distal volar radius. To expose the scaphoid fully,

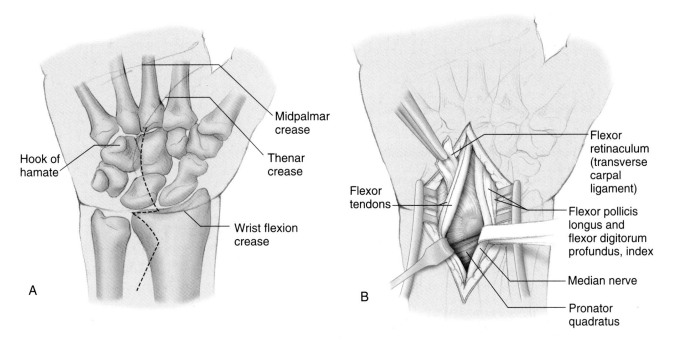

FIGURE 9-17 **Midline Palmar Approach.** *(From Cooney WP, Linscheid RL, Dobyns JH: The Wrist: Diagnosis and Operative Treatment. St Louis: Mosby, 1998, p 147.)*

the radioscaphocapitate and long radiolunate ligaments need to be incised, but care should be taken to note their location because repair is mandatory. This approach provides access to the entire volar radius, volar scaphoid, and scapholunate ligament.

The midline approach skin incision may begin in the palm as for a carpal tunnel release, or at the wrist crease just ulnar to the palmaris tendon to avoid damage to the palmar cutaneous nerve (**Fig. 9-17**). It remains on the ulnar side of the forearm until the mid forearm, at which point it may be directed radially if needed; this is to ensure adequate coverage of the median nerve in the distal forearm where it is not protected by the muscle bellies of the FDS tendons. The median nerve is identified, and the flexor retinaculum is divided from proximal to distal just radial to the hook of the hamate. The median nerve and flexor tendons are retracted, and the pronator quadratus is exposed. The pronator may be taken down from the radius and elevated ulnarly in the subperiosteal plane. Generally, this approach is used for a volar fasciotomy and complex carpal dislocations, and it likely would

be combined with a carpal tunnel release. This approach tends to spare the vasculature, but is not easily extendable to reach the radial border.

Combined Approaches

An exhaustive description of all possible approaches would be enervating to read; we focus on the principles that should guide surgical judgment. Most clinical scenarios can be planned using Figure 9-3 and **Table 9-1**, which show where the skin perforators arise, and what structures can be exposed using the described approaches.

With regard to the skin incision, one should not make two parallel incisions between skin perforators because the skin between the incisions would be ischemic. Referencing Figure 9-3 showing where the perforators arise in the distal forearm, we observe that we could make two incisions on either side of the radial artery/lateral intermuscular septum (FCR and dorsal radial approaches) because there is collateral flow on the volar side from

TABLE 9-1 Recommended Surgical Approaches According to Fracture Morphology

Approach	Fracture Type			
	Dorsal, Colles', Die Punch, Dorsoulnar	**Radial Styloid**	**Volar Plating**	**Volar-Ulnar Radius**
Central dorsal	+	–	–	–
Radial	–	+	+/–	–
Flexor carpi radialis	–*	+	+	+
Extended carpal tunnel release	–*	–	+	+
Combined dorsal/volar	+	+	+	+

*Able to reach die punch–type fracture.

the ulnar artery and on the dorsum from the AIA. Alternately, if the FCR and volar midline approaches are used, there are no perforators arising to the skin between the incisions resulting in ischemia. Undermining between incision lines above the plane of the vessels also should be limited or avoided because this would transect perforating vessels to the overlying skin bridge.

The same perforator principle is used for the radius, ulna, and carpus. The difference from the skin lies in that the blood supply to the bone is more segmental relying only on the periosteal plexus to supply immediately adjacent bone. The networks of arches with their perforators serve as vascular redundancy. The arches described earlier link the radial artery, AIA, and ulnar artery. The main arches around the carpus include the PRCA, deep palmar arch, DRCA, SRA, and DICA. As long as one arch remains intact on the volar and dorsal surfaces, the blood supply is likely to remain intact with certain exceptions. These exceptions are due to bones with a single perforating vessel or without intraosseous vascular connections between perforating vessels.

Panagis and coworkers[23] classified carpal bone vascularity into three groups based on number and location of perforating branches, presence of intraosseous vascular anastomosis, and existence of a large portion of the bone supplied by a single perforator. Group 1 included bones with perforators only on one surface, or a large portion of bone supplied by a single perforator. Group 1 included the scaphoid, in which the dorsal vessel enters at the dorsal ridge and travels proximally to supply the proximal bone without intraosseous connection to the palmar perforator; the capitate, in which in 50% of their series the head was supplied only via a palmar perforator; and some lunates, 20% of their series, which had only a single palmar perforator. Group 2 had at least two perforators at different sites, but lacked intraosseous anastomosis. This group included the trapezoid, which has dorsal and volar perforators, but no anastomosis, and the hamate, which has a volar perforator for the hook and a dorsal perforator for the body without anastomosis. Group 3 had at least two perforators with intraosseous anastomosis and included the trapezium, triquetrum, pisiform, and most lunates.

Discussion and Conclusion

It is important to be able to visualize the angiosomes of the distal forearm and wrist as a three-dimensional structure. The radial artery supplies the skin of the radial side of the forearm, and the ulnar artery supplies the ulnar side of the forearm. There is a dorsal strip of skin that is supplied distally by the dorsal branch of the AIA and proximally by the PIA. When these skin boundaries are segmented three-dimensionally, they form an elongated pyramid with the base of the pyramid on the dorsal skin and the tip at the volar skin flanked on either side by a semicircular tube (**Fig. 9-18**). The intersecting lines roughly divide the bone into angiosome segments.

The distal carpal row is richly supplied by the radial artery, ulnar artery, and AIA via the deep volar palmar arch and the DICA, but the capitate is at greater risk of avascular necrosis because of its perforating vessels. The scaphoid is supplied by the radial artery, and the pisiform is supplied by the ulnar artery. The lunate and triquetrum are supplied by the PRCA and DRCA, and have a more robust collateral circulation, but the lunate is at risk of avascular necrosis in patient subsets because of the origin of its perforators and their intraosseous course. The ulna is supplied largely from the ulnar artery, and the PIA with some collateral flow is supplied from the dorsal AIA. The radial styloid is supplied by the radial artery, and the central column of the radius

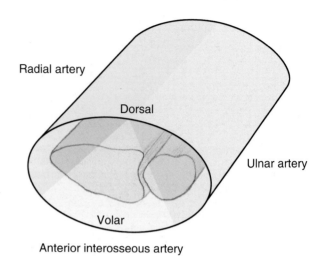

FIGURE 9-18 Angiosome Schematic.

is supplied by the AIA, but the ulnar artery gives contributions to the radius via the dorsal (DRCA, DICA) and volar (PRCA) arches.

When surgically approaching the distal radius and carpus, it is safe to use the volar or dorsal approach because the opposing side provides the collateral circulation. In combined approaches or in situations in which the vasculature is damaged away from the surgical approach, one must consider the remaining collateral circulation via the traversing arches and the locations of skin perforators. We have discussed in detail the vascular anatomy of the distal forearm and wrist, and related this anatomy to common approaches to the wrist. Key points and principles guiding the surgical dissection include the following:

- The periosteum should be stripped only to the level of the fracture line. This preserves the vascular plexus at the periosteum and prevents the avulsion of bony perforators. In some cases, there may be only one, as in the group 1 carpal bones—scaphoid, capitate, minority of lunates.
- Retrograde flow may be sufficient to keep bony fragments of the distal radius viable as evidenced by the success of vascularized bone grafts, but complicating factors, such as crush injuries, tobacco use, and diabetes, affect collateral flow and may lead to complications (e.g., 1,2 SRA and smoking).
- Perforators enter the bone at the bases of the second and fourth extensor compartments and should be spared.
- Common errors include stripping the vascular supply off of the scaphoid while obtaining exposure and injuring the volar RCA at the volar AIA and at the radial artery during a volar approach. Both of these errors result in devascularized bone.
- One should not make two incisions between skin perforators, and one should not undermine tissues above the level of the vessels between incisions.
- In patients with diabetes, history of smoking, or crush injuries, vascularity is compromised further.

Using these principles and knowledge of angiosome anatomy, a surgeon can design and execute the safest surgical approach possible to complicated wrist pathology.

REFERENCES

1. Taylor GI, Palmar JH: The vascular territories (angiosomes) of the body: experimental study and clinical applications. Br J Plast Surg 1987; 40:113-141.

2. Inoue Y, Taylor GI: The angiosomes of the forearm: anatomic study and clinical implications. Plast Reconstr Surg 1996; 98:195-210.

3. Dhar SC, Taylor GI: The delay phenomenon: the story unfolds. Plast Reconstr Surg 104:2079-2091, 1999.

4. Martin D, Bakhach J, Casoli V, et al: Reconstruction of the hand with forearm island flaps. Clin Plast Surg 1997; 24:33-48.

5. Rohrich RJ, Ingram AE Jr: Brachioradialis muscle flap: clinical anatomy and use in soft-tissue reconstruction of the elbow. Ann Plast Surg 1995; 35:70.

6. Braun FM, Haong PH, Merle M, et al: Technique and indications of the forearm flap in hand surgery: a report of thrity-three cases. Ann Chir Main 1985; 4:85-97.

7. Govila A, Sharma D: The radial forearm flap for reconstruction of the upper extremity. Plast Reconstr Surg 1990; 86:920-927.

8. Soucacos PN, Beris AE, Xenakis TA, et al: Forearm flap in orthopaedic and hand surgery. Microsurgery 1992; 13:170-174.

9. Muhlbauer W, Herndl E, Stock W: The forearm flap. Plast Reconstr Surg 1982; 70:336-342.

10. Sheetz KK, Bishop AT, Berger RA: The arterial blood supply of the distal radius and ulna and its potential use in vascularized pedicled bone grafts. J Hand Surg [Am] 1995; 20:902-914.

11. Haerle M, Schaller HE, Mathoulin C: Vascular anatomy of the palmar surfaces of the distal radius and ulna: its relevance to pedicled bone grafts at the distal palmar forearm. J Hand Surg [Br] 2003; 28:131-136.

12. Shibata M, Ogishyo N: Free flaps based on the anterior interosseous artery. Plast Reconstr Surg 1996; 97:746-755.

13. Hu W, Martin D, Baudet J: Thumb reconstruction by the anterior interosseous osteocutaneous retrograde island flap. Eur J Plast Surg 1994; 17:10.

14. Chen HC, Tang YB, Chuang D, et al: Microvascular free posterior interosseous flap and a comparison with the pedicled posterior interosseous flap. Ann Plast Surg 1996; 36:542-550.

15. Zancolli EA, Angrigiani C: Posterior interosseous island forearm flap. J Hand Surg [Br] 1988; 13:130-135.

16. Cavadas PC, Mir X: Single-stage reconstruction of the flexor mechanism of the fingers with a free vascularized tendon flap: case report. J Reconstr Microsurg 2006; 22:37-40.

17. Gelberman RH, Panagis JS, Taleisnik J, et al: The arterial anatomy of the human carpus, part I: the extraosseous vascularity. J Hand Surg [Am] 1983; 8:367-375.

18. Millender LH, Nalebuff EA: Arthrodesis of the rheumatoid wrist: an evaluation of sixty patients and a description of a different surgical technique. J Bone Joint Surg Am 1973; 55:1026-1034.

19. Potts H, Noble J: Surgical approaches to the dorsum of the wrist: brief report. J Bone Joint Surg Br 1988; 70:328-329.

20. Weil C, Ruby LK: The dorsal approach of the wrist revisited. J Hand Surg [Am] 1986; 11:911-912.

21. Bowers WH: The distal radioulnar joint. In Green DP, ed: Operative Hand Surgery. 2nd ed, vol 2. New York: Churchill Livingstone, 1988.

22. Russe O: Fracture of the carpal navicular: diagnosis, nonoperative treatment, and operative treatment. J Bone Joint Surg Am 1960; 42:759-768.

23. Panagis JS, Gelberman RH, Taleisnik J, et al: The arterial anatomy of the human carpus, part II: the intraosseous vascularity. J Hand Surg [Am] 1983; 8:375-382.

Dorsal Plate Fixation

10

Ronaldo S. Carneiro, MD, Cynthia Radi-Peters, OTR, CHT, and Renato Gonçalves, MD

The dorsal approach to treating distal radius fractures has fallen into disfavor during the past few years because of reports of problems with tendon irritation, ruptures, and fracture collapse that occurred with plates that were anatomically correct but had a relatively high profile.[1-3] Discouraged by these results, the focus turned to the volar approach,[4,5] and the dorsal plates went out of fashion even though new plates with a lower profile were introduced to the market. Lately, new literature has confirmed that the results of dorsal plating are comparable to those of the volar approach.[6,7] The use of low-profile, anatomically contoured plating systems results in a reduction of extensor tendon irritation while providing stable bony fixation. To our minds, the big advantage of the dorsal plate fixation for dorsally displaced fractures is the direct visualization of the dorsal defects that are created by the collapse and multifragmentation present in most of these injuries, especially in the senior population. We have been placing two different types of plates in the distal radius: a stainless steel, nonlocking plate (Locon-T by Wright Medical, Arlington, TN) and a titanium locking plate (Stryker Universal distal radius system by Stryker, Kalamazoo, MI). The Locon-T plate is 1.2-mm thick with the screws fully engaged. The distal radius T portion varies and can accommodate from 3 to 5 2.7-mm screws, depending on the size of the plate. The stem is 3.5-cm long and accepts 3.5-mm screws. The advantages of the stainless steel plate are malleability and a very anatomical design. The advantages of the titanium plates are the strength and the locking screws, with virtually no profile increase, both important in the treatment of osteopenic patients.

Indications

The ideal candidate for low-profile dorsal plating is a patient with a multifragmented dorsally displaced fracture of the distal radius with dorsal bony defects, due to a high-velocity injury or the presence of osteoporosis. The indications include unstable fractures that have previously undergone closed reduction and splinting with unsuccessful reduction or loss of reduction. This includes extra-articular fractures (AO type A), intra-articular shear fractures (AO type B), and comminuted intra-articular fractures with metaphyseal comminution (AO type C). Some authors use the criteria of more than 20 degrees of dorsal angulation, radial shortening of more than 2 mm, or articular incongruity between 1 and 2 mm.[6] The age range of patients for the procedure encompasses adolescents at the age of closure of the epiphyses to those in their nineties. It is often better to wait 5 to 7 days after injury to treat these fractures if there is no neurologic or vascular compromise. The reasons are better visualization of the fracture fragments, stabilization of health situations, decrease in the edema of the wrist and fingers, and better understanding of the procedure by

patients and their families. We have used the dorsal plates in all types of fractures of the distal radius, including complex intra-articular multifragmented fractures, classified as C1, C2, and C3 by the AO classification system. In C3.3 fractures there might be a call for additional stabilization of the radius shaft fracture component, and we obtain reduction with extra screws taken from the distal radius set or an occasional Kirshner wire.

Contraindications

The only absolute contraindication to dorsal fixation is a distal radius fracture with a large volarly displaced fragment, especially one with minimal dorsal defects. In that case the volar approach is clearly indicated. Relative contraindications have to do with the health status of the patient, which can commonly be corrected during the 7- to 10-day waiting period. Anticoagulation in the elderly always presents a challenge if the patient is on Coumadin or other drugs, so an internal medicine, cardiology, or neurology consultation should be obtained to manage those situations.

Surgical Technique

Under general or brachial block anesthesia, the forearm is prepped and draped to the elbow area. A fluoroscopy preliminary film is obtained to confirm the deformities and the initial impressions. Following that, traction is applied to the index and ring fingers by Chinese finger traps with cords that are attached to a traction apparatus clamped to the operating-hand-procedure side table (Schlein Hand Positioner with rail attachment; Allen Medical Systems, Acton, MA) (**Fig. 10-1**). In case of doubt and in severe multifragmented fractures, the fluoroscopy film is repeated after traction has been applied. This is a very useful maneuver because in some situations the real severity of the comminution is revealed in this post-traction film rather than in the resting position.

Under tourniquet control, a 5- to 6-cm dorsal longitudinal incision is made spanning the wrist joint and the distal forearm and deepened to the extensor retinaculum. The third dorsal space is incised obliquely following the direction of the extensor pollicis longus (EPL) tendon (**Fig. 10-2**). A hematoma is often present in the third dorsal space, and the identification of the tendon direction is facilitated by the presence of blood. At this point, we also open the second dorsal space longitudinally, exposing the extensor carpi radialis longus and brevis and freeing the tubercle of Lister. One of the interesting findings in severely comminuted fractures is that the EPL tendon can be caught between the displaced fracture fragments, and one has to extricate the tendon from the fragments (**Fig. 10-3**). In those cases, immediate visualization of the tendon is not easy and the surgeon might have to look for the tendon more distally and follow it to the fracture site. That happens in 2% of cases, in our empirical observation, but it

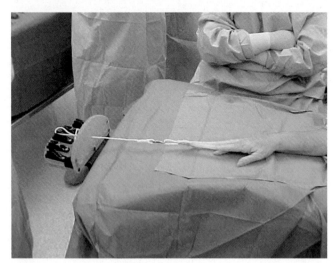

FIGURE 10-1 Setup for open reduction of distal radius fractures with traction apparatus in place.

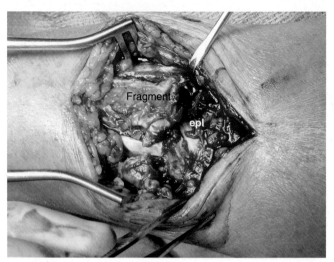

FIGURE 10-3 Tendon of the extensor pollicis longus (epl) caught between fracture fragments *(Fragment)* in a severely comminuted, dorsally displaced fracture of the distal radius.

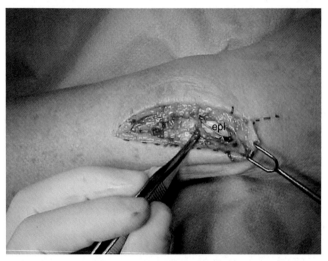

FIGURE 10-2 Exposure of the fracture through incision of the third dorsal space following the tendon of the extensor pollicis longus (epl).

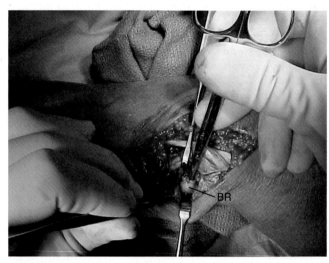

FIGURE 10-4 Tenotomy of the brachioradialis tendon (BR) exposed through the first dorsal space.

is significant because traction applied to the hand and wrist will push the tendon farther into the separation between the fragments, making the reduction of the fracture impossible prior to dissection and extraction of the tendon. This situation would be impossible to recognize if such a fracture were being treated using the volar approach.

If the radial fracture fragment is translated toward the radial side and it involves a large portion of the radius styloid, it may not be reducible by traction alone. In these situations, we perform a tenotomy of the brachioradialis tendon as it inserts into the displaced fragment. The first dorsal space tunnel is incised and the contents are exposed. At the floor of that space, one can encounter the tendon of the brachioradialis, which is separate from the extensor pollicis brevis and the abductor pollicis longus.[10] The brachioradialis tendon is tenotomized transversely, which greatly facilitates the reduction maneuvers for that fragment (**Fig. 10-4**).

The dorsal capsule is kept intact if at all possible. It is opened only in the rare instances in which there is a loose dorsal piece of

the distal radius that has sheared off the articular surface, and we deem it important to the stability and congruity of the joint. In those cases we use an extender provided in the Locon-T set to capture the fragment.

In sequence, a wide periosteal elevator is used to elevate the periosteum together with the floor of the fourth dorsal space, therefore avoiding entering the space and exposing the finger extensor tendons. With that maneuver, the fracture is completely exposed. Sometimes fragments are still not visualized well enough and they have to be dissected further with a scalpel. Lister's tubercle can be very prominent, and when that is the case, a rongeur is used to remove the dorsal part of the tubercle. A potential pitfall here is that in an osteopenic patient with multiple fragmentations, it is possible to remove one of the fragments together with the part of the tubercle that is being intentionally removed. Caution and a very shallow resection are strongly advised.

Usually in an elderly patient there is a large bone defect in the dorsal aspect of the radius (**Fig. 10-5**). For many years now, we have been using iliac crest bone allograft chips previously recon-

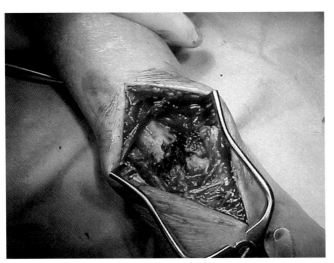

FIGURE 10-5 Large dorsal defect usually found in distal radius fractures in elderly patients.

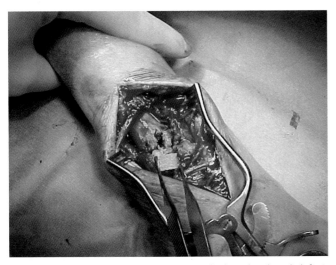

FIGURE 10-6 Bone allograft chips are applied to the dorsal defect, augmenting the bone stock and increasing internal support.

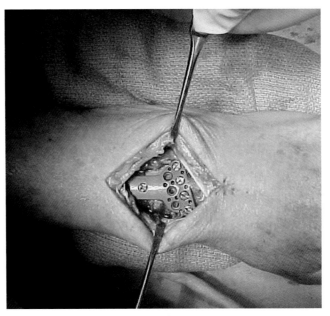

FIGURE 10-7 Stryker distal radius plates in place.

stituted in saline to fill this void (**Fig. 10-6**). The bone chips are excellent in this situation because they provide internal support and augment the bone stock, preventing collapse of the distal fragments.

A dorsal plate is chosen according to the size of the radius and the side affected, and it is temporarily applied to the reduced fracture. Usually we use Locon-T plates because they fit the fractures well, have variable sizing, and are malleable. The other plate that we have used is the Stryker plate, which has the advantage of having locking screws; therefore it is used in situations in which there is great comminution in a severely osteoporotic patient. Nevertheless, the Stryker plate is somewhat bulky and stiff, making it less versatile (**Fig. 10-7**).

With the Locon-T plate, one can choose a small, medium, or large size. The large is rarely used except in tall men. Most of the time, the small size fits women and smaller men comfortably. The radial side of the plate invariably has to be bent using one of the benders provided in the tray. This is easily accomplished because of the malleability of the plate. The pitfall is to forget this

step and at the end of the proximal fixation realize that the extensors of the wrist are caught *beneath* the plate.

The position of the plate is chosen under fluoroscopy. One of the advantages of the Locon-T plate is that it can be positioned all the way to the edge of the dorsal radius distally to treat a shearing fracture that does not have a large distal fragment. Once the size and position of the plate have been established, the first screw is applied. Often the plate is separated from the bone by a couple of millimeters, and placement of the first screw brings the plate into intimate contact with the dorsal cortex. One should be able to estimate the length of the screw to be applied by subtracting the cortex/plate separation ahead of time; otherwise the first screw will be too long and have to be replaced later. The first 3.5-mm screw is placed in the oblong screw hole, which is located in the shaft portion of the plate. Another film is obtained after the placement of the first screw so as to demonstrate the new position of the plate after tightening the screw. Often we have to move the plate distally or proximally when distal fragments are pushed volarly by the first screw and plate. Therefore, in most cases it is wise to place the first screw in the middle of the oblong hole so that one has the leeway to move the plate either way, if necessary (**Fig. 10-8**).

Following that, the proximal shaft screws are drilled with the provided 2.5-mm drill, measured, and applied. These are 3.5-mm self-tapping screws. Measuring the screws in the proximal fragment is easy because most of the time the volar cortex is intact. Usually we do not place the most proximal screw into the plate because as a rule it does not add to the stability. Also, placing it requires a longer skin incision and more muscle retraction to expose the hole, which adds to the postsurgery morbidity.

The distal screws are applied at this time. Distal measurements can be a problem because of the poor quality of bone in the elderly and the comminution of the fracture. Added to that difficulty is the fact that the drill used distally is a 2-mm drill. Therefore, after the placement of the first 2.7-mm screw distally, a lateral film should be performed to determine whether the screw is of adequate size. The other screws are applied following that guideline

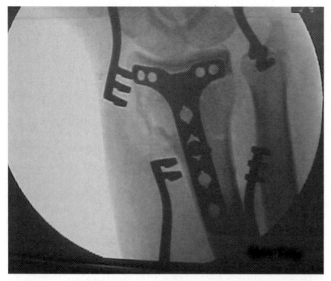

FIGURE 10-8 Locon-T; first screw applied.

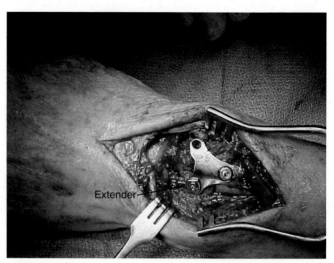

FIGURE 10-10 Plate extender *(Extender)* in place, securing a small, centrally located fracture fragment.

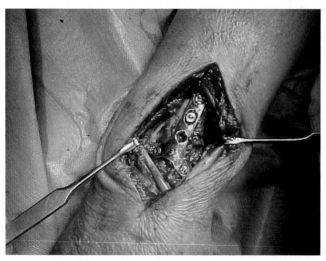

FIGURE 10-9 After fracture reduction, with screws applied, one screw hole was left empty because of the position of the fracture.

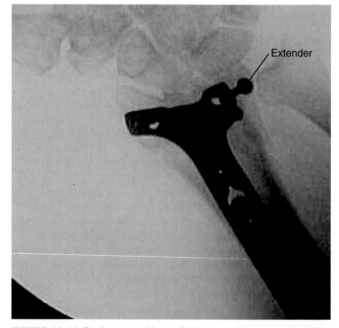

FIGURE 10-11 Radiograph of Locon-T plus extender *(Extender)* securing radially placed dorsal fragment.

(**Fig. 10-9**). As a very crude practical rule, the distal screws are roughly 4 mm longer than the most distal screw placed in the shaft; hence, an 18-mm distal shaft screw would correspond to a 22-mm distal fragment screw.

After all screws have been applied distally, assessment of the final fixation is made. Sometimes a small intra-articular dorsal fragment is left unsecured after the plate has been applied. In those cases we use the small extender that is provided in the tray. This extender fits distally and it has two holes, one that attaches to the plate with a regular 2.7-mm screw and one that is placed on top of the unsecured fragment and accepts a 1.8-mm screw. The extender can be attached to any dorsal screw hole and has helped on many occasions to secure a central fragment (**Fig. 10-10**) or a fragment in the radial or ulnar side of the distal radius (**Fig. 10-11**).

After placement of all screws, final films are obtained, and the extensor retinaculum is closed partially, leaving the EPL free dorsal to the repair. Skin is approximated using horizontal mattress sutures of 5-0 nylon, and a large dressing and a volar splint

are applied. A typical moderately severe case is illustrated in **Figures 10-12** through **10-16**.

Rehabilitation

Virtually all patients whose distal radius fractures are reduced surgically are treated as outpatients. The dressing is changed 2 days later in the office and a plaster splint is applied. The post-surgical regimen consists of immobilization for 3 weeks in a splint or cast. Range of motion exercises in the hand therapy department start after cast removal. We have attempted immediate mobilization as described in the literature[4] but have found that patients tolerate the exercises better and experience less swelling and pain if the therapy is started at 3 weeks. Strengthening starts at 5 to 7 weeks, and the patients are reviewed for the last time prior to discharge at 3 months.

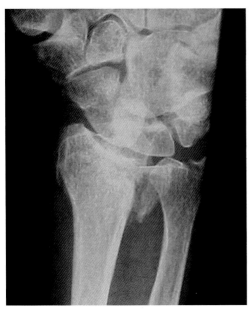

FIGURE 10-12 Radiograph of a typical fracture of the distal radius, posteroanterior view, with intra-articular component, multiple fragments, and shortening of more than 5 mm.

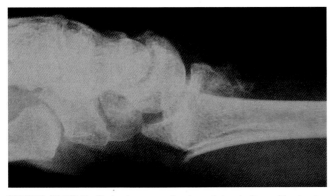

FIGURE 10-13 Radiograph, same fracture, lateral view with greater than 20 degrees of dorsal displacement.

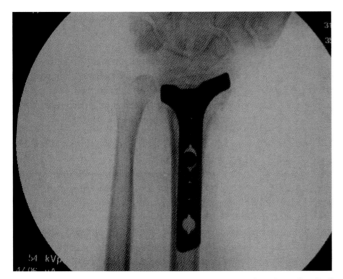

FIGURE 10-14 Postsurgery fluoroscopic posteroanterior view of typical fracture.

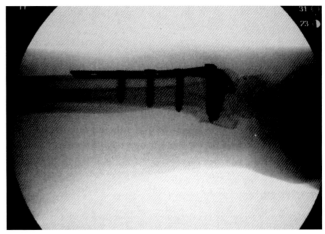

FIGURE 10-15 Postsurgery fluoroscopic lateral view of typical fracture. Notice that no screws were applied in the most proximal hole.

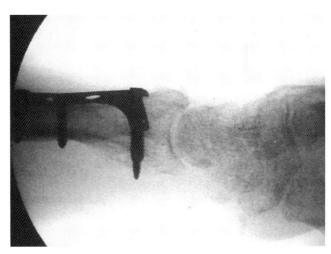

FIGURE 10-16 Postsurgery fluoroscopic view of typical fracture: 30-degree oblique lateral articular view.

Complications

Aside from the usual complications related to residual stiffness of flexion-extension and pronation-supination that are inherent in any treatment of distal radius fractures, the complications to be expected from the dorsal approach are irritation of the extensor tendons by tendinitis and possible rupture and loosening of the screws.[1,9] Tendinitis has not been a major concern when plates are employed. After the insertion of more than 100 plates, only two patients experienced tendinitis—one 2 months after surgery and one 2 years after surgery. The second one may have had an intersection syndrome unrelated to the plate. Both of them were treated with rest and nonsteroidal anti-inflammatory drugs and responded well.

Screw loosening at the distal fragment is a slightly bigger problem with Locon-T plates; we have seen it happen in roughly 5% of patients. We have removed only two screws that were very prominent during the past 7 years of using the plate. No plate removals were necessary. In contrast, there has been no screw-loosening problem with the Stryker plate. It is therefore a better option for the very osteopenic patient. The design of the screw hole in the Stryker plate permits locking with no increase in the profile and allows for locking the screws at various angles, which is a distinct advantage in situations where poor bone stock or a lot of comminution is present.

Other complications have to do with poor choice of the approach by the surgeon. If the volar fragment is bigger than the dorsal one, this approach should be avoided because the screws placed from the dorsal side will not be able to capture the volar fragment and reduce it satisfactorily. We have had at least three patients in the past 7 years who fell into the category of being poor candidates for the approach and suffered fracture collapse. One of them ended up having a radiocarpal fusion 1 year after surgery because of continued pain. The other two had no residual pain and they chose to accept the deformity without correction.

Results

We studied 28 consecutive patients (24 women and 4 men) who had severe distal radius fractures, were treated using the Locon-T dorsal plate, and underwent a follow-up of 3 years. All procedures were performed on an outpatient basis. The criteria for patient selection were as follows:

- Being 65 years of age or older (mean age 72.4 years; the youngest was 65, the oldest 86); 4 patients were older than 80, 20 were older than 70.
- Having severe fractures, which means two or more of the following criteria:
  - Having comminution (more than three fragments)
  - Having an intra-articular component: radiocarpal, radioulnar, or both
  - Having more than 5 mm of shortening
  - Having more than 20 degrees of dorsal tilt
  - Having osteopenia
  - Having a fracture that was not reducible by closed means or having recurrent deformity after attempted reduction.

The objectives of our treatment were:

- Acceptable reduction, taking into consideration that the relative length of the radius in the elderly is more important than tilt or intra-articular gaps[10]
- Early mobilization of fingers (immediate) and wrist (maximum 3 weeks of casting or splinting)
- Increase of bone stock
- Functional range of motion (at least 30 degrees of flexion, 30 degrees of extension, and full or nearly full pronation-supination)
- Comfort during the consolidation phase

The results were measured initially at 3 months, when the patients were discharged from therapy. The patients were recalled at 36 months and re-examined. Flexion-extension and pronation-supination figures were compared to two articles in the literature—one utilizing dorsal and volar approaches (Jupiter and colleagues[11]) and one employing a volar approach only (Orbay and colleagues[4]). These articles referred to 20 patients measured at 38 months and 26 patients measured at 16 months, respectively. The comparison is illustrated in **Table 10-1**.

Grip strength varied from 38 lb to 75 lb, and that corresponded with 84.4% to 150% (mean 92%) of the contralateral side. The lower percentage grip strength corresponded with a fractured nondominant wrist.

The postoperative radiologic evaluation did not show any loss of radius height or articular congruity from the 3-month mark to the 36-month re-evaluation. We strive mostly for radius length in comparison to tilt or intra-articular congruity, and we tend to accept zero degrees of tilt during the reduction as a successful result. The traction plus the addition of bone allograft makes that position readily achievable, and in the elderly it translates into ultimate good function. Therefore, our postoperative radiologic examinations take that fact into consideration. Even so, all radiologic evaluations showed a range of 0 degrees of volar tilt to 4 degrees; no ulnar-positive variance (except in one case that showed postoperative collapse due to poor indication of the dorsal approach) and less than 2 mm of articular incongruity in all cases.

Additional Comments

We have been using bone allograft chips in addition to the plate to create an internal support structure in these situations, with the goal of increasing the bone stock and helping the stable fixation of these fractures. It is our experience that the low-profile plates that are used in the distal radius area do not interfere severely with gliding of the extensor tendons.

Because the approach is simple and relatively quick, there is no justification for doing lesser procedures in the elderly with the excuse of saving anesthesia time. Our tourniquet time has ranged from 37 to 45 minutes in the past 70 cases. This is less time than is required for other approaches in our hands, except for closed pinning without the addition of bone graft, which has been abandoned because it is unreliable in the elderly.[8] Our surgical time corresponds with the experience of one surgeon (RSC) and is in sharp contrast to the reported tourniquet times of 105.3 minutes for dorsal plating with Pi plates reported by Grewal and colleagues.[9] Their study included six orthopaedic surgeons, and the reported tourniquet times may reflect variables other than simply the dorsal approach and plate design.

The fracture treatment time interval limit for the procedure is about 2.5 weeks in patients who are 50 years old or younger and 3.5 weeks for older patients. After that period of time, the surgery can still be performed, but it will take other maneuvers such as osteotomies to accomplish acceptable results.

TABLE 10-1 Comparison of Our Results in 28 Patients to Previously Published Studies[4,11]

	Carneiro, 3 mo (degrees)	Jupiter, 38 mo (degrees)	Orbay, 16 mo (degrees)	Carneiro, 36 mo (degrees)
Extension	54.6	65	58	55
Flexion	50	55	55	53.5
Pronation	85.4	75	80	86.4
Supination	72.9	75	76	85.7

None of my patients has suffered from sympathetic dystrophy, even though one has had a presympathetic dystrophy condition that is characterized by an increase in swelling and discoloration of the skin, with a sudden increase in pain and decrease of motion (a "flare reaction"). Our very attentive hand therapist brought this patient to my attention early, and she was treated with an oral steroid dose pack and experienced an excellent response.

Conclusion

The dorsal approach to distal radius fractures is a viable option for patients with severe dorsally displaced fractures. This approach has fallen into disfavor during the past few years, but the advent of new low-profile plates promises to revive this procedure, especially in the elderly population. The advantages are:

+ Less risk for sympathetic dystrophy due to dissection away from the median and ulnar nerves
+ Easier augmentation of bone stock
+ An approach that is quick and affords better visualization of dorsally displaced fracture fragments

The results are at least similar to those found when using the volar approach. Judging by the comparison, the results are better in terms of pronation-supination though slightly worse in terms of extension.

REFERENCES

1. Ring D, Jupiter JB, Brennwald J, et al: Prospective multicenter trial of a plate for dorsal fixation of distal radius fractures. J Hand Surg [Am] 1997; 22:777-784.
2. Ruch DS, Papadonikolikis A: Volar versus dorsal plating in the management of intra-articular distal radius fractures. J Hand Surg [Am] 2006; 31:9-16.
3. McKay SD, MacDermid JC, Roth JH, et al: Assessment of complications of distal radius fractures and development of a complication checklist. J Hand Surg [Am] 2001; 26:916-922.
4. Orbay JL, Fernandez DL: Volar fixation for dorsally displaced fractures of the distal radius: a preliminary report. J Hand Surg [Am] 2002; 27:205-215.
5. Musgrave DS, Idler RS: Volar fixation of dorsally displaced distal radius fractures using the 2.4 mm locking compression plates. J Hand Surg [Am] 2005; 30:743-749.
6. Simic PM, Robinson J, Gardner MJ, et al: Treatment of distal radius fractures with a low-profile dorsal plating system: an outcome assessment. J Hand Surg [Am] 2006; 31:382-386.
7. Kamth AF, Zurakowski D, Day CS: Low-profile dorsal plating for dorsally angulated distal radius fractures: an outcome study. J Hand Surg [Am] 2006; 31:1061-1067.
8. Harley BJ, Scherfenberger A, Beaupre LA, et al: Augmented external fixation versus percutaneous pinning and casting for unstable fractures of the distal radius: a prospective randomized trial. J Hand Surg [Am] 2004; 29:815-824.
9. Grewal R, Perey B, Wilmik M, et al: A randomized prospective study on the treatment of intra-articular distal radius fractures: open reduction and internal fixation with dorsal plating versus mini open reduction, percutaneous fixation and external fixation. J Hand Surg [Am] 2005; 30:764-772.
10. Koh S, Andersen CR, Buford WL, et al: Anatomy of the distal brachioradialis and its potential relationship to distal radius fractures. J Hand Surg [Am] 2006; 31:2-8.
11. Jupiter JB, Ring D, Weitzel PP: Surgical treatment of redisplaced fractures of the distal radius in patients older than 60 years. J Hand Surg. [Am] 2002; 27:714-723.

Dorsal Double Plating and Combined Palmar and Dorsal Plating for Distal Radius Fractures

11

Daniel A. Rikli, MD

If operative therapy is indicated to treat a distal radius fracture, the majority of cases can be treated by palmar plating. Extra- and intra-articular fractures can be managed by this method, which is straightforward, by using a simple surgical approach. The result is low morbidity and overall good clinical outcome, even in very osteoporotic bone. However, there is a subset of intra-articular fractures that require a dorsal approach to achieve anatomical reduction of the radiocarpal joint surface and direct fixation of specific key fragments. Moreover, a dorsal approach is always combined with a limited dorsal arthrotomy that allows for direct visualization of the radiocarpal joint surface and—importantly—the proximal carpal row, so as to rule out associated ligament tears. In a series of 100 consecutive distal radius cases that were plated at our institution, 75% were treated by using a palmar plate, 20% by dorsal double plating, and 5% by combined palmar and dorsal plating.

Biomechanical Background

The concept of plating for distal radius fractures is based on the three-column model.[1] The model says simply that the distal forearm consists of three columns (**Fig. 11-1**). The *radial column* is composed of the radial styloid process and the scaphoid facet; the *intermediate column* is formed by the lunate facet and the sigmoid notch; and the distal ulna is the *ulnar column* together with the triangular fibrocartilage and the ulnar part of the lunate facet and sigmoid notch. In extension fractures of the distal radius, the distal epiphyseal fragment is displaced toward the dorsal and radial directions. Separate buttressing of the intermediate and the radial columns by two individual plates to prevent dorsal (intermediate column plate) and radial (radial column plate) dislocation has been shown to be a stable mechanical construct with greater stiffness than a conventional 3.5-mm T-plate or a Pi plate (2.7 mm) in cadaver wrists that show a simulated dorsal metaphyseal defect.[2]

In vivo analysis of force transmission across the radioulnocarpal joint has revealed data that are consistent with the three-column model. Only a small amount of force is transmitted through the radial column. The radial column serves more as a radial osseous buttress and an insertion for the radiocarpal ligaments. In intra-articular fractures, the radial styloid most often is one single bone fragment without comminution or impaction of the joint surface. The greatest force is transmitted across the intermediate and the ulnar columns. In intra-articular fractures, the key articular fragments and impaction zones are found at the level of the intermediate column due to these compressive forces. The intermediate column, therefore, is the key to the radiocarpal joint. The ulnar column also transmits an amount of force that is com-

parable to that of the intermediate column. It is therefore very sensitive to radial shortening (relative ulnar overlength), which produces painful ulnar impaction. Thus, reconstruction of radial length is an important prognostic outcome factor. Moreover, the ulnar column is the pivot that serves as the center of rotation of the hand and carpus around the forearm, with a complex soft tissue stabilizing construct (TFC, ulnocarpal ligaments, ECU).[3]

In light of these biomechanical data and on the basis of clinical experience, it makes sense to look at the three columns separately. In distal radius fractures, all three columns should be stable or stabilized.

Three-Step Approach to High-Energy Intra-articular Distal Radial Fractures

High-energy impact to the wrist can lead to disruption of the three columns and to separation of the fragments, fragmentation of the column, impaction of articular fragments, osseous defects, cartilage damage and disruption, and avulsion of stabilizing ligaments. Soft tissue swelling is usually considerable, and bruising or even open wounds may be present. Acute median neuropathy may occur due to dorsal dislocation of the distal fragment or direct pressure of the shaft fragment on the nerve.

Analysis of the individual fracture personality on the basis of the initial emergency room radiograph when the fracture has been unreduced is difficult, and a clear treatment strategy often cannot be developed based on the initial imaging. So for complex, high-energy injuries, it may be advisable to perform a closed reduction and a joint-bridging external fixator as a first measure in the emergency situation (step 1). The advantages are as follows: closed reduction and external fixation are easy to perform, even by inexperienced staff; skin and soft tissue lesions can calm down over the coming days; and median nerve neuropathy usually resolves after preliminary closed reduction. A computed tomography (CT) scan of the wrist in traction allows accurate analysis of the fracture personality and provides more information about a definitive treatment strategy than does a CT scan of an unreduced fracture because some fragments are reduced under ligamentotaxis (step 2). When the swelling has subsided, usually after 3 to 7 days, the definitive osteosynthesis, according to the preoperative planning based on conventional radiographs and CT scans, can be performed (step 3). An external fixator in place is then a helpful intraoperative reduction tool.[4]

Analysis of the Fracture Personality

A thorough analysis of the fracture personality is the prerequisite for developing an adequate treatment strategy. Fernandez[5] has

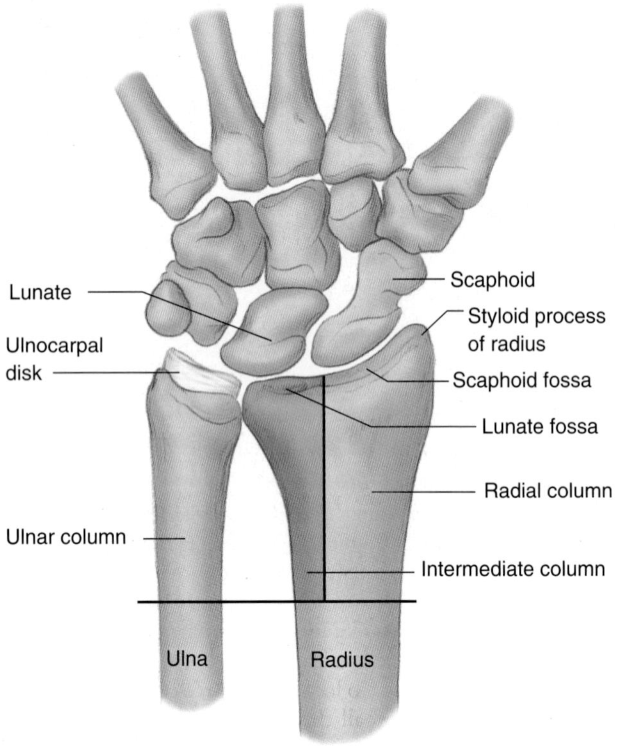

FIGURE 11-1 The Three-Column Model. Ulnar column with head of the ulna and TFCC; intermediate column with the lunate sulcus and ulnar notch (DRUJ); and radial column with scaphoid sulcus and radial styloid process. *(From Rikli DA, Businger A, Babst R: Dorsal double-plate fixation of the distal radius. Oper Orthop Traumatol 2005; 6:624-640. Used with permission.)*

proposed a pathomechanical classification that allows identification of the principal forces involved in the individual injury: bending, shear, avulsion, and compression. Categorizing the fracture into these groups helps to define the major treatment strategy: bending responds to ligamentotaxis; shear requires buttressing; avulsion needs reinsertion of ligaments; and compression affords individual reconstruction of the columns, often with formal revision of the intermediate column ("the key to the radiocarpal joint").

In high-energy intra-articular fractures, a preoperative CT scan in traction should be indicated deliberately. If a three-step approach is performed, as delineated earlier, a CT scan with an external fixator in place is the preferred investigation. In our experience and in accordance with Melone,[6] there are five key elements that should be analyzed in the CT image:

1. The radial shaft and its rotatory relationship to the articular block
2. The radial styloid (radial column), usually a big "chunk" of bone with little or no impression at the level of the joint surface
3. A palmar-ulnar fragment (intermediate column). This fragment may be undisplaced and have good contact with the cortex of the proximal shaft or the fragment may be hyperextended with no contact to the shaft cortex (and thereby difficult to control when using a dorsal approach). The palmar cortex may be comminuted and hence the support for the palmar-ulnar fragment is lacking.
4. A dorsoulnar fragment (intermediate column), a key element for osseous stability of the distal radioulnar joint and for force

transmission across the radiocarpal joint. It may be realigned with ligamentotaxis or may remain displaced
5. Any centrally impressed articular fragment that does not respond to ligamentotaxis due to impaction

All five of these key elements should be identified and considered when planning treatment.

Dorsal Double Plating

The indications for dorsal double plating are any situations in which a dorsal arthrotomy is warranted in order to revise the radiocarpal joint surface and the proximal carpal row. We do not perform palmar arthrotomies so as to avoid provoking carpal ligament instability. A dorsal arthrotomy may be indicated to reconstruct the articular surface at the level of the intermediate column, especially when impacted articular fragments are present. Such fragments may require direct manipulation. In a dorsal arthrotomy, disruption of interosseous ligaments (especially the scapholunate) can be ruled out or confirmed and be treated immediately at the time of fixation of the distal radius fracture. Furthermore, a dorsal approach is preferred when a displaced dorsoulnar fragment is present. This fragment, which is a key fragment of the radiocarpal articular surface and the sigmoid notch, can then be reduced anatomically and fixed specifically with a separate intermediate column plate. In some cases of corrective osteotomies, a dorsal approach may also be preferred.[7]

A single dorsal approach should not be used if a palmar articular fragment is in hyperextension or if there is considerable comminution at the level of the palmar cortex.

Indications

- Distal radius fractures with articular fragments impacted into the metaphysis that cannot be simply reduced indirectly (from the palmar aspect) and cannot be reduced closed by ligamentotaxis (AO classification C3, Pechlaner I-2, II-2a)
- Distal radius fractures with displaced dorsoulnar fragment (AO classification C1.1, C2.1, Pechlaner II-2c, II-2d)
- Distal radius fractures with associated bony or ligamentous injuries in the area of the proximal carpal row, requiring specific treatment

Contraindications
Absolute
- General medical contraindications for surgical intervention

Relative
- Distal radius fractures with palmar displacement of the distal fragment (Smith fracture, reverse Barton's fracture)

Approach and Operative Technique
Surgical Instruments and Implants
- Distal Radius 2.4 mm Locking Plates set (Synthes, Oberdorf, Switzerland)
- Possible need for small external fixator
- Image intensifier

Anesthesia and Positioning
- General or local anesthesia

+ Supine position, arm table; the arm table is not set at the height of the shoulder but at the level of the patient's chest. This brings the arm into a position of approximately 45 degrees abduction on the table and is easier to move from a supine to a prone position. A tourniquet may be used on the upper arm, nonsterile, but this is used only in exceptional cases (**Figs. 11-2** through **11-5**).

Postoperative Management

The goal of dorsal double plating is stable internal fixation to allow for immediate early function after treatment. At our institution the wrist is protected by a dorsal plaster splint for the first days and is followed by a removable Velcro splint for 4 to 6 weeks. The patient is encouraged to use his or her hands for daily activities, such as dressing, eating, holding a sheet of paper, and so forth. The splint is removed for active mobilization of the hand and wrist under the supervision of a physiotherapist two to three times a week. After the first radiological follow-up 6 weeks postoperatively, the splint is removed and unrestricted use of the wrist is allowed.

Results

We analyzed a series of 25 consecutive patients with intra-articular distal radius fractures treated with dorsal double plating (**Table 11-1**). The minimum follow-up was 12 months. There were 14 men and 11 women, for an average age of 52 years. No bone grafts or bone substitutes were used. All fractures united in an anatomical position. The average Disabilities of the Arm, Shoulder, and Hand (DASH) score was 7.2 (0 to 56) and the patient-rated wrist evaluation (PRWE) score was 8 (0 to 31). There was no significant loss of strength compared with the contralateral side as measured by a JAMAR dynamometer. The range of motion for flexion and extension was between 100 degrees and

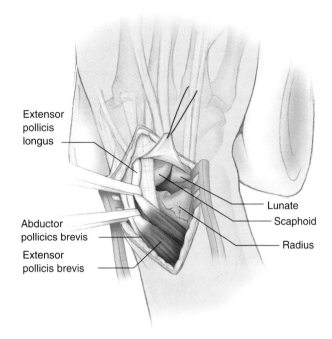

FIGURE 11-2 The radiocarpal joint is inspected from the intermediate column via a transverse arthrotomy along the dorsal edge of the radius. The proximal carpal row is inspected for any concomitant injuries (scapholunate ligament, TFCC, cartilage damage). The proximal carpal row can be pushed further in the distal direction with the aid of an elevator. In this way the radiocarpal joint can be reconstructed under direct vision without leaving a step in the area of the lunate surface. *(From Rikli DA, Businger A, Babst R: Dorsal double-plate fixation of the distal radius. Oper Orthop Traumatol 2005; 6:624-640. Used with permission.)*

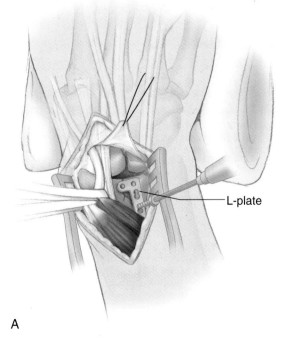

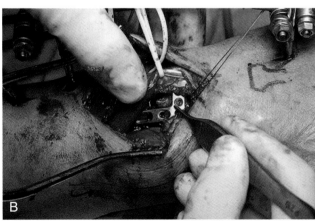

FIGURE 11-3 A Suitable L-plate Is Contoured. It usually has to be bent backward slightly and twisted. It is preferable to stabilize the plate temporarily by inserting a standard screw into the long hole in the proximal fragment adjacent to the fracture. *(From Rikli DA, Businger A, Babst R: Dorsal double-plate fixation of the distal radius. Oper Orthop Traumatol 2005; 6:624-640. Used with permission.)*

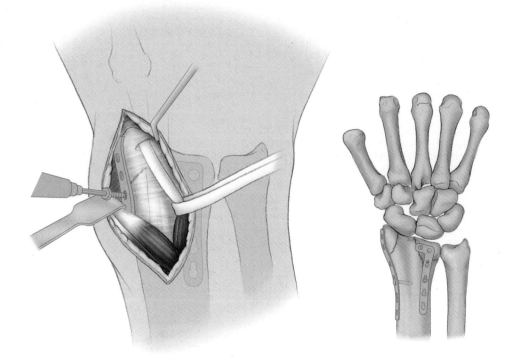

A

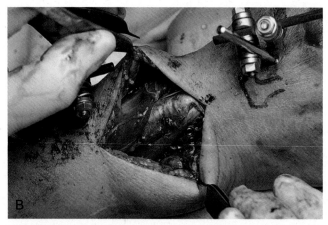

B

FIGURE 11-4 Correction of the reduction and of the positions of the plates can now be carried out without any problem. The osteosynthesis is then completed by inserting a standard screw into each of the most proximal plate holes. This prevents any further slipping of the plate. Locking head screws are then inserted into the distal plate holes. Two screws are sufficient in the radial plate. The most distal screw is usually very short, the proximal screw is long; it also supports the radiocarpal joint. The transverse plate arm in the area of the dorsoulnar plate is usually fixed with fixed-angle screws. This supports the reconstructed articular surface subchondrally. It must be ensured that the screws do not protrude into the joint. The threaded drill sleeve for the fixed-angle, locking screws must be screwed very carefully onto the plate. This is the only way to ensure that the screws sink completely into the plate and are securely anchored in the plate-hole threads. Check using the image intensifier. If the reconstruction is satisfactory and the implants are in the correct positions, the fixator is loosened and the wrist is passed through a full range of motion under image intensification in order to determine if the fixation is stable enough to allow early wrist motion. *(From Rikli DA, Businger A, Babst R: Dorsal double-plate fixation of the distal radius. Oper Orthop Traumatol 2005; 6:624-640. Used with permission.)*

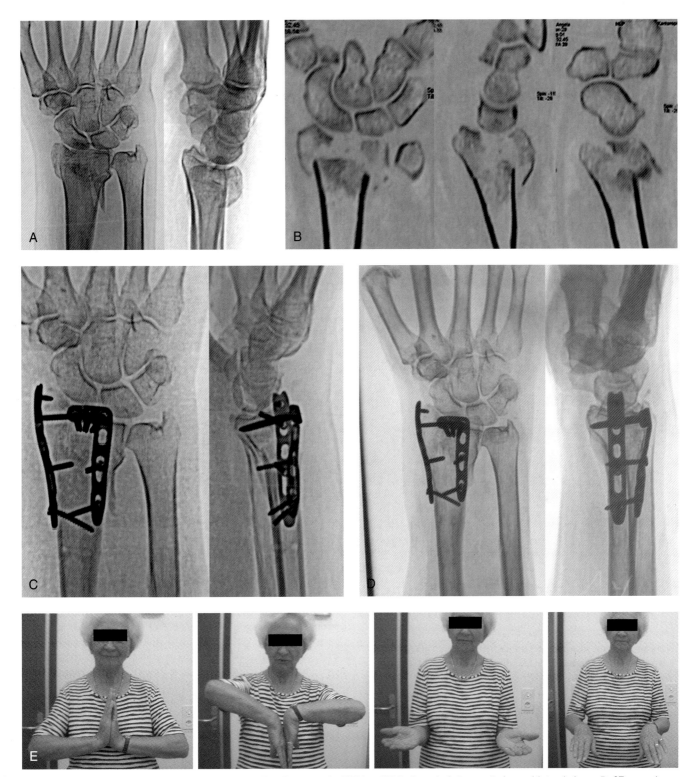

FIGURE 11-5 A Comminuted Intraarticular Distal Radius Fracture of a 75-Year-Old Patient. A, Anteroposterior and lateral views. **B**, CT-scan shows articular comminution, a displaced dorsoulnar fragment and metaphyseal bone defect. **C**, Postoperative x-rays after dorsal double plating. No bone graft, early rehabilitation. **D**, 1 year postoperatively. **E**, Clinical result 1 year postoperatively.

TABLE 11-1 Results of Dorsal Double Plating

Patients	25
Men/women	14/11
Age	52 (17-83)
A3 (early correction)	2
C1-C3	23
Dominant hand	17
Cancellous bone graft	0
Functional rehabilitation	25
Stewart score: very good	25
DASH score (points)	7.2 (0-56)
PRWE score (points)	8.0 (0-31)
Extensor tendon irritation	1
Reflex sympathetic dystrophy	1
Implant removal	6

DASH, disability of arm, shoulder, and hand; PRWE, patient-related wrist evaluation.

160 degrees; for pronation and supination, it was between 160 degrees and 180 degrees. One patient showed irritation of the extensor pollicis longus tendon due to adhesions at the level of the musculotendinous junction, but no extensor tendon ruptures occurred. There was one case of mild algodystrophy that resolved completely. In six patients the implants were removed.[7]

Combined Palmar and Dorsal Plating

The indications for combined palmar and dorsal plating are as follows:

The combination of a hyperextended palmar articular fragment (palmar ulnar fragment) or loss of palmar cortical bone support with:

1. A displaced dorsoulnar fragment (that is not amenable from the palmar approach and needs direct reduction under visualization of the radiocarpal joint surface and fragment-specific fixation)
2. Centrally impacted articular fragments that need direct manipulation under visualization of the radiocarpal joint surface
3. An associated scapholunate ligament tear that must be addressed specifically

Or any combination of these three conditions

Approach and Operative Technique

If the wrist is not in a joint-bridging external fixator (a three-step approach to high-energy injuries), an external fixator is placed first to preliminarily reduce the fracture by putting the wrist under traction. This measure is very helpful and is strongly recommended. Other traction devices may be used instead. It is preferable to start with the palmar approach, a modified Henry's approach between the tendon of the flexor carpi radialis and the radial artery. The palmar cortical buttress is reconstructed, and a hyperextended palmar articular fragment is reduced. This palmar-ulnar fragment is then fixed with a single 2.4-mm locking plate. The articular fragment is held with one or two short screws so as to avoid interfering with any dorsoulnar fragment that may remain in an imperfect position. The radial column is buttressed by using the same palmar approach and a radial column plate (2.4-mm locking plate). As an alternative, both the palmar-ulnar fragment and the radial column can be stabilized by a single palmar T-plate (2.4-mm locking plate). That way, a limited dorsal approach has been established. Only the intermediate column is visualized through the third extensor tendon compartment (similar to dorsal double plating). It is not necessary to approach the radial column because this column is already controlled from the palmar access (**Figs. 11-6** and **11-7**). The dorsoulnar fragment and any centrally impacted fragment are visualized, and a limited transverse arthrotomy is performed. This allows for direct inspection of the proximal carpal row (SL tear) and the radiocarpal joint surface at the level of the intermediate column. The fragments are then reduced and fixed with a separate 2.4-mm locking plate. Then the palmar fixation is completed. Any of these steps may be controlled by using intraoperative fluoroscopy as needed. At the completion of fixation, the external fixator is opened, and the wrist is driven through flexion-extension, radial-ulnar duction, and pronation-supination to demonstrate the stability of the construct. The wounds are then closed in layers and the external fixator pins are removed. A sterile dressing and a dorsal or palmar plaster slap is applied.

Rehabilitation

If the decision is made to go for open reduction and internal fixation of such complex fractures using a combined palmar and dorsal approach, the goal must be to achieve enough stability for early active motion. This is started on day one with the aid of a physiotherapist. Special attention is paid to treating postoperative swelling and controlling pain. The plaster slap is replaced by a removable Velcro splint as soon as the swelling has subsided. The patient is encouraged to use his or her hands for daily activities, such as dressing, eating, holding a sheet of paper, and so forth. The splint is removed for active mobilization of the hand and wrist under the supervision of a physiotherapist two to three times a week. After the first radiological follow-up 6 weeks postoperatively, the splint is removed and unrestricted use of the wrist is allowed.

Results

We analyzed the results of a consecutive series of 10 patients following combined palmar and dorsal plating for complex intra-articular distal radial fractures (**Table 11-2**). The average age was 47 years, and eight patients were heavy laborers. The minimum follow-up was 12 months. All had early active rehabilitation. All fractures united with no infectious complications. The range of motion in relation to the unaffected side was 80% for flexion, 95% for extension, 97% for pronation, and 94% for supination. Two patients had unsatisfactory clinical results and did not resume work; one had algodystrophy (associated SL tear, repaired), and one had a concomitant fracture-dislocation of the ipsilateral elbow. The DASH and PRWE scores of these two patients were

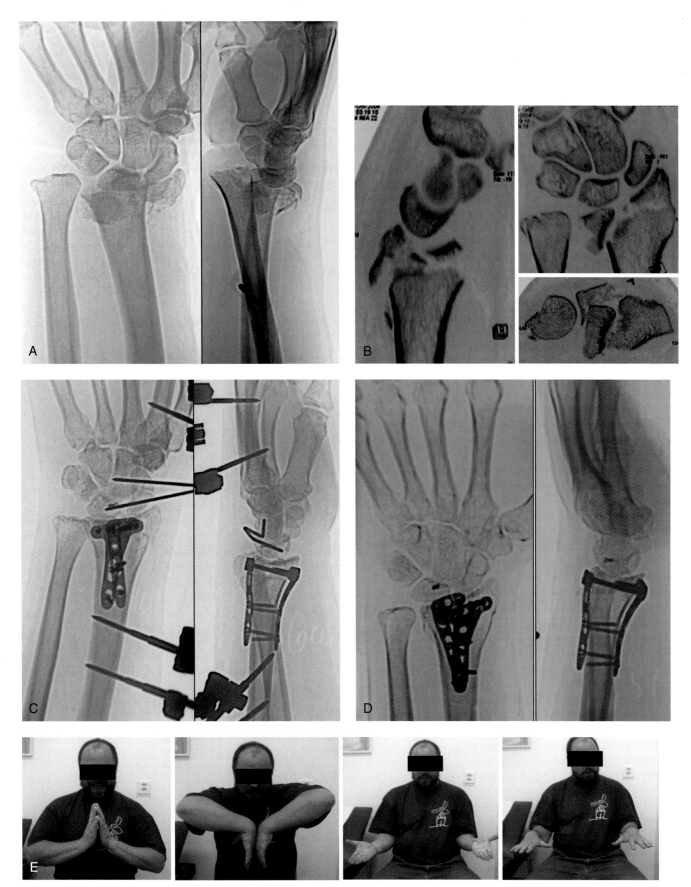

FIGURE 11-6 **A Comminuted Distal Radius Fracture of a 38-Year-Old Worker. A,** Anteroposterior and lateral views. **B,** CT scan in traction (external fixator) shows articular involvement, the intermediate column fragment is flipped 90 degrees in two planes. **C,** Immediately postop. An associated complete SL tear was repaired, temporary carpal transfixation, external fixator left in place for 8 weeks to protect ligament repair. **D,** 1 year post-operatively, slight DISI and diastasis of DRUJ. **E,** Clinical result 1 year postoperatively; slight pain, back to work.

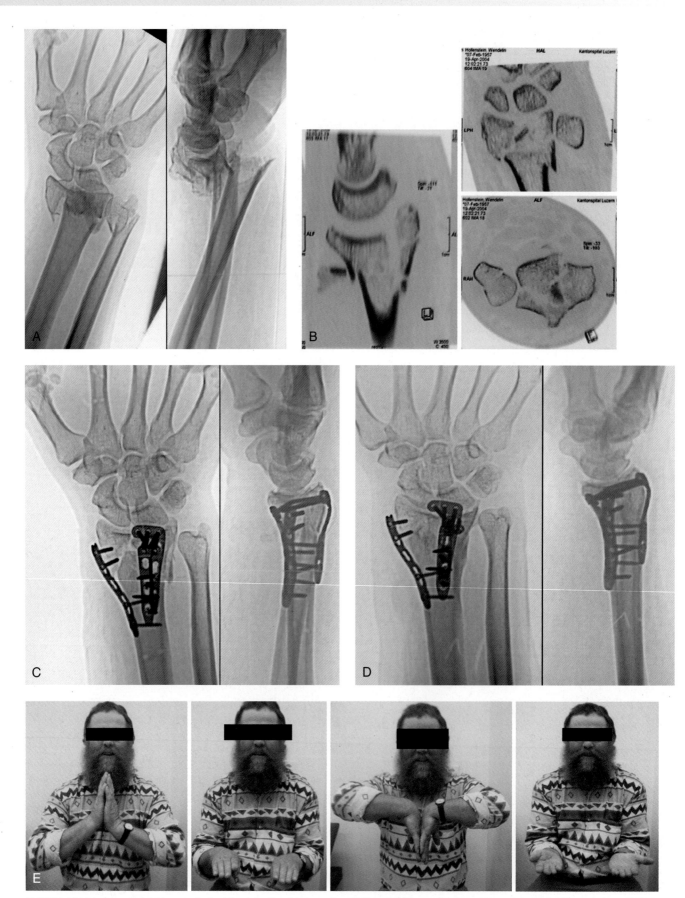

FIGURE 11-7 A Comminuted Intra-articular Distal Radius Fracture of a 40-Year-Old Farmer. A, Anteroposterior and lateral views. **B,** CT scan in traction (external fixator) shows impacted articular fragment, loss of palmar cortex and displaced dorsoulnar fragment. **C,** Immediately postop. **D,** Radiograph taken 1 year postoperatively. **E,** Clinical result 1 year postoperatively; pain-free, back to heavy labor.

TABLE 11-2 Results of Combined Palmar and Dorsal Plating

Patients	10
Men/women	10/0
Heavy labor	8
Age	47 y (av.)
Classification	C3
Bone graft	0
Functional rehabilitation	10
Resume work	8
Unsatisfactory	2
DASH score (pts) (Back to work)	0-12.5
PRWE score (pts) (Back to work)	0-33
Grip strength (% of contralat.) (Back to work)	72-99%
DASH score (pts) (Unsatisfactory)	91,132
PRWE score (pts) (Unsatisfactory)	62,120
Reflex sympathetic dystrophy	1

DASH, disability of arm, shoulder, and hand; PRWE, patient-related wrist evaluation.

91 and 132, and 62 and 120, respectively. Eight patients returned to premorbid heavy labor with a DASH between 0 and 12.5 and a PRWE of 0 and 33. This latter group achieved grip strength of between 72% and 99% of the contralateral side.[8]

Summary

There is a subset of patients with high-energy intra-articular distal radius fractures that may need a direct dorsal approach or a combined dorsal and palmar approach for direct reduction and fragment-specific fixation. A structured approach and thorough analysis of the individual fracture personality are prerequisites to success. The analysis of the fracture is based on the three-column concept and on CT imaging of the articular and extra-articular components of the fracture. The fracture should then be addressed with a clear operative strategy. Plate fixation should always result in anatomical reconstruction of the key articular fragments; restoration of length, axes, and rotation; and enough stability to allow for early active rehabilitation. If these goals are achieved, good clinical results, including a pain-free wrist and reasonable motion, can be expected, even in heavily comminuted high-energy injuries.

REFERENCES

1. Rikli D, Regazzoni P, Babst R: Die dorsale Doppelplattenosteosynthese am distalen Radius: ein biomechanisches Konzept und dessen klinische Realisation. Zentralbl Chir 2003; 128:1003-1007.
2. Peine R, Rikli D, Hoffmann R, et al: Comparison of three different plating techniques for the dorsum of the distal radius. J Hand Surg [Am] 2000; 25:29-33.
3. Rikli DA, Honigmann P, Babst R, et al: Intra-articular pressure measurement in the radioulnocarpal joint using a novel sensor: in vitro and in vivo results. J Hand Surg [Am] 2007; 32:67-75.
4. Rikli DA, Regazzoni P: The double plating technique for distal radius fractures. Tech Hand Up Extrem Surg 2000; 4:107-114.
5. Fernandez DL: Distal radius fracture: the rationale of a classification. Chir Main 2001; 20:411-425.
6. Melone CP: Open treatment for displaced articular fractures of the distal radius. Clin Orthop 1984; 202:103-111.
7. Rikli DA, Businger A, Babst R: Dorsal double-plate fixation of the distal radius. Oper Orthop Traumatol 2005; 17:624-640.
8. Rikli D, Droeser R, Babst R: Combined dorsal and palmar plating for complex intraarticular distal radial fractures. Abstract from Annual Congress of Swiss Society of Surgery. Vortrag Schweizerischer Chirurgenkongress, Lugano, June 2006.

Fragment-Specific Fixation of Distal Radius Fractures

12

Leon S. Benson, MD and Robert J. Medoff, MD

Of the various types of distal radius fractures, those with intra-articular extension have the most to gain from operative intervention. Many of these fractures are inherently unstable and not amenable to conservative methods of reduction and cast immobilization. Treatment that fails to correct residual incongruity of the joint and leaves a significant step-off or gap in the articular surface can result in chronic osteoarthritis and pain.[1-4] Furthermore, unreduced fragments that alter the geometry and normal kinematics of the radiocarpal or distal radioulnar joint can cause painful movement, restricted motion, and joint instability. Ideally, treatment should be directed at stable restoration of normal anatomy of the articular surface.

Although intra-articular fractures of the distal radius do not occur as a single, homogeneous pattern, the majority of these injuries contain a subset of five basic fracture elements: the radial column, ulnar corner, dorsal wall, volar rim, and free intra-articular fragments (**Fig. 12-1**). Occasionally, these fracture elements themselves may have further comminution. In addition to these cortical elements, these fractures may have other associated pathological processes, such as compressive damage to the metaphyseal bone, fractures of the distal ulna, and soft tissue injuries of the triangular fibrocartilaginous complex (TFCC), distal radioulnar joint (DRUJ), and radioulnar syndesmosis. In more complex fracture patterns, appropriate treatment of distal radius fractures often must be customized to the specific components and mechanism of the particular injury. Although recently there has been a rise in the popularity of fixed-angle volar plates for the treatment of distal radius fractures, this method of treatment can be inadequate for fractures with small distal fragments or injuries with complex, multiarticular patterns.[5] Treatment starts with careful analysis of the injury and initial postreduction radiographs.[6] When needed, computed tomography (CT) can supplement standard radiographs to help with the interpretation of the fracture pattern. These topics have been covered in previous chapters.

Fragment-specific fixation is a treatment approach in which each independent major fracture fragment is stabilized with an implant specifically designed for that particular fracture element (**Fig. 12-2**).[7-10] One objective of fragment-specific fixation is to restore a stable, anatomical joint surface by direct and independent fixation of each major fracture fragment. As a general rule, fragment-specific fixation is a load-sharing construct in which each fracture element is pieced back together into a unified composite structure. Fragment-specific implants are intentionally designed to be extremely low profile and conform to the local surface topography at the site of application, avoiding the need for bulky plates that can irritate tendons or large distal screw holes that can cause further comminution of small distal frag-

ments. Another goal of treatment is to achieve enough stability to allow motion immediately after surgery.

In some ways, fragment-specific fixation has certain similarities to simple, multiple Kirschner wires (K-wires). In each technique, individual fragments are reduced and secured to the proximal shaft. In each technique, a goal of treatment is to restore normal anatomy to the articular surface. Furthermore, each technique avoids extensive dissection and wide osseous exposure of the distal surface and eliminates fixation that depends on thread purchase in small distal fragments. Fragment-specific fixation, however, has some significant differences to fixation with multiple K-wires because it achieves a stable, load-sharing construct of the fracture components, allowing immediate motion without a cast postoperatively. In addition, fragment-specific fixation avoids potential problems of pin tract irritation and pin site infection, as well as the need to perform a second procedure to remove K-wires.

Fragment-Specific Implants

The radial border of the distal radius is often involved as a major component of distal radius fractures. In most cases this area breaks as the radial column, a single piece of bone that includes the scaphoid facet, the radial styloid, and the osseous pillar that extends proximally to the distal attachment of the brachioradialis tendon. The radial column is typically a large fragment that includes the orthogonal surfaces of the dorsal, radial, and volar cortices and is often a significant fracture element. Although trans-styloid pinning of the radial column is a simple technique, it usually results in rather tenuous fixation because stability is dependent on the stiffness of the K-wire as well as the purchase by the tip of the wire in the far cortex of the proximal fragment. Bending or small amounts of angulation of the K-wire at the site of purchase in the far cortex can result in significant shortening and displacement of the radial column fragment.

The radial pin plate is a fragment-specific implant designed specifically for stable fixation of the radial column fragment. Mechanically, this implant acts as an outrigger to add a second point of constraint to the pin at its entry site on the surface of the unstable radial column fragment. As a result, proximal drift of the K-wire is prevented because pin failure from bending or angulation at the site of purchase in the far cortex is eliminated. The radial pin plate creates a rigid pin construct that triangulates fixation to both near and far cortices of the proximal fragment. Because this maintains the length of the radial column, the carpus is held out to length, preventing collapse of the proximal carpal row into remaining unstable fragments within the lunate facet.

Although the primary function of the radial pin plate is to provide rigid fixation of the radial column, the radial pin plate has

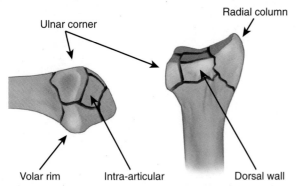

FIGURE 12-1 Fragment-specific classification. Articular fractures of the distal radius tend to propagate along recurrent pathways, resulting in generation of five basic fracture components: the radial column, ulnar corner, dorsal wall, free intra-articular, and volar rim. In addition to these distal radius fracture elements, impaction of the metaphyseal bone, DRUJ and distal ulna injuries, and intracarpal pathologic processes may affect the natural history of a particular fracture pattern.

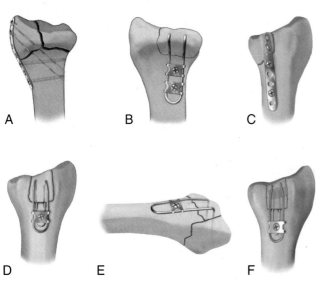

FIGURE 12-2 Fragment-specific implants. **A,** Radial pin plate for radial column fixation. **B,** Volar buttress pin for volar rim fixation. **C,** Ulnar pin plate for ulnar corner fixation. **D,** Small fragment clamp for dorsal wall fixation. **E,** Dorsal buttress pin for dorsal wall and free intra-articular fragment fixation. **F,** Small fragment clamp/buttress pin for combined dorsal wall and free intra-articular fragment fixation.

a secondary role that can also help with stabilization of many articular fractures. Although the plate is thin, because it is applied along the plane of the radial border, it is extremely stiff in resisting bending moments caused by flexion and extension movements of the wrist. Moreover, the radial pin plate is slightly overcontoured to the curve of the radial border and flattens like a leaf spring against the bone as it is secured to the proximal fragment. This causes the plate to push the distal fragment toward the ulna, locking intra-articular fragments in place and improving DRUJ stability by seating the ulnar head within the sigmoid notch of the radius. Because this property of the radial pin plate is quite effective in securing intra-articular fragments in whatever position they happen to be, it is generally a good idea to ensure that articular fragments are first fully reduced before securing the radial pin plate to the proximal fragment.

Although radial shear fractures are relatively uncommon, it should be noted that these injuries do not generate a typical radial

column fragment. In this fracture pattern, the carpus translates radially, causing a failure in shear across the tip of the radial styloid. Radial shear fractures have a characteristic radiographic image that shows a small triangular fragment that involves only the tip of the styloid; unlike the true radial column fracture, the fracture line does not extend proximally into dorsal, radial, and volar cortical surfaces. These injuries are associated with significant shear damage to the articular surface and often have free chondral fragments present in the joint as well as ligamentous tears within the carpus. In addition, injury to the TFCC and/or ulnar styloid is often observed with this pattern of injury. Although a radial pin plate can effectively stabilize radial shear fractures, in healthy bone satisfactory fixation can often be simply achieved with one or two screws.

The ulnar pin plate is a fragment-specific implant that is designed for dorsal fixation of the ulnar corner fragment. This fragment includes the dorsal portion of the sigmoid notch and is typically the result of axial impaction of the lunate against the dorsal surface of the lunate facet. The ulnar corner fragment displaces proximally and dorsally and can cause problems with DRUJ function. Although sometimes this fragment can be quite small, the fracture line nearly always extends to the radial side of the dorsal insertion of the DRUJ capsule. The ulnar pin plate should be used with an interfragmentary pin that penetrates the ulnar corner fragment and is directed proximally and slightly radially to engage the volar cortex of the shaft proximally. Like any plate placed dorsally along the ulnar border of the radius, a 15-degree torsional bend should be added proximally to the plate to match the twist of the dorsal surface of the radial shaft. In addition, the ulnar pin plate may also be used for fixation along the central or radial aspect of the dorsal wall.

Dorsal wire forms (buttress pin, small fragment clamp, and combined wire forms) are prebent 0.045-inch K-wires designed for stabilization of dorsal and free articular fragments. These implants are easily adapted for variations in the size and location of independent fragments. The buttress pin can be simply inserted like a clip and then used as a joystick to reduce and fix a dorsal fragment. Alternatively, the buttress pin can be easily applied through a dorsal defect behind free articular fragments to sandwich them against the proximal carpal row. Other dorsal wire forms include the small fragment clamp that can grab and stabilize dorsal wall fragments and the combination small fragment clamp/buttress pin that can address combined dorsal wall and free articular fragments. These implants may be supplemented with dorsal bone graft to provide additional support behind the distal articular surface.

The volar buttress pin is an implant that is designed for unstable fragments that involve the volar rim. Fragmentation of the volar rim is usually the result of either a volar shear or axial loading mechanism. If the volar rim fragment is small, plate fixation can be inadequate; flexion or axial loading of the wrist can cause this fragment to displace over the edge of the plate, carrying the carpus with it into the palmar soft tissues. Alternatively, if the volar rim fragment is dorsiflexed with a depressed teardrop angle, plate fixation may further aggravate the angular deformity by pushing up on the volar surface of the fragment. The volar buttress pin is often a simple, effective solution for these complicated problems. Like the dorsal buttress pin, the legs of the volar buttress pin can be driven like a clip into the volar rim fragment and the implant then used as a joystick to manipulate and correct the position and angular deformity of the fragment. Once reduction is achieved, the wire form is simply fixed proximally with two screws and washers or a small wire plate.

Fragment-specific implants can also be used to treat certain types of distal ulna fractures when indicated. The ulnar pin plate can be used to stabilize displaced fractures through the base of the ulnar styloid or ulnar head. Wire forms can also be used when indicated on the ulnar side.

Of course, it is possible to augment standard volar or dorsal plating techniques with fragment-specific implants when needed. For instance, a dorsal wire form can supplement a fixed-angle volar plate by securing an unreduced or unstable dorsal or free articular fragment. As another example, a radial column plate can be used as supplemental fixation to a volar plate to add stability to a radial column fragment or to push the distal fragment radially to close the DRUJ.

Fragment-specific fixation has the flexibility to address many different types of fracture patterns. Initially, this simple ability to mix and match implants to the characteristics of the fracture may seem a bit overwhelming. However, fragment-specific fixation is really nothing more than a complete set of tools that has the capability to address a variety of different fracture patterns. For many patterns, there are standardized algorithms that can be used for treatment and will be discussed in the next sections.

Surgical Approaches
Video

Radial Palmar Exposure

The surgical approach to apply a radial pin plate and volar buttress pin can be called "radial palmar" not only because of the implant locations but also because of the incision (**Fig. 12-3**). Typically, a 7-cm linear incision is made on the "radial palmar" aspect of the distal forearm, extending proximally from the level of the radial

styloid.[11] The incision is about halfway between the true midlateral line of the forearm and its palmar surface. Another way to situate the incision is to feel the radial artery pulse and make the incision a little radial to this landmark.

Longitudinal blunt dissection is carried out through the subcutaneous fat, and the numerous branches of the radial sensory nerve and the termination of the lateral antebrachial cutaneous nerve are identified and retracted. Although some patients may have quite a network of large and small sensory branches, these nerves can be retracted safely while still gaining adequate exposure to reduce and stabilize the fracture. Keep in mind that whenever K-wires or drill bits are used, soft tissue guides must be employed to prevent inadvertent damage to these sensory nerves (or other soft tissues structures).

The first extensor compartment is next identified and released to mobilize the abductor pollicis longus and extensor pollicis brevis tendons either dorsally or palmarly for exposure of the fracture segments. The extensor pollicis brevis usually has a separate subsheath that can be released. It is prudent to leave the last centimeter or so of the first extensor compartment sheath intact to reduce the likelihood of tendon subluxation postoperatively. The first compartment extensor tendons can be retracted dorsally, which will allow easy visualization of the brachioradialis tendon as it inserts at the base of the radial styloid in the midlateral plane.

The brachioradialis should be released for two reasons. Its insertion obscures access to the radial column fracture site and it must be released completely to allow mobilization of this segment. Additionally, the brachioradialis produces a deforming force on the radial column fracture and release of this tendon insertion reduces the tendency for subsidence of the fracture. The brachioradialis insertion becomes the floor of the first extensor compart-

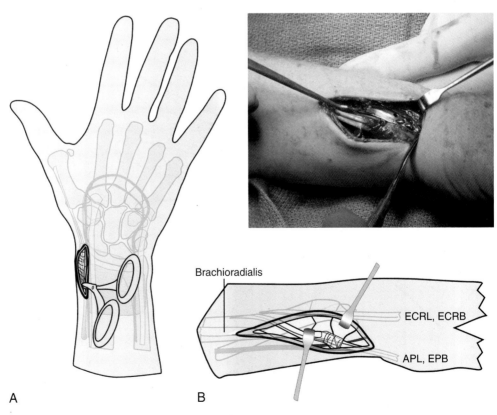

FIGURE 12-3 Radial palmar incision. **A**, Initial exposure with incision between the radial artery and the first dorsal compartment tendons. The tip of a tenotomy scissors is placed along the superficial surface of the first dorsal compartment sheath proximally and swept distally to elevate a skin flap that includes the sensory nerves along the radial border of the wrist. **B**, Completion of the radial column exposure by releasing the first dorsal compartment sheath proximally, leaving the distal 1 cm intact and reflecting the insertion of the brachioradialis. APL, abductor pollicis longus; EPB, extensor pollicis brevis; ECRL, extensor carpi radialis longus; ECRB, extensor carpi radialis brevis. **Inset**, Surgical photograph with radial pin plate applied through radial palmar incision.

Brachioradialis

ECRL, ECRB

APL, EPB

A

B

ment, and at the margins of the radial styloid prominence it blends into the first extensor compartment tendon sheath.

Once the brachioradialis has been released, dissection should be directed at the palmar side of the first extensor compartment's palmar sheath. Dissection should hug the palmar surface of the tendon sheath and stay radial to the radial artery, which is within a centimeter of the sheath, running parallel. The radial artery runs adjacent to the incision's ulnar margin, although at the distal part of the wound the artery starts to angle toward the base of the thumb metacarpal; and, for this reason, care should be exercised when dissecting in the distal part of the incision, where the artery starts to run *across* the incision line rather than parallel to it. As dissection proceeds toward the radial styloid's cortical surface, the artery and the radial insertion of the pronator quadratus can be swept ulnarly. It is possible to use a blunt elevator to expose the radial styloid and the entire palmar surface of the distal radius. A wide blunt retractor is ideal to safely retract the pronator quadratus, the median nerve, and flexor tendons palmarly and ulnarly so that the entire radial and palmar aspect of the distal radius can be visualized directly.

Closure of the wound is accomplished via suturing the subcutaneous layer and skin closure. Care should be taken to protect radial sensory nerve branches from entrapment during closure. The first extensor compartment tendons are allowed to return to their native positions, but repair of the tendon sheath is unnecessary. It should also be noted that repair of the brachioradialis is similarly not warranted.

Dorsal Exposure

Access to the dorsal aspect of the distal radius is required to address dorsal wall and ulnar corner fragments, as well as impacted free articular fragments. A dorsal exposure can also be used to aid in the reduction of particularly impacted radial styloid fragments

or help elevate and use bone grafts in depressed articular segments. The dorsal incision is longitudinal and typically 5 cm long, located about 1 cm radial to the ulnar head and ending about 1 cm distal to the radiocarpal joint line (**Fig. 12-4**). Although there are fewer sensory nerves deep to this incision compared with the radial palmar region, care should be taken to pursue blunt dissection until the extensor retinaculum is encountered. There are usually a few large veins that can be either retracted or cauterized. The retinaculum overlying the fourth extensor compartment is next opened longitudinally, and the common digital extensor (and extensor indicis proprius and extensor digiti quinti) tendons can be retracted ulnarly to expose the dorsal metaphyseal area. The extensor pollicis longus should be mobilized by releasing the retinaculum proximally in a longitudinal fashion; often the retinaculum overlying Lister's tubercle can be left in place and the extensor pollicis longus can be satisfactorily retracted radially. Occasionally, it can be helpful to fully release the extensor pollicis longus from Lister's tubercle, thereby allowing it to be retracted farther radially. This is particularly helpful when the dorsal wall fragment extends radially and involves Lister's tubercle as part of the fracture pattern.

Exposure of the dorsal fracture fragments requires patience and attention to detail. Although this part of the surgery does not need to take more than 10 minutes, two critical issues must be addressed to allow placement of the appropriate hardware. First, the soft tissue around the dorsal fragments must be released enough to enable both good direct visualization as well as adequate mobility of the individual fragments so that they can be reduced. Use of a small elevator is helpful to pry apart any hematoma, incipient fracture callus, and periosteal attachments so that dorsal fracture pieces can be clearly identified. Sometimes it is even necessary to free up the retinacular extensions of the second compartment tendons (wrist extensors) as well as transpose the

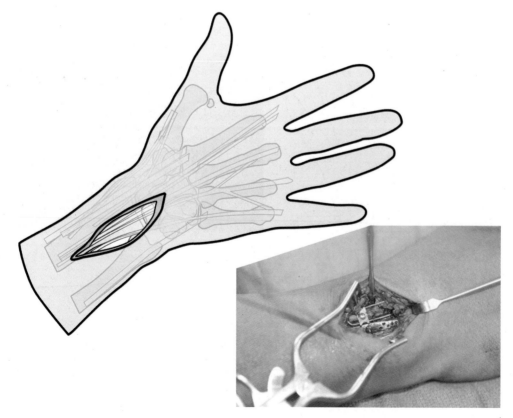

FIGURE 12-4 Dorsal incision. Longitudinal incision is made dorsally and extends about 1 cm beyond the distal border of the radius. Retinaculum is incised over the fourth dorsal compartment. **Inset,** Dorsal incision showing placement of ulnar pin plate and dorsal buttress pin.

extensor pollicis longus radially so that the dorsal wall and region around Lister's tubercle can be more easily treated.

The second critical issue relating to the exposure of dorsal fracture segments relates to identifying the proximal fracture perimeter. Fragment-specific fixation implants depend on a base of fixation that is anchored in the solid cortical bone proximal to the fracture; with the dorsal exposure, the shaft of the radius proximal to all fracture lines must be accessible. This can be facilitated by placing a narrow Hohmann retractor in the radial aspect of the wound, wrapping around the proximal, radial margin of the radial shaft. This maneuver will nicely demonstrate the step-off between the shaft of the radius and dorsal fracture fragments, which are usually buckled into each other and elevated dorsally by hematoma and comminution.

The terminal sensory branch of the posterior interosseous nerve is easily seen running just ulnar along the base of Lister's tubercle. Many surgeons will choose to intentionally transect this nerve at the most proximal margin of the wound to reduce the likelihood of developing a painful neuroma due to compression from either scar formation or metal implants.

Once fracture reduction and fixation have been accomplished, closure of the dorsal wound is routinely accomplished in two layers, with absorbable sutures for the subcutaneous fat layer followed by skin closure.

Fracture Patterns
Extra-articular Fracture

This is the typical "Colles'" pattern, which is a purely metaphyseal fracture that does not have a radiocarpal fracture extension. Whereas many fractures can be treated with a closed reduction and cast, this fracture type can benefit from internal fixation if there is palmar displacement or if dorsal displacement is significant and cannot be reliably controlled with other methods. Additionally, radial column shortening often occurs in older patients or when the initial injury mechanism includes axial loading; and if radial shortening progresses more than 5 mm, operative correction may be warranted in select cases.

Internal fixation of the metaphyseal fracture segment can be accomplished through a single, radial palmar incision. A secure construct and anatomical reduction can be achieved by using a radial pin plate and a volar buttress pin (**Fig. 12-5**). The radial pin plate restores radial column length, and the volar buttress pin prevents dorsal or palmar translation. The volar buttress pin also has the effect of anatomically reducing the thick cortical margin on the palmar surface of the radius, which helps resist the tendency for proximal subsidence of the metaphyseal segment. It should also be noted that a key effect of the radial pin plate is application of a medially directed vector on the metaphyseal segment, which not only aids in restoration of radial length but just as importantly reduces the DRUJ and allows the cortical perimeter of the distal radius to be anatomically reduced, adding stability to the whole construct. This fracture can be visualized like the top of a rectangular box that has been sawed off and the box top then slides a little sideways and has one or two sides overhanging the base. Exact realignment of the box top allows all four sides of the top to contact the base edges and provides four sides of support.

The radial styloid and entire metaphyseal fracture piece (which are together just one piece) can be reduced with the aid of an elevator inserted into the fracture site. Once the metaphyseal part is reduced, a smooth 0.045-inch K-wire is drilled through the

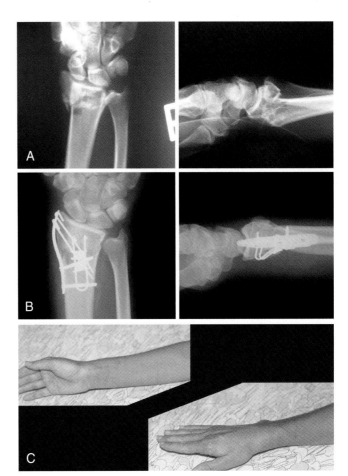

FIGURE 12-5 Extra-articular fracture fixed with a radial pin plate and volar buttress pin. **A,** Injury radiographs. **B,** Radiographs at 2 weeks with biplanar fixation with radial pin plate and volar buttress pin. Radial pin plate resists flexion and extension movements of wrist, maintains length to the radial border, and pushes distal fragment ulnarly to seat ulnar head within sigmoid notch. Volar buttress pin maintains orientation of the joint surface in the sagittal plane, resists radial and ulnar deviation, and helps to maintain length. **C,** Clinical appearance at 17 days after surgery.

radial styloid tip and secured into the cortical bone of the radial shaft, proximal to the fracture site. Anchoring the wire into cortical bone is critical to creating a strong construct. A radial pin plate is then placed over the K-wire, with the tip of the plate situated at the tip of the radial styloid. Checking the plate's position with intraoperative mini-fluoroscopy should confirm that the gentle curve of the radial pin plate matches the shape of the distal radius in the anteroposterior projection. Small adjustments may be necessary to situate the plate so that it exactly matches the contour of the radial styloid region. Bending the plate manually is usually not necessary and means that the plate is not seated correctly relative to the native curve of the radial styloid region. Additional proximal dissection of the brachioradialis is often required to allow the radial pin plate to sit on the cortical margin of the radial shaft in the midlateral line. Also, the placement of the radial styloid K-wire will determine where the plate sits at its distal tip. Having the wire situated too dorsally or too palmarly will cause the proximal end of the pin plate to ride off the radial shaft. The shape of the distal radius and, in particular, of the styloid region, can be misleading, because the styloid area looks quite prominent palmarly and there is a tendency to place the K-wire starting point too palmar. A good anteroposterior landmark is the first extensor tendon sheath. Placement of the K-wire exactly at the dorsal, outer margin of the tendon sheath's dorsal slip will usually result in the radial pin plate being seated in the exact midlateral line of the distal radius. If the plate is situated correctly, the first compartment tendons will cross over the plate in its distal third, with the pin holes of the plate being dorsal to the tendons and the screw holes of the plate being palmar to them.

Once the pin plate is correctly located, it is fixed to the radius shaft by placing two screws proximal to the fracture site. These are 2.3-mm screws that are predrilled with a 1.75-mm drill bit. Careful attention is required to make sure that the screws gain good purchase in the far (ulnar) cortex of the radial shaft and that the screws are not exiting through a fracture line. Tightening of these screws will compress the plate to the radial column and, by buttressing the radial side of the fracture and pushing the metaphyseal segment medially, will restore not only radial length but also DRUJ congruity. The 0.045-inch K-wire is then trimmed with a wire cutter, bent 180 degrees at its distal end, and tamped proximally so that it engages another pin hole in the pin plate and resists backing out. The length of the wire should be cut so that when taking into account the process of terminally seating into the pin plate it will just penetrate the proximal cortical margin of the radius. Gaining a cortical "bite" proximally is an important feature that adds strength to the pin plate construct. A second 0.045-inch K-wire is then placed in a similar fashion by drilling it through one of the remaining open pin holes in the plate, thereby traversing the distal fracture segment a second time and also gaining a proximal cortical purchase. This wire is also trimmed, bent 180 degrees at its distal end, and advanced to sit flush against the surface of the pin plate.

At this point, additional fixation can be applied to the palmar surface of the distal radius. There are rare circumstances in which a single radial pin plate may suffice, but this would be suitable for a small radial shear type fracture (that usually exits at the radiocarpal articular margin). For a metaphyseal, extra-articular fracture, the fracture segment is better secured with additional fixation. Placement of an implant at 90 degrees to the plane of the pin plate will tremendously strengthen the entire construct and prevent the fracture from subsiding, reangulating, or translating. Given the strength of the radial pin plate, another plate on the palmar surface of the distal radius is typically not necessary. Use of a volar buttress pin will prevent the fracture from shifting but is simple to apply.

To apply the volar buttress pin, a 0.045-inch K-wire or the 1.75-mm drill is used to place two unicortical pilot holes in the palmar surface of the fracture segment, usually 10 to 15 mm apart. The axis of the drill should be angled with the tip pointing proximally to match the shape of the subcortical bone of the distal radius and the "teardrop" contour of the radial styloid. The two pilot holes describe a line segment that is near perpendicular to the long axis of the radius. A volar buttress pin of appropriate length is then situated with each leg placed into one of the pilot holes. The buttress pin can be handled with a needle holder or wire bending forceps. If necessary, it is simple to modify the contour of the curve of the wire form with the three-point bender to match the flare of the distal radius. The legs of the buttress pin usually have to be shortened a little and cutting the radial leg slightly shorter than the ulnar one facilitates placement of the buttress pin legs into the pilot holes one side at a time. The volar buttress pin is then pressed down against the palmar surface of the radius; fluoroscopy should confirm that in the lateral projection the shaped buttress pin matches the contour of the palmar

cortex of the distal radius. The buttress pin is then fixed with a 2.3-mm screw and washer combination; often a second screw and washer is warranted to resist axial load on the implant. Firm fixation of the proximal loop of the implant should be obtained. When necessary, a blocking screw and washer rotated 90 degrees can be used just proximal to the proximal end of the implant to prevent shortening. Fluoroscopic assessment in the anteroposterior projection should show that the volar buttress pin legs are contained with the metaphyseal or subchondral bone, distal to the fracture line, and that the proximal extension of the buttress pin is situated over the radial shaft.

At this point, fluoroscopy can be used to recheck the fracture reduction and hardware placement. There should be no hardware prominent outside the cortical margins of the radius and full passive range of motion of the wrist in rotation, radial and ulnar deviation, and flexion and extension should be confirmed. Occasionally, bone graft can be applied after final irrigation of the wound, although often the reduction will be anatomical and secure enough that additional bone graft is unnecessary and has no place to reside.

As an alternative, extra-articular fractures may also be effectively treated with a radial pin plate along the radial column and dorsal fixation with either an ulnar pin plate or dorsal buttress pin (**Fig. 12-6**). Like the previous technique, these combinations

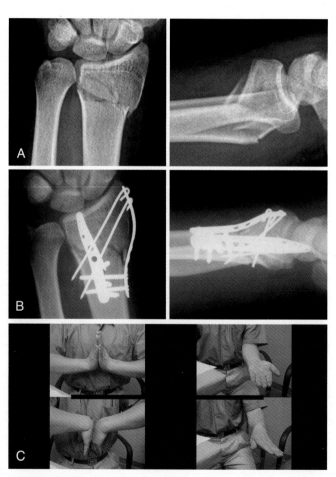

FIGURE 12-6 Extra-articular fracture fixed with a radial pin plate and ulnar pin plate. **A,** Injury radiographs. **B,** Biplanar fixation with a radial pin plate through a limited radial palmar approach and an ulnar pin plate through a limited dorsal approach. **C,** Clinical appearance at 8 weeks after surgery.

also create a 90/90-degree construct. Either a second dorsal incision can be used, or both implants can be placed through a single dorsal incision by elevating a radial skin flap and supinating the forearm to gain access to the radial column.

Volar Shear Fracture

The volar shear fracture is sometimes also referred to as an anterior marginal fracture or a "volar Barton" fracture. An oblique fracture line starts at the radiocarpal articular surface and exits on the palmar cortex of the radial metaphysis. The "shear" fragment has the wrist capsule and the extrinsic ligaments attached to it, and the entire carpus may sublux palmarly as the shear fragment displaces. Stabilization of this fracture segment requires a palmarly situated support, and this can be accomplished with a plate or volar buttress pin. A plate may be more appropriate if the fracture line exits proximally enough that the fracture fragment is large. In this case, it is easy to place a fixed-angle plate so that the distal margin of the plate supports the shear fragment. Placement of locking pins or screws at the plate's distal margin adds extra fixation to the shear fragment, although simply securing the plate to the palmar cortex of the radius so it can act as a buttress is the key mechanical feature that reduces this fracture pattern.

Sometimes the volar shear fragment will be very small, appearing more like a fracture through the very distal "lip" of the radius. In these cases, a volar plate can be awkward because the plate's edge has to be exactly at the edge of the radiocarpal joint to capture the fracture piece. It is easier to use a volar buttress pin in these situations. Two pilot drill holes (using a 0.045-inch K-wire or the 1.75-mm drill bit) can be made in the fracture segment and the volar buttress pin legs then inserted into the fracture fragment. Again, cutting one leg slightly longer than the other simplifies placement by allowing each leg to independently engage a hole as it is inserted. By securing the proximal end of the volar buttress pin to the radius shaft with one or two screw/washer constructs, the volar buttress pin can easily capture and reduce the marginal shear fragment.

Dorsal Shear Fracture

The dorsal shear fracture, or posterior marginal fracture, is equivalent to a "dorsal Barton" fracture and requires stabilization from the dorsal side (**Fig. 12-7**). Through a dorsal approach, this fracture can be secured by using an ulnar pin plate, or if the fracture segments do not extend too far proximally, a variety of wire forms can be applied to reduce the fracture. It is critical to gain solid purchase in good bone proximally, so if the fracture segment is large a pin plate (or even two pin plates) may be a better choice.

A dorsal shear component is often associated with many axial loading injuries with intra-articular involvement. In these more complex fracture patterns, other components of the fracture can divert attention from the dorsal pathological process, and it is possible to easily miss the dorsal subluxation of the carpus on the lateral projection of the wrist. It is important to check intraoperatively that the dorsal margin of the distal radius is stable and reduced. Any significant dorsal subluxation requires reduction and stabilization and typically mandates a dorsal exposure. Although it is possible to capture the dorsal fragment with locked screws anchored in a palmarly situated plate, the dorsal fragments are often comminuted and are characterized by thin cortical margins. Dorsally located wire forms or pin plates have a much better mechanical advantage in holding down the shear component, thereby reducing the carpus back into a normal position relative to the forearm axis.

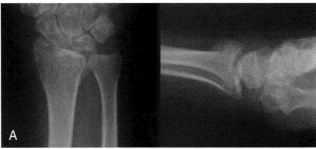
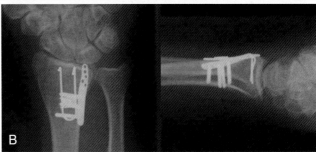

FIGURE 12-7 Dorsal shear fragment fixed with an ulnar pin plate and dorsal buttress pin. **A,** Injury radiographs. **B,** Internal fixation with an ulnar pin plate and dorsal buttress pin. Because of the uninvolved volar rim, the ulnar pin plate in this case could be used as a simple dorsal buttress plate.

Radial Shear Fracture

A pure radial shear fracture corresponds to the "chauffeur's fracture" eponym, in which the fracture line starts at the radial carpal margin and exits via an oblique path through the radial column cortex. This fracture can be associated with a carpal ligamentous pathological process, most commonly a scapholunate dissociation. The radial styloid fracture segment can be directly visualized through the radial palmar exposure and easily reduced using a radial pin plate. If the styloid segment is small, a three-hole radial pin plate may be all that is required. More commonly, however, the radial styloid involvement extends 2 cm more proximally and a five-hole radial pin plate affords better security. Whereas a pure radial shear pattern is not particularly common relative to the other more comminuted fracture patterns, if the radial styloid piece is indeed the only fracture segment present, then use of a single radial pin plate is all that is necessary.

Three-Part Articular Fracture

Three-part articular fractures are common low-energy injuries that are the result of a combination of dorsal bending and axial loading mechanisms. These fractures are characterized by a large radial column fragment and a smaller fragment at the ulnar corner of the dorsal radius. Although treatment with a fixed-angle volar plate is often effective, at times it is not adequate to reduce or stabilize the ulnar corner fragment. Fragment-specific fixation, on the other hand, provides a simple, direct approach that allows fixation of both radial column and dorsal fragments.[12] In addition, the fragment-specific approach to this pattern often requires a much more limited surgical exposure with less soft tissue dissection and is particularly appropriate for younger patients with higher functional demands.

The combination of a radial pin plate with either an ulnar pin plate or dorsal buttress pin is the most common fragment-specific approach for the treatment of three-part articular fractures (**Fig. 12-8**). Typically, this is done through a two-incision approach,

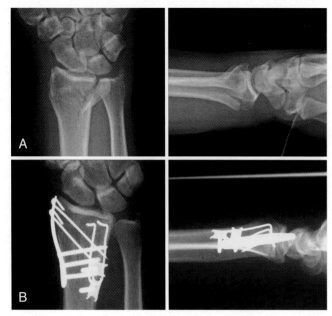

FIGURE 12-8 Three-part fracture treated with radial pin plate and dorsal buttress pin. **A,** Injury radiographs. **B,** Radiographs at 1 month show fixation of radial column with radial pin plate and simple fixation of ulnar corner with dorsal buttress pin.

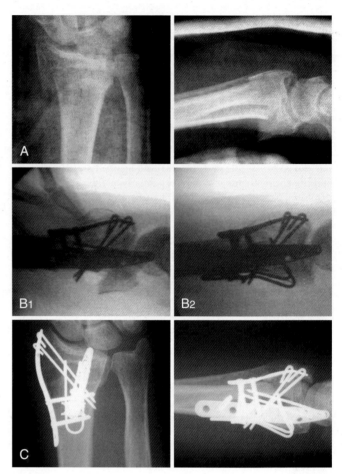

FIGURE 12-9 Multipart articular fracture fixed with radial pin plate, volar buttress pin, and ulnar pin plate. **A,** Radiographs after attempted closed reduction. **B,** Intraoperative films. **B1,** Note displacement of an independent volar rim fragment after stabilization of the radial column and dorsal fragments, with depression of the teardrop angle, increase in the anteroposterior distance, and a nonuniform joint interval. **B2,** Application of volar buttress pin with reduction of the volar rim and restoration of the anteroposterior distance, teardrop angle, and a uniform joint interval. **C,** Final postoperative radiographs.

using the radial palmar incision for application of the radial pin plate and a limited dorsal incision for applying the buttress pin or ulnar pin plate. Alternatively, this pattern may be approached through a single dorsal incision by elevating a subcutaneous flap radially and supinating the forearm to gain access to the radial column.

Complex Articular Fracture

Complex articular fractures are ideally suited for the fragment-specific approach (**Figs. 12-9** and **12-10**). The key to fractures with many pieces is that the reduction is achieved in little steps. Reduction and fixation of one part will have an influence on the ability to reduce another fragment, and, consequently, some "tweaking" of the reduction is required. The entire distal radius is like a puzzle that has several interlocking pieces, and sometimes it is necessary to alternate between different fracture pieces and "nudge" the reduction in different spots until the whole radius can be anatomically puzzled back together.

The radial palmar exposure is accomplished first, with release of the brachioradialis to help relax its deforming force on the radial styloid. Release of the radial insertion of the pronator quadratus will allow exposure of the palmar aspect of the radius, so that the palmar marginal cortex and the "teardrop" area can be fully inspected and manipulated. It is often helpful to reduce the radial styloid fragment with respect to length and angulation and then provisionally pin it in place with a single 0.045-inch K-wire placed through the tip of the styloid and anchored proximally in unfractured cortical bone. If a volar rim fragment is present, it is usually stabilized next.

Next, the dorsal exposure is achieved and the ulnar corner fragment is identified, cleaned, and reduced. It is important to properly reduce this fragment because bringing it back out to length will have the effect of restoring the correct palmar tilt to the distal radius. Sometimes, manipulation of the ulnar corner will need to be performed together with reduction of the dorsal

wall fragment (if a dorsal wall fragment is also present). When the ulnar corner fragment is reduced, a 0.045-inch K-wire should be drilled through its most distal and ulnar edge from the dorsal side. The K-wire needs to be directed proximally, palmarly, and somewhat radially, so that it engages cortical bone on the palmar radial shaft proximal to the fracture site. An ulnar pin plate (either three or five hole) is then placed over the K-wire and fixed to the dorsal surface of the radius. The plate can be twisted slightly with wire bending forceps so that it sits flush with the dorsal surface of the radius. Two screws (2.3-mm diameter) are used to fix the ulnar pin plate proximally, and then the K-wire is trimmed for length, bent over, and advanced so that it sits flush in the two most distal pin holes of the plate. If room allows, a second K-wire is then drilled through another open hole of the pin plate and similarly trimmed to length and bent over so that it engages two pin holes of the plate. Alternatively, the tips of the K-wires may be trimmed directly through the volar incision. Both K-wires should be just long enough that their proximal tips engage cortical bone of the radial shaft.

Fluoroscopy can be used to check hardware position and reduction of the ulnar corner. Particular attention should be paid to assessing the congruency of the DRUJ. Once the ulnar corner

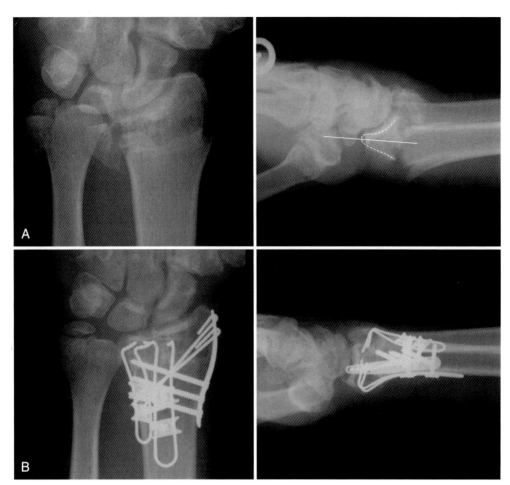

FIGURE 12-10 Highly comminuted intra-articular fracture pattern. **A,** Injury radiographs reveal presence of radial column, dorsal wall, ulnar corner, and volar rim fragments. Note outline of teardrop with depressed teardrop angle and dorsal subluxation of the carpus. There is a new fracture through the base of the ulnar styloid in addition to a preexisting ulnar styloid nonunion. **B,** Radiographs at 2 months after fragment-specific fixation.

has been reduced, attention can be returned to the radial styloid region. The provisional K-wire previously placed can be removed and relocated so that it is exactly in the tip of the radial styloid. A radial pin plate (usually five-hole length) is then placed over the K-wire and seated along the midlateral aspect of the radial column. By securing the plate with two 2.3-mm screws, it will push the radial styloid not only distally (restoring length) but also ulnarly, which has the effect of closing down any articular surface gaps and additionally restoring the correct inclination angle to the distal radius.

An alternative to fixation of dorsal wall or dorsal ulnar corner fragments is to use a dorsal buttress pin for fixation of larger fragments. In this technique, the fragment is reduced and two 0.045-inch K-wires inserted through the fragment parallel to the joint surface. The position and orientation of these pilot K-wires can be checked by initially placing a buttress pin upside down on the dorsal surface so that the legs point vertically up off the bone. The position and orientation of the legs is noted, and the pilot K-wires are inserted and checked with fluoroscopy. The buttress pin can then be contoured to fit any dorsal curve and the legs cut, leaving one leg longer than the other. The pilot K-wires are individually withdrawn and replaced with a corresponding leg of the buttress pin, and the wire form is fully seated. The buttress pin is secured proximally with one or two screws and washers or a small wire plate.

Any other fragments that are not reduced at this point can now be addressed. Sometimes a dorsal wall fragment will be

present, which can be stabilized with a small fragment clamp (wire form). Sometimes the third fragment will be the palmar ulnar corner, which can be buttressed upward with a volar buttress pin (secured with a proximal screw and washer). Restoration of the radial column can be performed as an intermediate step, after definitive fixation of the ulnar corner, or the radial column fixation can be reserved as a final maneuver, after stabilization of both the ulnar corner fragment and whatever other articular fragment is present.

The technique of fragment-specific fixation is characterized by some inherent "tinkering" with the fracture fragments and the hardware. The nature of multifragmented articular fractures is such that anatomical reduction of the entire distal radius requires puzzling little pieces back together, and sometimes a perfect reduction of one fragment will actually preclude another piece from being seated into place. Consequently, it may be necessary to make minor adjustments, alternating between individual pieces, so that the entire construct can be eventually reduced perfectly. It may be necessary, for example, to back out the radial styloid K-wire while reducing the ulnar corner if the K-wire blocks the ability of the ulnar corner fragment from being fully reduced. Similarly, if the ulnar pin plate is not holding the ulnar corner and/or the dorsal wall fragment fully out to length, the radial styloid fragment will not reduce properly when the radial column is addressed. Although the fracture-specific fixation method is characterized by a stepwise approach to the distal radius fracture, making numerous, alternating adjustments throughout the course of the surgery is essential to ultimately achieving an anatomical reduction of all the individual fracture fragments.

Volar Rim Fragment

A particularly challenging fracture fragment is the volar rim fragment along the palmar ulnar corner of the radius. This fracture segment is in the exact opposite position from the dorsal ulnar corner fragment. It is less common and typically has a square footprint that can be seen through the radial-palmar exposure. It can be readily stabilized because its palmar surface is thick cortical bone. Malposition of this fragment has the same implications as malposition of the dorsal ulnar corner: incongruity of the DRUJ and loss of forearm rotation. In addition, failure to stabilize this important fragment can result in progressive displacement with palmar subluxation of the carpus.

Visualization of the palmar corner fragment is best achieved by using a blunt, narrow retractor via the radial palmar exposure. This fracture fragment can be stabilized using a single volar buttress pin, although drilling the pilot holes in the fragment (for seating the volar buttress pin legs) can be difficult. Use of a soft tissue guide while drilling is mandatory, and sometimes making a separate small incision ulnar to the median nerve can be helpful. Careful, blunt dissection through a 1-cm incision, located longitudinally between the median nerve and ulnar neurovascular bundle, can be used to place the soft tissue sleeve to more easily drill two holes into the palmar corner fragment. Firm fixation of the volar buttress pin with two screws and washers is needed to avoid shortening of this fragment; when needed, a blocking screw and washer rotated 90 degrees in line with the wire form can help prevent sliding.

Ulnar Styloid Fracture

Whether an ulnar styloid fracture merits fixation is a topic beyond the scope of this chapter. If it is decided to internally fix this piece, it can be easily accomplished using the "ulnar sled" or a three-hole ulnar pin plate. Either of these fixation constructs is easy to apply and provides rigid fixation of the styloid.

Exposure of the ulnar styloid is accomplished through whichever method the surgeon prefers. The styloid itself can be stabilized by drilling two small holes in its tip with a 0.045-inch K-wire and then sliding the legs of the ulnar sled down into these holes. The outer wire margin of the ulnar sled can then be fixed to the ulnar neck with a single screw and washer. Alternatively, if an ulnar pin plate is used, a 0.045-inch K-wire is first drilled through the tip of the styloid fracture, anchoring the proximal tip of the K-wire in the cortical bone of the ulnar shaft or neck. The tip of the plate is bent 90 degrees and the distal most pin hole of a three-hole ulnar pin plate is then placed over this K-wire. The plate is fixed to the ulnar cortex using one or two 2.3-mm screws.

Implant Fixation: Technical Tips

The fragment-specific approach is characterized by making multiple small adjustments, and some technical pointers may be helpful. First, soft tissue drill sleeves should always be used when drill bits or K-wires are placed to avoid wrapping up tendons or superficial nerves. Having two such drill sleeves available makes their use convenient and timely and thereby makes it less likely that this important safety step will be skipped. A narrow blunt retractor (e.g., Army-Navy) is particularly useful in safely retracting the palmar soft tissues (including the median nerve and flexor tendons) when exposing the palmar aspect of the distal radius.

Careful use of this retractor will allow visualization of even the most medial aspect of the palmar distal radius.

K-wires specifically designed for use in fragment-specific fixation have stripes on them, marking every 5 mm. Paying close attention to the stripes will allow precise placement of the K-wires so that, at final implantation, they are long enough to engage proximal cortical bone but short enough that they do not protrude too far. Note that K-wires placed through the dorsal approach that protrude palmarly, can not only be felt but can also be seen through the radial palmar incision. By using an end-cutting wire cutter, it is a simple matter to trim off the prominent end of such a K-wire through the radial palmar incision, which precludes having to remove the K-wire and start over. Be sure to keep track of the trimmed wire end; it has a tendency to fly off the wire cutter jaws and embed itself in the pronator quadratus muscle belly.

When placing the radial pin plate, the insertion point for the trans-styloid K-wire is crucial. If this K-wire is placed too dorsally or too palmarly, it will cause the radial pin plate to sit improperly on the midlateral aspect of the radial shaft. This will not only change the force vector applied by the pin plate so that it does not push the radial styloid fragment medially but also make it likely that the proximal end of the plate will not sit on the radial shaft and make it impossible to secure with cortical screws. The anchoring K-wire for the radial pin plate should be in the midlateral plane, and location of this exact plane can be difficult owing to the irregular shape of the distal radius. A good landmark for placement of this K-wire is the periosteal attachment of the dorsal sheath of the first extensor compartment. Additionally, if the radial pin plate is seated properly, the first compartment tendons will pass over it obliquely, with the pin holes of the plate being located dorsal to the tendon pathway and the proximal screw holes of the plate lying underneath or just palmar to the tendons.

When bending K-wires to terminally implant their distal ends into pin holes of a pin plate, it can be useful to overcrimp the K-wire, thereby creating a hook effect that helps the wire "lock" into two adjacent pin holes. This creates extra grip for the K-wire and reduces the likelihood of loosening in the postoperative period.

Securing a volar buttress pin with a single screw and washer can be sufficient to hold reduction of a particular fracture segment. However, if the piece being held is large or is preventing the entire carpus from subluxing, consideration should be given to using two screw/washer constructs or placement of a screw proximal to the wire form (in the manner of a "blocking screw") so that the wire form cannot slide proximally.

Depressed articular segments can be nicely elevated and held in place using buttress pins, either from the dorsal or palmar side. However, it is prudent to add cancellous bone graft in the subchondral zone, which will help reduce fracture resorption and resist the tendency for subsidence. Remember that the patient's premorbid bone quality as well as the degree of comminution will have a major influence on the tendency for collapse of bone, and bone graft should be added liberally when needed.

Sometimes adjustments need to be made to the radial styloid reduction after a radial pin plate has already been secured to the shaft of the radius. These situations often relate to improving the radial column length a little bit more after other fracture segments have been reduced. Instead of removing the radial pin plate and starting over, a helpful trick can be to simply remove the distal K-wires from the pin holes, manually apply traction to restore length of the radial column, and re-drill new K-wires directly through pin holes. This method can also be used to make minor adjustments in the rotation or palmar tilt of the radial styloid.

In addition to the specialized wire-bending forceps, K-wire bending pliers, and wire impactors that typically come with fragment-specific fixation implant trays, there are other commonly found operative instruments that will aid in managing difficult distal radius fractures. Straight and curved small curets are useful for manipulating fracture voids, removing fracture debris, and applying bone graft. Dental picks as well as narrow impactors are invaluable for mobilizing and holding tiny cortical fracture fragments. An "end-cutting" wire cutter is useful for trimming K-wires that have already been implanted but protrude a little too far on the palmar surface of the radius.

Postoperative Care

Immediately after wound closure, a soft dressing is applied over the incision and the patient placed into a removable volar brace. Alternatively, the forearm can be placed into a forearm-based plaster splint that does not limit elbow motion and stops short of the distal palmar crease to allow full finger motion. If a plaster splint is used, this is converted at day 3 to a Velcro-type wrist splint, but patients are instructed that it is a "transitional" device to help them feel safe when they are out of the home for the first week. They are specifically encouraged *not* to wear it when sleeping or pursuing simple household activities. Occupational therapy can be started on postoperative day 3, and most patients are encouraged to stop at the hand therapy clinic before going home from the first dressing change.

Therapy orders specify active and careful passive motion of the wrist joint in all planes, and immediate elbow and finger motion is mandatory. Patients tend to have significant dorsal hand swelling, especially if both a radial palmar and a dorsal incision were required, although swelling typically improves dramatically within the first week. Recovery of forearm rotation can be accomplished almost immediately, and this provides enormous functional benefits that tend to facilitate early recovery of wrist motion in the other planes.

Patients are directed to attend therapy sessions twice per week. In addition to a dressing change on postoperative day 3, office visits are scheduled on postoperative day 10 for suture removal and then once every 2 weeks thereafter until their motion and function have reached 85% of normal. This goal is typically reached within the first 6 weeks after surgery.

Complications

Injury to normal structures is always a possibility in any operation, especially during surgical exposures that are in close proximity to nerves and arteries.[13] It is important to carefully protect the radial artery and vein during the radial-palmar approach and be aware that the artery crosses obliquely over the distal portion of the incision. Although release of the arm tourniquet is rarely necessary before wound closure, if the artery or any of its small branches are particularly troublesome to mobilize, release of the tourniquet to check for bleeding may avoid a postoperative hematoma.

The radial sensory and terminal branches of the lateral antebrachial cutaneous nerves have numerous branches that need to be retracted or mobilized during the initial part of the radial-palmar approach. Although it is quite common for patients to note a "strip" of numbness along the midlateral wrist ending at the dorsal aspect of the thumb metacarpal, this numbness tends to resolve by itself within a few months and requires no treatment.

Development of a painful, radial sensory neuroma is possible but extremely uncommon.

When both the radial palmar and dorsal incisions are required, it might seem as though the incisions could produce local ischemia to the soft tissue island between them. In reality, this problem has never been reported, although it is prudent to make sure that the radial palmar and dorsal incisions are longitudinal and meticulously located so that they are almost 180 degrees apart relative to the diameter of the wrist. It is probable that the close location of the radial artery and its branches to the radial palmar incision creates a zone of vascularity that adds an extra margin of safety for soft tissue viability.

Despite the location of the radial pin plate under the first compartment extensor tendons, symptomatic tendinitis related to this pin plate is very rare. Occasionally a K-wire loosens and starts to back out, causing pain and prominence in the skin. Being meticulous about K-wire length and making sure that the proximal end of the K-wire fully engages *cortical* bone will prevent loosening. Additionally, it is possible to overbend the distal tip of the K-wire so that when it engages the pin plate through two adjacent pin holes, the K-wire actually grips tightly between the pin holes and strongly resists loosening. In cases where K-wires have loosened and become symptomatic (typically from the radial pin plate), they can usually be removed easily in the office setting.

The screws used to anchor pin plates and wire forms are self tapping, and, consequently, if they are prominent, the sharp cutting tips can potentially injure soft tissues. In particular, if self-tapping screws are placed on the palmar side of the radius and the sharp tip protrudes dorsally, it is theoretically possible to erode and rupture any of the digital extensors. Careful attention to screw length will prevent this. K-wires should be trimmed to length so that they protrude modestly past cortical margins but not enough to be externally palpable or irritate local structures.

Release of the carpal tunnel at the time of fracture fixation is rarely indicated. However, if the patient has pronounced median paresthesias before surgery, then a carpal tunnel release coincident with fracture surgery may be prudent. Patients who present with preoperative symptoms of median nerve compression often have high-energy injuries or fracture patterns that either impale the median nerve or stretch it over severe palmar angulation. It is certainly worthwhile to look for any median nerve pathology while obtaining the preoperative history and physical examination so that clues to median nerve compromise can be identified ahead of time. The radiographic appearance of the fracture before initial closed reduction attempts and the mechanism of injury can also be valuable predictors of potential median nerve compromise.

One simple cause of loss of reduction may be simply related to failure to recognize a major fracture component. Carpal subluxation or shortening can occur either on the dorsal side from a dorsal wall or ulnar corner fragment that is left untreated or on the palmar side from a missed volar rim fragment. Careful evaluation of radiographs both at the time of injury as well as during operative stabilization can help identify major components of the fracture pattern so that major sources of instability are not missed.

Clinical Outcome Data

There have been only a few published reports regarding the outcome of fragment-specific fixation to date. Use of fixed-angle plates as the sole implant to stabilize comminuted distal radius fractures has gained popularity, and good results have been reported.[14] Use of a fixed-angle plate as the only approach to distal radius fractures is certainly attractive due to the simplicity of operative planning and ease of application. A prospective, controlled study directed comparing the surgical morbidity and clinical outcomes of comminuted intra-articular fractures treated with fixed-angle plates and a fragment-specific approach has not yet been published, and these types of studies would be needed to clearly advocate one method over another.

Some authors, however, have noted that the stability of highly comminuted distal radius fractures depends also on reduction and fixation of smaller fragments in addition to the major fracture segments.[15] Additionally, biomechanical studies have demonstrated that pin plates, wire forms, and K-wires as used in a fragment-specific approach are more stable than K-wire–supplemented external fixation.[16] Using cadaver models, Taylor and coworkers showed that fragment-specific constructs were comparable in strength to fixed-angle plates and that ulnar corner fractures of the distal radius were much better addressed via a fragment-specific approach.[17] Grindel and coworkers showed that fragment-specific implants used with a fixed-angle plate provided a stronger construct than use of a fixed-angle plate alone.[18] In addition to the biomechanical evidence supporting the stability of fragment-specific fixation, it should also be realized that comminuted distal radius fractures present with a wide variation in stability and fracture geometry and that a fragment-specific approach uniquely enables internal fixation to be tailored to the exact needs of the fracture.

Konrath and colleagues reported on 27 patients with a 2-year minimum follow-up treated by fragment-specific fixation.[19] Pin plates and various wire forms were used in all patients. There was a high level of patient satisfaction, and only one fracture lost reduction; there were no tendon ruptures. Schnall reported on two groups of patients treated with fragment-specific fixation.[20] Group 1 consisted of 20 patients with high-energy trauma, and group 2 consisted of 17 patients treated at another institution.

Average time to return to work in group 1 was 6 weeks and all fractures united. In group 2, there was no significant loss of reduction and grip strength averaged 67% that of the contralateral limb.

A research group for one of the authors (L.S.B.) recently performed a retrospective evaluation of 81 patients, representing 85 intra-articular distal radius fractures, with a minimal follow-up of 1 year (mean follow-up, 32 months).[21] All patients were treated with fragment-specific fixation and were evaluated at final follow-up with physical examination, repeat radiographs, and outcome scoring according to Gartland and Werley as well as a Disabilities of the Arm, Shoulder, and Hand (DASH) outcome survey. Patients were allowed to start motion in the immediate postoperative period and underwent supervised occupational therapy for at least the first month after surgery.

Within the first 6 weeks after operation, 62% of patients achieved a 100-degree arc of motion in the flexion/extension plane as well as normal forearm rotation. Comparison of radiographs between final follow-up and immediately after surgery demonstrated that fracture alignment was maintained and that no cases of post-traumatic arthritis had developed. The average DASH score was 9 and, using Gartland and Werley scoring, 61% of patients had excellent and 24% had good results. Grip strength of the operated side recovered to 92% of that of the uninjured side and the flexion/extension range of motion of the fractured wrist, when compared with the normal side, averaged 85% and 92%, respectively. Analysis of the fracture reductions obtained with the fragment-specific approach showed that palmar tilt was on average within 4 degrees of the normal side and that ulnar variance changed on average by 1.2 mm. Average changes for radial height and inclination angle were within 1 mm and 1 degree of the uninjured side, respectively. Articular congruity was unchanged. There were no infections or complications relating to nerve, artery, or tendon injuries. Several patients required a second operation to address symptomatic hardware; overall, the rate of

TABLE 12-1 Fragment-Specific Fixation: Average Clinical Motion and Grip

	AO Type A		AO Type C Volar Displaced		AO Type C Nonvolar Displaced	
Follow-up period	1 mo	1.5 yr	1 mo	9 mo	1 mo	1 yr
Palmar flexion	38	79	51	55	42	76
Dorsiflexion	43	85	58	65	45	80
Radial deviation	8	14	11	13	10	16
Ulnar deviation	16	27	21	22	17	26
Pronation	65	88	87	75	69	87
Supination	54	87	80	75	59	84
MCP extension	−3	−5	−4	−4	−3	−5
MCP flexion	87	99	104	98	89	100
Injured grip	10	11	24	29	14	27
Uninjured grip	27	13	44	36	33	34

MCP, metacarpophalangeal.

TABLE 12-2 Fragment-Specific Fixation: Average Radiographic Measurements

	AO Type A			AO Type C Volar Displaced			AO Type C Nonvolar Displaced		
	Injury	Postop	Final (1 yr)	Injury	Postop	Final (1 yr)	Injury	Postop	Final (1 yr)
Radial height	6.0	11.2	12.6	6.2	13.2	11.0	5.1	11.0	11.4
Radial inclination	10.1	11.2	12.6	6.2	26.5	22.2	9.7	24.3	25.6
Ulnar variance	2.0	−1.2	−0.4	2.8	0.3	−0.2	2.1	−1.0	−1.0
Articular step-off	0.5	0.0	0.0	2.3	0.3	0.4	2.2	0.2	0.1
Articular separation	0.6	0.0	0.0	3.6	0.0	0.2	3.1	0.1	0.1
Volar tilt	−21.5	4.2	2.6	23.6	8.5	9.0	−24.2	5.1	6.0
Anteroposterior distance	18.5	18.7	17.4	21.6	19.3	19.0	21.0	18.6	18.7
Radiocarpal interval	2.1	2.0	2.6	2.1	1.9	1.9	2.0	2.0	1.8
Teardrop angle	34.2	62.3	62.3	67.7	67.3	70.0	25.5	63.1	63.8
Radiocarpal arthritis (0-3)	0.0	0.0	0.0	0.4	0.3	0.4	0.0	0.0	0.2
DRUJ arthritis (0-3)	0.0	0.0	0.0	0.0	0.0	0.4	0.0	0.0	0.1

hardware removal after the primary procedure was 6%. One patient required a second operation 9 months after the primary procedure to perform a distal ulna resection to address painful forearm rotation.

The clinical experience from the other author (R.J.M.) is quite similar. Over an 8-year period, 187 unstable distal radius fractures were treated with internal fixation; of these, 136 fractures had fragment-specific fixation. There were 24 A3 fractures (unstable bending injuries), 16 C1 fractures (three-part articular fractures), 4 shear fractures (AO type B2 and B3), and 92 comminuted articular fractures (AO type C2 and C3). In all but three patients, motion was started immediately after surgery. Resistive loading was not allowed until signs of radiographic healing was evident on follow-up radiographs. By 1 month, patients regained an average motion of over 80 degrees of flexion/extension arc, 60 degrees of supination, and 70 degrees of pronation. Finger motion returned rapidly. In addition, grip strength at 1 month averaged 50% of the uninvolved side, increasing to an average of 90% of the uninvolved side by final follow-up (**Table 12-1**).

Radiographs on these patients showed near-anatomical restoration of the joint surface, with correction of radiographic parameters postoperatively that remained essentially unchanged until union (**Table 12-2**). All fractures united. Three fractures had failure of fixation, and two patients had a dorsal extensor tendon rupture, although the cause of one tendon rupture was from an untreated but displaced dorsal fragment. Final DASH scores were 8 ± 10 for AO type A fractures, 30 ± 21 for displaced AO type C fractures with volar displacement, and 13 ± 18 for displaced AO type C fractures with axial or dorsal displacement (with a range from 0 to 100 with 0 being the best DASH score possible). Patient-Rated Wrist Evaluation (PRWE) scores were 1 ± 2 for AO type A fractures and 2 ± 2 for AO type C fractures (with a range from 0 to 10 with 0 being the best PRWE score possible) (**Table 12-3**).

TABLE 12-3 Fragment-Specific Fixation: Clinical Outcome Scores

Fracture Type	Avg DASH	Avg PRWE
AO type A (2 year)	8 ± 10	1 ± 2
AO type C volar displaced (6 months)	30 ± 21	2 ± 2
AO type C nonvolar displaced (1 year)	13 ± 18	2 ± 2

DASH, Disabilities of the Arm, Shoulder, and Hand (DASH) outcome survey; PRWE, Patient-Rated Wrist Evaluation (PRWE) score.

Conclusion

Fragment-specific fixation is an entirely different concept for treatment of distal radius fractures than traditional plates and screws. Fragment-specific fixation really starts with analysis of the fracture pattern, with careful examination of the radiographs to identify the presence and displacements of various fracture components, the mechanism of injury, and the presence of any associated pathological process along the ulnar column. The surgical approach needs to be selected so that direct exposure of each fracture element can be obtained; occasionally, this means exposures that are capable of 360-degree access around the wrist to reach independent palmar-, radial-, dorsal-, and ulnar-based fragments. Stabilization of each major fracture component is done in a staged and progressive manner, allowing each piece of the puzzle to be fit and locked together as a dynamic, load-sharing construct. Ultimately, the goal of fragment-specific fixation is the restoration of an anatomical, articular surface with enough stability to start early or even immediate motion after surgery.

Fragment-specific fixation is a highly flexible technique that can allow "minimal implant surgery" for simple bending fractures yet can provide all of the tools necessary for stable restoration of highly complex articular injuries. The technical difficulty of fragment-specific fixation is directly proportional to the complexity of the fracture pattern. Extra-articular fractures and simple three-part articular fractures can be typically treated with straightforward surgical techniques; highly comminuted articular injuries often require a piecemeal approach to sequentially interlock the various fracture components back together and consequently are more demanding. Although treatment of the more complex articular fractures often requires a higher level of surgical skill and expertise, these are often the very same fracture patterns in which fragment-specific fixation is the only reasonable option capable of reconstructing the articular surface.

The best appeal of fragment-specific fixation may be that it allows the flexibility to treat almost any type of fracture pattern of the distal radius and can allow the surgeon to develop a fixation plan based on the character of the injury. Sometimes, hidden or unsuspected components of the injury only become evident during surgery as fragments are pieced together; with fragment-specific fixation, these surprises can be directly addressed.

Finally, fragment-specific fixation has been shown to provide enough stability to allow early motion after surgery. Although the long-term outcomes for simple extra-articular fractures may not be significantly different, early motion certainly allows earlier return to work and faster recovery, with less downtime from immobilization. The benefit of early use of the injured arm for normal daily activities can have a profound positive impact on recovery psychology as well as re-integration into a more normal home and work lifestyle; most patients are extremely pleased with the acceleration in recovery. For complex, intra-articular fractures, restoration of a stable articular surface combined with early motion appears to have significant benefits for both short-term as well as long-term outcome.

REFERENCES

1. Knirk J, Jupiter J: Intra-articular fractures of the distal end of the radius in young adults. J Bone Joint Surg Am. 1986; 68:647-659.
2. Catalano L, Cole R, Evanoff R, et al: Displaced intra-articular fractures of the distal aspect of the radius: long-term results in young adults after open reduction and internal fixation. J Bone Joint Surg Am. 1997; 79:1290-1302.
3. Missakian M, Cooney W, Amadio P, Glidewell H: Open reduction and internal fixation for distal radius fractures. J Hand Surg [Am]. 1992; 17:745-755.
4. Trumble T, Schmitt S, Vedder N: Factors affecting functional outcome of displaced intra-articular distal radius fractures. J Hand Surg [Am]. 1994; 19:325-340.
5. Medoff R: Plating of distal radius fractures. In Trumble T, Budoff J, eds: Wrist and Elbow Reconstruction & Arthros-

copy: A Master Skills Publication. Rosemont, IL: American Society for Surgery of the Hand, 2006.
6. Medoff R: Essential radiographic evaluation for distal radius fractures. Hand Clin. 2005; 21:279-288.
7. Leslie B, Medoff R: Fracture specific fixation of distal radius fractures. Tech Orthop. 2000; 15:336-352.
8. Medoff R: Fragment specific fixation of distal radius. In Trumble T, Budoff J, eds: Wrist and Elbow Reconstruction & Arthroscopy: A Master Skills Publication. Rosemont, IL: American Society for Surgery of the Hand, 2006.
9. Bae D, Koris M: Fragment-specific internal fixation of distal radius fractures. Hand Clin. 2005; 21:355-362.
10. Barrie K, Wolfe S: Internal fixation for intraarticular distal radius fractures. Tech Hand Up Extrem Surg. 2002; 6:10-20.
11. Swigart C, Wolfe S: Limited incision open techniques for distal radius fracture management. Orthop Clin North Am 2001; 30:317-327.
12. Shumer E, Leslie B: Fragment-specific fixation of distal radius fractures using the Trimed device. Tech Hand Up Extrem Surg. 2005; 9:74-83.
13. Cooney W, Dobyns J, Linscheid R: Complications of Colles' fractures. J Bone Joint Surg Am. 1980; 62:613-619.
14. Orbay J, Fernandez D: Volar fixed-angle plate fixation for unstable distal radius fractures in the elderly patient. J Hand Surg [Am]. 2004; 29:96-102.
15. Harness N, Jupiter J, Orbay J, et al: Loss of fixation of the volar lunate facet fragment in fractures of the distal part of the radius. J Bone Joint Surg Am. 2004; 86:1900-1908.
16. Dodds S, Cornelissen S, Jossan S, Wolfe S: A biomechanical comparison of fragment-specific fixation and augmented external fixation for intra-articular distal radius fractures. J Hand Surg [Am]. 2002; 27:953-964.
17. Taylor K, Parks B, Segalman K: Biomechanical stability of a fixed-angle volar plate versus fragment-specific fixation system: cyclic testing in a C2-type distal radius cadaver fracture model. J Hand Surg [Am]. 2006; 31:373-381.
18. Grindel S, Wang M, Gerlach M, et al: Biomechanical comparison of fixed-angle volar plate versus fixed-angle volar plate plus fragment-specific fixation in a cadaveric distal radius fracture model. J Hand Surg [Am]. 2007; 32:194-199.
19. Konrath G, Bahler S: Open reduction and internal fixation of unstable distal radius fractures: results using the Trimed system. J Orthop Trauma. 2002; 16:578-585.
20. Schnall S, Kim B, Abramo A, Kopylov P: Fixation of distal radius fractures using a fragment specific system. Clin Orthop Relat Res 2006; 445:51-57.
21. Benson L, Minihane K, Stern L, et al: The outcome of intra-articular distal radius fractures treated with fragment-specific fixation. J Hand Surg [Am]. 2006; 31:1333-1339.

Volar Plate Fixation

Alejandro Badia, MD and Prakash Khanchandani, MS

13

Fractures of the distal end of the radius have been estimated to account for nearly 20% of all fractures seen routinely in an emergency department.[1] Despite this, until very recently the distal radius fracture was not treated as aggressively as other less common periarticular fractures. Perhaps Abraham Colles' perception that this fracture had good outcomes no matter what was done had permeated our thinking. The reality is that frequent poor outcomes in wrist injury fueled a gradual, albeit delayed, pursuit of a better treatment option.[2]

Distal radius fractures are usually sustained by elderly osteoporotic patients after a fall or by younger patients as a result of high-energy trauma. Both of these fractures deserve stable internal fixation: the former is due to osteoporotic bone that demands sound fixation principles, and the latter requires the ability to reduce intra-articular comminuted fragments in a stable manner that maintains the reduction and permits early mobilization. Until the advent of volar fixed-angle plating, no technique could satisfy these requirements in a consistent manner.

Rationale and Basic Biomechanics

Although the concept of volar plating could be initially attributed to Lanz and Kron[3] back in 1976 for plate fixation after osteotomy of malunited distal radius fractures, the volar approach remained restricted to fixation of volar rim fractures in the acute setting only.[4] Volar plating was first recommended for fixation of both typical and atypical distal radius fractures by Georguoulis and associates in 1992.[5] This was published in a little-known journal and was not widely accepted for dorsally displaced fractures until the landmark paper by Orbay and Fernandez in 2002.[6] Volar plating offers many advantages when used in dorsally displaced fractures. The key to its success is to ensure that this was a locking plate, hence creating a fixed-angle device that would maintain the reduction and eliminate screw toggle (**Fig. 13-1**). Volar plating also provides the opportunity to release the pronator quadratus muscle, which is often trapped in the fracture and can be a cause of pronation contracture. A nonlocking plate when used in buttress mode can resist only moderate axial and bending forces. Thus, a simple nonlocking volar plate used in a dorsally displaced fracture without any bony contact in the opposite cortex is subject to much higher axial and bending loads, leading to failure. Therefore, a stable and strong volar fixation of a dorsally displaced fracture is only possible with a fixed-angle locking plate that can resist such high forces. Fixed-angle implants transfer load stress from the fixed distal fragment to the intact radial shaft, thus enhancing peg/plate/bone construct stability (**Fig. 13-2**), unlike rigid internal fixation devices that rely mainly on the frictional force between plate and bone to achieve fixation.[7]

The ideal volar implant should have a design compatible with the volar articular surface of the radius and should provide concomitant angular and axial stability while stabilizing the dorsal surface.[8] The distal volar plate (DVR Hand Innovations, Depuy Orthopedics, Warsaw, Indiana) has two parallel rows, and the orientation planes of their respective pegs specifically match the complex three-dimensional shape of the radial articular surface. The primary row pegs are directed obliquely from proximal to distal to support the dorsal aspect of the articular surface. They are angled accurately to provide support for the radial styloid and the dorsal ulnar fragment. These pegs are most effective in supporting the dorsal aspect of the subchondral plate and hence avoid the re-displacement of the dorsally displaced fractures. Concurrently, their action induces a volar force that tends to displace the fragments in a volar direction, an effect that must be opposed by a properly configured volar buttressing surface. To enhance fracture fixation in cases of severe comminution, volar instability, or osteoporosis, an additional row of pegs originating from a more distal position on the plate and having an opposite inclination to the proximal row was conceived. The distal row is directed in a relatively proximal direction and crosses the proximal row at its midline and is intended to support the more volar and central part of the subchondral bone. It prevents the dorsal rotation of a volar marginal fragment and volar rotation of severely osteoporotic or unstable distal fragments with central articular comminution, thus neutralizing volar displacing forces of the pegs in the proximal row.

Newer generation of volar plates have now introduced the concept of variable-angle locking screws and/or pegs. This provides the distinct advantage of being able to vary the plate placement with the locking screws adjusting to the necessary angle to be placed in the strongest subchondral bone. One of the newest generation plates, APTUS (Medartis, Basel, Switzerland), utilizes a revolutionary multidirectional infinitely variable locking system facilitated by the Trilock concept—a spherical three-point wedge locking mechanism. Other variable locking systems utilize variable hardness of materials whereby the threaded peg literally cuts its own thread. The biomechanical soundness of these newer systems remains to be seen, and clinical studies are forthcoming.

Indications and Contraindications

Volar plating is indicated in nearly all unstable fractures of the distal radius. It is used in young and active patients for optimal reconstruction of the articular surface and restoration of bony anatomy while allowing nearly immediate, but protected, active range of motion. It is also ideally suited for polytraumatized patients facing potential rehabilitation problems or elderly patients who particularly benefit from a quicker recovery. The inherent biomechanical advantages previously mentioned lead us to indicate this approach for virtually all cases.

An unstable distal radius fracture has been defined as a fracture that, after an attempt at closed reduction, demonstrates

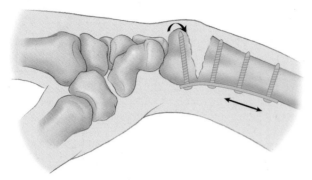

FIGURE 13-1 Schematic diagram showing volar fixation maintaining the anatomy of the radius but screw toggle leads to plate motion relative to the shaft, which can lead to late failure.

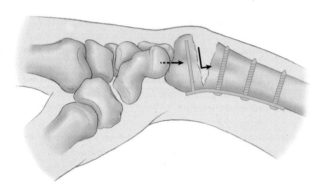

FIGURE 13-2 Schematic diagram showing fixed-angle implant transferring load stress from the fixed distal fragment to the proximal radial shaft.

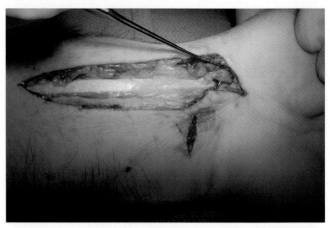

FIGURE 13-3 Identifying the superficial radial artery in the distal Henry approach between the flexor carpi radialis and radial artery proper. The zigzag extension of the incision across the creases minimizes hypertrophic scarring and improves exposure for more distal fractures.

radiographic evidence of more than 15 degrees of angulation in any plane, articular step-off of more than 2 mm, and/or radial shortening of more than 2 mm.[6] However, fractures with severe comminution or pronounced initial articular displacement or that are simply osteoporotic are also termed "unstable" despite possible initial good alignment.

Malunions and the rare nonunions after distal radial fractures can also be considered for this procedure with slight modification of technique.

The ideal timing for the surgery is within 1 week of injury, although this implant can be used in a patient even after a malunion of the fracture after other forms of managements. There is no time limit for the procedure as such, and volar plating can be used even after consolidation for correction of the deformities.

The absolute contraindications for volar plating are severely contaminated open injuries and compartment syndrome. The relative contraindication is open distal radial epiphysis in which smooth wires are preferable. The rare distal shear fracture is also poorly suited for volar plate fixation because the fragments may not be substantial enough to permit purchase of the volarly placed pegs. These severe comminuted fractures can be managed with external fixation maintaining relative wrist alignment, arthroscopic reduction, and excision of small osteochondral fragments with subchondral fixation by K-wires supporting the reduction. Age or medical status should not be a contraindication unless the patient absolutely cannot undergo surgery of any type. In these scenarios, one must accept the resultant malunion unless an attempt is made to use simple K-wire fixation utilizing local anesthesia.

Surgical Technique

Web V

13-

Unless the patient suffered polytrauma, or is medically unstable, the internal fixation procedure is performed in the outpatient setting. Regional anesthesia, usually a three-nerve block at the elbow level, is performed along with intravenous sedation to control tourniquet discomfort. Axillary regional blocks are more difficult to perform and have occasional complications. Bier blocks can have profound systemic complications and take longer to take effect. This is not as practical in the ambulatory setting of a busy surgery center running two rooms sequentially.

The patient is placed in the supine position with the arm extended on the hand table. A simple fracture less than 7 to 14 days old can be managed through a standard flexor carpi radialis (FCR) approach (distal Henry) (**Fig. 13-3**). On the other hand, complex intra-articular fractures, nascent malunions, and 2- to 3-week old fractures require a more extensile exposure, facilitated via the extended FCR approach.[9] This approach allows an intrafocal reduction by using the fracture plane itself to reduce the articular major fragments. The radial shaft (proximal fragment) is rotated into pronation (**Fig. 13-4**), allowing fracture reduction, and the shaft is then supinated back into anatomical position. The first step is to release the sheath of the FCR and identify the pronator quadratus between the FCR sheath floor and radial artery, which seats deep to the flexor pollicis longus and flexor digitorum superficialis muscle bellies. An L-shaped incision is made in the fascia of the pronator quadratus to allow proximal and ulnar reflection to expose the fracture site and distal shaft of the radius. A more thorough exposure of the volar surface of the radius, including the volar rim of the lunate fossa, is then performed. At this point, the brachioradialis must be released subperiosteally to improve exposure and allow reduction of the radial column. Specifically, the sheath of the first dorsal compartment is opened starting proximally, the abductor pollicis longus is retracted, and the insertion of the brachioradialis on the radial styloid is identified. A step-cut tenotomy can alternatively be performed to facilitate later repair if desired. Releasing this radial septum eliminates the major deforming forces on the radial column, and reduction can be achieved much more easily. Reduction of less complex fractures is now done by longitudinal traction on the fingers by the assistant and volar flexion of the wrist; the plate is applied manually once bony length and volar tilt is restored. Insertion of a Freer elevator or narrow osteotome into the fracture site and levering the metaphysis dorsally and distally may be helpful to restore length and critical volar tilt (**Fig. 13-5**). The longitudinal slot in most plates is used for the initial diaphyseal screw so that later plate adjustment can be easily made if needed. While traction and wrist flexion is maintained, the distal locking screw/peg is now inserted. With most fractures, this will suffice to hold the reduction transiently while plate placement/reduction is checked on fluoroscopy. If this is satisfactory, the remainders of the locking screws distally are placed, followed by the shaft fixation for further strength. Gross examination of the plate placement also is necessary to ensure there is not impingement of the distal radioulnar joint or the radial soft tissues, which can cause postoperative discomfort (**Fig. 13-6**). Fractures with die-punch

components or reduction difficulty due to early healing may require the extended FCR approach. This requires that the proximal radius is mobilized, elevated, and pronated out of the field to access the dorsal and articular aspect of the fracture. This facilitates proper débridement of the fracture hematoma or callus and hence reduction of the complex articular injuries. The dorsal periosteum and any organized hematoma/early callus is then excised with a rongeur. The same technique is used in cases of osteoporotic bone, whereas malunions or nonunions require a modified technique that incorporates a dorsal opening wedge osteotomy by a volar approach. In these cases, it is imperative to use the extended FCR approach to expose the dorsal aspect of the distal radius, allowing release of the dorsal periosteum and soft tissues, achieving of the required correction, and application of the cancellous autografts. The fixed-angle plate is fixed first to the proximal frag-

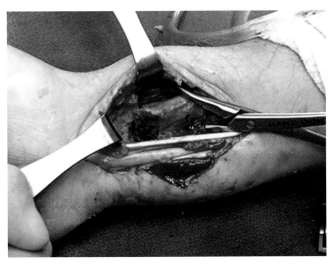

FIGURE 13-4 The extended flexor carpi radialis approach is illustrated by the pronation maneuver of the proximal shaft, which gives an intrafocal view of the fracture, enabling reduction.

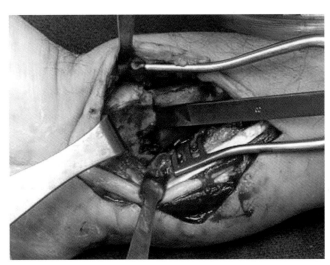

FIGURE 13-5 Less complex fractures allow reduction using a lever and external traction by the assistant. Once length is obtained, the volar tilt is restored by flexion of the wrist via dorsal ligamentotaxis.

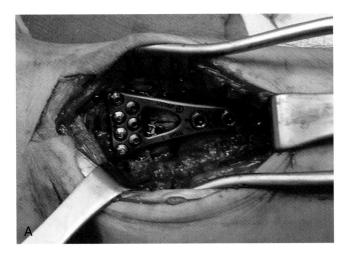

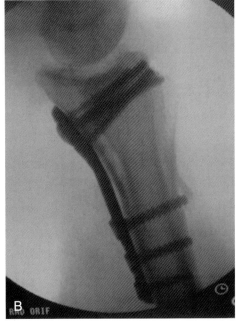

FIGURE 13-6 **A,** Placement of the Contour VPS™ plate (Orthofix). Any soft tissue impingement is ruled out. **B,** Final fluoroscopy shows correct plate placement maintaining anatomical reduction via adequate-length screws for fixation.

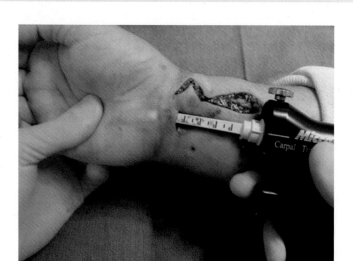

FIGURE 13-7 Division of transverse carpal ligament by one-portal endoscopic technique. Note the transillumination of the skin where the ligament has already been divided.

ment and the distal fragment is reduced to it with traction and direct manipulation of the distal fragment to obtain the necessary volar tilt. Our preferred strategy is to attach the plate to the distal fragment first and then lever the distal fragment into correction by relying on the variable-angle peg fixation. This allows restoration of volar tilt in a much more controlled manner.

We believe that the median nerve should be decompressed due to swelling from both the fracture itself and the operative procedure. Routine endoscopic carpal tunnel release using an Agee[10] endoscopic blade is performed (**Fig. 13-7**). In grossly displaced fractures, the carpal tunnel release is done after reduction of the fracture so to normalize carpal anatomy and prevent iatrogenic injury to the median nerve.[11] However, the majority of endoscopic releases in the fracture scenario are performed before reduction to get the endoscopic equipment away from the field. The concept of releasing the carpal tunnel and decompressing the nerve has two advantages: (1) the nerve release obviously helps relieve current median nerve symptoms and prevent the development of late post-traumatic carpal tunnel syndrome and (2) decompressing the carpal canal allows one to free the nine tendons constrained within the tunnel, worse so because of trauma. Consequently, the flexion/extension of the fingers is much easier, and less painful, in the immediate recovery phase. We are convinced this helps minimize the development of sympathetic-mediated pain syndromes.

Volar plating can also be combined with arthroscopic débridement to accurately assess the reduction and perhaps improve on it. Die-punch fractures can be elevated and reduced just before volar plate placement if necessary. The concept of arthroscopic-assisted fixation has been used by a few surgeons and offers the advantage of more accurate articular reduction and improved joint débridement.[12,13] An added benefit is that concomitant soft tissue injuries, such as triangular fibrocartilage complex or intercarpal ligament injuries, can be diagnosed and managed at the time of internal fixation of the distal radius. This arthroscopic assistance is usually reserved for younger patients with high-energy injuries or the most severe fracture patterns with articular comminution. The typical elderly patient is not indicated for arthroscopy because underlying degenerative changes are present and the wrist demands are not as great.

Once final fluoroscopy pictures are taken, the wound is closed with several subcutaneous sutures followed by skin-absorbable horizontal mattress stitches. The pronator quadratus is usually not closed over the plate because this would require tension on that tissue that could increase postoperative discomfort and even lead to contracture and limited pronosupination. Geissler reported that, in fact, patients had slightly worse rotation after closure of the pronator quadratus, as compared with allowing in situ scarring (data presented at American Association for Hand Surgery annual meeting, Tucson, AZ, 1996).

A bulky dressing with gauze and cast padding over a nonadherent wound covering is applied followed by a volar plaster splint with the wrist in slight dorsiflexion. Immediate finger range of motion is encouraged as the regional block wears off. Light use of the hand via simple activity of daily living exercises is encouraged in the immediate postoperative phase of recovery.

Rehabilitation

Active finger motion and forearm rotation are encouraged immediately after the surgery, and a short arm postoperative splint dressing is used for an average of 7 days. After the first postoperative visit a custom-made removable short arm splint is used for an average of 3 additional weeks. Severe osteoporotic or comminuted fractures can be casted for a total of 4 weeks to allow early bone consolidation. Rehabilitation is adjusted to the patient's clinical course. Patients are instructed to remove this splint three times daily for active range of motion exercises in addition to their regular therapy sessions. Functional use of the hand with light daily exercises is encouraged, and a weight limit of 5 lb is recommended for the injured hand until union is achieved. Patients are expected to recover full digital motion by the first postoperative visit (1 week) and full forearm rotation at the second visit by the end of the month. At 6 to 8 weeks, patients should have regained most of their wrist motion. A more prolonged rehabilitation program is used for patients with highly comminuted intra-articular injuries, fractures with associated injury to the distal radioulnar joint, or ligament injuries that required pinning. These are patients who typically underwent arthroscopy due to the fracture pattern, mechanism of injury, or younger age with greater activity demands.

Results and Complications

Harness and colleagues[14] noted that volar plating, however, was unable to control a very distal volar lunate facet fragment, regardless of the type of implant. They reported on a cohort of patients with a volar shearing fracture of the distal end of the radius in whom the unique anatomy of the distal cortical rim of the radius led to failure of support of a volar ulnar lunate facet fracture fragment.

Brief Literature Review

Rozental and Blazar[15] studied 41 patients with a mean age of 53 years with an average follow-up of 17 months. All fractures were stabilized with volar locking plates. Radiographs in the immediate postoperative period showed a mean radial height of 11 mm, mean radial inclination of 21 degrees, and mean volar tilt of 4 degrees. At fracture healing the mean radial height was 11 mm, mean radial inclination was 21 degrees, and mean volar tilt was 5 degrees. The average score on the Disabilities of the Arm, Shoulder, and Hand (DASH) questionnaire was 14, and all patients achieved excellent and good results on the Gartland and Werley scoring system, indicating minimal impairment in activities of daily living. Nine patients experienced postoperative complications. There were four instances of loss of reduction with fracture collapse, 3 patients required hardware removal for tendon irritation, 1 patient developed a wound dehiscence, and 1 patient had metacarpophalangeal joint stiffness.

Orbay and Fernandez,[16] using a volar approach, treated a consecutive series of 29 patients with 31 dorsally displaced, unstable distal radial fractures with a new fixed-angle internal fixation device. At a minimal follow-up time of 12 months the fractures had healed with highly satisfactory radiographic and functional results. The final volar tilt averaged 5 degrees; radial inclination, 21 degrees; radial shortening, 1 mm; and articular incongruity, 0 mm. Wrist motion at final follow-up examination averaged 59 degrees of extension, 57 degrees of flexion, 27 degrees of ulnar deviation, 17 degrees of radial deviation, 80 degrees of pronation, and 78 degrees of supination. Grip strength was 79% of the contralateral side. The overall outcome according to the Gartland and Werley scales showed 19 excellent and 12 good results.[6]

In a later study, these authors reported their experience treating distal radius fractures in 23 patients older than 75 years using a volar fixed-angle plate with an average follow-up of 63 weeks. Final volar tilt averaged 6 degrees and radial tilt 20 degrees, and radial shortening averaged less than 1 mm. The average final dorsiflexion was 58 degrees, with volar flexion, 55 degrees; pronation, 80 degrees; and supination, 76 degrees. Grip strength was 77% of the contralateral side. There were no plate failures or significant loss of reduction, although there was settling of the distal fragment in three patients (1 to 3 mm). Orbay and Fernandez found that this technique minimized morbidity in the elderly population by successfully handling osteopenic bone, allowed early return to function, provided good final results, and was associated with a low complication rate.

Case Examples
Case 1

A C2 type fracture in a young female (**Fig. 13-8**) was managed by volar plating (**Fig. 13-9**). The patient demonstrated excellent range of motion at the final follow-up visit (**Fig. 13-10**).

Case 2

A motorcycle injury in a young active individual resulted in grossly comminuted fractures of the distal radius and ulna (**Fig. 13-11**). The injury was treated by an external fixator elsewhere (**Fig. 13-12**). The external fixator was removed and fixation was achieved using an extended flexor carpi ulnaris approach and a DVR plate (**Fig. 13-13A**). A good fixation of the fracture was achieved, and the distal end of the ulna was excised (**Fig. 13-13B, C**). At final follow-up 2 years later, the fracture had healed well and the patient had functional range of motion, despite not having been compliant with the physical therapy. He returned to work as a contractor but did not purchase a new motorcycle.

Summary

Improvement in the design of volar plates for the distal radius fracture has allowed us to indicate this treatment methodology for virtually all displaced fractures, regardless of the pattern. Volar placement of a plate, assuming there is a locking mechanism, on better-quality cortical bone allows for improved stability and avoids soft tissue problems. Newer-generation plates with variable-angle locking allow even the occasional wrist surgeon to obtain good fixation that allows earlier return of function in patients presenting with this common, and potentially disabling, injury.

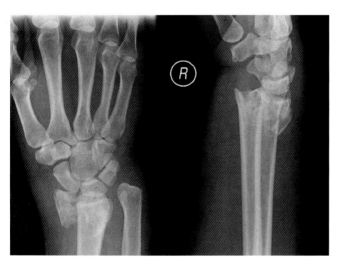

FIGURE 13-8 Preoperative radiographs showing a C2 type distal radius fracture in a young female involved in a motor vehicle accident.

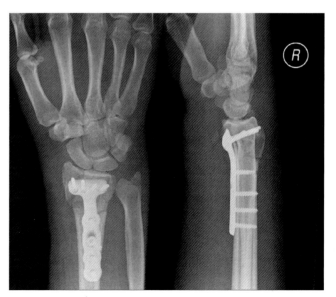

FIGURE 13-9 Postoperative radiographs of the patient in Figure 13-8 show rigid fixation of the fracture with the DVR plate. Because of the high-energy injury and severe displacement, this young patient had an arthroscopic confirmation of reduction with synovectomy at the time of surgery.

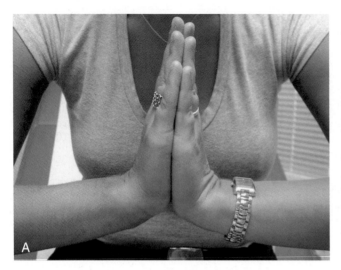

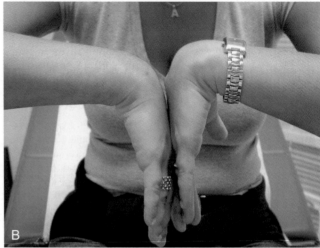

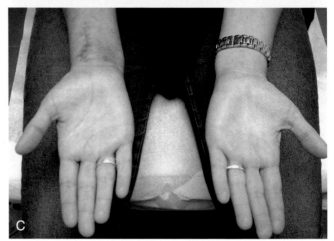

FIGURE 13-10 A to **C,** Range of motion of the patient in Figures 13-8 and 13-9 at final follow-up.

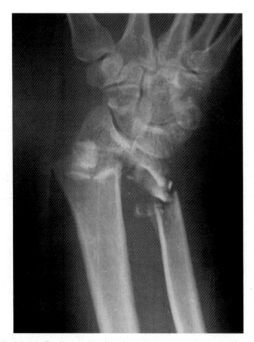

FIGURE 13-11 Radiograph showing open severely comminuted fractures of distal radius and ulna after a high-energy motorcycle injury.

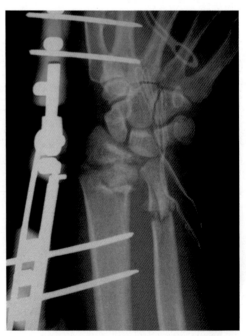

FIGURE 13-12 Radiograph of the fracture in Figure 13-11 managed by an external fixator elsewhere. Note the deformity is not corrected nor is the fracture reduced, but the fixator did improve length and facilitate later definitive surgery.

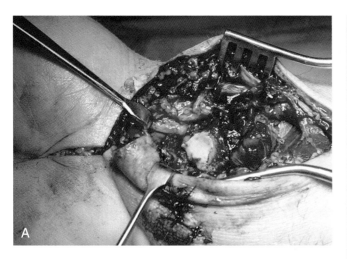

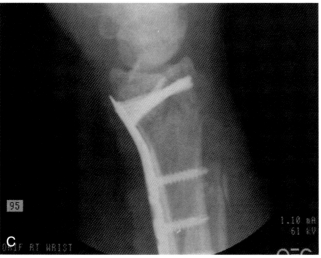

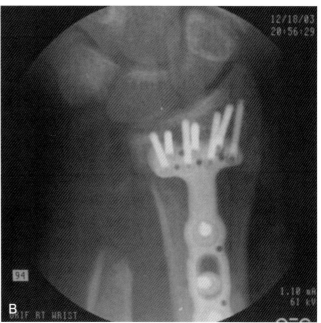

FIGURE 13-13 **A,** Intraoperative photograph during open reduction of fracture in Figure 13-11 showing multiple fracture fragments and soft tissue disruption, a characteristic of high-speed injury. **B** and **C,** Intraoperative fluoroscopy demonstrating good fixation of the severely displaced radius. The distal end of the ulna was excised owing to such severe comminution, and an extensor carpi ulnaris tenodesis was performed.

REFERENCES

1. Jupiter JB: Current concepts review: fractures of the distal end radius. J Bone Joint Surg. 1991; 73:461-469.

2. Cooney WP, Dobyns JH, Linscheid RL: Complications of Colles fractures. J Bone Joint Surg. 1980; 62:613-619.

3. Lanz U, Kron W: A new technic for the correction of malunited distal radius fractures. Handchirurgie. 1976; 8:203-206.

4. Smith RS, Crick JC, Alonso J, Horowitz M: Open reduction and internal fixation of volar lip fractures of the distal radius. J Orthop Trauma. 1988; 2:181-187.

5. Georgoulis A, Lais E, Bernard M, Hertel P: Volar plate osteosynthesis in typical and atypical distal radius fractures. Akt Traumatol. 1992; 22:9-14.

6. Orbay JL, Fernandez DL: Volar fixation for dorsally displaced fractures of the distal radius: a preliminary report. J Hand Surg [Am]. 2002; 27:205-215.

7. Egol KA, Kubiak EN, Fulkerson E, et al: Biomechanics of locked plates and screws. J Orthop Trauma. 2004; 18:488-493.

8. Badia A, Touhami A: Volar plating of distal radial fractures. Atlas Hand Clin. 2006; 11:137-148.

9. Orbay JL, Badia A, Indriago IR, et al: The extended flexor carpi radialis approach: a new perspective for the distal radius fracture. Tech Hand Upper Extrem Surg. 2001; 5:204-211.

10. Agee JM, McCarroll HR Jr, Tortosa RD, et al: Endoscopic release of the carpal tunnel: a randomized prospective multicenter study. J Hand Surg [Am]. 1992; 17:987-995.

11. Badia A: Median nerve compression secondary to fractures of distal radius. In Luchetti R, Amadeo P, eds: Carpal Tunnel Syndrome. New York: Springer, 2006, pp 247-252.

12. Geissler WB, Freeland AE: Arthroscopically assisted reduction of intraarticular distal radius fractures. Clin Orthop Relat Res. 1996; 327:125-134.

13. Osterman AL, Vanduzer ST: Arthroscopy in the treatment of distal radial fractures with assessment and treatment of associated injuries. Atlas Hand Clin. 2006; 1:231-241.

14. Harness NG, Jupiter JB, Orbay JL, et al. Loss of fixation of the volar lunate facet fragment in fractures of the distal part of the radius. J Bone Joint Surg [Am]. 2004; 86:1900-1908.

15. Rozental TD, Blazar PE: Functional outcome and complications after volar plating for dorsally displaced, unstable fractures of the distal radius. J Hand Surg [Am]. 2006; 31:359-365.

16. Orbay JL, Fernandez DL: Volar fixed-angle plate fixation for unstable distal radius fractures in the elderly patient. J Hand Surg [Am]. 2004; 29:96-102.

Volar Rim and Barton's Fracture

14

Asif M. Ilyas, MD, Chaitanya S. Mudgal, MD, MS (Orth), MCh (Orth), and Jesse B. Jupiter, MD

In 1838 John Rhea Barton described a specific fracture pattern of the distal radius characterized by a shearing injury to a portion of the articular and metaphyseal surface and subluxation of the carpus: "The fragment may be, and usually is, quite small, and is broken from the end of the radius … and through the cartilaginous face of it, and necessarily into the joint."[1] Although some disagreement has existed about whether Barton's original article limited the fracture to a dorsal or a volar displacement, it is now well accepted that the volar articular marginal shearing pattern is more common.[2] Therefore, to avoid confusion we will describe Barton's fractures as either volar or dorsal (**Fig. 14-1**).

Volar rim and volar or dorsal Barton's fractures are considered among marginal articular shearing type fractures. In the case of these marginal fractures, the shearing mechanism and obliquity of the fracture line result in volar and proximal subluxation of the carpus. The volar surface of the distal radius is relatively flat. However, the very distal margin slopes volarly in the form of a ridge from which the volar radiocarpal ligaments take origin. It is also important to understand that when viewed in cross section, the distal radial cortical margin slopes volarly from radial to ulnar and, in fact, has a slight dorsal turn just before terminating in the volar edge of the semilunar notch, giving it a somewhat convex appearance. The ulnar volar margin of the lunate facet slopes volarly from a proximal to distal direction. Thus, the volar lunate facet extends more distally than expected and effective support of this area with a plate can be challenging (**Fig. 14-2**).[3-5] In addition, anatomical studies demonstrate that the short radiolunate ligament originates from the volar margin of the lunate facet and attaches to the volar surface of the lunate. It is proposed that this ligament may play a vital role in the stability of the radiocarpal articulation.[6] Radiographic assessment of the volar lunate facet is best accomplished with a lateral projection inclined 10 degrees proximally, thereby providing a distinct profile of the articular surface and assessment of the "teardrop," or U-shaped, outline of the volar rim of the lunate facet (see **Fig. 14-2C**).[7] Normally, a line drawn down the central axis of the teardrop creates an angle of 70 degrees to the central axis of the radial shaft (see **Fig. 14-2D**).[7] A volar lunate facet fragment that is displaced or rotated can be identified by displacement of the teardrop and disruption of the teardrop angle. This will create a functional incompetence of the short radiolunate ligament, leading to radiocarpal instability.

In comparison to its volar counterpart, dorsal Barton's fractures are less common injuries and are often included in the spectrum of radiocarpal dislocations or complex articular fractures. The mechanism of injury is similar to volar injuries but with a dorsally directed shearing force, resulting in dorsal cortical compromise and proximal migration of the carpus. The definition of a Barton's fracture is a shearing marginal articular fragment and

requires maintenance of an intact opposite cortex.[8] Confusion between a true dorsal Barton's fracture versus either a radiocarpal fracture-dislocation or a complex articular fracture can be clarified by reviewing the AO classification of distal radius fractures (**Table 14-1**).[9] Type B fractures are partial articular fractures of the distal radius and encompass dorsal Barton's (type B2) and volar Barton's (type B3) fractures and include maintenance of an intact opposite cortex. In comparison, the AO type C fracture patterns are complete articular fractures of the distal radius with multiple articular and metaphyseal fragments and therefore are not shear fractures and should not be considered a Barton fracture.

Indications

When defining the indications for treatment of any distal radius fracture, the two most important factors are the stability of the fracture and the functionality of the patient. Involvement of the patient in the decision-making process is critical to optimize outcome. Associated injuries are also helpful in the decision-making process and include carpal injuries, polytrauma or other associated limb injury, median neuropathy, and open fractures.

Traditionally, closed treatment of marginal fractures of the distal radius has been limited to undisplaced fractures. Yet even undisplaced fractures need to be followed closely radiographically until union because the very unstable nature of this injury predisposes to displacement in a cast. In our experience, any displacement is to be viewed with great suspicion and these fractures are best treated operatively. External fixation is also ill suited for the treatment of marginal fractures and can potentially promote greater displacement.

The traditional variables of instability (age >60, extent of initial deformity, dorsal comminution, and associated ulna fracture) cannot be applied readily to these fractures.[10] Our indications for open reduction and internal fixation of marginal fractures of the distal radius include:

- Subluxation or dislocation of the radiocarpal joint
- Displaced or rotated volar lunate facet fragments
- Intra-articular incongruity of more than 2 mm
- Associated carpal injury, polytrauma, neuropathy, and open fractures
- Failure of nonoperative treatment

Contraindications

Patients with medical conditions that prohibit the use of anesthesia or those with an insensate hand or a lack of motor control of the hand and wrist may not be suitable candidates for open reduction and internal fixation.

157

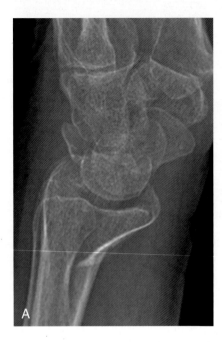
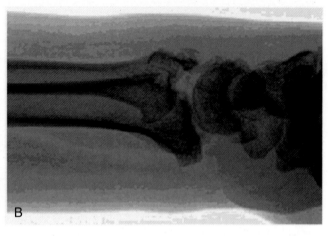

FIGURE 14-1 **A,** Volar Barton's fracture. **B,** Dorsal Barton's fracture.

TABLE 14-1 AO Classification of Distal Radius Fractures

Type A	Extra-articular
A1	Extra-articular ulna fracture with radius intact
A2	Extra-articular radius fracture with ulna intact
A3	Extra-articular multifragmented radius fracture
Type B	Partial articular
B1	Sagittal plane fracture of radius
B2	Dorsal rim (Barton's) fracture of radius
B3	Volar rim (Barton's) fracture of radius
Type C	Complete articular
C1	Simple articular and metaphyseal fracture of radius
C2	Simple articular fracture with multifragmented metaphysis
C3	Multifragmented articular fracture

Web Video ## Surgical Technique

14-1

In most instances of operative fixation of distal radius fracture we prefer regional anesthesia. We routinely use a pneumatic tourniquet, fluoroscopic imaging, and perioperative intravenous antibiotics. It is important to have a complete array of instrumentation available before embarking on surgical fixation. Our preferred implants are fixed-angle locked volar plates.

In most instances the volar approach is our preferred approach. The surgical approach is made through the floor of the flexor carpi radialis sheath or, alternatively, through the distal portion of the extensile approach of Henry between the flexor carpi radialis and the brachioradialis. The flexor pollicis longus is retracted ulnarly, and the pronator quadratus is incised in an inverted L-shaped manner, taking care to elevate it subperiosteally from the radial

border and also to avoid injury to the volar radiocarpal ligaments distally. In making the transverse limb of this "L" the surgeon must be aware of a rim fragment being displaced volarly. This alters the anatomical perspective, and an injudiciously placed incision in the pronator quadratus may transect the volar ligaments. We therefore recommend this incision be done through the fat stripe just distal to the pronator quadratus and then proximal to the volar edge of the distal radius. Or, we identify the location of the joint initially with a 25-gauge hypodermic needle and make the incision just proximal to it.

In addition, to approach more ulnar fragments such as the volar lunate facet fragment, the volar ulnar approach is utilized. This interval lies between the ulnar nerve and artery and the flexor tendons of the fingers. To help visualization and mobilization of the interval, the approach is extended distally with release of the carpal tunnel.[8]

When dorsal fixation is required, an incision is made in line with the third metacarpal just ulnar to Lister's tubercle. The extensor pollicis longus tendon is identified, freed from its sheath, and mobilized from the third dorsal compartment. The second and fourth dorsal compartments are then mobilized in a subperiosteal fashion in a radial and ulnar direction, respectively, exposing the dorsal distal radius.

We will review our technique for five types of marginal fractures: (1) volar Barton's fractures, (2) volar shearing fracture with a volar lunate facet fragment, (3) volar marginal shearing fracture with a dorsal cortical fracture, (4) dorsal Barton's fracture, and (5) radiocarpal fracture-dislocations.

Volar Barton's Fracture

Web V

14-

The vast majority of volar Barton's fractures can be reduced with a combination of dorsiflexion over a bolster, manual digital traction applied by an assistant, and manipulation under direct vision with a Freer elevator. Should there be any articular depression, then this can be elevated by working through the fractured surface. A T-shaped volar plate of sufficient length is applied to ensure fixation of two bicortical screws proximal to the fracture in the

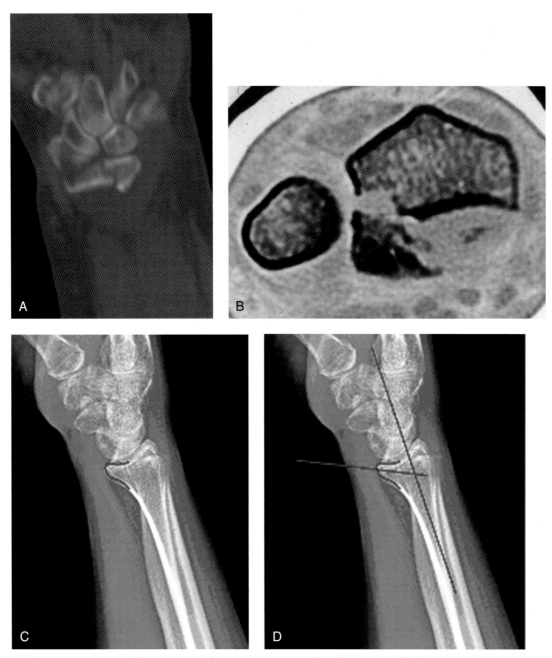

FIGURE 14-2 A, Coronal CT depicting the fractured volar lunate facet fragment. **B,** CT of distal radius depicting the fractured volar lunate facet fragment. **C,** Ten-degree lateral projection showing the "teardrop" or lunate facet in profile. **D,** The teardrop angle is formed by a line drawn down the central axis of the teardrop and a second line drawn down the axis of the radial shaft. Normally the angle is approximately 70 degrees.

radius. The plate is undercontoured and applied so that on tightening the proximal screws the plate assists in reducing the fracture by pushing it distal and buttressing it. Reduction of the articular surface is confirmed with the wrist imaged in the lateral view and the x-ray beam inclined 10 degrees from distal to proximal.[7] Although placement of distal screws is not always necessary, we routinely use them because we see no disadvantage to their careful placement (**Fig. 14-3**). In closure, the pronator quadratus is carefully closed over the plate if possible. Postoperatively the wrist is placed in a splint for 5 to 10 days, after which sutures are removed and active wrist motion is initiated.

Volar Shearing Fracture with a Volar Lunate Facet Fragment

Before approaching volar shearing fractures, obtaining a preoperative computed tomographic (CT) scan is prudent to specifically look for a volar lunate facet fragment (see **Fig. 14-2A, B**). Jupiter and associates demonstrated that a significant number of volar marginal shearing fractures have two or more such articular fragments.[11] Intraoperatively, every effort is made to confirm the presence or absence of these fragments. If required, the surgical approach is directed ulnar, through the interval between the flexor tendons and the ulnar neurovascular structures, so as to

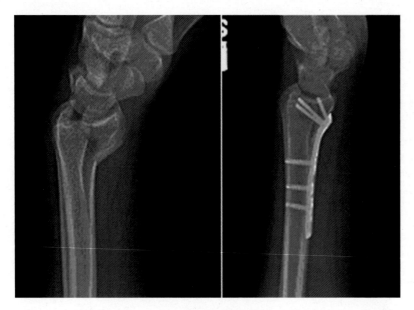

FIGURE 14-3 Postoperative radiographs of volar Barton's fracture.

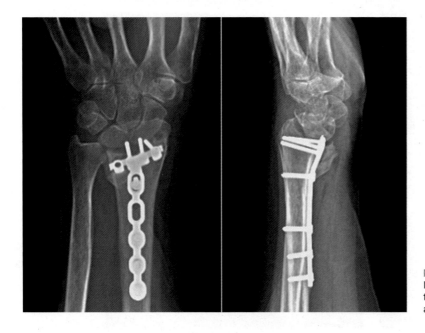

FIGURE 14-4 Inadequate fixation of a very distal volar lunate facet fracture with secondary volar subluxation of the carpus. Although the width of the plate appears to be adequate, it failed to support this very distal fragment.

adequately visualize this area because it may not always be visible or accessible through a standard volar approach. Extension of the incision distally with release of the carpal tunnel will aid in visualization and soft tissue mobilization. Implants are placed to achieve stable buttressing of the volar lunate facet/corner. If a single implant does not span the entire width of the radius, then the surgeon should support this fragment with an additional small plate. In situations in which the fragment is extremely small, a Kirschner wire (K-wire) is passed through the fragment to exit dorsally. Alternatively, a suture passed through the volar short radiolunate ligament and through drill holes in the volar distal radial metaphysis in the form of a figure of eight can provide fixation of this fragment.[12] Reduction of the volar lunate facet fragment is checked with the wrist imaged in the lateral view and the x-ray beam inclined 10 degrees from distal to proximal and thereby confirming reconstitution of the "teardrop" or the volar rim of the lunate facet.[7] Stable fixation of this fragment is critical

in prevention of its displacement during the rehabilitation phase. Displacement of this fragment is usually associated with volar subluxation of the carpus, a reduction in ultimate range of motion in the wrist, and degenerative changes in the radiocarpal articulation (**Fig. 14-4**).

Volar Marginal Shearing Fracture with a Dorsal Cortical Fracture

This particular subset of volar shearing fractures of the distal radius is usually seen in older women and includes a portion of the distal radial articular surface with an oblique metaphyseal fracture line extending dorsally (**Fig. 14-5**). The articular fragment tends to displace volarly and in doing so takes the carpus with it, subluxing volarly and proximally. Plate fixation with an undercontoured volar buttress plate is to be avoided in the treatment of this injury because it leads to displacement of the entire

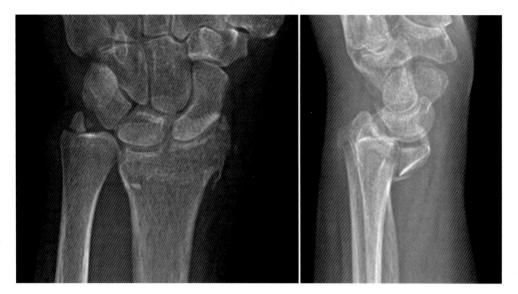

FIGURE 14-5 Radiographs of volar shearing fracture of the distal radius with dorsal cortical extension.

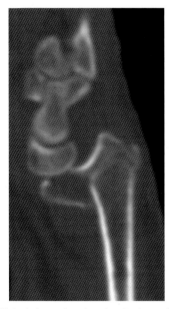

FIGURE 14-6 CT depicting volar shearing fracture with subluxation of the carpus and extension of the fracture line into the dorsal cortex.

juxta-articular portion of the distal radius in a dorsal direction, such that the articular surface may be angulated dorsally.[13] It is therefore critical to be aware of this possibility. In the preoperative assessment of these patients, we recommend radiographs taken in standard planes without any plaster splints that may obscure an occult fracture line. Furthermore, if concern still exists, then a CT scan to rule out or confirm an occult dorsal cortical fracture is highly recommended (**Fig. 14-6**). In situations in which a dorsal cortical fracture line is identified, a fully contoured volar plate is applied. The distal screw holes are utilized, and no attempt is made to undercontour the plate. The volar fragment is provisionally fixed to the radius with a K-wire, and this construct is neutralized with a volar locking plate. This allows anatomical reduction of the articular fracture and prevents dorsal angulation of the entire articular surface (**Fig. 14-7**).

Dorsal Barton's Fracture

Before approaching dorsal Barton's fractures, a preoperative CT scan is prudent to evaluate the number of dorsal fragments, evaluate for the presence of volar avulsion fragments, and assess for a possible radial styloid fracture. The dorsal surface is approached through the floor of the third dorsal compartment. Dorsal comminution is the rule, and marginal fragments are mobilized along with the dorsal capsule so that they could be reflected distally. With in-line traction and a slight flexion moment being performed by the assistant, the fracture can be readily reduced. Metaphyseal defects can be filled with bone graft or substitutes of the surgeon's preference. A dorsal plate is applied as a buttress plate. In cases of comminution or severe subchondral bone loss a locking dorsal plate is preferred to support the articular surface (**Fig. 14-8**). Reduction of the articular surface is confirmed with the wrist imaged in the lateral view with the x-ray beam inclined 20 degrees from distal to proximal.

In cases of severe metaphyseal defect and/or soft tissue injury, an external fixator can also be applied to provide additional stability for 3 to 4 weeks. Also, in cases with avulsion fractures of the volar distal radius, internal fixation volarly is indicated for stability of the carpus. Either the standard volar approach can be utilized or the approach can be through the interval between the flexor tendons and the ulnar neurovascular structures. Fixation can be accomplished with volar plating or fragment-specific fixation.

Radiocarpal Fracture-Dislocations

Radiocarpal fracture-dislocations can result in either a volar or a dorsal dislocation of the carpus, but the dorsal pattern is most common. Fixation of these injuries requires a four-stage approach (**Fig. 14-9**). First, the standard volar approach is utilized and the radiocarpal joint is examined through the capsular violation. The joint is irrigated and débrided of any entrapped osteochondral fragments. Avulsion fractures, most commonly of the radial styloid, are then internally fixed with either a radial or volar plate or, alternatively, with lag screws placed through the styloid into the proximal ulnar cortex of the radius. Second, volar capsular violations are repaired with the aid of suture anchors and any remaining avulsed marginal fractures are also fixed and may require utilization of the volar ulnar approach. Third, when the

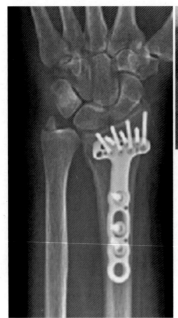
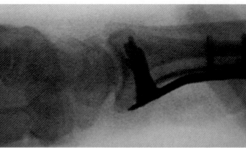

FIGURE 14-7 Volar locking plate fixation of a volar shearing fracture with dorsal cortical extension.

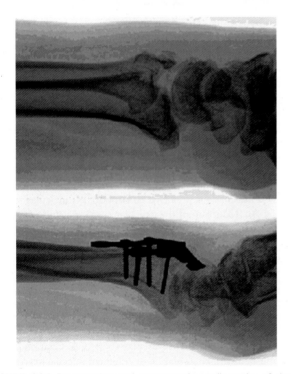

FIGURE 14-8 Preoperative and postoperative radiographs of dorsal Barton's fracture.

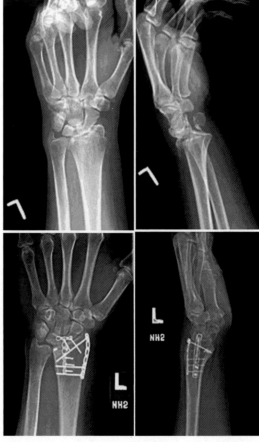

FIGURE 14-9 Preoperative and postoperative radiographs of radiocarpal fracture-dislocation.

dorsal rim of the distal radius is involved a second dorsal incision is made and the radiocarpal joint is approached through the floor of the third dorsal compartment. Impacted articular rim fragments are elevated, defects are bone grafted, and a dorsal buttress plate can be applied. Last, the fourth stage involves fixation of the ulnar styloid, if fractured and if intraoperative examination of the distal radioulnar joint suggests instability.

Results

Review of the literature finds that operative fixation of these fractures is effective. But the use of the Barton eponym has made

critical study of the morphology of articular margin fractures of the distal radius imprecise. Jupiter and colleagues studied 49 volar intra-articular fractures in patients who underwent T-plating; there were 31 excellent, 10 good, and 8 fair results by Gartland and Werley scoring.[11] Interestingly, these authors reported the high incidence of at least two or more fragments of the volar articular surface and stressed the importance of recognizing this preoperatively to aid in planning of the approach and appropriate type of fixation.

Harness and coworkers examined outcomes in 7 patients who had loss of fixation of the volar lunate facet after volar plating of a distal radius fracture.[3] Five of these patients elected to undergo revision fixation. In this subgroup, there were 2 excellent, 2 fair, and 1 poor outcome. Both patients who elected not to undergo revision fixation were classified as having a good outcome. When the two groups were compared, there was no significant difference in the range of motion, but patients who had revision fixation were noted to demonstrate decreased grip strength. Whereas articular restoration appears paramount, and revision fixation would seem intuitive, the results of this study appear to suggest otherwise. However, the small sample size in this study precludes drawing any firm conclusions from these data.

Harness and coworkers also examined volar rim fractures with unrecognized extension of the dorsal cortex of the distal radius in 5 patients. The use of an undercontoured plate resulted in a loss of normal volar tilt and an average dorsal tilt of 6 degrees.[13] They stressed the importance of identifying compromise of the dorsal cortex and recommended the use of a contoured volar locking plate in those circumstances.

Lozano-Calderón and colleagues studied dorsal articular margin fractures in 20 patients, 7 of whom needed combined dorsal and volar fixation. There were 6 excellent, 12 good, and 2 fair results based on the modified Gartland and Werley scoring system.[14] These researchers warned of the inherent instability of dorsal articular margin fractures owing to their predilection toward dorsal radiocarpal subluxation or dislocation and also of associated volar ligament injuries, volar avulsion fractures, or articular impaction. A combined dorsal and volar exposure is often necessary for these injuries to treat the central articular impaction and the radiocarpal instability.

Mudgal and colleagues reviewed their series of radiocarpal fracture-dislocations and illustrated the rarity of these injuries but their predilection toward dorsal dislocation, a high-energy mechanism, and sensory impairment.[15] Using volar and dorsal fixation they achieved 5 excellent and good, 2 fair, and 2 poor results in patients free of any associated intercarpal injuries. In the 2 patients with associated intercarpal injuries, the results were 1 fair and 1 poor, indicating that these fractures when associated with intercarpal injuries may have significantly compromised outcomes.

Based on a review of available data, it thus appears that good or excellent outcomes can be achieved in a majority of volar rim and Barton's fractures of the distal radius if identification of all fracture fragments is performed and appropriate fixation is utilized.

REFERENCES

1. Barton JR: Views and treatment of an important injury of the wrist. Med Exam. 1838; 1:365-368.

2. Thompson GH, Grant TT: Barton's fractures–reverse Barton's fractures: confusing eponyms. Clin Orthop Relat Res. 1977; 122:210-221.

3. Harness NG, Jupiter JB, Orbay JL, et al: Loss of fixation of the volar lunate facet fragment in fractures of the distal part of the radius. J Bone Joint Surg [Am]. 2004; 86:1900-1908.

4. Mekhail AO, Ebraheim NA, McCreath WA, et al: Anatomic and x-ray film studies of the distal articular surface of the radius. J Hand Surg [Am]. 1996; 21:567-573.

5. Andermahr J, Lozano-Calderon S, Trafton T, et al: The volar extension of the lunate facet of the distal radius: a quantitative anatomic study. J Hand Surg [Am]. 2006; 31:892-895.

6. Berger RA, Landsmeer JM: The palmar radiocarpal ligaments: a study of adult and fetal human wrist joints. J Hand Surg [Am]. 1990; 15:847-854.

7. Medoff RJ: Essential radiographic evaluation for distal radius fractures. Hand Clin. 2005; 21:279-288.

8. Fernandez DL, Jupiter JB, eds. Fractures of the Distal Radius: A Practical Approach to Management. New York: Springer, 2002.

9. Cohen MS, McMurtry RY, Jupiter JB: Fractures of the distal radius. In Browner BD, Jupiter JB, Levine AM, Trafton PG, eds: Skeletal Trauma, 2nd ed. Philadelphia: WB Saunders, 1998, p 1385.

10. LaFontaine M, Hardy D, Delince PH: Stability assessment of distal radius fractures. Injury. 1989; 20:208-210.

11. Jupiter JB, Fernandez DL, Toh CL, et al: The operative management of volar articular fractures of the distal end of the radius. J Bone Joint Surg Am. 1996; 78:1817-1828.

12. Chin KR, Jupiter JB: Wire-loop fixation of volar displaced osteochondral fractures of the distal radius. J Hand Surg [Am]. 1999; 24:525-533.

13. Harness N, Ring D, Jupiter JB: Volar Barton's fractures with concomitant dorsal fracture in older patients. J Hand Surg. 2004; 29:439-445.

14. Lozano-Calderón SA, Doornberg J, Ring D: Fractures of the dorsal articular margin of the distal part of the radius with dorsal radiocarpal subluxation. J Bone Joint Surg Am. 2006; 88(7):1486-1493.

15. Mudgal CS, Psenica J, Jupiter JB: Radiocarpal fracture-dislocation. J Hand Surg [Br]. 1999; 24:92-98.

Pediatric Distal Radius Fractures

15

Scott H. Kozin, MD

Pediatric distal radius fractures are common. In fact, forearm fractures account for 40% of all pediatric fractures and the distal radius and distal ulna are the most common sites within the forearm.[1-3] High-risk activities for these fractures include horseback riding, skateboarding, and snowboarding.[4] In addition, overweight adolescents have poorer balance than those of healthy weight, which may explain their propensity for fracture.[5] Most distal radius fractures are Salter-Harris II fractures and are treated without surgery. In general, acceptable reduction is angulation less than 20 degrees with 2 years of growth remaining. In the young child, complete bayonet apposition is acceptable. However, operative intervention is indicated in certain fracture types. In this chapter the focus is on those pediatric distal radius fractures that require surgery with an emphasis on indications, technique, and clinical pearls.

Pertinent Anatomy

The pediatric skeleton is unique in multiple ways. The presence of the physis or growth plate provides longitudinal growth. The physis is divided into four distinct zones: germinal, proliferative, hypertrophic, and provisional calcification. The hypertrophic and provisional calcification zones are relatively weaker than the germinal and proliferative layers.[6,7] Classically, fracture lines tend to pass through the hypertrophic and provisional calcification zones. However, high-energy injuries may undulate through all four zones of the physis.[6-9]

The presence of the secondary ossification center is another distinguishing feature that can complicate fracture detection. The distal radius epiphysis is absent at birth and appears at approximately 1 year of age. Specifically, the appearance is between 0.5 and 2.3 years in boys and between 0.4 and 1.7 years in girls.[10] The configuration of the epiphysis also changes with age. Initially, the epiphysis is transverse in shape and becomes more triangular with time. The radial physis closes at approximately 16 years of age in girls and 17 years of age in boys.[11] The distal radius and ulnar physis contribute 75% to 80% of the forearm growth and 40% of the entire upper extremity.[12]

Indications

The principal surgical indications for pediatric distal radius fractures are irreducible fractures, displaced intra-articular fractures, and Galeazzi fracture-dislocations. Irreducible fractures require open reduction to extricate the offending structure from the fracture site. In children, the interposed structure is usually periosteum. Intra-articular fractures are relatively uncommon in children and often secondary to high intensity sports. The fracture pattern is usually a Salter-Harris III or IV fracture. Similar to adults, articular congruity must be restored to prevent traumatic arthritis

and to decrease the chances of a physeal arrest. Galeazzi fractures are less common in children than adults. The treatment principles in adults and children are similar with reduction of the radius and the distal radioulnar dislocation. Unfortunately, the pediatric Galeazzi fracture-dislocation is often treated as an isolated radius fracture without appreciation of the distal radioulnar joint (DRUJ) component. Subsequently, the patient fails to regain forearm rotation and the distal radioulnar injury is recognized late.

Additional indications for surgery are open fractures and fractures associated with nerve injuries, such as carpal tunnel syndrome (**Figs. 15-1** and **15-2**). The treating physician must be aware that children and adolescents do not routinely complain of numbness. In addition, sensation is difficult to examine in the pediatric patient and two-point discrimination is unreliable until about 9 years of age. Therefore, the physician must have a high index of suspicion for nerve compression after treatment of markedly displaced fractures. The treatment principles for open fractures and fractures associated with nerve injuries are similar to those for adults and will not be specifically addressed in this chapter.

Surgical considerations are influenced by a variety of parameters unique to children. First, the timing of surgery is different in children compared with adults. Children heal more quickly than adults and form abundant callus faster. Therefore, surgery performed within the first week after injury is preferable. Second, the potential for remodeling is present in children. Fractures about the physis will remodel, especially in young children and particularly in the sagittal plane of motion. Consequently, considerable angulation is acceptable in the young child and less angulation in the adolescent approaching skeletal maturity. Third, growth plate fractures injure the physis and additional manipulation or surgery may further damage the growth potential. Repeat manipulations are particularly harmful to the physis and should be avoided. Children who present later than 1 week after injury or have partially lost reduction pose particular problems. In these cases, the surgeon must compare and contrast the risk/benefit ratio of surgical intervention on the growth plate with the remodeling capacity of the child.

Contraindications

Contraindications for surgery stem from the indications just listed. The main point that distinguishes children from adults is the remodeling capacity of the immature skeleton. Displaced fractures that would require surgery in adults are often acceptable in children, especially growth plate fractures and fractures that present late. The surgeon must avoid unnecessary surgery that could do additional harm, particularly in the very young child.

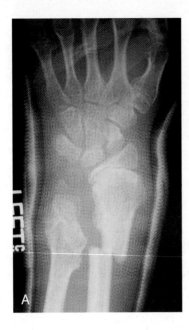

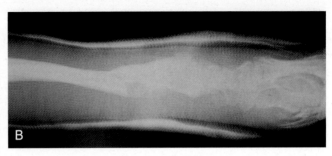

FIGURE 15-1 A 16-year-old boy with multiple hereditary exostosis sustained a displaced left distal radius fracture. Closed reduction and casting was performed. Anteroposterior (**A**) and lateral (**B**) radiographs after closed reduction. *(Courtesy of Shriners Hospital for Children, Philadelphia, PA.)*

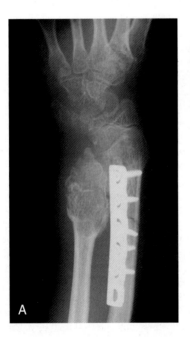

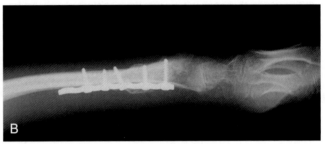

FIGURE 15-2 The patient developed acute carpal tunnel syndrome requiring emergent open reduction and internal fixation along with carpal tunnel release. Anteroposterior (**A**) and lateral (**B**) radiographs after open reduction and internal fixation. *(Courtesy of Shriners Hospital for Children, Philadelphia, PA.)*

Surgical Technique

Standard Set-up

The child is placed in the supine position. General anesthesia is used. An adult or pediatric tourniquet (Delfi Medical Innovations, Vancouver, Canada) is placed on the upper arm depending on the size of the child. The pediatric size avoids irritation in the antecubital fossa. All bony prominences are padded. Preoperative antibiotics are administered. The extremity is prepped and draped in sterile fashion.

Intra-articular Fractures

Displaced Salter-Harris III and IV fractures require surgery to restore anatomical alignment of the joint surface.[13] The goal of

internal fixation is intraepiphyseal fixation with avoidance of the physis. If fixation must cross the physis, smooth pins are preferable to limit further physeal injury. Mini-fluoroscopy is invaluable to assess joint alignment and implant fixation. External fixation may be necessary to augment the fixation and to unload the joint surface until satisfactory healing has occurred.

The specific approach depends on the fracture configuration (**Fig. 15-3**). Computed tomography (CT) can further delineate the fracture pattern. In general, the approach is directed at the fracture fragment. A dorsal fragment requires a dorsal longitudinal incision along Lister's tubercle. Sharp dissection is performed to the extensor retinaculum. Skin flaps are elevated from this level. The third compartment is opened, and the extensor pollicis longus is transposed in a radial direction. The posterior interos-

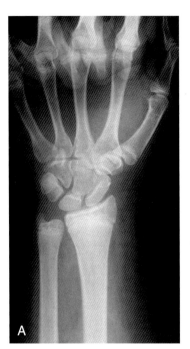

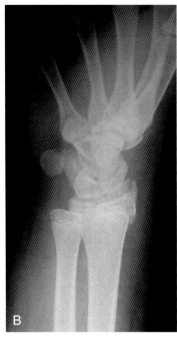

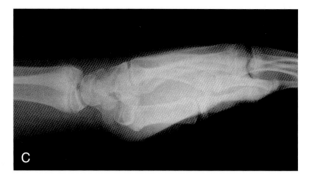

FIGURE 15-3 A 14-year-old boy with a history of Blount's disease fell from a bicycle sustaining an intra-articular Salter-Harris III fracture. Anteroposterior (**A**), oblique (**B**), and lateral (**C**) radiographs. *(Courtesy of Shriners Hospital for Children, Philadelphia, PA.)*

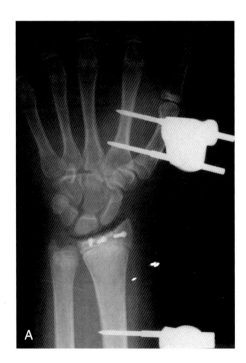

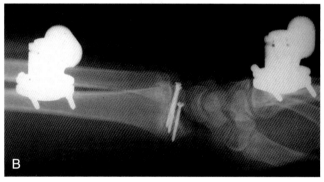

FIGURE 15-4 Open reduction and internal fixation using intraepiphyseal screws. Adjuvant external fixation was applied to protect fixation until union. Anteroposterior (**A**) and lateral (**B**) radiographs after fixation. *(Courtesy of Shriners Hospital for Children, Philadelphia, PA.)*

seous nerve is identified and resected to prevent postoperative neuroma formation. The second and fourth compartments are retracted, and a longitudinal capsulotomy is performed.

Any hemarthrosis within the joint is evacuated. The capsulotomy may require extension into a T-configuration to increase exposure. The distal radial surface is exposed, and a reverse retractor is placed on the volar lip. The joint surface is examined, and the fracture line is delineated. Hematoma is removed from the fracture site. The fracture is then reduced, and provisional fixation is obtained using K wires drilled from dorsal to palmar.

Fluoroscopic imaging is used to confirm joint reduction and wire position—preferably intraepiphyseal fixation with avoidance

of the physis. Direct joint inspection avoids intra-articular wire placement. In sequential fashion, the pins are removed and replaced with compression screws across the fracture (**Fig. 15-4**). The placement of screws across the physis is avoided. At this point, the fixation is assessed and a determination made regarding the necessity of an external fixator to unload the joint surface until healing has occurred. In children, I have a low threshold to apply an external fixator because compliance is unlikely. The fixator is placed using standard open incisions. Distraction is applied until the scaphoid and lunate are elevated from the articular surface to eliminate compressive forces until union. Standard closure is performed with absorbable suture, and the external fixator is securely

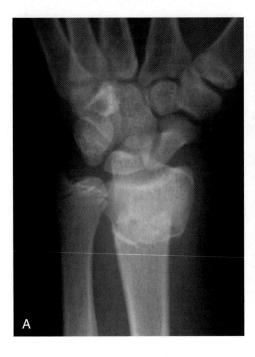
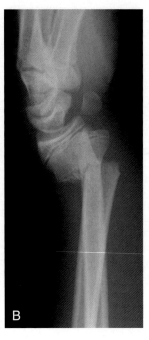

FIGURE 15-5 A 15-year-old boy fell and sustained a Galeazzi fracture-dislocation. **A,** Anteroposterior view with shortening. **B,** Lateral radiograph demonstrates the volar position of the ulna relative to the radius. *(Courtesy of Shriners Hospital for Children, Philadelphia, PA.)*

tightened. The tourniquet is deflated to ensure capillary refill. A long arm splint is applied. The external fixator is removed 5 to 6 weeks after surgery. Active and active-assisted range of motion is instituted. Formal therapy is usually not required.

Arthroscopically assisted reduction has been described to directly visualize the articular surface.[14,15] However, this technique is relatively demanding and requires additional equipment. I prefer direct visualization of the joint surfaces.

Pediatric Galeazzi Fractures

The most common pattern of pediatric Galeazzi fracture is when there is dorsal displacement of the distal radius fracture and volar displacement of the distal ulna (**Fig. 15-5**). A less common type is when there is volar displacement of the distal radius and dorsal displacement of the distal ulna.[16] Regardless of the pattern, recognition of the disrupted DRUJ is mandatory. A true lateral radiograph is necessary to assess the status of the DRUJ. The injury pattern can also involve the distal ulnar physis and then is called a Galeazzi-equivalent fracture.

Unlike in adult Galeazzi fractures, closed reduction can be successful as long as the DRUJ congruity is reestablished. This tenet is especially true in children with incomplete fractures of the radius. The reduction maneuver involves realignment of the distal radius fragment and rotation of the forearm to restore DRUJ congruity. The direction of forearm rotation depends on the position of the distal ulna; pronation is used for volar displacement and supination is used for dorsal displacement. A long arm cast is required for 6 weeks. Post-reduction radiographs must demonstrate anatomical reduction or additional treatment is required. Questionable reduction requires a CT scan for verification. Adolescents with complete fractures of the distal radius are treated like adults with Galeazzi fractures and require internal fixation.

Open reduction and internal fixation is accomplished via a volar trans–flexor carpi ulnaris (FCR) approach. Stable internal fixation is required. The radial artery and FCR tendon are identified by palpation. The limb is exsanguinated, and the tourniquet

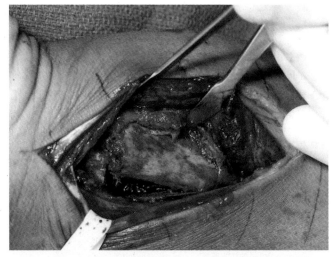

FIGURE 15-6 Exposure of the fracture site reveals considerable displacement. *(Courtesy of Shriners Hospital for Children, Philadelphia, PA.)*

is inflated. A longitudinal incision is made measuring directly over the FCR tendon beginning just proximal to the wrist crease. Sharp dissection is performed down the tendon sheath, which is incised in a longitudinal direction. The tendon is retracted in a radial direction, and the underlying subsheath is incised with the knife to reveal the volar compartment muscles and tendons. These structures are swept in an ulnar direction with a moist sponge directly over the pronator quadratus.

The pronator quadratus is elevated from the radius in an extraperiosteal manner leaving a 2-mm sleeve along the radial border. The radius and fracture site are clearly exposed (**Fig. 15-6**). Hematoma is removed from the fracture site. The fracture is reduced under direct visualization (**Fig. 15-7**). Fixation can be accomplished using a variety of plates. The fixation device selected should consider the close proximity of the growth plate. Fixed-

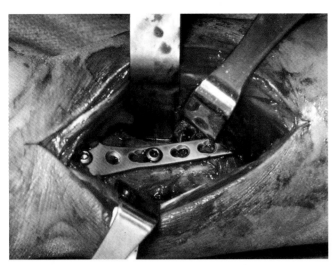

FIGURE 15-7 Open reduction and internal fixation with T-plate. *(Courtesy of Shriners Hospital for Children, Philadelphia, PA.)*

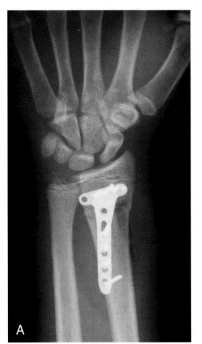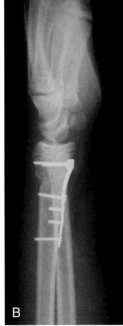

FIGURE 15-8 Radiographs after internal fixation with T-plate that avoids the physis. **A,** Anteroposterior view with anatomical reduction. **B,** Lateral view with distal radioulnar joint reduction. *(Courtesy of Shriners Hospital for Children, Philadelphia, PA.)*

angle devices provide rigid fixation distal to the fracture site and can avoid the physis. Mini-fluoroscopy is used to assess fracture reduction and internal fixation placement (**Fig. 15-8**).

At this point, the status of the DRUJ is assessed. Usually, anatomical restoration of the radius results in DRUJ reduction. On rare occasion, the DRUJ is irreducible because of interposed tissues.[17-19] Periosteum or tendon (e.g., extensor carpi ulnaris or extensor digiti quinti) can be blocking reduction. Exploration of the DRUJ is necessary to remove the offending agent. A separate ulnar approach to the DRUJ is necessary.

Closure is performed with careful repair of the pronator quadratus followed by layered skin closure. The FCR tendon sheath is not repaired. The tourniquet is deflated to ensure capillary refill.

A long arm splint is applied to maintain reduction of the DRUJ. The splint is changed to a long arm cast 2 weeks after surgery. The cast is removed 6 weeks after surgery, and wrist and forearm range of motion exercises are started.

Irreducible Fractures

Irreducible fractures are secondary to soft tissue interposition within the fracture site. With dorsal displacement, the volar periosteum or pronator quadratus can be trapped within the fracture. A volar trans-FCR approach is performed, as described earlier. The pronator quadratus is elevated from the radius leaving a 2-mm sleeve along the radial border for later closure. The radius fracture site is clearly exposed. The interposed material is removed from the fracture site, which is usually periosteum. The fracture is reduced under direct visualization. Fixation is usually accomplished with percutaneous K-wire fixation across the physis. Another option is plate fixation that avoids the physis. The surgeon must remember that the goal is fracture reduction and not necessarily rigid fixation. Therefore, large dominating plates should be avoided. Mini-fluoroscopy is used to assess fracture reduction and fixation placement. After the procedure a long arm cast is applied until fracture union. In general, open reduction delays healing by 1 or 2 weeks compared with closed reduction.

Clinical Pearls

The standard hardware may not be appropriate in children considering their small size and proximity of the fracture to the growth plate. Smaller implants are necessary because standard fixation devices overwhelm the bone and create an unnecessary stress riser. In addition, devices that are T-shaped are often necessary to obtain adequate distal fixation and to avoid fixation across the physis. Locking plates with variable-angle fixation offer several advantages, including distal fixation, avoidance of the physis, and biomechanical strength.

Results

The actual results of pediatric and adolescent distal radius fractures are difficult to decipher based on the literature. In general, most children do well with closed or open treatment as long as the treatment approach adheres to the standard guidelines previously discussed. However, a study that shows consistently good outcomes is often not worthy of formal publication. Instead, most reports discuss complications of distal radius fractures, such as growth arrest, missed fracture-dislocations, and instability.[20-24]

Another confounding factor is that the standard measurements of outcome in adults after wrist fracture (e.g., Disabilities of the Arm, Shoulder, and Hand [DASH] and Mayo wrist scores) are not applicable to the growing child. Children are unable to comply with the measure and are very adaptable to mild impairment. This reality complicates the construction of valid outcome measurements in children. Extensive pediatric outcome research is underway that may improve our ability to critically assess the outcomes after injuries in children, including distal radius fractures.

Complications

Growth plate closure occurs in 4% to 5% of all Salter-Harris distal radius fractures.[20,21] All growth plate fractures require a radiograph 3 to 6 months after healing to ensure continued growth. Failure to recognize a growth plate arrest can lead quickly to deformity (**Figs. 15-9** and **15-10**). The deformity varies according to the location and extent of the physeal bar. Peripheral bars lead to angular deformity as unequal growth occurs. In contrast, small central bars cause tenting of the articular surface and larger bars prevent any longitudinal growth, which results in shortening of the radius relative to the ulna. Advanced imaging studies better delineate the size and location of the physeal bar (**Fig. 15-11**). Management depends on the location of the bar, size of the bar, and the amount of remaining growth. Radioulnar discrepancy of less than 1 cm is well tolerated at long-term follow-up.[21] Options include resection of the bar, formal epiphysiodesis, corrective osteotomy, and distraction osteogenesis. In addition, the ulna may be addressed by epiphysiodesis and/or shortening (**Fig. 15-12**).

Malunion after distal radius fractures is common, but remodeling with growth results in gradual correction. Angulation less than 20 degrees will remodel over 2 years; greater angulation requires additional growth. If the patient is close to skeletal maturity, little remodeling can be expected. Corrective osteotomy with bone grafting is indicated in patients with pain or limited motion. The goal is to restore alignment to alleviate pain, enhance motion, correct midcarpal instability, or prevent degenerative arthritis.[22] The surgery should correct both the sagittal and coronal alignment (**Fig. 15-13**). A distal radius corrective osteotomy can be addressed from a dorsal or volar approach. Similar to adults, the

volar approach and volar locking systems have gained popularity to avoid prominent hardware. A trans-FCR exposure is performed. The malunion site is identified. The distal portion of a fixed-angle plate is contoured and applied parallel to the physis and articular surface (**Fig. 15-14**). Mini-fluoroscopy is used to avoid the physis. The plate protrudes from the proximal radius but acts as a guide to correction. The radius is cut parallel to the physis and articular surface at the level of malunion. The osteotomy is opened using a laminar spreader, and the plate is used as a guide to correction. The proximal plate is affixed to the radius

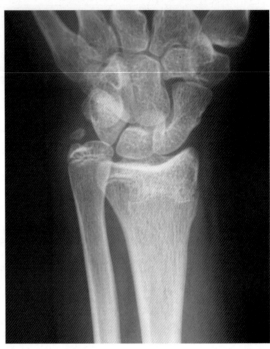

FIGURE 15-10 Anteroposterior radiograph shows shortening of the radius with markedly positive ulnar variance. *(Courtesy of Shriners Hospital for Children, Philadelphia, PA.)*

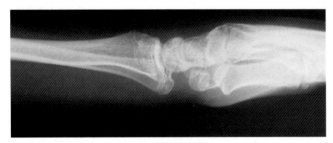

FIGURE 15-9 A 14-year-old girl presented 6 months after a distal radius Salter-Harris II fracture with radius deformity and prominent ulna. Lateral radiograph reveals loss of volar tilt. *(Courtesy of Shriners Hospital for Children, Philadelphia, PA.)*

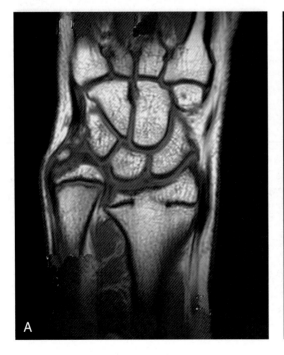

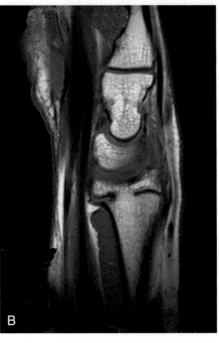

FIGURE 15-11 A 13-year-old girl with a radius fracture presented with growth arrest and ulnar abutment. **A,** Coronal MR image shows central bar in midportion of growth plate. **B,** Sagittal MR image shows position of the physeal bar. *(Courtesy of Shriners Hospital for Children, Philadelphia, PA.)*

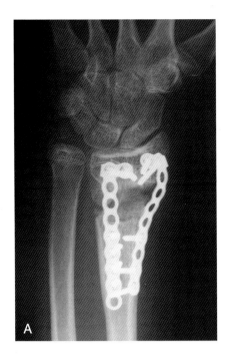

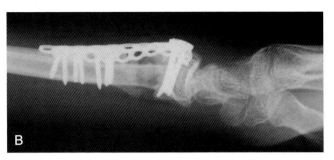

FIGURE 15-12 Patient shown in Figure 15-17 after a corrective osteotomy, bone grafting, and ulnar epiphysiodesis. **A,** Anteroposterior radiograph shows restoration of radial length. **B,** Lateral radiograph demonstrates reestablishment of volar tilt. *(Courtesy of Shriners Hospital for Children, Philadelphia, PA.)*

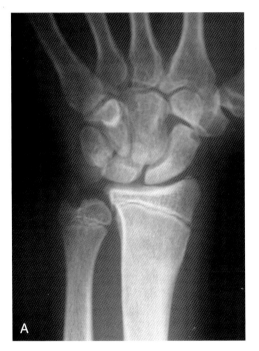

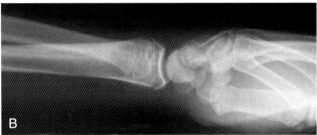

FIGURE 15-13 A 16-year-old boy with symptomatic malunion of the distal radius. **A,** Anteroposterior radiograph reveals loss of radial inclination. **B,** Lateral radiograph shows mild loss of radial tilt but considerable carpal malalignment. *(Courtesy of Shriners Hospital for Children, Philadelphia, PA.)*

using a bone reduction clamp. Correction is assessed via mini-fluoroscopy, and adjustments made accordingly. The plate is then firmly secured to the radius using bicortical screw fixation (**Fig. 15-15**). Cancellous bone graft is placed within the osteotomy site. The graft can be harvested from the ulna or iliac crest depending on the size of the defect. I do not use bone graft substitutes because ample autologous bone is available. Radiographs are taken to verify correction of the coronal and sagittal alignment (**Fig. 15-16**).

Intra-articular malunion can occur after a Salter-Harris III or IV fracture. Fortunately, this malunion is uncommon because treatment is very difficult. The surgeon must weigh the risk/

benefit ratio between intra-articular osteotomy and acceptance of the malunion. An advanced imaging study, preferably a CT scan, can delineate the magnitude of incongruity and is essential in the decision-making process.

A missed Galeazzi fracture-dislocation is a formidable problem. The ulna is subluxated and forearm rotation is limited. Treatment depends on time from the injury and the status of the DRUJ. Early recognition can be treated with corrective osteotomy of the radius and reduction of the DRUJ. Later recognition requires assessment of the articular surfaces of the distal ulna and sigmoid notch. Articular degeneration is a contraindication for reduction. In these cases, a salvage procedure, such as a Darrach

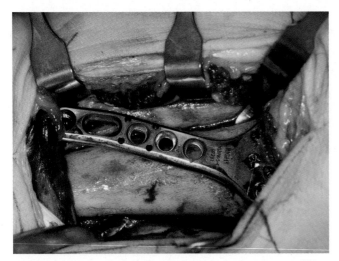

FIGURE 15-14 Volar approach with fixation of volar plate parallel to the physis. Plate protruding from the radius demonstrated a degree of malunion. *(Courtesy of Shriners Hospital for Children, Philadelphia, PA.)*

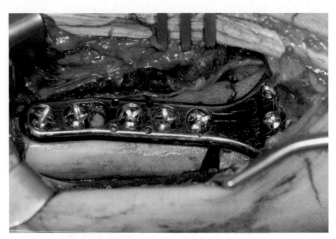

FIGURE 15-15 Plate was reduced to the proximal radius to correct the volar tilt and maintain radial inclination. *(Courtesy of Shriners Hospital for Children, Philadelphia, PA.)*

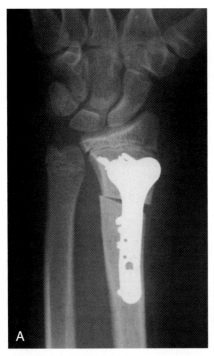
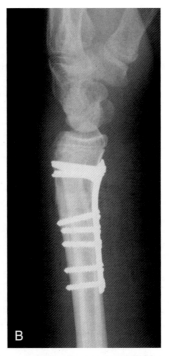

FIGURE 15-16 Intraoperative radiographs after corrective osteotomy and before bone graft. **A,** Anteroposterior radiograph reveals a locking plate proximal to the physis and normal radial inclination. **B,** Lateral radiograph shows good position of plate and screws and restoration of radial tilt. *(Courtesy of Shriners Hospital for Children, Philadelphia, PA.)*

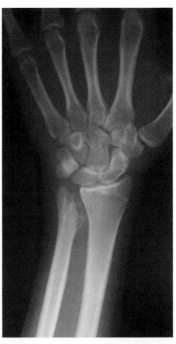

FIGURE 15-17 A 16-year-old wrestler with a chronic volar Galeazzi fracture-dislocation and articular degeneration was treated with matched distal ulnar resection and tenodesis. Anteroposterior radiograph demonstrates matched resection with some bony regrowth. *(Courtesy of Shriners Hospital for Children, Philadelphia, PA.)*

or Sauvé-Kapandji, is required (**Fig. 15-17**). Fortunately, this injury occurs in children close to skeletal maturity and progressive ulnar-negative variance is not a concern because ulnar-negative variance up to 1 cm is usually asymptomatic.[21] However, in the young child the length of the ulna needs to be addressed by distraction osteogenesis.

Persistent pain after distal radius fracture may be related to an associated chondral injury, triangular fibrocartilage (TFC) tear,

or scapholunate ligament injury. These injuries are rare in children. Most TFC and scapholunate ligament tears are partial and can be treated by arthroscopic inspection and débridement. Arthroscopic treatment can result in long-term improvement.[23,24] In cases of peripheral TFC tears, open or arthroscopic repair is warranted.[24]

Volar fixation with plate and screws can result in prominent hardware along the dorsum of the distal forearm and wrist area.

The child presents with extensor tenosynovitis of the irritated tendons. This finding is a forewarning of future problems, including tendon rupture. Treatment requires plate and screw removal, which can be difficult with titanium implants. Another option is dorsal exposure and burring the prominent screw head(s).

REFERENCES

1. Lawton L: Fractures of the distal radius and ulna in management of pediatric fractures. In Letts M, ed: Management of Pediatric Fractures. New York: Churchill-Livingstone, 1994.

2. Landin LA: Fracture patterns in children: analysis of 8682 fractures with special reference to incidence, etiology, and secular changes in a Swedish urban population, 1950-79. Acta Chir Scand Suppl. 1983; 202:1-109.

3. Thomas EM, Tuson KW, Brownie PS: Fractures of the radius and ulna in children. Injury. 1975; 7:120-124.

4. Matsumoto K, Sumi H, Sumi Y, Shimizu K: Wrist fractures from snowboarding: a prospective study for 3 seasons from 1998 to 2001. Clin J Sport Med. 2004; 14:64-71.

5. Goulding A, Jones IE, Taylor RW, et al: Dynamic and static tests of balance and postural sway in boys: effects of previous wrist bone fractures and high adiposity. Gait Posture. 2003;17:136-141.

6. Bright RW, Bursein AH, Elmore SM: Epiphyseal plate cartilage: a biomechanical and histological analysis of failure modes. J Bone Joint Surg Am. 1974; 56:688-703.

7. Moen CT, Pelker RR: Biomechanical and histological correlations in growth plate failure. J Pediatr Orthop. 1984; 4:1180-1184.

8. Smith DG, Geist RW, Cooperman DR: Microscopic examination of naturally occurring epiphyseal plate fracture. J Pediatr Orthop. 1985; 5:306-308.

9. Wattenbarger JM, Gruber HE, Phieffer LS: Physeal fractures: I. Histologic features of bone, cartilage, and bar formation in a small animal model. J Bone Joint Orthop. 2002; 2:703-709.

10. Garn SM, Rohmann CG, Silverman FN: Radiographic standards for postnatal ossification and tooth calcification. Med Radiogr Photogr. 1967; 43:45-66.

11. Greulich W, Pyle SI: Radiographic Atlas of Skeletal Development of the Hand and Wrist. Stanford, CA: Stanford University Press, 1959.

12. Ogden JA, Beall JK, Conlogue GJ, et al: Radiology of postnatal skeletal development: IV. Distal radius and ulna. J Skeletal Radiol. 1981; 6:255-266.

13. Peterson HA: Triplane fracture of the distal radius: case report. J Pediatr Orthop. 1996; 16:192-194.

14. Geissler W, Freeland A, Weiss AP, et al: Techniques of wrist arthroscopy. Instructional course lecture. J Bone Joint Surg Am. 1999; 81:1184-1197.

15. Doi K, Hattori Y, et al: Intra-articular fractures of the distal aspect of the radius: arthroscopically assisted reduction compared with open reduction and internal fixation. J Bone Joint Surg Am. 1999; 81:1093-1110.

16. Walsh HP, McLaren CA, Owen R: Galeazzi fractures in children. J Bone Joint Surg Am. 1987; 69:730-733.

17. Kozin SH, Wood MB: Early soft tissue complications after fractures of the distal part of the radius. J Bone Joint Surg [Am]. 1993; 75:144-153.

18. Letts RM: Monteggia and Galeazzi fractures. In Letts RM, ed: Management of Pediatric Fractures. New York: Churchill-Livingstone, 1994.

19. Kraus B, Horne G: Galeazzi fractures. J Trauma. 1985; 25:1093-1095.

20. Lee BS, Esterhai JL Jr, Das M: Fracture of the distal radial epiphysis: characteristics and surgical treatment of premature, post-traumatic epiphyseal closure. Clin Orthop Relat Res. 1984; 185:90-96.

21. Cannata G, De Maio F, Mancini F, et al: Physeal fractures of the distal radius and ulna: long-term prognosis. J Orthop Trauma. 2003; 17:172-179.

22. Watson K, Taleisnik J: Midcarpal instability caused by malunited fracture of the distal radius. J Hand Surg [Am]. 1984; 9:350-357.

23. Earp BE, Waters PM, Wyzykowski RJ: Arthroscopic treatment of partial scapholunate ligament tears in children with chronic wrist pain. J Bone Joint Surg [Am]. 2006; 88:2448-2455.

24. Bae DS, Waters PM: Pediatric distal radius fractures and triangular fibrocartilage complex injuries. Hand Clin. 2006; 22:43-53.

Complications of Locked Volar Plates

16

David Nelson, MD

Volar plating with locked plates has dramatically reshaped the treatment of distal radius fractures. Along with any new technique come new complications, and locked volar plating is no exception. Complications of locked volar plating reported in the literature, at national and international presentations, in online discussion forums, in my personal cases, and in cases submitted for review to me have included:

- Irritation/rupture of dorsal tendons from pastpointing of distal screws
- Placement of the distal screws into the radiocarpal joint
- Irritation/rupture of volar tendons from prominent plates, incomplete reduction, or backing out of distal screws
- Subsidence of fragments and/or dorsal subluxation of the carpus from failure to engage the dorsal ulnar fragment
- Subsidence of fragments and volar subluxation of the carpus from failure to stabilize the volar rim of the lunate facet
- Failure to support the subchondral bone by placement of the distal screws too proximally
- Prominent hardware that is clinically palpable volarly due to implant placement too far radially

Another complication that is much less common includes the inability to remove a plate/screws because of bony adherence to titanium implants. A complication that has been reported but is controversial is tendinitis due to titanium; it remains a controversial area because of contradictory basic science studies.

Along with Drs. Jorge Orbay and Randy Bindra, I have performed 14 cadaveric dissections and examined 39 prepared distal radii. This work served as the basis for the anatomical explanations for these complications. The clinical observations were based on estimated collective case lists of more than 600 personal clinical cases, as well as other cases submitted to me for review.

Analysis of Complications
Tendon Irritation or Rupture from Pastpointing of Distal Screws

The earliest complication reported and the most common is tendon irritation or outright rupture resulting from screws extending beyond the dorsal cortex, or pastpointing.

The dorsal cortex of the distal radius can be thought of as being composed of two surfaces, one radial and one ulnar to Lister's tubercle. In the MR image shown in **Figure 16-1** the two surfaces form a dihedral angle of approximately 140 degrees (see also **Fig. 16-3**), neither of which is parallel to the plane of a lateral radiograph. Therefore, the lateral radiograph will not profile

either of the dorsal distal radial surfaces. Even if the profile of Lister's tubercle is ignored, a lateral view of the distal radius will not be able to determine if the screw is extending beyond the dorsal cortex. This brings up several additional points.

First, the classic AO teaching has included the concept of "bicortical purchase," that is, surgeons attempted to obtain fixation into the proximal and distal cortices of the bone being plated. A new approach is needed, however, with locked volar plates for the distal radius. The "proximal cortex" that needs to be engaged by the screw with a locked plate is the *plate*, not the volar cortex. The "distal cortex" in the distal radius is not the dorsal cortex, which is actually very thin.

Indeed, the thinness of the dorsal cortex is easily appreciated during surgery when using the dorsal approach. In addition, together with the common finding of a high degree of comminution in distal radius fractures, this makes the dorsal cortex an unsuitable point of fixation for the screws. The true source of stability in locked volar plating of the distal radius is support of the *subchondral bone*. As originally pointed out by McQueen, the subchondral bone is always thick and strong, even in severely osteoporotic patients. If the distal screws are in contact with the subchondral bone, the articular surface will be supported. If the distal screws are placed even a few millimeters proximal to the subchondral bone, subsidence is possible. Therefore, in the context of locked volar plating, the "distal cortex" is actually the subchondral bone, not the dorsal cortex.

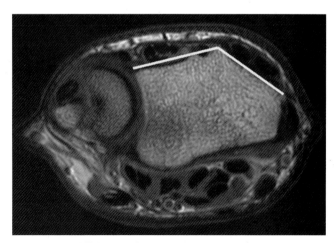

FIGURE 16-1 MR image of the distal radius, indicating the dihedral angle of the dorsal surfaces of the radius. The two surfaces are angled about 40 degrees, and neither of them is in line with the lateral radiograph. Note the close apposition of the tendons to the dorsal surface of the radius.

The second point is that extensor tendons are less than 1 mm away from the dorsal cortex, separated from it by only a thin layer of periosteum. Pastpointing by only 1 mm will bring the screw into contact with the tendons. The earliest locked volar plates used standard orthopaedic screws. Their cutting flutes are on the order of 2 to 3 mm and are particularly dangerous. Many of the current generation of locked volar plates use custom distal locking screws, with a taper on the leading end on the order of 1 mm and much smaller cutting flutes. Traditional orthopaedic practice has been to have the screw pastpoint beyond the cutting flutes and/or screw tip taper to obtain optimal purchase on the far cortex. This practice in locked volar plating will bring the screw tip into contact with the extensor tendons. Even screws designed without a formal cutting flute will have a tapering thread, to start the thread into the bone. This leading edge of the thread can be problematic if it comes in contact with the tendons, which are forced against the dorsal cortex whenever the patient performs simultaneous wrist flexion and finger extension.

The third point, returning to an analysis of the distal radial anatomy and the lateral radiograph, is that even oblique views of the distal radius, such as obtained with intraoperative mini-fluoroscopy, cannot easily define the location of the dorsal cortex, because some tendons, particularly the extensor pollicis longus (EPL), lie in a slight indentation in the dorsal cortex (**Fig. 16-2**).

Therefore, even fluoroscopic views may not precisely determine the location of the tip of the screw with respect to the dorsal cortex and the adjacent tendon. Screw tips should stop short of the dorsal cortex by 2 to 4 mm to be sure that they do not pastpoint and come in contact with the extensor tendons.

A fourth point is that there is no *need* to attempt to place the screws beyond or even close to the dorsal cortex. As observed earlier, the "distal cortex" is the subchondral bone. An examination of the lateral radiograph (see **Fig. 16-8**, later) shows that the subchondral bone stops several millimeters shy of the dorsal cortex. A screw can fully support the subchondral bone and yet stop 2 to 4 mm short of the dorsal cortex.

Case Examples

A 65-year-old woman fell and sustained a distal radius fracture. A locked volar plate was placed and intraoperative fluoroscopy indicated proper distal screw placement: just below the subchondral bone, out of the joint, and screw tips just below the dorsal cortex. Plain films were taken (**Fig. 16-3A**) and demonstrated a slight ulnar placement of the plate but good purchase on the dorsal ulnar corner and adequate purchase of the radial styloid on the posteroanterior view and good placement of the distal screws—just below the subchondral bone, out of the joint, and screw tips just below the dorsal cortex—on the lateral facet view.

Follow-up plain films in the office, probably with a slightly different rotation, indicated that the screw tips were just penetrating the dorsal cortex but seemed appropriate at the time on review by several orthopaedic surgeons (see **Fig. 16-3B**).

However, the patient complained about wrist stiffness and pain more than most patients. There was absolutely no localizing tenderness along the dorsal radius to suggest screw prominence, and there was no irritation with finger range of motion. After several visits without improvement in symptoms or change in the physical examination to suggest screw prominence, computed tomography (CT) was performed (see **Fig. 16-3C**).

The CT scan clearly shows that the screws are extending beyond the dorsal cortex. The screws are 2.7 mm in diameter, so they are extending about 3 mm dorsal to the radius. Note the dihedral angle of the two dorsal surfaces, as well as the fact that the tendons seem to be lying in a depression such that fluoroscopic views might not reveal their prominence.

The patient was taken to the operating room, where the screws were found to be just a few millimeters beyond the dorsal cortex.

In a different case (**Fig. 16-4A**), note how much tendon damage was done by a screw in precisely the wrong place—directly below the EPL tendon, with only 1 mm of pastpointing (see **Fig.**

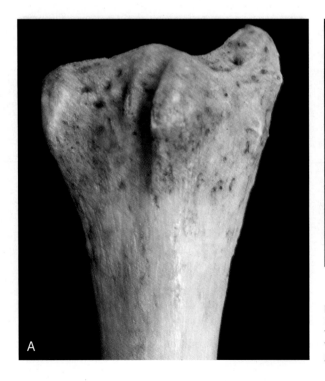

A

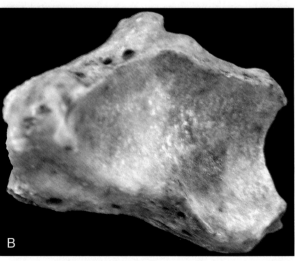

B

FIGURE 16-2 A, Dorsal view of a distal radius (prepared specimen). Note the groove for the EPL tendon, just ulnar to Lister's tubercle. **B,** End view of a distal radius (prepared specimen). Note the prominence of Lister's tubercle and the depth of the EPL groove compared with the surrounding bone.

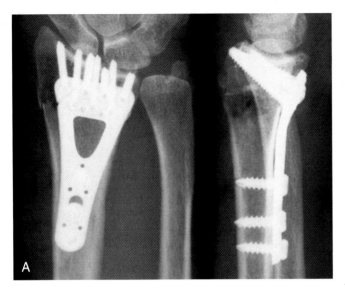

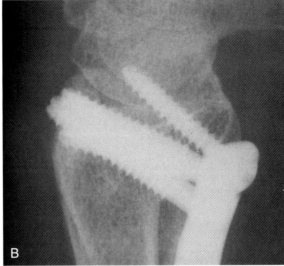

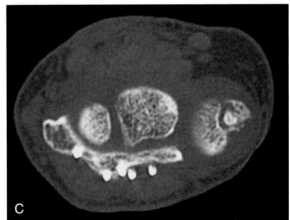

FIGURE 16-3 **A,** Posteroanterior and lateral facet views of a distal radius treated with a volar plate. Screws do not project beyond the dorsal cortex. **B,** Close-up view of lateral radiograph in same patient with slight rotation. Screws are at or beyond the dorsal cortex. **C,** CT of the distal radius showing screws are definitely beyond the dorsal cortex.

16-4B). Even *minimal* pastpointing can be disastrous if screws are positioned in the wrong place!

Each screw in the distal row of the locked volar plate requires unique consideration. The radial styloid screw is at the greatest angle, with its axis oriented radially. The length of this screw requires a fluoroscopic view of the dorsoradial surface of the radius, not the dorsal surface, and is always the shortest screw. The screw in the most ulnar position has the greatest requirement for accuracy of placement, owing to the nature of the dorsal ulnar corner fragment. The central screw holes require the most accurate determination of length compared with the dorsal cortex, unless one is attempting rigid internal fixation of the EPL tendon. One should bear in mind these unique characteristics as the fluoroscopic evaluation of the distal row is performed while pronating and supinating the forearm.

To summarize, in locked volar plating for distal radius fractures, in terms of "bicortical purchase," the "proximal cortex" is the plate and the "distal cortex" is the subchondral bone. There is (1) no need to engage the dorsal cortex, (2) the tendons are in close apposition to the dorsal cortex (<1 mm), (3) it is difficult to determine the precise location of the dorsal cortex and the tendons in relationship to the tip of the screws, and (4) slight pastpointing (~1 mm) can lead to tendon injury. It is recommended to have the screw tips 2 to 4 mm short of the dorsal cortex on the lateral radiograph.

Placement of the Distal Screws into the Radiocarpal Joint

The distal screws should support the subchondral bone, requiring the placement of the plate as distally as possible and yet not into the joint. Is the plate distal enough with the subchondral bone optimally supported? Is the plate too distal with a screw into the joint? This is the intraoperative quandary we face each time we place a locked volar plate. Intraoperative fluoroscopy is routinely used to assess the location of the screws. In conventional fracture management, true posteroanterior and lateral radiographs have normally been obtained. These views were adequate before the advent of locked volar plating. However, the need for screw placement immediately under the subchondral bone, yet not into the joint, has led to a need for a level of precision not previously required (on the order of 1 or 2 mm), and true lateral radiography has been found frequently to be misleading. How can we obtain the accuracy the new technique demands? The anatomy of the distal radius provides the answer.

In the posteroanterior view of a normal distal radius, the articular surface is curved, but if it is approximated as a straight line, it is tilted approximately 21 degrees. The true lateral of the radius, therefore, does not profile the scaphoid and lunate facets but views them at a 21-degree angle. If the forearm is tilted by approximately 21 degrees, the facets can be seen in true lateral profile and the view is called the *lateral facet view*.

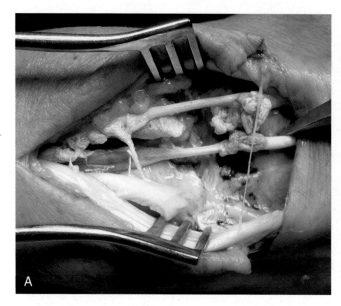

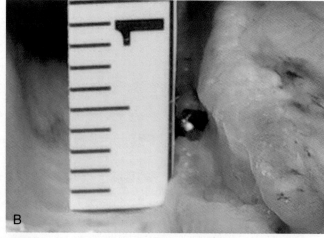

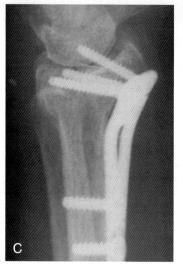

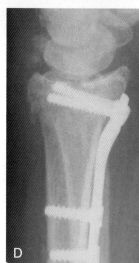

FIGURE 16-4 A, Dorsal intraoperative view shows significant injury to extensor tendons. **B,** Magnified dorsal view of same patient with tendons retracted. Tip of screw in the groove for the EPL shows that only 1 mm of pastpointing caused the tendon injuries noted in **A. C,** Lateral radiograph of distal radius. Note the appearance of screw penetration of the joint. **D,** Facet lateral to distal radius. Note the screws are actually not in the joint.

Clinical Pearl: To determine whether a screw will be into the joint, place a Kirschner wire (K-wire) through the drill guide locked into the screw hole in the plate. Remove the guide and plate, leaving the K-wire in place. Obtain a fluoroscopic view of the K-wire *end-on.* This view will precisely determine if the screw will be in the joint.

Figure 16-4C is a true lateral view, appearing to show penetration of the joint space by several screws and flagrant violation of the joint space by the radial styloid screw. However, the screw position resolves with a facet lateral view (**Fig. 16-4D**), with the majority of the screws nicely supporting the subchondral bone. A combination of the posteroanterior and the facet lateral views shows that the radial styloid screw is also out of the joint space.

Clinical Pearl: When using fluoroscopy in the operating room, do not tilt the patient's arm, but tilt the fluoroscopy arm for both lateral facet views and posteroanterior facet views. Rotating the patient's wrist while the C-arm is tilted will also provide excellent oblique facet views.

Clinical Pearl: Do not completely tighten the rotation clamps on the mini-C-arm, but keep them just loose enough so that you can tilt the arm when you need to. I find it is easy to control the angle of the mini-C-arm with one hand on the upper portion of the arm and a toe hooked on the lower portion of the arm.

Irritation or Rupture of Volar Tendons from Prominent Plates or Backing Out of Distal Screws

Some of the early locked volar plates and some of the first versions of current plates were more prominent than some of the other current generation plates. The Synthes volar 2.4/2.7 distal radius plate, colloquially called the "volar π plate,"* was a great innovation but had the disadvantages of both raised margins around the screw holes and sharp edges because the width needed to be trimmed to size. When selecting a locked volar plate, be sure that it is properly precontoured, low profile, and smooth on its distal margin.

Plate placement can also affect the tendons. If the plate is placed too distally, the flare of the volar rim of the joint will cause the plate to be prominent along its distal margin. The plate should not extend beyond the *watershed line* (yellow line in **Fig. 16-5A**), a term coined by Orbay that refers to the line at the highest (most volar) margin of the radius. This will be the part of the radius (or plate) that is closest to the flexor tendons and therefore at greatest risk of injuring them.

---

*The term "π plate" was never used by Synthes but was created by surgeons as more descriptive.

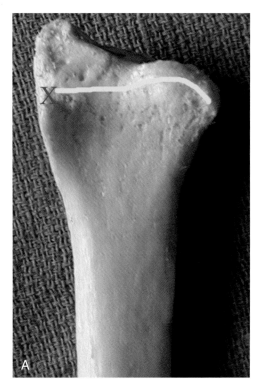 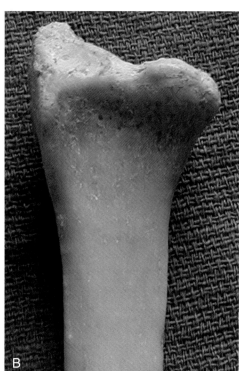

FIGURE 16-5 Volar views of prepared distal radius. **A,** The watershed line (*yellow*) and the volar radial tuberosity (*red X*). **B,** The lunate facet buttress (*red X*). *Note:* the lighting was changed to highlight the structures.

If the plate is placed too radially, a tuberosity called the *volar radial tuberosity,** will raise up the radial margin. The tuberosity is easily palpated approximately 2 cm proximal to the volar tuberosity of the scaphoid (which is known to most surgeons in conjunction with the Watson test) and on the most radial aspect of the wrist. A plate placed too radially can become both clinically palpable ("Doc, is this bump supposed to be here? It wasn't there before the surgery!") and possibly a problem for the tendons (usually the flexor pollicis longus). If the plate is placed too ulnarly and has a flat profile across its distal margin, a bony feature called the *lunate facet buttress* will raise up the ulnar margin. The lunate facet buttress is a bony area just proximal to the lunate facet. The lunate facet projects several millimeters volarly more than the scaphoid facet (see **Fig. 16-2B**) and is supported by the lunate facet buttress, which varies in size from a millimeter to several millimeters. Some plates (Hand Innovations, Orthofix, and Acumed) are contoured to fit over the lunate facet buttress and still have the plate flat on the volar surface of the radius. The more distally a plate is placed and the larger the buttress is, the more relevant a contour in the plate becomes.

Figure 16-5A is a volar view of a radius, with the lighting coming from the left to highlight the volar radial tuberosity (indicated by the red "X") and, extending proximally, the *volar radial ridge*. The yellow line represents the watershed line. **Figure 16-5B** is the same specimen, with the lighting coming from the top to highlight the lunate facet buttress (indicated by the red "X").

Case Example

A 31-year-old man fell off a boat onto a dock and sustained a distal radius fracture. He had had a prior distal radius fracture

at age 15 with some residual deformity. A locked volar plate that is well contoured to fit a normal distal radius was placed. The volar surface of the radius was flatter than normal, and because the plate was contoured to fit a normal radius it did not fit well distally. The pronator quadratus was securely closed over the plate.

Postoperatively, at 3 to 4 months, the patient complained of volar wrist pain with wrist extension and when he was carrying something very heavy. He developed paresthesias at 5 months. Surgical exploration was carried out at 7 months because of continuing symptoms.

Damage was found to two tendons (**Fig. 16-6**) but no rupture. There was a hole in the pronator quadratus, and the plate was visible and felt to be prominent. The intraoperative assessment was that the properly precontoured plate did not fit the abnormal radius and that the screw holes felt "sharp" to evaluation. The plate was removed, and the symptoms resolved. (In addition, I have spoken to the manufacturer and confirmed that this was an early-generation design. The design has undergone a number of improvements, such that there is now less chance for screw hole "sharpness.")

Case Example

A 61-year-old female bus driver fell in the schoolyard and sustained a volar Barton fracture (**Fig. 16-7A, B**). A volar π plate was placed to buttress the fracture (**Fig. 16-7C, D**).

The fracture was incompletely reduced, and the plate's distal edge was therefore prominent. She developed a wrist ache with forceful use beyond 2 hours, which was attributed to her radioscaphoid arthritis. She also developed subsidence of the scaphoid into the radius with cystic degeneration within a year, had an ache in her wrist, and retired as a bus driver.

---

*These terms have been proposed by Jorge Orbay, Randy Bindra, and the author in a paper submitted to the *Journal of Hand Surgery.*

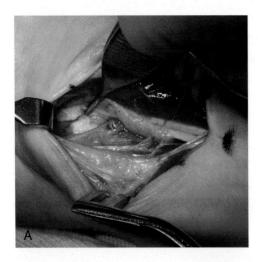

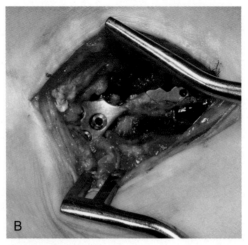

FIGURE 16-6 A, Volar view of a fracture during plate removal. Note the tendon injury. **B,** Another volar view. Note the hole in the pronator quadratus, with a visible plate.

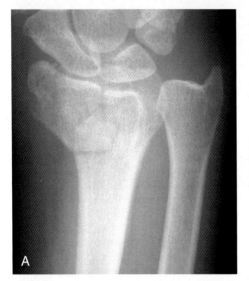

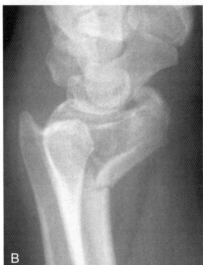

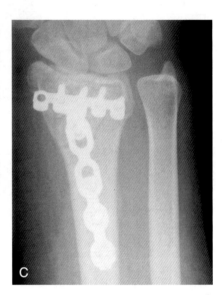

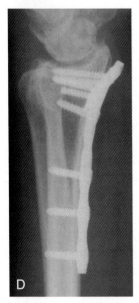

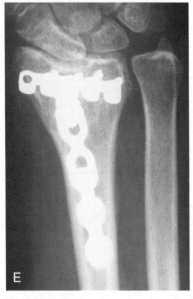

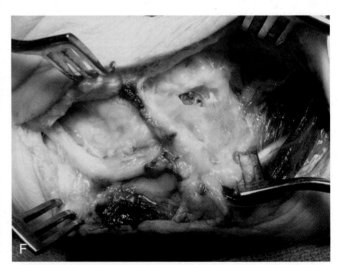

FIGURE 16-7 Posteroanterior (**A**) and lateral (**B**) radiographs of a volar Barton fracture. **C,** Posteroanterior radiograph after treatment with a volar π plate. **D,** Lateral postoperative radiograph. Note the incomplete reduction, with resulting prominence of the distal edge of the plate. Even without the incomplete reduction the plate was placed beyond the watershed line and would have been prominent. **E,** Posteroanterior radiograph obtained 6 years later. Note the subsidence of the scaphoid facet. **F,** Intraoperative view during plate removal. Note the hole in the dense scar tissue overlying the plate.

Six years after surgery she presented with the sudden onset of an inability to flex her thumb interphalangeal joint, wrist swelling, and wrist tenderness. Radiographs showed no progression of the subsidence of the scaphoid into the radius (see **Fig. 16-7E**) and resolution of the cystic degeneration. The plate continued to be prominent volarly.

The diagnosis was made of a flexor pollicis longus rupture due to rubbing on the distal edge of the prominent plate. At surgery, the plate was found to be covered by a dense layer of scar tissue, except at one point. The most radial distal screw (there was one empty hole to the radial side of this screw) was easily seen through a rent in the scar tissue (see **Fig. 16-7F**).

The tendon was grafted with a strip of flexor carpi radialis, because there was no palmaris longus. The bone had overgrowth on the plate, but the titanium screws and plate were not firmly bonded to the bone and were removed without problem. The patient regained excellent range of motion of the thumb.

The plate was removed. It is a second-generation volar π plate. The screw holes are surrounded by a raised lip that is high profile, and the distal margin of the plate has a sharply squared-off end. The screws have cruciate heads. Cruciate heads can form razor-sharp edges if the screwdriver slips out of the head while seating the screw. The current-generation Synthes locked volar plates are much improved, and all have rounded edges, are lower profile, and use hex or torx screw heads.

There seems to be an advantage to covering the plate with the pronator quadratus (PQ) to interpose the muscle between the plate and the flexor tendons. During the initial dissection, most surgeons incise the PQ distally at the edge of the muscle fibers. This line is referred to as the *PQ line.** After plate placement, most surgeons repair the PQ muscle. However, the thinness of the fascia of the muscle makes this an exercise in futility, because the sutures typically rip out before the next layer is closed. One technique that has proved to be quite secure is to release the PQ during the original dissection not along the margin of the muscular fibers (the *PQ line*), but 1 to 2 mm beyond the *PQ line*, into the fibrous tissue proximal to the volar capsule. This fibrous tissue, termed the *fibrous transition zone*, has been determined in cadaveric dissections not to be part of the mobile volar wrist capsule (composed of the radioscaphoid, radiocapitate, long radiolunate, and short radiolunate ligaments) but to be immobile and attached to the distal margin of the radius. It is believed that incising the fibrous transition zone should not add unnecessarily to wrist capsular scarring or wrist joint stiffness. Continue the dissection radially 1 to 2 mm into the fibrous tissue at the base of the first dorsal compartment. If this is done there will be a 1- to 2-mm thick, strong margin along the edge of the PQ muscle. This margin will securely hold the sutures and the PQ will remain in place, serving as an interpositional layer between the plate and the flexor tendons.

Clinical Pearl: During the initial dissection, incise the PQ muscle 1 to 2 mm distal to the PQ line. Continue the dissection radially 1 to 2 mm into the fibrous tissue at the base of the first dorsal compartment. This will create a strong 1- to 2-mm margin at the edge of the PQ muscle and allow a secure repair.

*These terms have been proposed by Jorge Orbay, Randy Bindra, and the author in a paper submitted to the *Journal of Hand Surgery.*

Subsidence of Fragments and/or Dorsal Subluxation of the Carpus from Failure to Engage the Dorsal Ulnar Fragment

The dorsal ulnar corner of the radius cannot be neglected because it serves as the attachment point for the dorsal portion of the distal radioulnar joint (DRUJ) ligament. Forearm rotation exerts a very strong force on the dorsal ulnar fragment and can easily displace it. The dorsal ulnar fragment is usually not well visualized on either the postero-anterior or the lateral view, and oblique views are needed to assess it. Good screw purchase may be a challenge for such fragments with the volar approach. One should be prepared mentally for this challenge: either get good fixation with the most ulnar screw in the distal row or place a small dorsal, fragment-specific plate.

Case Example

A 20-year-old man fell from a mountain bike and sustained bilateral wrist injuries. Radiographs demonstrated bilateral distal radius fractures and a right scaphoid fracture. The left wrist is shown in **Figure 16-8A**.

The radiographs indicated a fracture of the dorsal ulnar corner, so oblique views were obtained to assess its displacement (see **Fig. 16-8B**). The oblique view much better demonstrated the size and displacement of the dorsal ulnar corner. The opposite wrist had a very similar distal radius fracture in addition to the scaphoid waist fracture. Open reduction and internal fixation was performed for all three fractures.

A locked volar plate was supplemented with a dorsal 0.062-inch K-wire to hold the left radius. Once the radius was fixed, DRUJ stability was assessed and found to be unstable. This was attributed to the ulnar styloid fracture. This was fixed with a 0.045-inch K-wire and figure-of-eight wire in a tension band configuration (see **Fig. 16-8C**). The patient was seen at 1 week and follow-up radiographs were obtained.

The follow-up views demonstrated displacement of the dorsal ulnar corner, in a manner identical to the original injury (see **Fig. 16-8D**). A critical review of the immediate postoperative films shows that the dorsal ulnar corner was not fixed with the volar plate and that the K-wire fixation was not stiff enough alone to resist the deforming forces. One could also speculate that the instability of the DRUJ was entirely or in part due to the dorsal ulnar corner rather than the ulnar styloid fracture. It was thought that the instability had a chance of progressive subsidence, and further fixation was required. (The opposite wrist had an identical subsidence and reoperation was also done on it.)

The patient was returned to the operating room where a dorsal plate was placed through a dorsal incision (see **Fig. 16-8E**). This reduction was maintained and at 1 year the patient had good motion with little to no pain.

Clinical Pearl: If there is a dorsal ulnar fragment you need to stabilize, determine the future axis of the ulnarmost screw by placing a K-wire through the drill guide locked into the ulnar screw hole in the plate. Leave the K-wire in place, and remove the guide and plate. Obtain a fluoroscopic view of the K-wire end-on. This view will determine precisely if the screw will be in the fragment.

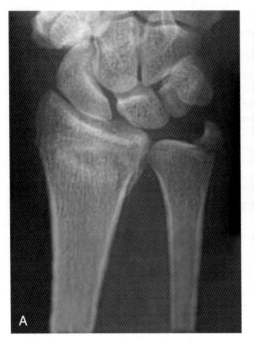

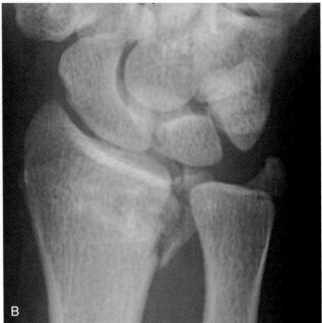

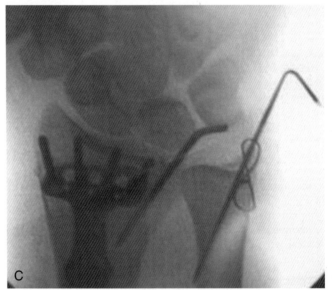

FIGURE 16-8 A, Posteroanterior radiograph of distal radius fracture. (The patient also has distal radius and scaphoid fractures on the opposite hand.) **B,** Oblique radiograph demonstrates the dorsal ulnar corner fracture. **C,** Slightly obliqued posteroanterior radiograph showing the lack of purchase of the dorsal ulnar corner by the plate and screws; it was supplemented with a Kirschner wire. The fracture appears reduced.

Subsidence of Fragments and Volar Subluxation of the Carpus from Failure to Stabilize the Volar Rim of the Lunate Facet

Small volar rim fragments are difficult to stabilize, and experience has shown that they are easily underestimated. Common mistakes are to place the plate too ulnarly or too proximally or to choose a technique or plate that cannot stabilize the volar rim of the lunate.

Figure 16-9A is the lateral view of a dried radius from the ulnar side. The key point is that the lunate facet projects quite a bit volarly (see also Figs. 16-1 and 16-2B) and that the center of the facet is directly over the *volar* aspect of the radius. It is not over the center of the medullary canal. The load from the carpus places a force on the lunate facet that has a component that is distinctly volarly directed. This, combined with the extent of volar

projection of the lunate facet, makes lunate rim fractures very unstable (**Fig. 16-10**).

No locked volar plate extends to the volar lip of the lunate facet. The one that comes the closest is the Synthes 2.4 LCP Volar Juxta-Articular Distal Radius Plate. Most designs do not want to extend that far past the watershed line and risk injuring the flexor tendons, and how far a plate should extend distally is controversial. However, in the case of a fracture of the volar lip of the lunate facet, some kind of stabilization is required and some violation of the watershed line is needed. Various techniques have been used or proposed, including using the Synthes Juxta-Articular plate, placing a standard plate more distally, using a fragment-specific approach, or using K-wires. The effectiveness of each approach depends on the fragment size, the technique used, and the actual shape of the implant. The Synthes Juxta-Articular plate or the fragment-specific approaches are probably the most common, but each has its limitations. The

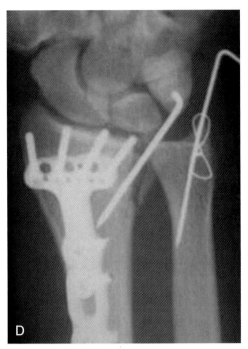 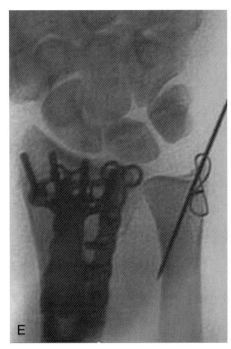 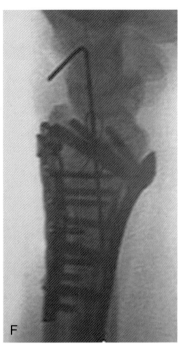

FIGURE 16-8, cont'd **D**, Slightly obliqued posteroanterior radiograph at 1 week. Note the displacement of the fracture fragment. **E** and **F**, Postero-anterior and lateral radiographs after revision surgery. Note the fragment-specific plate on the dorsal ulnar corner of the radius.

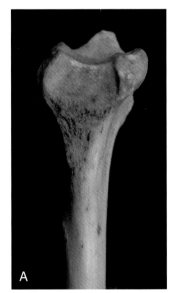 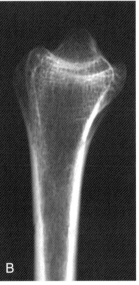

FIGURE 16-9 **A**, lateral view of a dried radius from the ulnar side. **B**, radiograph of the specimen approximately the same projection (the scaphoid and lunate facets are overlapping in the dried radius but offset in the radiograph.

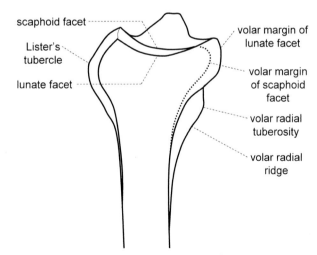

FIGURE 16-10 Anatomical drawing of the radius identifying structural features.

Synthes plate unnecessarily extends beyond the watershed line for the scaphoid facet, which does not need support. The fragment-specific approach is less stable and more complex to apply.

Case Example

A 19-year-old man fell and sustained a distal radius fracture. Radiographs showed a very distal volar lip fracture of the radius and slightly rotated radial styloid fracture, with just enough volar subluxation of the lunate to suggest volar instability.

A CT scan and CT reconstruction with the carpus removed confirmed the size, shape, and location of the fragments, as well as the volar subluxation of the lunate. It was believed that a standard locked plate would not stabilize this fracture, and a fragment-specific technique was used.

Another clinical case, with a more complex fracture, was stabilized with a similar technique.

Placement of the Distal Screws Too Proximally and Failing to Support the Subchondral Bone

Older patients with severe osteoporosis are a challenge to treat. Locked volar plates take advantage of the two strongest areas of bone, which are the volar cortex just proximal to the metaphyseal bone and the subchondral bone. The bone is quite fragile. However, the radiograph clearly demonstrates that these two areas are the most dense, with little bone showing in the dorsal cortex of the metaphyseal bone or a few millimeters proximal to the subchondral bone. Although distal screws can support the joint several millimeters away from the subchondral bone in younger patients, they need to be placed distally in the osteoporotic patient. If the screws are several millimeters away from the subchondral bone, they may settle through the cancellous metaphyseal bone until they reach the subchondral bone. I am not aware of any case in which the distal screws have settled through the subchondral bone.

Prominent Hardware That Is Clinically Palpable Volarly from Implant Placement Too Far Radially

Palpate the volar radial tuberosity in your own wrist. It is 2 cm proximal to the volar tuberosity of the scaphoid (the part of the scaphoid where you push for the Watson test) at the most radial border of the wrist. It is quite subcutaneous, with little overlying fat. Plates that are placed too radially can be easily palpated by the patient. Care must be taken, before the drilling for the first screw, to assess the plate placement. Most plate systems have methods to hold the plate in place while the placement is assessed radiographically, either K-wire holes or drill guides that accept K-wires. Once the position of the plate is tentatively determined, remove the retractors, replace the skin edges, and palpate the skin over the volar radial tuberosity. Move the plate if required.

Inability to Remove a Plate/Screws Because of Bony Adherence to Titanium Implants

There have been reports of titanium screws being so firmly bonded to the bone that the heads shear off, the driver tip shears off, or the head strips out. Surgeons have had to resort to breaking the implants and burring off any projecting screw remnants. This point remains controversial. Some authors recommend the use of stainless steel implants to avoid bonding and screw breakage, and others claim that there is no chemical bonding between bone and titanium. It is interesting to observe the competing claims of two groups with very different agendas: the trauma companies deny that bonding to their titanium implants exists, whereas the total joint companies tout the strength of the bonding to their titanium implants. Many surface treatments, from polishing to chemical treatment or hydroxyapatite coating, have been tried to avoid or enhance bonding. The controversy does not seem to have a resolution at this time, and there does not seem to be a clear reason to avoid titanium locked volar plates. In the one case of late titanium plate removal in my experience, at 6 years after implantation (see case cited earlier involving a second-generation Synthes titanium plate [see **Fig. 16-7F**]), all screws were easily removed once the bony overgrowth covering the screw heads was removed.

Tendinitis Due to Titanium

Tendinitis due to titanium is even more controversial than the inability to remove titanium screws due to bonding. Some authors of animal studies report finding titanium synovitis that is more than that found with stainless steel, whereas others report the opposite. The influence of synovial fluid on the formation of tendinitis is also controversial. At this time there does not seem to be a clear reason to avoid titanium locked volar plates.

Clinical Pearls

1. Nothing is so humbling as reviewing your own cases 2 or so years later. Be brutal in your criticisms.
2. Perform a cadaveric dissection. When you know you do not have to repair anything and the exposure can be exceedingly wide, a lot of new lessons will be learned. Our normal exposure windows hide as much as they reveal.
3. Obtain and study a distal radius. You cannot reconstruct a bone if all you look at are shadows (radiographs) and microviews (surgical exposures). I have kept one on my desk for 14 years (seen in **Figs. 16-2A, 16-2B, and 16-9**), and this one bone has taught me a treasure trove of lessons.

ACKNOWLEDGMENTS

The author would like to acknowledge the contributions of Drs. Jorge Orbay and Randy Bindra for the development of the new anatomical terms and the contributions of clinical material by Drs. Kendrick Lee, Stefan Zachary, and Rob Medoff.

DISCLOSURE

I have designed a locked volar plate and receive royalties related to that plate.

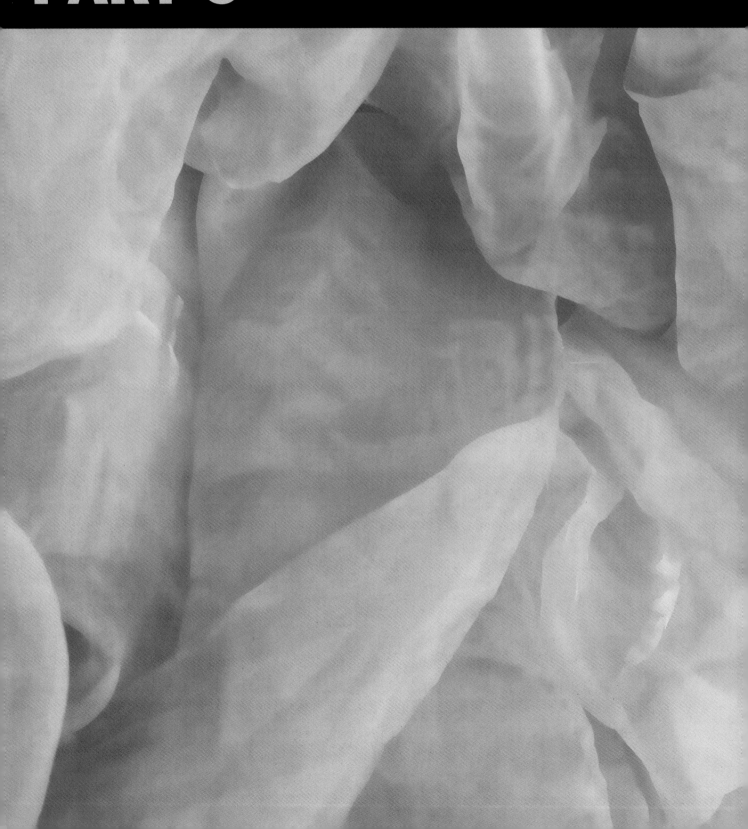

PART 5 ALTERNATIVES TO INTERNAL FIXATION

Kapandji Pinning of Distal Radius Fractures

17

Ruby Grewal, MD, MSc and Graham J. W. King, MD, MSc

Distal radius fractures are among the most common upper extremity injuries. They account for one sixth of all fractures treated in the emergency department[1] and this incidence is expected to increase as the population ages. Thompson and colleagues report that the incidence of distal radius fractures continues to rise with age in women older than 50 and in men older than 65.[2]

Many different treatment methods have been advocated depending on the fracture type and stability. Various authors have attempted to identify factors that predict instability in distal radius fractures. Mackenney and coworkers found that the most consistent predictors of instability were patient age, metaphyseal comminution, and ulnar variance.[3]

Most stable fractures can be successfully treated with closed reduction and casting. However, when the reduction cannot be maintained with casting alone, the surgeon must consider additional treatment modalities. The treatment method chosen will depend on the fracture pattern and the preferences of the treating surgeon. Options include percutaneous pinning, open reduction and internal fixation, or external fixation. These modalities can also be used together as needed to ensure stable fixation.

Percutaneous pinning is a widely used technique that helps to maintain reduction while also having the advantage of being minimally invasive and inexpensive.

Many methods of percutaneous pinning have been described in the literature, including trans-styloid pinning, intrafocal pinning, and pinning into the distal fragments.[4-10]

One technique of percutaneous pinning—intrafocal pinning—utilizes Kirschner wires (K-wires) inserted directly into the fracture site to manipulate and reduce the distal fragment.

This technique was originally described by Kapandji in 1976 as a method of treating unstable extra-articular distal radius fractures.[11] His original report described a technique whereby two threaded K-wires were inserted into the fracture site and then used to directly manipulate and lever the distal fracture fragment into the desired position. Once reduction was achieved, the wires were advanced into the proximal fragment; the pins do not fix the distal fragment but rather buttress it in place. In the original description, patients were not immobilized postoperatively. Kapandji originally advocated this technique for younger patients, whose fractures were only minimally comminuted. It was contraindicated in patients with osteoporotic bone or severe comminution and in fractures with intra-articular extension. In the original publication, little information was available regarding the clinical results of this procedure.[11]

In 1987, Kapandji reported his experience with the original technique and recommended adding a third dorsal ulnar pin.[12] He expanded the indications to include fractures with multiple fragments.[12] Since then, many authors have described modifications to the original technique,[11] and the clinical indications have expanded from those originally described.[13-21]

Literature Review

There are several published case series reporting a large percentage of overall good to excellent results using intrafocal pinning. Epinette and associates reported 83% good and excellent results in 70 cases, including elderly patients and fractures with undisplaced intra-articular extension.[13] Docquier and colleagues also reported a high percentage of good and excellent clinical and radiographic results using this technique for articular and extraarticular fractures.[14] Peyroux and coworkers reported the outcome of 159 cases (81% extra-articular) with 93% good and excellent clinical results.[15]

Dowdy and associates retrospectively reviewed the results of 17 patients treated with intrafocal pinning.[16] All K-wires were cut below the skin, and the injured area was immobilized for 6 weeks. Sixteen of 17 patients were pleased with their outcomes. The average visual analog score on the pain scale was 0.44/10, and function was 8.6/10. There was a trend for older osteopenic patients to lose their postoperative reduction, but this was not statistically significant.[16] Patients aged 65 and older also had significantly less restoration of volar tilt than those younger than 65 years of age ($P = .04$). Dowdy recommended that Kapandji pinning alone should be avoided in patients with severe osteopenia.

In the largest series published to date, Nonnenmacher and coworkers reported the results of 350 intra-articular and extraarticular distal radius fractures in patients aged 12 to 89 treated with this technique.[17] They used three intrafocal pins, which were buried below the skin and removed at 6 weeks. Plaster immobilization was not used, and patients were allowed to begin range of motion postoperatively. The subjective results were good and excellent in 90% of patients, and functional outcomes were reported as good and excellent in 99%. No patients reported poor subjective or functional outcomes. The radiologic results were also evaluated as 93% good to very good, 6% average, and 1% poor.[17]

The experience with intrafocal pinning in older patients has grown in recent years. Greating and coworkers reported on the results of 24 fractures with minimal intra-articular involvement in patients aged 16 to 94.[18] They utilized immobilization in patients for 6 weeks after the surgery. In 13 fractures, the clinical outcomes were excellent in 7, good in 4, and fair in 2 based on the Mayo wrist score. The two fair results were in patients younger than age 65. They also report good and excellent radiologic results (using Sarmiento and colleagues' criteria[22]) in 79% of patients younger than 65 and in 60% of patients older than 65. They concluded that this technique provides acceptable clinical results in elderly patients despite some loss of reduction after pinning.

Trumble and coworkers published a review of their experience with intrafocal pinning supplemented with external fixation.[19] They reviewed 61 patients with either intrafocal pinning alone or in combination with external fixation. They included fractures with undisplaced intra-articular extension and all age groups. There were 96% good to excellent results in young patients (<55 years) with displaced extra-articular distal radius fractures (minimal comminution) treated with intrafocal pin fixation alone. In patients older than 55 years of age, they reported 94% good to excellent results in patients who received supplemental external fixation and they also reported that range of motion, grip strength, and pain relief were significantly better when external fixation was used in this age group, even when only one cortex demonstrated comminution. Their final recommendation was that older patients, or younger patients with involvement of more than two surfaces of the radial metaphysis (or >50% of the metaphyseal diameter), require external fixation in addition to percutaneous pin fixation for optimal results.[19]

In a retrospective review by Board and associates comparing closed reduction and casting to intrafocal wiring in patients older than 55 years, it was found that functional results were good to excellent in 19 of 23 patients who received intrafocal pinning versus 12 of 23 who received plaster alone, supporting the use of this technique in older patients.[20]

Hollevoet recently published a study assessing anterior fracture displacement in Colles' fractures after intrafocal pinning in women older than age 59 years (without supplemental external fixation).[21] It was demonstrated that the intrafocal pins were not sufficient to prevent anterior fracture displacement in almost one third of patients. Five weeks after fracture, 36 of 89 (40.4%) patients had more than 20 degrees of palmar shift or tilt or more than 10 degrees of dorsal angulation; 37 patients (41.6%) had more than 2 mm of ulnar-positive variance; and 6 (6.7%) had more than 5 mm of ulnar-positive variance. The clinical implications of this displacement were not discussed. They concluded that intrafocal wiring of Colles' fractures in elderly, osteoporotic patients may not be sufficient to prevent anterior fracture displacement.[21]

Indications

Intrafocal pinning is indicated for unstable displaced distal radius fractures in which it is not possible to obtain or maintain a reduction with cast immobilization (**Fig. 17-1**). The ideal candidate for Kapandji pinning is a younger patient with good quality bone. Ideally, the fracture should be extra-articular with minimal comminution and easily reducible with closed methods. Since the original description of this technique,[11] the indications have expanded to include older patients,[13] fractures with undisplaced intra-articular extension,[13] and fractures with multiple fragments.[12]

This technique works best in the acute setting while the fracture fragment is still mobile. If the procedure is delayed, this technique is not contraindicated but it may become more difficult or impossible to successfully manipulate the distal fragment into the correct position with closed methods.

Contraindications

The intrafocal technique is contraindicated in fractures with significant intra-articular displacement and/or volar cortical comminution.[8,18,23] It is also contraindicated if a reduction cannot be achieved by closed means.[18,23] Relative contraindications to this technique are poor bone quality and osteoporosis.[17] We also avoid intrafocal pinning in patients with severe osteopenia, marked dorsal radial comminution, an associated ipsilateral distal metadiaphyseal ulna fracture, and both volar and dorsal comminution.[16] In these circumstances, the Kapandji pins may require supplementation with an external fixator.[16,24]

Surgical Technique

Web Vi

17-1

At our institution, this procedure is performed with the patient under general anesthesia or with a brachial plexus block with tourniquet control. The patient is positioned supine, with the affected extremity suspended from sterile finger traps with 10 to 15 pounds of countertraction. Fluoroscopy is available to ensure that adequate anteroposterior and lateral images can be obtained during the procedure.

Attention is directed toward first correcting the dorsal tilt. Two 0.062-inch K-wires are percutaneously inserted into the dorsal aspect of the wrist. A dorsal radial pin is inserted between the third and fourth extensor compartments, and a dorsal ulnar pin is inserted between the fourth and fifth extensor compartments. The K-wires are then manually advanced through the dorsal cortex and into the fracture site just short of the volar cortex. The image intensifier facilitates locating the fracture site. These two wires are then levered distally under image control to correct the dorsal tilt (**Fig. 17-2**). A 0.062-inch K-wire is then inserted percutaneously on the radial aspect of the wrist, between the first and second dorsal compartments, and manually advanced into the fracture site. The K-wire is then levered distally to restore the radial inclination (**Fig. 17-3**). When an adequate reduction is achieved fluoroscopically, the wires are then advanced through the intact volar and ulnar cortex using a powered wire driver. The final reduction and pin position should then be confirmed radiographically (**Fig. 17-4A**). Excessive pin protrusion through intact cortex should be avoided to prevent impingement on adjacent structures. The K-wires can then be cut just below the skin but superficial to the extensor tendons to avoid rupture. Alternatively the K-wires can be bent over and cut above the skin. The arm is immobilized in a short arm cast for 6 weeks (see **Fig. 17-4B**). Early digital motion and forearm rotation are encouraged. At 6 weeks, the K-wires are removed under local anesthetic in the clinic. Range of motion exercises of the wrist are then initiated and supervised by a hand therapist (see **Fig. 17-4C**).

Clinical Pearls

When performing intrafocal pinning for distal radius fractures, the K-wires should be inserted through the skin, just distal to the fracture so that when the wire is tilted distally, as the fracture is reduced, the skin will not be tethered. During the reduction process, avoid bending the K-wire by pushing on the wire immediately adjacent to the skin. In addition, the reduction process should be monitored with live fluoroscopy to avoid either undercorrecting or overcorrecting the displacement.

Potential Pitfalls

Although the procedure is not technically demanding, there are some potential pitfalls to avoid. When advancing the K-wires into the volar cortex, one must ensure that the K-wire does not enter the volar compartment because this may cause nerve or tendon irritation. It is also possible to over-reduce the fracture, cause volar translation of the fragment, or displace an intra-articular fracture. As mentioned previously, these pitfalls can be avoided by monitoring the reduction process with fluoroscopy. One should also

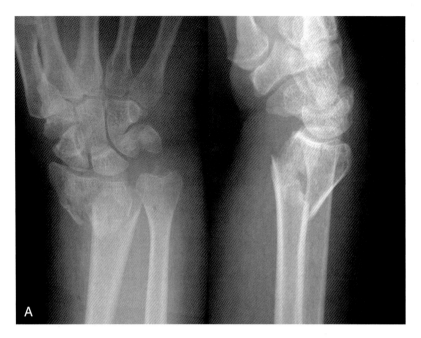

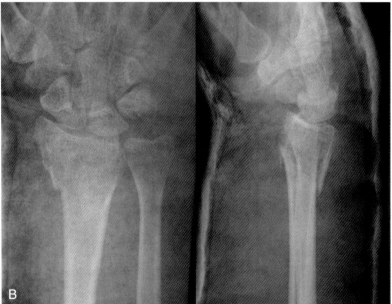

FIGURE 17-1 A 46-year-old woman slipped on ice, fell onto her outstretched hand, and sustained an extra-articular distal radius fracture. Pre-reduction (**A**) and post-reduction (**B**) anteroposterior and lateral radiographs.

consider supplementing intrafocal pinning with an external fixator if the patient is older than 55 years of age or if there is comminution involving more than two surfaces of the radial metaphysis (or >50% of the metaphyseal diameter)[19,24] (**Fig. 17-5**).

Controversies

There are many modifications of the intrafocal pinning technique. Some prefer to leave the K-wires above the skin for ease of removal, whereas others prefer to bury them below the skin, to reduce the risk of infection. Some insert the K-wire percutaneously, whereas others believe strongly that a small incision should be made to ensure all essential neurovascular and tendinous structures can be retracted aside. The other controversial aspect is postoperative immobilization. Although Kapandji's original description did not include postoperative immobilization, in more recent reports the fractures are usually immobilized to prevent

displacement, particularly if using this technique for more challenging cases.

Salvage Procedures

The benefit of this technique is that it does not preclude the use of more traditional techniques such as open reduction and internal fixation. If the fracture cannot be reduced or if the fragments are over-reduced or displaced during the reduction procedure, one can always perform an open reduction and internal fixation.

Personal Results

We reviewed the experience with extra-articular distal radius fractures at the Hand and Upper Limb Center in London, Ontario, from June 1997 to June 2004. Twenty-eight patients were treated with the intrafocal pinning technique described by Kapandji and were available for 1-year follow-up. All patients

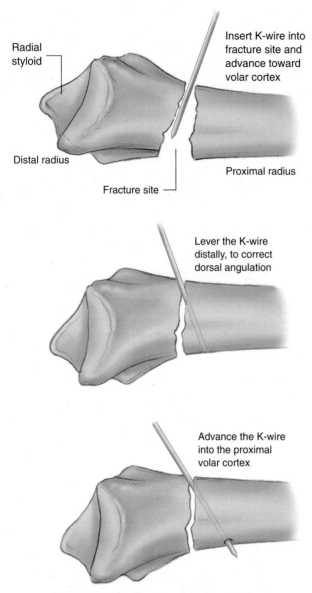

FIGURE 17-2 Restoration of dorsal angulation.

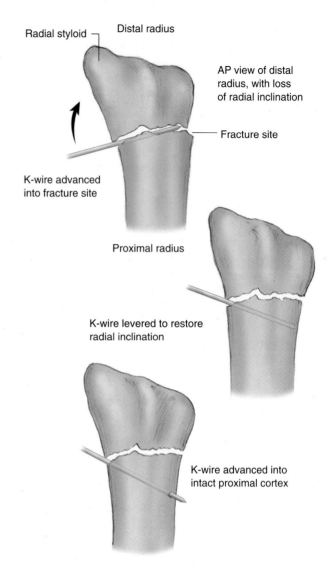

FIGURE 17-3 Restoration of radial inclination.

were followed at 6 weeks, 3 months, 6 months, and 1 year. At each visit, objective clinical data (range of motion and grip strength), radiographs, Disabilities of the Arm, Shoulder, and Hand (DASH) scores, Patient-Rated Wrist Evaluation (PRWE) scores, and SF-36 scores were obtained.

There were 5 men and 23 women in this group. The average age was 46.9 ± 15.3 years (range 18 to 72). One patient was involved in a workers' compensation claim. Seventeen patients were treated with Kapandji pinning and cast immobilization alone, 9 patients were treated with Kapandji pinning plus external fixation, and 2 patients had an open reduction and internal fixation supplemented with intrafocal pinning. Of the nine external fixators in this series, eight were used in patients older than the age of 55. There were 3 patients older than the age of 55 who were treated with Kapandji pinning and casting alone.

Clinical Outcomes

The mean PRWE score[25] was 17.5 (score 0 to 100, with 100 worst possible score), and the mean DASH score[26] was 16.1

(score 0 to 100, with 100 worst possible score). The SF-36[27] physical component summary score was 44.4, and the mental component summary score was 51.1 (U.S. population norm = 50).

The average range of motion was 52.3 degrees of wrist flexion, 65.9 degrees of wrist extension, 16.6 degrees of radial deviation, 27.4 degrees of ulnar deviation, 74.0 degrees of pronation, and 72.6 degrees of supination. The grip strength on the affected side was 80% of that of the unaffected side at 1 year.

Radiographic Outcomes

Radial inclination, dorsal tilt, and ulnar variance were measured before reduction, after final reduction, and at 1 year. The mean loss of dorsal angulation over 1 year was 1 ± 4.5 degrees ($P = .3$), the mean loss of radial inclination was 0.2 ± 1.8 degrees ($P = .6$), and there was a mean loss of 1 ± 1.0 mm of radial length from the time of reduction to 1-year follow-up ($P < .001$).

We also evaluated the quality of the reduction according to guidelines of the American Society for Surgery of the Hand (ASSH).[28] They indicate that the alignment of a distal radius fracture is considered unacceptable if the dorsal angulation is

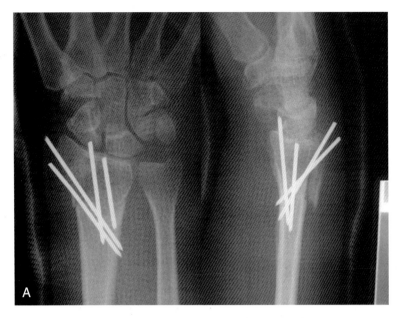

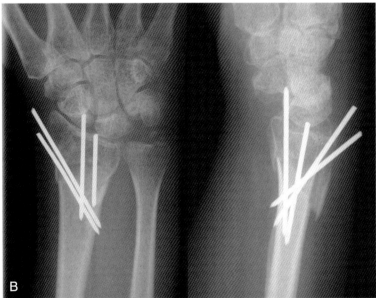

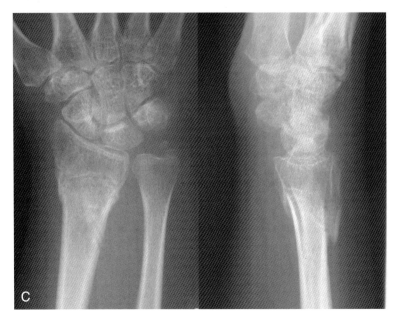

FIGURE 17-4 Same case as in Figure 17-1. **A**, Postoperative anteroposterior and lateral radiographs. **B**, Radiographic appearance at 7 weeks: fracture is healed and pins ready for removal. **C**, Anteroposterior and lateral radiographs at 3 months after the injury.

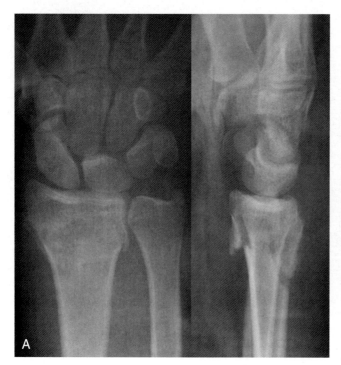

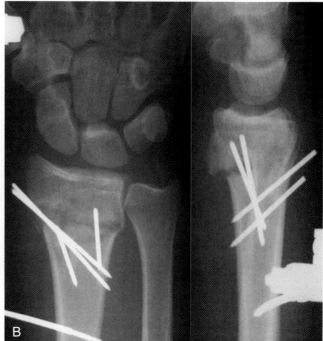

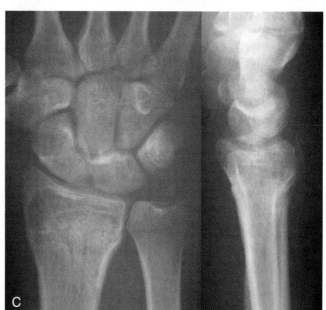

FIGURE 17-5 A 22-year-old man fell while snowboarding and sustained an extra-articular distal radius fracture with volar comminution. **A,** Preoperative anteroposterior and lateral radiographs. **B,** Postoperative anteroposterior and lateral radiographs showing Kapandji pins and external fixation. **C,** Healed fracture with Kapandji pins and external fixator removed. Patient regained full motion at 3 months.

more than 10 degrees, if the radial inclination is less than 15 degrees, or if there is more than 2 mm of ulnar-positive variance. According to these criteria, 5 of the 28 patients (17.9%) had "unacceptable reductions." Four of these patients had unacceptable ulnar variance (3.0, 4.5, 4.8, and 5.0 mm), and 1 had excessive volar angulation (23 degrees). Two of the patients with excessive ulnar variance were older than 55 (despite addition of a supplemental external fixator), and one had an infected nonunion.

Complications

The most common complications reported with Kapandji pinning are loss of fracture reduction, extensor tendon rupture, radial sensory nerve irritation, and reflex sympathetic dystrophy.[8] Early pin removal, fracture displacement after pinning, and infection are

also described.[8] In the largest series on Kapandji pinning,[17] complications reported include 1 patient with distal radioulnar joint instability, reflex sympathetic dystrophy (8%), need for early pin removal (7%), radial sensory nerve irritation (6%), ulnar neuropathy of the wrist (n = 1), extensor tendinitis (2%), and some displacement of fracture fragments after pinning (14%). It was found that secondary displacement of the fracture did not usually affect the final clinical result.[17]

In our experience, loss of fracture reduction over time was uncommon, perhaps because all fractures in older patients were supplemented with external fixation. There were four complications in our cohort. There was one patient with reflex sympathetic dystrophy (requiring a stellate ganglion block), one extensor pollicis longus rupture (requiring surgical repair), and one patient requiring early pin removal because of volar migration of the K-wire. In addition, there was one infected nonunion, which occurred despite the wires being buried below the skin.

REFERENCES

1. Owen RA, Melton LJ, Johnson KA, et al: Incidence of Colles' fracture in a North American community. Am J Public Health. 1982; 72:605-607.
2. Thompson PW, Taylor J, Dawson A: The annual incidence and seasonal variation of fractures of the distal radius in men and women over 25 years in Dorest, UK. Injury. 2004; 35:462-466.
3. Mackenney PJ, McQueen MM, Elton R: Prediction of instability in distal radial fractures. J Bone Joint Surg Am. 2006; 88:1944-1951.
4. Duncan S, Weiland AJ: Minimally invasive reduction and osteosynthesis of articular fractures of the distal radius. Injury. 2001; 32:14-24.
5. Habernek H, Weinstabl R, Fialka C, Schmid L: Unstable distal radius fractures treated by modified Kirschner wire pinning: anatomic considerations, technique, and results. J Trauma. 1994; 36:83-88.
6. Munson GO, Gainor BJ: Percutaneous pinning of distal radius fractures. J Trauma. 1981; 21:1032-1035.
7. Naidu SH, Capo JT, Moulton M, et al: Percutaneous pinning of distal radius fractures: a biomechanical study. J Hand Surg [Am]. 1997; 22:252-257.
8. Rayhack JM: The history and evolution of percutaneous pinning of displaced distal radius fractures. Orthop Clin North Am. 1993; 24:287-300.
9. Ring D, Jupiter JB: Percutaneous and limited open fixation of fractures of the distal radius. Clin Orthop Relat Res. 2000; 375:105-115.
10. Rodriguez-Merchan EC: Plaster cast versus percutaneous pin fixation for comminuted fractures of the distal radius in patients between 46 and 65 years of age. J Orthop Trauma. 1997; 11:212-217.
11. Kapandji A: L'osteosynthese par double enbrochage intrafocal: traitement fonctionnel des fractures nonarticulaires de l'extrémité inferieure du radius. Ann Chir Main. 1976; 30:903-908.
12. Kapandji A: Intra-focal pinning of fractures of the distal end of the radius 10 years later. Ann Chir Main. 1987; 6:57-63.
13. Epinette JA, Lehut JM, Cavenaile M, et al: Pouteau-Colles fracture: double-closed 'basket-like' pinning according to Kapandji: apropos of a homogeneous series of 70 cases. Ann Chir Main. 1982; 1:71-83.
14. Docquier J, Soete P, Twahirwa J, Flament A: Kapandji's method of intrafocal nailing in Pouteau-Colles fractures. Acta Orthop Belg. 1982; 48:794-810.
15. Peyroux LM, Dunaud JL, Caron M, et al: The Kapandji technique and its evolution in the treatment of fractures of the distal end of the radius: report on a series of 159 cases. Ann Chir Main. 1987; 6:109-122.
16. Dowdy PA, Patterson SD, King GJ, et al: Intrafocal (Kapandji) pinning of unstable distal radius fractures: a preliminary report. J Trauma. 1996; 40:194-198.
17. Nonnenmacher J, Kempf I: Role of intrafocal pinning in the treatment of wrist fractures. Int Orthop. 1988; 12:155-162.
18. Greating MD, Bishop AT: Intrafocal (Kapandji) pinning of unstable fractures of the distal radius. Orthop Clin North Am. 1993; 24:301-307.
19. Trumble TE, Wagner W, Hanel DP, et al: Intrafocal (Kapandji) pinning of distal radius fractures with and without external fixation. J Hand Surg [Am]. 1998; 23:381-394.
20. Board T, Kocialkowski A, Andrew G: Does Kapandji wiring help in older patients? A retrospective comparative review of displaced intra-articular distal radius fractures in patients over 55 years. Injury. 1999; 30:663-669.
21. Hollevoet N, Verdonk R: Anterior fracture displacement in Colles' fractures after Kapandji wiring in women over 59 years. Int Orthop. 2006; Jul 25 [Epub ahead of print].
22. Sarmiento A, Zagorski JB, Sinclair WF: Functional bracing of Colles' fractures: a prospective study of immobilization in supination and pronation. Clin Orthop Relat Res. 1980; 146:175-183.
23. Stoffelen DV, Broos PL: Closed reduction versus Kapandji pinning for extra-articular distal radial fractures. J Hand Surg [Br]. 1999; 24:89-91.
24. Weil WM, Trumble TE: Treatment of distal radius fractures with intrafocal (Kapandji) pinning and supplemental skeletal stabilization. Hand Clin. 2005; 21:317-328.
25. MacDermid JC, Turgeon T, Richards RS, et al: Patient rating of wrist pain and disability: a reliable and valid measurement tool. J Orthop Trauma. 1998; 12:577-586.
26. Beaton DE, Katz JN, Fossel AG, et al: Measuring the whole or the parts? Validity, reliability, and responsiveness of the disabilities of the arm, shoulder and hand outcome measure in different regions of the upper extremity. J Hand Ther. 2001; 14:128-146.
27. McHorney CA, Ware JE Jr, Raczek AE: The MOS 36-Item Short-Form Health Survey (SF-36): II. Psychometric and clinical tests of validity in measuring physical and mental health constructs. Med Care. 1993; 31:247-263.
28. eRADIUS International Distal Radius Fracture Study Group. Basic knowledge (Indications for reduction in distal radius fractures). ASSH Specialty Day at AAOS (Trumble, 1999). Available at: http://www.eradius.com. Accessed December 2006.

18

Use of the T-Pin in the Treatment of Extra-articular Distal Radius Fractures

John S. Taras, MD, Kimberly Z. Accardi, MD, and Joshua M. Abzug, MD

Distal radius fractures are among the most common fractures treated by orthopaedic surgeons. Numerous techniques and implants have been devised to stabilize these fractures. The T-Pin (Union Surgical, LLC, Philadelphia, PA) is a novel instrument designed to stabilize extra-articular distal radius fractures utilizing minimal surgical dissection. The T-Pin allows for early active wrist range of motion, thus promoting earlier return to functional activities. Here we discuss the instrumentation, the techniques of insertion and extraction, and the postoperative care required for the use of the T-Pin in the treatment of extra-articular distal radius fractures.

Historical Perspective

Fractures of the distal radius are one of the most common fractures treated by orthopaedic surgeons. Owen stated that distal radius fractures represent one in six fractures in patients older than 50 years of age.[1] Various procedures and fixation techniques have evolved to treat this common fracture based on many factors, which include the patient's age, bone quality, and ability to tolerate the procedure and the type of fracture. Treatment modalities have included immobilization as originally described by Colles,[2] pins in plaster, external fixation, percutaneous pinning with casting, and open reduction with internal fixation with a number of different implants.

Since Abraham Colles described the comminuted and displaced distal radius fracture in 1814, orthopaedic surgeons have sought to stabilize the fracture after reduction.[3] Many fractures treated in plaster have a tendency to redisplace.[4] For this reason, percutaneous pinning evolved as a relatively simple fixation method for extra-articular fractures prone to redisplacement with cast treatment alone. Various methods of pinning have been developed. The described techniques include two pins placed through the radial styloid[5]; two crossed pins, one inserted at the radial styloid just dorsal to the first extensor compartment and the second inserted on the dorsal ulnar aspect of the distal radius between the fourth and fifth extensor compartments[3,6]; three to four intrafocal pins within the fracture site[7]; transulnar oblique pinning in which a threaded wire is inserted in the distal ulna and passed obliquely through the distal ulna to the distal radius so that it engages the radial styloid fragment[8]; one radial styloid pin and a second across the distal radioulnar joint[9]; and multiple transulnar to radius pins, including the distal radioulnar joint.[10] Despite improved maintenance of reduction with pinning, many of these series report 25% to 33% of patients having a significant loss of reduction.

The T-Pin is a threaded pin designed specifically to treat acute distal radius fractures. The T-Pin technique has the advantages of (1) a short operative time, (2) being relatively inexpensive, (3) having utility for patients with medical conditions for whom general anesthesia poses a greater risk, and (4) allowing early active wrist motion. The T-Pin is threaded and affords better purchase of the fracture fragments than commonly used smooth pins (Fig. 18-1). Currently, we are undergoing a prospective multicenter study to further evaluate the efficacy of the procedure.

Indications and Contraindications

The main indication for use of the T-Pin is an unstable extra-articular dorsally displaced distal radius fracture (Fig. 18-2). This technique is useful for active patients because it is a relatively brief procedure and allows for a quick return of function. The brief nature of the procedure, especially the limited incisions (1 to 2 cm) required to insert the pins, makes this procedure useful in the elderly and medically unstable populations because it can be performed under local anesthesia with intravenous sedation.

The contraindications to this procedure include intra-articular fractures having displacement and/or severe comminution. Low-demand patients who have fractures amenable to treatment by immobilization alone would also not be considered candidates for this procedure.

Surgical Technique

Web Video

18-1

Patients are placed supine on the operating table. Typical anesthesia for the case is conscious sedation with a local field block and fracture hematoma block. We use bupivicaine 0.5% without epinephrine. A tourniquet is then applied to the operative extremity, and the extremity is prepped and draped in a sterile fashion. The limb is exsanguinated, and the tourniquet is inflated to 250 mm Hg. Our typical tourniquet time is approximately 20 minutes.

Under fluoroscopic guidance, closed reduction of the fracture is performed. A 0.620-inch Kirschner wire (K-wire) can be placed percutaneously into the distal fragment to use as a joystick to regain the normal anatomical volar tilt. Typically two 1- to 2-cm longitudinal incisions are made (1) at the distal aspect of the radial styloid between the first and second dorsal extensor compartment, dorsal to the abductor pollicis longus/extensor pollicis brevis tendons and (2) proximal to the fracture site on the radius (Fig. 18-3). Alternatively, for the younger patient with good bone stock, two pins can be placed at the radial styloid alone through a single incision (Fig. 18-4). The soft tissues are bluntly dissected to bone for safe placement of guidewires. Dissection is carried down to visualize the pin insertion site, and adjacent extensor tendons are protected by retraction or by use of the tissue protec-

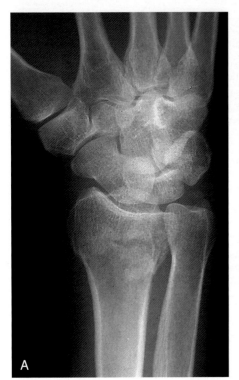

FIGURE 18-1 Various lengths of the T-Pin.

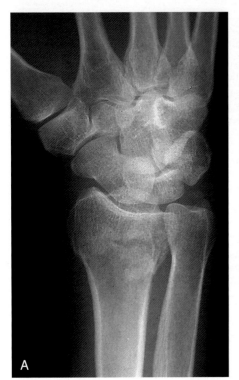

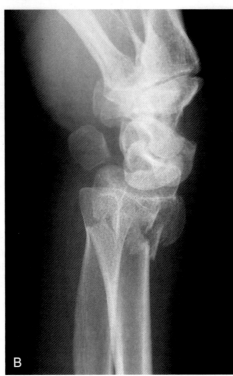

FIGURE 18-2 Preoperative anteroposterior (**A**) and lateral (**B**) radiographs of a typical fracture amenable to the T-Pin procedure.

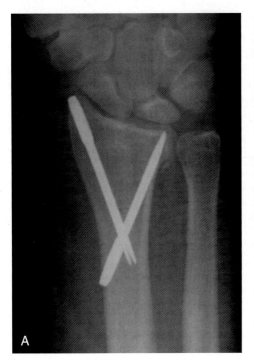

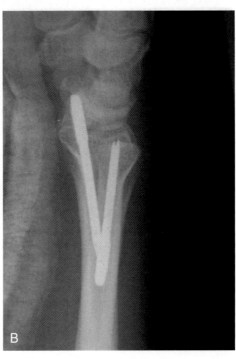

FIGURE 18-3 Anteroposterior (**A**) and lateral (**B**) radiographs showing pin placement pattern with proximally and distally directed pins.

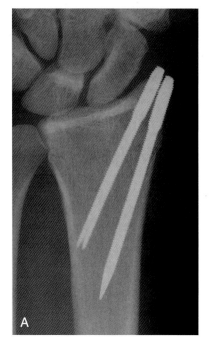 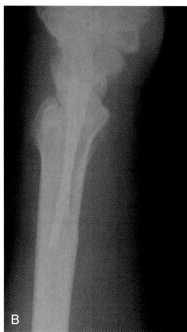

FIGURE 18-4 Anteroposterior (**A**) and lateral (**B**) radiographs showing typical pin placement patterns with two radial styloid pins.

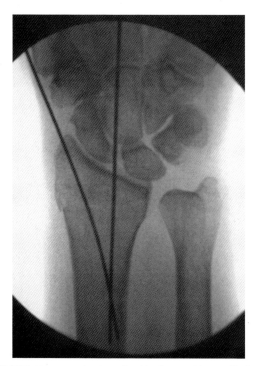

FIGURE 18-5 Fluoroscopic view of guidewires making cortical contact, with the radial styloid pin bowing slightly.

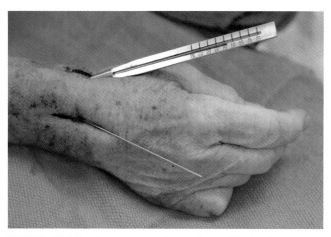

FIGURE 18-6 Depth gauge used over the guidewire to measure length.

The pin tray supplies pin lengths from 40 to 70 mm in 5-mm increments. To avoid having the guide pin kink and bend near the tip, we back out the guide pin 10 mm after measuring its depth.

The cannulated T-Pin is secured onto the power driver and inserted over the guidewire (**Fig. 18-7**). The T-Pin is driven along the guidewire until the trailing threads are nearly flush with the bone. The split tissue protector opens to allow removal for final seating of the pin without having to disengage the driver. The surgeon disengages the power driver and removes the guidewire, leaving only the T-Pin in place. The break-off driving mechanism of the pin is easily removed by bending the smooth shaft by hand.

Stability of the fixation is checked under fluoroscopy (**Fig. 18-8**). The tourniquet is deflated and the skin closed with nylon sutures. The postoperative dressing includes sterile gauze and a volar splint.

tion guide provided on the tray. The fracture is initially stabilized with smooth 1-mm guidewires at the aforementioned insertion sites, and placement is adjusted under fluoroscopic guidance. A technical point to note is that the guidewire will deflect off the inner cortices and bend, whereas the more rigid T-Pin will not; therefore, guidewire insertion should stop when cortical contact is made (**Fig. 18-5**). A measuring guide is then applied along each guidewire indicating the length of the T-Pin required (**Fig. 18-6**).

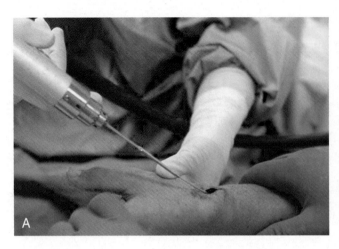

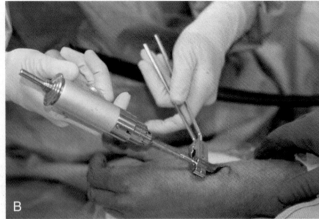

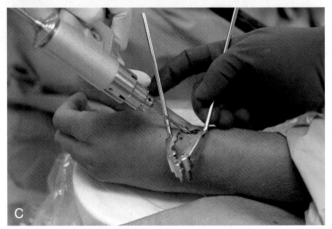

FIGURE 18-7 **A** to **C,** T-Pin insertion over the guidewire utilizing a split soft tissue protector.

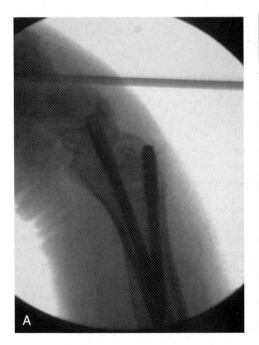

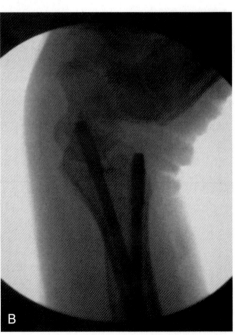

FIGURE 18-8 **A** and **B,** Stability of the fixation is checked under fluoroscopy.

Complications

Potential complications include infection, loss of reduction, nerve irritation, tendon rupture, and pin migration.

Rehabilitation

The postoperative dressing is a plaster volar short arm splint that allows for unrestricted finger range of motion. The patient is given the usual instructions of elevation of the extremity, use of ice, and splint care and told to return for a follow-up visit on postoperative day 1 to 3. At this first postoperative visit the patient is fitted with a custom-molded, forearm-based static wrist splint, which can be removed for bathing and exercises. Therapy is initiated under the guidance of a hand therapist for active and passive digital range of motion, edema control, and gentle wrist active range of motion (**Fig. 18-9**). For severely osteoporotic bone, wrist range of motion is deferred until 2 to 3 weeks postoperatively. By initiating wrist range of motion on or before the third postoperative day, we believe it is possible to restore a greater degree of motion and quicker restoration of function compared with results achieved from delayed initiation of range of motion.

At 2 weeks after surgery, sutures are removed and the patient is advanced to a program of active, active assisted, and gentle passive wrist extension and flexion. Initial recommended wrist range of motion limits are 30 degrees of extension and 30 degrees of flexion. At this point, the patient may also begin pain-free light-resisted grip exercises.

After 6 weeks, a decision is made whether to remove the pins. Our current practice is to remove the pins in active adults younger than 60 years of age. We tend to leave the pins in place in those patients with a sedentary lifestyle or those older than 60 years of age. Pins are removed with a removal tool designed to fit the flutes in the distal threads of the T-Pin, which is included in the pinning tray (**Fig. 18-10**). A 4.0-mm hollow mill is useful for cleaning scar tissue or bone from the distal threads of the T-Pin to allow easy placement of the removal tool. Once full fracture healing has occurred after the pin has been removed, as assessed by no tenderness from palpation at the fracture site, an unrestricted program

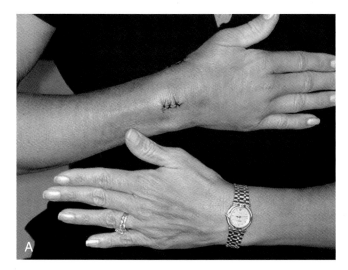

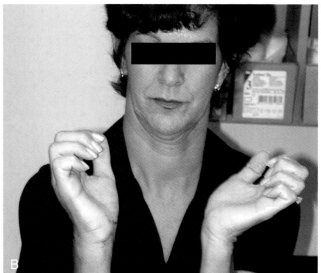

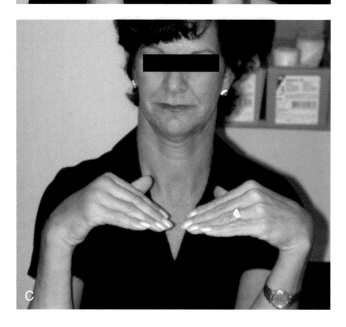

FIGURE 18-9 **A,** The minimally invasive nature of the procedure is demonstrated here by the limited incisions. **B** and **C,** Range of motion is initiated at the first postoperative visit.

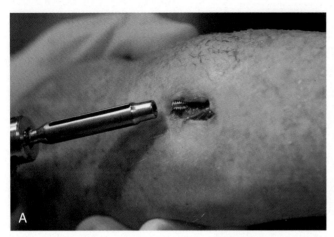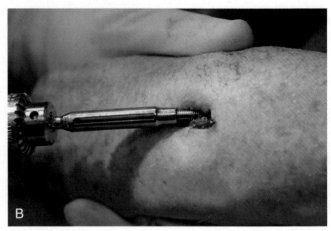

FIGURE 18-10 **A** and **B**, T-Pin removal instruments.

of range of motion and strengthening can begin. The protective splint is discontinued at this time.

REFERENCES

1. Owen RA, Melton LJ 3rd, Johnson KA, et al: Incidence of Colles' fracture in a North American community. Am J Public Health. 1982; 72:605-607.

2. Colles A: On the fracture of the carpal extremity of the radius. Edinb Med Surg J. 1814; 10:182.

3. Stein H, Katz S: Stabilization of comminuted fractures of the distal inch of the radius: percutaneous pinning. Clin Orthop Relat Res. 1975; 108:174-181.

4. Fernandez D, Palmer AK: Fractures of the distal radius. In Green D, Hotchkiss R, Pederson W, eds: Green's Operative Hand Surgery. New York: Churchill Livingstone, 1999.

5. Lenoble E, Dumontier C, Goutallier D, et al: Fracture of the distal radius: a prospective comparison between trans-styloid and Kapandji fixations. J Bone Joint Surg Am. 1995; 77: 562-567.

6. Clancey G: Percutaneous Kirschner-wire fixation of Colles fractures. J Bone Joint Surg Am. 1984; 66:1008-1014.

7. Kapandij A: Treatment of non-articular distal radius fractures by intrafocal pinning with pins. In Saffer P, Cooney WP, eds: Fractures of the Distal Radius. Philadelphia: Lippincott Williams & Wilkins, 1995.

8. DePalma A: Comminuted fractures of the distal end of the radius treated by ulnar pinning. J Bone Joint Surg Am. 1952; 34:651-662.

9. Mortier JP, Kuhlmann JN, Richet C, Baux S: Horizontal cubito-radial pinning in fractures of the distal radius including a postero-internal fragment. Rev Chir Orthop Reparatrice Appar Mot. 1986; 72:567-572.

10. Rayhack JM, Langworthy JN, Belsole RJ: Transulnar percutaneous pinning of displaced distal radial fractures: a preliminary report. J Orthop Trauma. 1989; 3:107-114.

Bridge Plating of Distal Radius Fractures

19

P. A. Martineau, MD, K. J. Malone, MD, and D. P. Hanel, MD

Distal radius fractures represent one sixth of all fractures seen and treated in emergency departments.[1] The treatment goals for the management of these fractures include restoring congruity to the radiocarpal and distal radioulnar joint (DRUJ) surfaces and maintaining radial length. Currently, there are a number of established surgical options for displaced distal radius fractures as well as newer novel approaches being developed for the surgical management of these injuries.[2-13] The choice of surgical technique for reduction and fixation will depend on fracture displacement, joint surface involvement, patient age, bone quality, handedness, occupation, and avocation. Recent advances in the biological and biomechanical understanding of wrist fractures have prompted a more aggressive approach to the fixation of the distal radius. As surgical treatment in general, and plating in particular, ensures more consistent correction of displacement and maintenance of reduction, there has been an increasing trend for operative treatment of these fractures in both the elderly and the young populations. In no area of fracture management has there been such a recent explosion of new treatment modalities as there has been in distal radius fixation.

Two subsets of patients with distal radius fractures continue to represent unique treatment challenges: (1) patients with high-energy wrist injuries with fracture extension into the radial diaphysis and (2) patients with multiple injuries that require load bearing through the injured wrist to assist with mobilization and nursing care. There exist few publications specifically addressing the management of distal radius injuries in the multiply injured patient and/or the problem of distal radius fractures with diaphyseal extension.[14,15] High-energy fractures of the distal aspect of the radius with extensive comminution of the articular surface and extension into the diaphysis represent a major treatment challenge. Standard plates and techniques may be inadequate for the management of such fractures.

Patients with multiple injuries, especially those with injuries to the pelvis and lower extremities, require use of the upper extremities for transfers and weight bearing. There exists no evidence that the newer fixation techniques can support such activities. Although it is possible that augmentation of distal radius fixation with a spanning external fixator could improve weight bearing through the upper extremity, this has not been clinically proved. However, it is known that external fixation of fractures presents a set of problems that can be particularly vexing for patients being cared for in intensive care units. These include the burden of pin care and an increased incidence of pin tract contamination and infection.[16,17] The ideal fixation device in this setting would assist with and maintain reduction, require no nursing care, and allow the use of the extremity for mobilization.

The use of internal distraction plating or bridge plating for distal radius fractures was first introduced by Burke and Singer.[18] The technique was further expanded by Ruch and coworkers, who described the use of a 12- to 16-hole 3.5-mm dynamic compression plate (DCP) (Synthes, Paoli, PA) placed in the floor of the fourth dorsal extensor compartment to span from the intact radius diaphysis to the third metacarpal.[14,19] The bridge plating technique provides strong fixation and allows for distraction across impacted articular segments. The technique can be combined with a limited articular fixation approach for those fracture patterns with intra-articular extension. Recently, bridge plating of the distal radius was further refined by Hanel and colleagues.[15] The authors described a variant of the bridge plating technique using 2.4-mm AO plates passed extra-articularly through the second dorsal compartment and secured onto the dorsal radial aspect of the radius diaphysis and the second metacarpal. They reviewed the senior author's experience with bridge plating in a series spanning a 10-year period at a level 1 trauma center. The patients earlier in the series were treated using a 22-hole 2.4-mm titanium mandibular reconstruction plate (Synthes, Paoli, PA) and later in the series with a 2.4-mm stainless steel plate specifically designed for use as a distal radius bridge plate (DRB plate) (Synthes, Paoli, PA). The mandibular reconstruction plate is made of titanium and has square ends and scalloped edges and threaded holes to accept locking screws. The DRB plate that we presently continue to use is made of stainless steel, has tapered ends to facilitate sliding the plate within the extensor compartment, and also has locking screws. The described bridge plating technique is technically easy and achieves the goals of maintenance of fracture reduction, allows weight bearing through the injured extremity, and is associated with few complications (**Table 19-1**).

Indications

This technique is indicated in patients with any type of distal radius fracture with extension into the radial metadiaphysis as well as polytrauma patients with associated lower extremity injuries requiring early weight bearing through the upper extremities, those with multiple injuries, especially those with injuries to the pelvis and lower extremities, and those who require use of the upper extremities for transfers and weight bearing.

Contraindications

General orthopaedic contraindications include medical comorbidity precluding surgical procedure and active infection. The only specific contraindication is metacarpal fracture of index and middle fingers, which would compromise the distal fixation of the bridge plate.

201

TABLE 19-1 Indications for Bridge Plating of Distal Radius Fractures

Indication	Explanation
Metadiaphyseal comminution of the radius	Extensive comminution in metadiaphyseal region is difficult to treat with standard implants used for distal radius fractures.
Need for weight bearing through the upper extremity	Patients with associated lower limb injuries may require the need for early weight bearing through the upper extremities.
Polytrauma	Nursing care of the multiply injured patient may be easier with spanning internal fixation than with external fixation.
Augmented fixation	In osteoporotic bone, bridge plating can be used to augment tenuous fixation.
Carpal instability	Carpal instability, particularly radiocarpal, isolated, or in combination with a distal radius fracture, may be held in a reduced position with the help of spanning internal fixation.

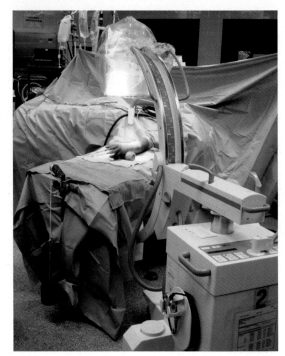

FIGURE 19-1 Picture of our setup for this procedure, with longitudinal traction applied through finger traps and the C-arm coming in from above or below the hand table.

Technique and Surgical Approach

19-1

With the patient anesthetized and supine on the operating table, the involved extremity is draped free and centered on a radiolucent hand table. Finger traps are applied to the index and middle fingers, and 4.5 kg of longitudinal traction is applied through a rope and pulley system. Under image intensification, the closed reduction maneuver described by Agee is performed[20] (**Fig. 19-1**). Longitudinal traction is first used to restore length and to assess the benefit of ligamentotaxis for the restoration of articular step-off (**Fig. 19-2**). Next, the hand is translated palmarly relative to the forearm to restore sagittal tilt and to assess the integrity of the volar lip of the radius (**Fig. 19-3**). Finally, pronation of the hand relative to the forearm is performed to correct the supination deformity. Once the initial reduction maneuver is completed, the bridge plate is then applied.

The DRB plate is superimposed on the skin from the radial diaphysis to the distal metadiaphysis of the second metacarpal. The position of the plate is verified with image intensification, and markings are placed on the skin at the level of the proximal and distal four screw holes of the plate (**Fig. 19-4**). The subcutaneous tissues are infiltrated with 0.25% bupivacaine with epinephrine to promote hemostasis. A 5-cm incision is made at the base of the second metacarpal and continued along the second metacarpal shaft. In the depths of this incision, the insertions of the extensor carpi radialis longus (ECRL) and the extensor carpi radialis brevis (ECRB) are identified as they pass beneath the distal edge of the second dorsal wrist compartment to insert on the second and third metacarpal bases, respectively. A second incision is made just proximal to the outcropper muscle bellies (abductor pollicis longus [APL]) and the extensor pollicis brevis (EPB), in line with the ECRL and ECRB tendons. The interval between the ECRL and ECRB is developed, and the diaphysis of the radius is exposed (**Fig. 19-5**). The DRB plate is introduced beneath the muscle bellies of the outcroppers extraperiosteally and advanced distally

between the ECRL and ECRB tendons (**Fig. 19-6**). Some resistance may be encountered as the plate emerges distally, but this can usually be easily overcome with gentle manipulation of the plate. Occasionally, the plate will not pass through the compartment. In these cases, a guidewire or stout suture retriever is passed along the compartment from distal to proximal. The plate is secured to the distal end of the wire and delivered into the hand. In the rare instance that these measures fail, a third incision is made directly over the metaphysis of the radius, the proximal one half of the second compartment is incised, and the plate is passed under direct vision. The third, or periarticular, incision may also be used to assess the articular surface, reduce die-punch fragments, and introduce bone graft (**Fig. 19-7**).

After passing the bridge plate, it is then secured to the second metacarpal by placing a nonlocking fully threaded 2.4-mm cortical screw through the most distal plate hole. The proximal end of the plate is then identified in the forearm. If the radial length has not been restored, then the plate, secured to the second metacarpal, is pushed distally until the length is reestablished and a fully threaded 2.4-mm nonlocking screw is placed in the most proximal plate hole. By using nonlocking screws the plate is effectively lagged onto the intact bone. Plate alignment along the longitudinal axis of the radius is guaranteed by securing the most distal and most proximal screw holes first. The remaining holes are secured with fully threaded locking screws inserted with bicortical purchase (**Fig. 19-8**).

It has been our experience that as the plate is passed along the radial diaphysis, through the second compartment and along the second metacarpal, extra-articular alignment, radial inclination, volar tilt, and radial length are restored. Intra-articular reduction may be further adjusted by using limited periarticular incisions to allow for direct manipulation of articular fragments, placement of subchondral bone grafts, repair of intercarpal ligament injuries,

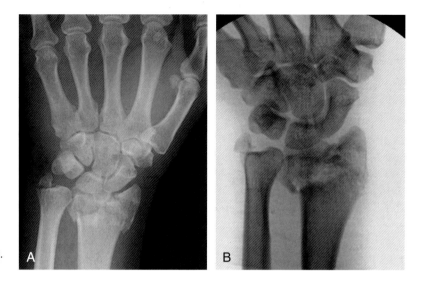

FIGURE 19-2 Anteroposterior radiographs of the wrist. **A,** Injury film. **B,** After distraction is applied.

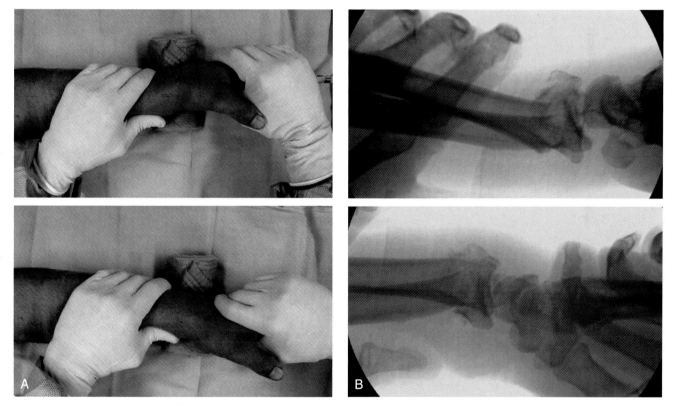

FIGURE 19-3 **A,** Clinical pictures showing the wrist deformity before (*top*) and after (*bottom*) application of the Agee reduction maneuver, which is a combination of longitudinal traction and volar translation of the carpus. **B,** Radiographs showing the wrist deformity before (*top*) and after (*bottom*) application of the Agee reduction maneuver.

and augmentation of fracture fixation with Kirschner wires (K-wires) and periarticular plates. Displaced volar medial fracture fragments that are not reduced with this technique require a separate volar incision and appropriate buttress support.

The stability of the DRUJ is assessed after radius reconstruction. If the DRUJ is stable, the limb is immobilized in a long arm splint with the forearm in supination for the first 10 to 14 days postoperatively. If the DRUJ is unstable, and there are no contraindications to prolonging the operation, repair or reconstruction of the DRUJ and triangular fibrocartilage complex

is undertaken. If, however, the patient's condition does not allow prolonging the operation, the ulnar head is reduced manually into the sigmoid notch and the ulna is transfixed to the radius with a minimum of two 1.6-mm K-wires passed proximal to the DRUJ.

Postoperative Rehabilitation

Digit range of motion exercises start within 24 hours of surgery. Load bearing through the forearm and elbow is allowed immediately, as well as the use of a platform crutch when the patient is

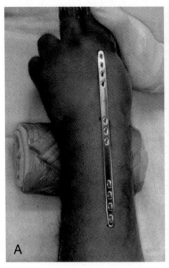
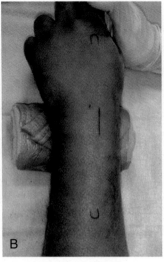
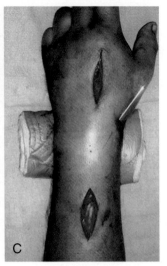

FIGURE 19-4 A, The plate is placed over the forearm and hand. Radiographs can be taken to confirm the position of the plate. The plate should be centered over the second metacarpal distally and the radius proximally. This will be along the course of the ECRL. **B,** The outline of the plate. **C,** The incisions made over the second metacarpal and the radius.

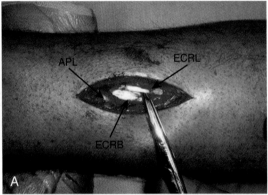
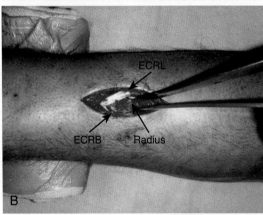

FIGURE 19-5 A, The ECRL and ECRB tendons just proximal to the APL in the forearm. **B,** The development of the interval between the ECRL and ECRB tendons to gain access to the radius shaft.

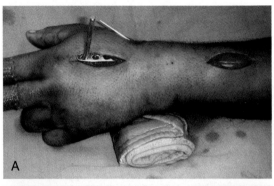
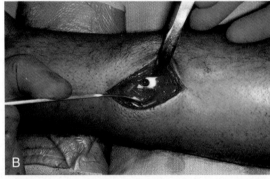

FIGURE 19-6 A, Insertion of the plate through the distal wound. The interval between the ECRL and ECRB distally can be developed for plate passage within the second dorsal compartment. **B,** The proximal aspect of the plate over the radius and in between the ECRL and ECRB. It is important to ensure that the plate runs within the second compartment and not superficial to the first and third compartment tendons.

physiologically stable. At 1 month postoperatively the platform is removed and weight bearing is allowed through the hand grip of regular crutches. Lifting and carrying is restricted to approximately 4.5 kg until the fracture has healed.

DRUJ stability and forearm motion are assessed 2 weeks after reduction. If the patient can supinate the forearm with little effort and the DRUJ is stable, then splinting is discontinued. Axial loading through the extremity is allowed at this point for transfers and for all weight-bearing needs. If the patient has difficulty maintaining supination, or if the DRUJ was reconstructed acutely, then a removable long arm splint is fabricated. If the DRUJ was transfixed with K-wires, then the wires are removed on the third postoperative week and DRUJ stability is reassessed.

Supplemental K-wires for articular fixation are removed 6 weeks postoperatively. The DRB plate and screws are removed usually no earlier than 12 weeks after injury.

Clinical Pearls

If a mandibular reconstruction plate was used, at the time of hardware extraction the screws are removed and the plate is twisted axially 720 degrees to break up the soft tissue adhesions and callus that grow around and onto the scalloped edges of the titanium plate. This maneuver is not usually required when the smooth-edged stainless steel DRB plate is used. A removable short arm splint is worn for 2 to 3 weeks after plate removal. Hand therapy at this point is directed at regaining motion and strength.

Results

The bridge plating technique for distal radius fractures was reviewed in a retrospective study consisting of 62 consecutive patients treated in this fashion and representing 10-year experience with the technique at a level 1 trauma center.[15] Patients managed with bridge plating either for distal radius fractures with extensive metadiaphyseal comminution or patients with distal radius fractures associated with other injuries requiring weight bearing through the affected extremity represented 13% of distal radius fractures requiring operative fixation during this time period. Fracture healing occurred in all 62 patients. In each case radial length was within 5 mm of ulnar-neutral variance, radial inclination was more than 5 degrees, and palmar tilt was at least neutral. There were also no articular gaps or step-offs greater than 2 mm, and the DRUJ was stable in all cases. Similarly, Ruch and coworkers showed 14 of 22 patients obtained excellent radiographic and functional results and another 6 of 22 patients obtained good results in their prospective cohort of patients with comparable pathological processes.[14]

All fractures united by an average of 110 days. Radiographs showed an average palmar tilt of 4.6 degrees and an average ulnar variance of neutral (0 degrees), whereas loss of radial length averaged 2 mm. Flexion and extension averaged 57 degrees and 65 degrees, respectively, and pronation and supination averaged 77 degrees and 76 degrees, respectively. The average Disabilities of the Arm, Shoulder, and Hand (DASH) scores were 34 points at 6 months, 15 points at 1 year, and 11.5 points at the time of final follow-up (at an average of 24.8 months). According to the Gartland-Werley rating system, 14 patients had an excellent result, 6 had a good result, and 2 had a fair result.

The plate was removed on average 112 days after placement. One outlying patient had the bridge plate in place upwards of 19 months because he did not wish to take time off work to have the plate removed. The plate in this case eventually failed at 16 months, but the patient continued to work until the broken hardware became increasingly prominent and symptomatic. Finally, at the time of plate removal the patient sustained an ECRL rupture that was treated with ECRL-to-ECRB tenodesis. There were no other documented complications in the series. In addition, there

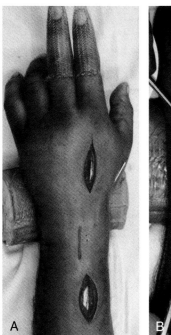
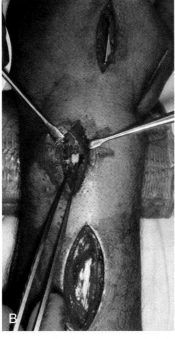

FIGURE 19-7 A, A third incision is marked out just ulnar to Lister's tubercle. **B,** The EPL tendon has been released from its compartment, and bone graft is inserted through the dorsal fracture line just ulnar to the bridge plate.

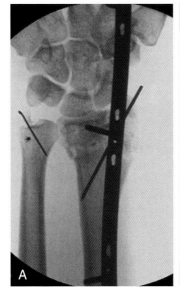
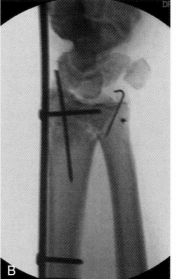
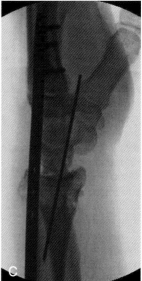

FIGURE 19-8 Final anteroposterior **(A)**, oblique **(B)**, and lateral **(C)** radiographs.

were no cases of excessive postoperative finger stiffness of reflex sympathetic dystrophy. This reflects the overall infrequent complications reported in the literature for bridge plating of the distal radius. In fact, Burke and Singer[18] reported no complications and Ruch and associates[14] reported no hardware failures and only 3 patients who developed long finger extensor lag of 10 to 15 degrees.

Excluding bridge plate removal, only 1 patient required a secondary operative procedure for fracture care. The patient underwent bridge plate removal at 4 weeks after injury and conversion to a 3.5-mm nonspanning DC plate by a separate surgeon closer to her home. The fracture went on to heal uneventfully and her range of motion at 1 year after injury was reported as 80% of her contralateral side. This patient eventually returned to all her previous activities.

Forty-one of the 62 patients have returned to their previous levels of employment. Of the remaining 21 patients, 8 were unemployed at the time of injury and remain so. Thirteen patients sustained multiple injuries requiring considerable changes in occupation and lifestyle. Only one of these 13 patients considers the wrist fracture to be the limiting factor in failing to return to work.

Overall, these results compare favorably with the findings of Burke and Singer[18] and Ruch and associates.[14] The bridge plates were removed at a mean of 110 days in the Ruch cohort versus 112 days in the senior author's series. Ruch and associates[14] reported 35 degrees of flexion, 45 degrees of extension, 69 degrees of pronation, and 72 degrees of supination at 6 months with a mean grip strength of 41% of the contralateral side. At 1 year, flexion and extension averaged 57 and 65 degrees, respectively; pronation and supination averaged 77 and 76 degrees, respectively; and grip strength improved to 69% of the contralateral side. DASH scores in their study decreased from 33.8 points at 6 months, to 15.4 points at 1 year, and 11.5 points at the time of final follow-up at an average of 24.8 months. Using the rating system of Gartland and Werley[21] at 1 year postoperatively, 63.6% of results were graded as excellent, 27.2% were graded as good, and 9.0% as fair. The authors of each of these studies proposed that distraction plating allows fracture reduction and fixation over a broad metadiaphyseal area while effectively diverting compression forces away from the fracture site.

Discussion

In the treatment of patients with extensive metadiaphyseal comminution there existed no other implants in our armamentarium that could effectively bridge the fracture and allow for early weight bearing through the extremity at the time the patients in our series were treated. There are currently several plates that have recently been developed with longer diaphyseal limbs. These new implants may circumvent the need for bridge plating in a select group of patients with isolated injuries and adequate distal bony purchase. However, in patients with multiple injuries, the need to bear weight through the affected extremity places excessive stress on the implants securing the fracture and therefore risks loss of reduction and hardware failure. Even with the advent of newer and longer implants, the subset of patients with extensive metadiaphyseal comminution and/or associated lower limb injuries may continue to benefit from spanning internal fixation.

Before the introduction of this technique, treatment of these injuries was limited to cast immobilization or external fixation with or without K-wire augmentation. Both of these methods are associated with unacceptably high complication rates. Lafontaine and coworkers showed that the end results of comminuted distal radius fractures treated by closed methods resembled the prereduction radiographs more than any other radiographs during treatment even when the reduction successfully restored wrist anatomy.[22] Szabo and Weber reported a greater than 50% complication rate when using external fixation alone, with the most frequent complications being pin tract infections.[23] This latter complication becomes an even more frequent occurrence in the patients confined to intensive care units.

The biomechanical stability of spanning plates is strong and predictable. Behrens and Johnson, studying the rigidity of external fixator configurations, demonstrated that rigidity is directly proportional to how close the longitudinal fixator bar is to the bone and the fracture.[24] A bridge plate, resting directly against the radius proximally and metacarpals distally, therefore, optimizes the conditions to obtain the strongest possible fixator construct. A DRB plate fixed with a minimum of three screws at either end of the plate confers significantly more stability than would an external fixator used to stabilize a comparable fracture.[25]

With prolonged immobilization and distraction there may be concerns that wrist stiffness will result and fracture nonunion will occur.[14,15] However, in the senior author's series, there were no nonunions and a functional range of motion was attained within a year of plate removal in all cases.[15]

The technique described here varies from that described by Burke and Singer.[18] The bridge plate used in this description is smaller, using 2.4-mm screws instead of 3.5-mm screws, and is converted to a fixed-angle device by the use of locking screws. The plate is placed in the second dorsal compartment rather than the fourth and secured to the second metacarpal rather than the third metacarpal. Becton and colleagues first suggested this position while presenting a fixation plate specific to the task.[26] However, we do not use the implant Becton and colleagues suggested because it is too short for most of the fractures we encounter and cannot be converted to a fixed-angle device. However, similar to Becton and colleagues, we note that the dorsal radial aspect of the radial diaphysis, the floor of the second extensor compartment, and the dorsal radial aspect of the second metacarpal are collinear. Passing a fixation plate along these surfaces through the intact retinaculum of the second dorsal compartment while applying longitudinal traction effectively restores radial length, radial inclination, and volar tilt of the radial styloid and scaphoid facet. Depression fractures of the lunate facet and volar shearing fractures, especially those involving the critical volar ulnar corner of the radius, may require separate manipulation and fixation. Burke and Singer[18] cite a significant intra-articular component of the fracture as the major advantage to a fourth dorsal compartment approach in these injuries. However, we use indirect reduction techniques, percutaneous wires, limited dorsal incisions, and open reduction of volar shearing fractures as needed to address the articular component of the fractures and maintain reductions.

Conclusion

The use of bridge plating in the treatment of distal radius fractures avoids the complications of external fixation. A bridge plate can remain implanted for extended periods of time, without deleterious effects on functional outcome. All patients in our series went on to heal with acceptable metadiaphyseal and intra-articular alignment. In patients with multiple traumatic injuries, bridge plating allowed earlier postoperative load bearing across the affected wrist. This enabled independent transfers and the use of ambulatory aids. Application of bridge plates is simple, and surgical time is comparable with the application of an external fixator.

REFERENCES

1. Graff S, Jupiter J: Fracture of the distal radius: classification of treatment and indications for external fixation. Injury. 1994; 25:S-D14-S-D25.

2. Drobetz H, Bryant AL, Pokorny T, et al: Volar fixed-angle plating of distal radius extension fractures: influence of plate position on secondary loss of reduction—a biomechanic study in a cadaveric model. J Hand Surg [Am]. 2006; 31:615-622.

3. Gradl G, Jupiter JB, Gierer P, Mittlmeier T: Fractures of the distal radius treated with a nonbridging external fixation technique using multiplanar K-wires. J Hand Surg [Am]. 2005; 30:960-968.

4. Handoll HH, Madhok R: Surgical interventions for treating distal radial fractures in adults. Cochrane Database Syst Rev. 2003; CD003209.

5. Hastings H 2nd, Leibovic SJ: Indications and techniques of open reduction, internal fixation of distal radius fractures. Orthop Clin North Am 1993; 24:309-326.

6. Kamath AF, Zurakowski D, Day CS: Low-profile dorsal plating for dorsally angulated distal radius fractures: an outcomes study. J Hand Surg. 2006; 31:1061-1067.

7. Konrath GA, Bahler S: Open reduction and internal fixation of unstable distal radius fractures: results using the Trimed fixation system. J Orthop Trauma. 2002; 16:578-585.

8. McQueen MM: Non-spanning external fixation of the distal radius. Hand Clin. 2005; 21:375-380.

9. McQueen MM, Simpson D, Court-Brown CM: Use of the Hoffman 2 compact external fixator in the treatment of redisplaced unstable distal radial fractures. J Orthop Trauma. 1999; 13:501-505.

10. Orbay JL, Touhami A: Current concepts in volar fixed-angle fixation of unstable distal radius fractures. Clin Orthop Relat Res. 2006; 445:58-67.

11. Rikli DA, Regazzoni P: The double plating technique for distal radius fractures. Tech Hand Up Extrem Surg. 2000; 4:107-114.

12. Schnall SB, Kim BJ, Abramo A, Kopylov P: Fixation of distal radius fractures using a fragment-specific system. Clin Orthop Relat Res. 2006; 445:51-57.

13. Tornetta P 3rd, Klein DM, Stein AB, McQueen M: Distal radius fracture. J Orthop Trauma. 2002; 16:608-611.

14. Ruch DS, Ginn TA, Yang CC, et al: Use of a distraction plate for distal radial fractures with metaphyseal and diaphyseal comminution. J Bone Joint Surg Am. 2005; 87:945-954.

15. Hanel DP, Lu TS, Weil WM: Bridge plating of distal radius fractures: the Harborview method. Clin Orthop Relat Res. 2006; 445:91-99.

16. Ahlborg HG, Josefsson PO: Pin-tract complications in external fixation of fractures of the distal radius. Acta Orthop Scand. 1999; 70:116-118.

17. Parameswaran AD, Roberts CS, Seligson D, Voor M: Pin tract infection with contemporary external fixation: how much of a problem? J Orthop Trauma. 2003; 17:503-507.

18. Burke EF, Singer RM: Treatment of communited distal radius with the use of an internal distraction plate. Tech Hand Up Extrem Surg. 1998; 2:248-252.

19. Ginn TA, Ruch DS, Yang CC, Hanel DP: Use of a distraction plate for distal radial fractures with metaphyseal and diaphyseal comminution: surgical technique. J Bone Joint Surg Am. 2006; 88(Suppl 1):29-36.

20. Agee JM: Distal radius fractures: multiplanar ligamentotaxis. Hand Clin. 1993; 9:577-585.

21. Gartland JJ Jr, Werley CW: Evaluation of healed Colles' fractures. J Bone Joint Surg Am. 1951; 33:895-907.

22. Lafontaine M, Hardy D, Delince P: Stability assessment of distal radius fractures. Injury. 1989; 20:208-210.

23. Szabo RM, Weber SC: Comminuted intraarticular fractures of the distal radius. Clin Orthop Relat Res. 1988; (230):39-48.

24. Behrens F, Johnson W: Unilateral external fixation: methods to increase and reduce frame stiffness. Clin Orthop Relat Res. 1989; (241):48-56.

25. Wolf JC, Weil WM, Hanel DP, Trumble TE: A biomechanic comparison of an internal radiocarpal-spanning 2.4-mm locking plate and external fixation in a model of distal radius fractures. J Hand Surg [Am]. 2006; 31:1578-1586.

26. Becton JL, Colborn GL, Goodrich JA: Use of an internal fixator device to treat comminuted fractures of the distal radius: report of a technique. Am J Orthop. 1998; 27:619-623.

Arthroscopic-Assisted Treatment of Distal Radius Fractures

20

Sidney M. Jacoby, MD and A. Lee Osterman, MD

The advent of wrist arthroscopy in the early 1990s marked the beginning of a novel and valuable adjunct in the treatment of distal radius fractures.[1] Anatomical reduction, stable internal fixation, and preservation of soft tissues are cornerstone concepts in fracture reconstruction. Distal radius fractures represent a unique subset of upper extremity injuries because they often involve not only articular margins but also surrounding soft tissue structures critical to normal wrist function. As arthroscopic technology has evolved at a rapid pace, so, too, has the utility of wrist arthroscopy in the treatment of various subtypes of distal radius fractures.

Arthroscopic-assisted reduction/internal fixation (ARIF) provides a unique, magnified and illuminated view of the distal radial joint surface that allows precise reduction of fracture fragments. Comminuted fractures involving the distal articular surface are particularly difficult to manage because they have an inherent tendency toward instability, either by shortening or collapse, and are less amenable to closed manipulation and casting. Arthroscopy allows the surgeon to explore the biconcave distal radius articular surface and remove chondral defects, loose bodies, and fracture fragments in both the radiocarpal and distal radioulnar joints. In addition to assisting with percutaneous pinning, external fixation, or limited open reduction techniques, arthroscopic visualization and repair of associated intercarpal soft tissue injuries is a crucial component to improving outcomes.

Precise reduction of the distal radial articular surface is critical in preventing the late sequelae of post-traumatic arthrosis. Numerous studies have shown that a poor result is likely if more than 1 mm of articular incongruity is present at the radiocarpal joint (**Figs. 20-1 to 20-3**).[2-6] Subchondral hematomas in the radiocarpal joint have also been shown to cause the early onset of mild osteoarthritis and worse outcomes after 1 year, even without a fracture line as demonstrated by arthroscopy.[7] Arthroscopic irrigation and débridement of hematoma may therefore ultimately improve outcome by removing a possible impetus for early post-traumatic degenerative changes.

ARIF affords a well-lit, magnified view of the distal radial joint surface with minimal morbidity. It has been shown to be superior to C-arm and plain radiographs for assessing both displacement between articular fragments as well as the diagnosis of soft tissue lesions.[8,9] In a study performed by Edwards and coworkers of intra-articular distal radial fractures that underwent closed manipulation and percutaneous pinning followed by sequential assessment of reduction by C-arm, radiography, and wrist arthroscopy, 33% of cases judged to have had optimal reduction by C-arm and radiography were found to have an articular displacement of more than 1 mm by adjunctive arthroscopy.[8] It has also been shown that arthroscopic-assisted reduction and external fixation of distal radius fractures permits a more thorough inspection of the ulnar-sided components of the injury when compared with fluoroscopic-assisted reduction and external fixation of distal radius fractures alone. In addition, a prospective cohort study showed that at follow-up examination, patients who underwent arthroscopic-assisted procedures had a greater degree of supination, flexion, and extension than patients undergoing fluoroscopic-assisted surgery.[10] It is now recognized that intraoperative fluoroscopic imaging does not provide sufficient precision to visualize a 1-mm step-off in the radial articular surface despite often satisfactory postoperative radiographs.[1,11]

Indications and Contraindications

Although the main indication for ARIF of a distal radius fracture is an intra-articular step-off of more than 1 mm, arthroscopy is particularly useful in the management of unstable or displaced intra-articular fractures as well as comminuted articular fractures. Additional fracture patterns amenable to ARIF include radial styloid fractures, lunate die-punch fractures, three-part T fractures, and Melone four-part fractures.[12] Other reasons to perform arthroscopy may include radiographic signs of concomitant injury, including diastasis of intercarpal joint spaces, subluxation of the distal radioulnar joint (DRUJ), or a broken carpal arch. ARIF may be contraindicated in the setting of forearm compartment syndrome, untreated median nerve compression, severe soft tissue injury, open joint injuries, unreduced carpal dislocations, infection, and complex regional pain syndrome.[13]

Timing of Surgery, Setup, and Portals

ARIF can be performed under either axillary block or general anesthesia between 3 and 7 days after the index traumatic event. Waiting a few days allows the surgeon to avoid difficulty with visualization secondary to active bleeding. Conversely, if arthroscopy is performed after 7 days, the fracture begins to consolidate and manipulation of the fragments is more challenging.

Before introducing the arthroscope, a pneumatic tourniquet (set at 250 mm Hg) is applied to the upper arm and an Esmarch bandage is wrapped around the forearm to diminish fluid extravasation into the muscle compartments. Lactated Ringer's solution is used for irrigation because of its rapid absorbability.[14]

The operating room setup and arthroscopic portals are virtually identical to those used in an elective wrist arthroscopy. Either a horizontal or a vertical arthroscopic setup may be used (**Fig. 20-4**).[15] Swelling often makes it difficult to palpate the extensor intervals, so the use of bony landmarks including the bases of the second and third metacarpals, Lister's tubercle, radial styloid, and distal ulna is useful. Traction provides ligamentotaxis, which aids in fracture fragment reduction. A useful technique to avoid iatrogenic cartilage damage during the introduction of arthroscopic

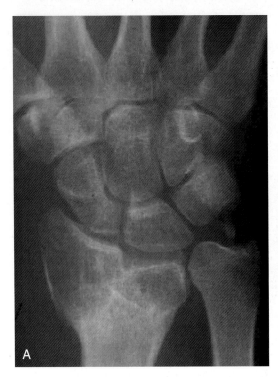

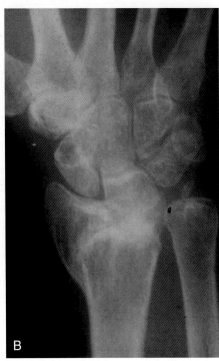

FIGURE 20-1 Anteroposterior (**A**) and oblique (**B**) radiographs of a distal radius fracture with more than a 2-mm articular incongruity results in traumatic arthritis.

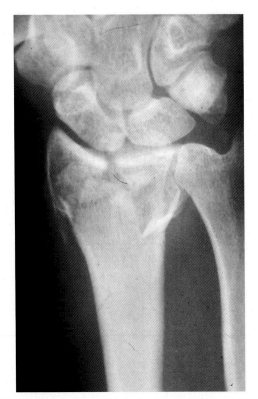

FIGURE 20-2 Radiograph of distal radius fracture with more than 2-mm radial ulnar diastasis.

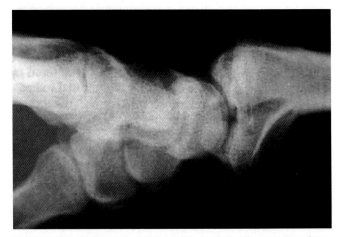

FIGURE 20-3 Radiograph of distal radius fracture with more than 2-mm dorsal volar diastasis.

The arthroscopic sheath is usually introduced in the 3-4 portal, and an outflow cannula is established in the 6-R portal. The first image obtained on entry into the joint is usually that of fibrin clot and debris. Lavage is particularly useful and nearly always necessary to clear the joint and provide unobstructed visualization for precise fragment manipulation and reduction. Washing out fracture hematoma and debris may also contribute to the increased range of motion and functional outcome associated with ARIF.[16,17]

Midcarpal arthroscopy offers significant information to the arthroscopic examination, particularly in the setting of soft tissue injuries suspected with distal radius fractures. Hofmeister and associates showed that a pathological process leading to additional surgical intervention was found on midcarpal examination in more than 60% of patients undergoing arthroscopy for evaluation of soft tissue injuries in the setting of distal radius fractures.[18]

instrumentation is the use of a 20-gauge needle in the proposed 3-4 portal before making a skin incision.[14] If the needle passes unobstructed without engaging bone, the portal is likely in the correct position. Fluoroscopy can also aid in needle placement and portal establishment.

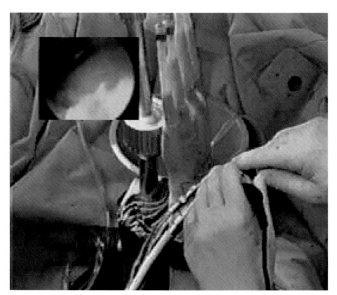

FIGURE 20-4 Setup for arthroscopic-assisted internal fixation. Note vertical traction tower, arthroscope, and C-arm fluoroscopy.

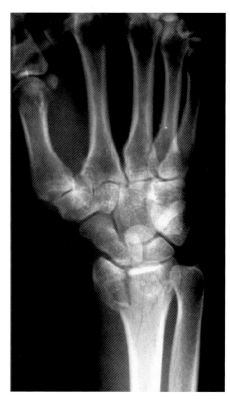

FIGURE 20-5 Radiograph of two-part radial styloid fracture.

Surgical Technique

Distal radius fracture fragments are sometimes reduced with longitudinal traction and external manipulation alone. However, depressed and displaced fragments often require mobilization with either a probe in the joint or instruments such as a Freer elevator placed through a separate skin incision over the fracture. Kirschner wires (K-wires) are also extremely useful because they may be placed in fracture fragments, and, under arthroscopic guidance, depressed fragments may be elevated and realigned via a joystick type maneuver. Once the fracture fragments are appropriately reduced, the surgeon may visualize the articular surfaces with the unparalleled view afforded by the arthroscope.

Two-Part Radial Styloid Fractures

Most radial styloid fractures can also be reduced by closed manipulation. Adequate reduction may be evaluated fluoroscopically, arthroscopically, or by a combination of the two (**Figs. 20-5 to 20-8**). Because radial styloid fractures have a propensity for rotation, K-wire joysticks can be used to manipulate fracture segments. The K-wires may be inserted through a 14-gauge needle, drill sleeve, or drill tap to protect the surrounding neurovascular structures (radial artery and superficial branch of the radial nerve). Arthroscopic assessment of adequate reduction of the articular surface is best evaluated by placing the scope in the 4-5 portal. Once adequate reduction is obtained, the K-wires may be driven across the fracture or another means of fixation, such as a cannulated screw, may be used for fixation (**Fig. 20-9**). Arthroscopic assistance is also useful in assessing for associated soft tissue injuries in the setting of radial styloid fractures. Scapholunate tears have been identified in up to 50% of radial styloid fractures, and arthroscopic assistance is therefore useful in assessing for these intercarpal injuries.[15]

Three-Part Fractures

The arthroscopic-assisted approach to management of three-part fractures (**Figs. 20-10 and 20-11**) includes preliminary reduction of the radial styloid as previously described. The reduced styloid segment may then be used as a landmark to reduce the medial

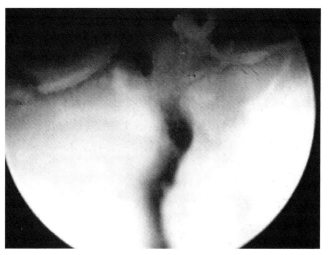

FIGURE 20-6 Arthroscopic view of articular surface of radial styloid fracture.

fragment (**Fig. 20-12**). Articular gaps may be reduced with the aid of a bone tenaculum, and depressed articular fragments may be elevated with the aid of a bone awl or a percutaneously placed Steinman pin. In select cases, bone grafting may be required.[19,20] Once again, arthroscopic assistance allows superior assessment of articular surface reduction and assessment of associated soft tissue injuries.[21]

Four-Part Fractures

Melone four-part fractures are characterized by further splitting of the medial segment into volar and dorsal fragments (**Fig. 20-13**).[22] Initial traction allows ligamentous reduction of fracture

Video

0-1

Web Video

20-2

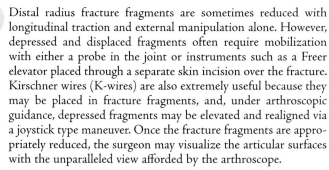

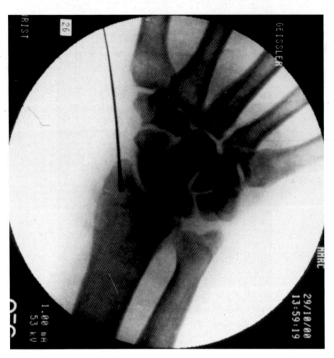

FIGURE 20-7 Fluoroscopic view of ARIF of radial styloid fracture.

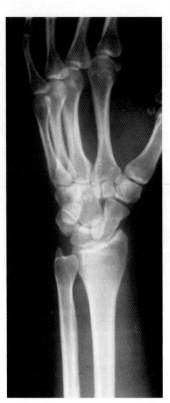

FIGURE 20-8 Follow-up radiograph of patient with radial styloid fracture treated with ARIF.

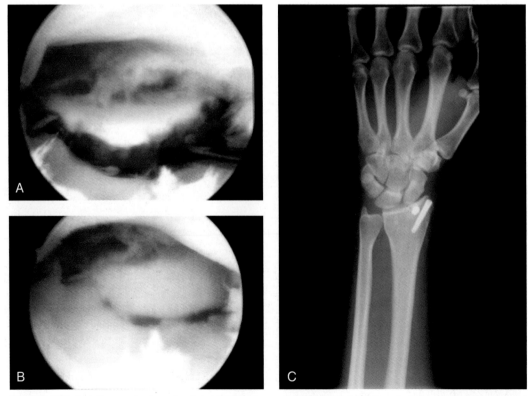

FIGURE 20-9 A, Arthroscopic view of radial styloid fracture with fracture mobilization. **B,** Arthroscopic view of radial styloid fracture ensuring reduction with less than 1-mm step-off. **C,** ARIF of radial styloid fracture with screw fixation.

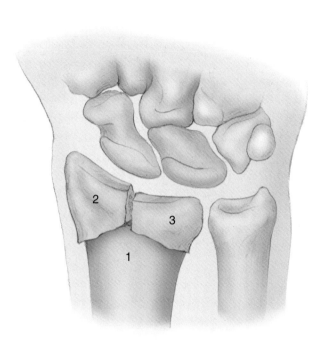

FIGURE 20-10 Schematic drawing of three-part distal radius fracture.

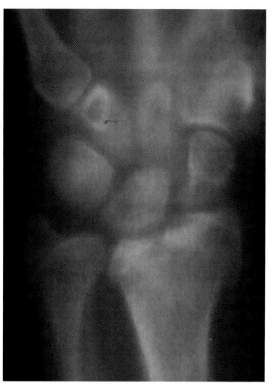

FIGURE 20-11 Three-part intra-articular distal radial fracture.

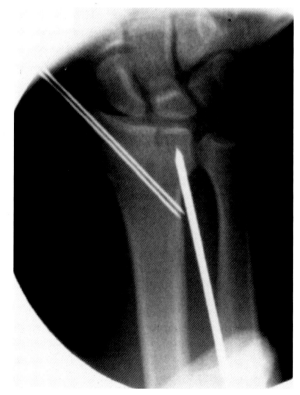

FIGURE 20-12 Intraoperative fluoroscopy with radial styloid component reduced and pinned and joystick in ulnar column fragment for reduction.

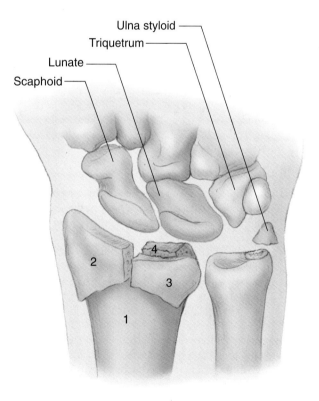

FIGURE 20-13 Diagram of four-part intra-articular distal radius fracture, with ulnar styloid fracture.

segments. Attention is first directed toward reduction of the radial styloid, which then serves as a guide for further fragment reduction. A limited open volar incision is usually required to allow adequate mobilization and reduction of the volar fragment. Buttress plate fixation (usually a 2.7-mm condylar plate) allows stabilization of the volar fragment, which may then be used as a fulcrum to reduce the dorsal fragment. Arthroscopic visualization again assists in evaluating adequate reduction of the dorsal fragment.

Management of Associated Injuries

Distal radius fractures exhibit a high incidence of associated injuries, including chondral and soft tissue injuries to the DRUJ, scapholunate interosseous ligament, lunotriquetral interosseous ligament, as well as the soft tissue structures on the ulnar side of the wrist, including the triangular fibrocartilage complex (TFCC). Geissler and colleagues reported that as many as 68% of patients with intra-articular fractures of the distal end of the radius had associated soft tissue injuries of the wrist.[23] The most commonly associated injury was a tear of the TFCC (49%), followed by injury to the scapholunate interosseous ligament (32%) and injury to the lunotriquetral interosseous ligament (15%). Twenty percent of patients had multiple soft tissue injuries, and chondral lesions of the carpal bones occurred in 23% to 44% of patients with displaced distal radius fractures. Subsequent studies have demonstrated similar results.[15,19,24] Arthroscopy, therefore, allows the treating surgeon to promptly identify and treat associated injuries that may otherwise be missed altogether or diagnosed at a later date requiring secondary reconstruction.

Chondral Lesions

Numerous studies have shown that distal radius fractures evaluated arthroscopically revealed cartilage lesions in both the carpus and distal radius articular surfaces in as many as 18% to 44% (average 27%) of patients.[1,7,23,25-27] These lesions include subchondral hematomas, cartilage impaction lesions, as well as chondral fractures. The significance of chondral injury was demonstrated by Lindau, who showed that in one third of patients with dislocated distal radius fractures and chondral defects, early onset of mild osteoarthritis was found in the same area as the identified lesion and worse outcomes were seen at 1-year follow-up.[7]

Scapholunate Injuries

Intercarpal ligaments play a crucial role in the biomechanics of normal wrist function.[28] If a complete rupture of the scapholunate or lunotriquetral intercarpal ligaments remains untreated, the resulting chronic alteration in wrist kinematics will lead to a predictable pattern of wrist arthrosis. Early primary treatment clearly yields superior results; therefore, early precise diagnosis is critical.[13] Arthroscopy allows direct visualization and magnification of the carpus and is currently the preferred imaging modality of many surgeons to evaluate for internal derangement of the wrist.[29,30]

In the setting of distal radius fractures, scapholunate interosseus ligament injuries have been reported to occur in 18% to 54% (average 31%) of patients undergoing arthroscopy.[1,15,19,23,25-27] Geissler and colleagues described a widely accepted arthroscopic classification system of tears of the intracarpal ligaments.[23] Grade I tears represent attenuation/hemorrhage of the ligament with no incongruence of carpal alignment. Grade II tears, as seen from the midcarpal space, represent partial tears of the ligament and add the element of incongruency to grade I. Grade I and II tears have

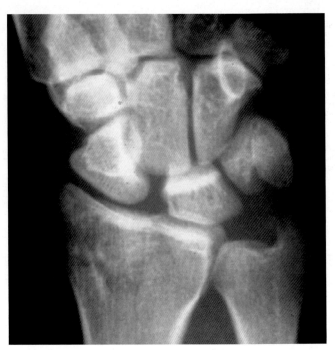

FIGURE 20-14 Radiograph of three-part distal radius fracture with schapholunate dissociation.

the potential to progress to degenerative wrist disease, but there is no current consensus regarding the optimal treatment, which could include either immobilization or arthroscopic pin fixation for 6 to 8 weeks in an effort to promote ligament healing.

Grade III tears are characterized by incongruence or step-off of carpal alignment when viewed from both the radiocarpal and midcarpal joints. A small arthroscopic probe (1 mm) may be passed through a gap between the carpal bones demonstrating a complete tear of the intracarpal ligament. Grade IV lesions represent gross instability of carpal bones with incongruence and the ability to pass a 2.7-mm arthroscope through the gap between the carpal bones—a "drive-through lesion" (**Figs. 20-14 to 20-16**).

In studies that grade scapholunate injuries associated with distal radius fractures, grade II tears are the most commonly reported subtype of scapholunate lesion (roughly 50%). Overall, scapholunate tears are associated with radial styloid and lunate impaction fractures, dorsal displacement of the radius greater than 20 degrees, and static dorsal intercalated segment instability (DISI) on prereduction films. When carpal incongruence is apparent through both radiocarpal and midcarpal portals, and a probe can be passed from the radiocarpal to the midcarpal joint through the scapholunate ligament (grade III tears and greater), ARIF may be indicated. This is best performed by scapholunate ligament débridement and transfixion with K-wires (**Fig. 20-17**). Grade III and IV tears requiring pinning are reported to occur in 25% to 37% of patients (**Figs. 20-18 and 20-19**).[19,23] In some cases, direct arthroscopic repair is not possible and treatment options could include open repair, open repair combined with capsulodesis, or stabilization with tendon transfer.[31]

Lunotriquetral Injuries

Lunotriquetral ligament injuries are reported in 12% to 15% of patients undergoing arthroscopy in the management of distal radius fractures. These injuries may be associated with a basiulnar styloid fracture or volar intercalated segment instability

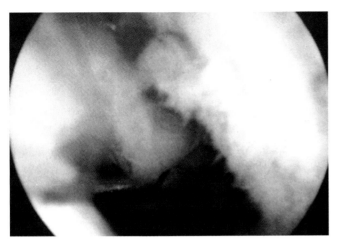

FIGURE 20-15 Arthroscopic view of a grade IV scapholunate tear, a "drive-through lesion."

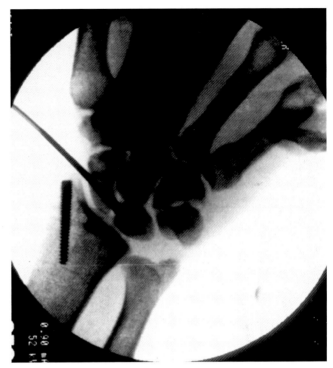

FIGURE 20-17 Fluoroscopic view after ARIF with cannulated screw in radial styloid fracture and percutaneous K-wire pinning of scapholunate tear.

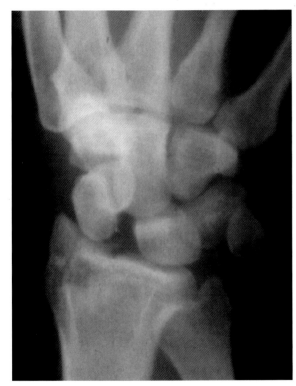

FIGURE 20-16 Distal radius fracture with scapholunate dissociation.

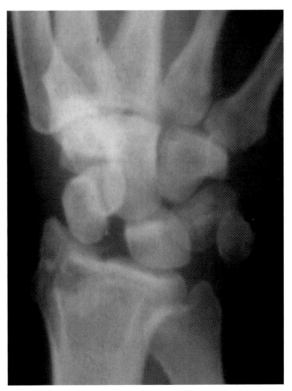

FIGURE 20-18 Radiograph of radial styloid fracture with suspected grade IV scapholunate injury.

(VISI) pattern on the prereduction radiograph. Geissler and colleagues reported lunotriquetral tears in a series of 9 of 60 patients (15%).[23] Seven of these 9 patients (77%) had grade III complete tears. The other 2 patients had partial tears of the lunotriquetral ligament. In our series, only 5% of patients with identified lunotriquetral tears were considered unstable enough to require pinning with K-wires (**Fig. 20-20**), but other series report lunotriquetral transfixation in up to 75% of patients with identified lunotriquetral tears in the setting of distal radius fractures.[19,26]

Concurrent Injuries

Roughly 20% of patients may have combined soft tissue injuries in association with arthroscopically evaluated distal radius frac-

tures. Combined injuries most commonly involve TFCC and scapholunate injuries, followed by TFCC and lunotriquetral injuries, and scapholunate and lunotriquetral injuries.[19,26] Slade and coworkers have reported combined fractures of the scaphoid and distal radius treated by percutaneous and arthroscopic

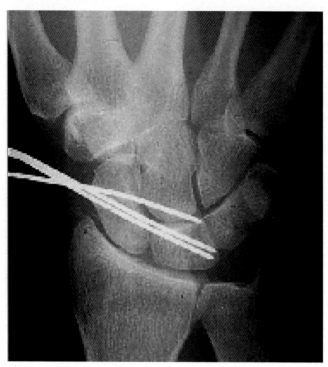

FIGURE 20-19 Radiograph of radial styloid fracture with associated scapholunate tear after ARIF.

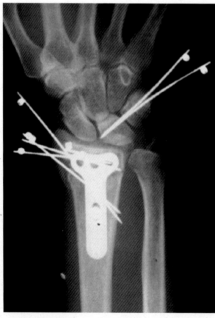

FIGURE 20-20 Radiograph of distal radius fracture with associated lunatotriquetral grade III tear treated with ARIF and pinning.

techniques.[32] They recommend percutaneous reduction of the scaphoid fracture and provisional stabilization with a guidewire placed along its central axis, percutaneous/arthroscopic reduction and rigid fixation of the distal radius fracture to permit early motion, and, lastly, fixation of the scaphoid fracture with implantation of a cannulated headless compression screw. Fractures of the ulnar styloid are frequently associated with distal radius fractures as well. Arthroscopy helps to provide a treatment rationale in approaching management of the ulnar styloid fracture. Loss of

the trampoline effect by a probe of the TFCC indicates laxity of the articular disc and may be indicative of DRUJ instability. If there is no demonstrable laxity of the TFCC and a stable DRUJ, the ulnar styloid fracture likely does not need to be stabilized. If, on the other hand, there is laxity of the articular disc and/or DRUJ instability, the ulnar styloid fracture should be fixed with pins or screws.

Complications

Complications of ARIF have been minimal in reported case series. A small percentage of patients may have settling of the fracture fragments resulting in loss of volar tilt. Five to 10 percent of patients may develop complications related to percutaneous pin placement, including loosening, infection, and sensory nerve irritation, but these findings may not be directly related to ARIF itself.[19] In addition, the development of complex regional pain syndrome in two patients after ARIF has been reported.[1]

Outcomes

There is now enough scientific evidence to validate the effectiveness and safety of ARIF in the management of distal radius fractures. Unfortunately, there are no prospective randomized double-blinded studies comparing ARIF with open reduction and internal fixation (ORIF) without arthroscopic assistance. Several studies have, however, compared results of ARIF versus ORIF in the treatment of distal radius fractures.[17,23,29] These studies uniformly describe increased range of motion, better outcomes, and better articular reduction with arthroscopic assistance when compared with ORIF without arthroscopic assistance.

Several concepts must be considered when assessing outcomes with respect to the use of arthroscopy in the management of selected distal radius fractures. The orthopaedic literature has proved that there is a direct relationship between the quality of anatomical reconstruction (which implies the recognition of all injuries) and the subsequent stability of that reconstruction. A stable construct allows for preservation of motion, minimizes the risk of post-traumatic arthrosis, and finally optimizes long-term functional outcome. Multiple studies have shown that the use of arthroscopy is effective in not only identifying and evaluating distal radius fractures and their associated injuries but also facilitating anatomical reduction and reconstruction.[17,19]

Conclusion

Fractures of the distal radius are among the most common fractures treated by orthopaedic surgeons. Contrary to historical dogma, the outcome of these fractures is not uniformly good regardless of the treatment initiated. As previously noted, orthopaedic literature has consistently shown that there is a direct relationship between the quality of anatomical reconstruction and long-term functional outcome. A contemporary approach to the management of intra-articular distal radius fractures should therefore involve arthroscopic assistance in some form. We recommend intraoperative arthroscopy to assist in the treatment of select intra-articular distal radius fractures, with or without initial radiographically evident displacement. The unique advantages afforded by ARIF help to ensure the most anatomical fracture reduction and the ability to treat associated injuries.

REFERENCES

1. Cognet JM, Bonnomet F, Ehlinger M, et al: Arthroscopy-guided treatment of fractures of the distal radius: 16 wrists.

Rev Chir Orthop Reparatrice Appar Mot. 2003; 89:515-523.

2. Axelrod TS, McMurtry RY: Open reduction and internal fixation of comminuted, intra-articular fractures of the distal radius. J Hand Surg [Am]. 1990; 15:1-11.

3. Knirk JL, Jupiter JB: Intra-articular fractures of the distal end of the radius in young adults. J Bone Joint Surg Am. 1986; 68:647-659.

4. Trumble TE, Culp RW, Hanel DP, et al: Intra-articular fractures of the distal aspect of the radius. Instr Course Lect. 1999; 48:465-480.

5. Trumble TE, Schmitt SR, Vedder NB: Factors affecting functional outcome of displaced intra-articular distal radius fractures. J Hand Surg [Am]. 1994; 19:325-340.

6. Fernandez DL, Geissler WB: Treatment of displaced articular fractures of the radius. J Hand Surg [Am]. 1991; 16:375-384.

7. Lindau T, Adlecreutz C, Aspenberg P: Cartilage injuries in distal radial fractures. Acta Orthop Scand. 2003; 74:327-331.

8. Edwards CC, Haraszti CJ, McGillivary GR, Gutow AP: Intra-articular distal radius fractures: arthroscopic assessment of radiographically assisted reduction. J Hand Surg [Am]. 2001; 26:1036-1041.

9. Kordasiewicz B, Pomianowski S, Orlowski J, Rapala K: Interosseous ligaments and TFCC lesions in intraarticular distal radius fractures—radiographic versus arthroscopic evaluation. Ortop Traumatol Rehabil. 2006; 8:263-267.

10. Ruch DS, Vallee J, Poehling GG, et al: Arthroscopic reduction versus fluoroscopic reduction in the management of intra-articular distal radius fractures. Arthroscopy. 2004; 20:225-230.

11. Nijs S, Broos PL: Fractures of the distal radius: a contemporary approach. Acta Chir Belg. 2004; 104:401-412.

12. Trumble TE, Schmitt SR, Vedder NB: Factors affecting functional outcome of displaced intra-articular distal radius fractures. J Hand Surg [Am]. 1994; 19:325-340.

13. Wiesler ER, Chloros GD, Mahirogullari M, Kuzma GR: Arthroscopic management of distal radius fractures. J Hand Surg [Am]. 2006; 31:1516-1526.

14. Geissler W, Freeland A: Arthroscopic management of intra-articular distal radius fractures. Hand Clin. 1999; 15:455-466.

15. Lindau T, Arner M, Hagberg L: Intra-articular lesions in distal fractures of the radius in young adults: a descriptive arthroscopic study in 50 patients. J Hand Surg [Br]. 1997; 22:638-643.

16. Geissler WB: Intra-articular distal radius fractures: the role of arthroscopy? Hand Clin. 2005; 21:407-416.

17. Doi K, Hattoi Y, Otsuka K, et al: Intra-articular fractures of the distal aspect of the radius: arthroscopically assisted reduction compared with open reduction and internal fixation. J Bone Joint Surg Am. 1999; 81:1093-1110.

18. Hofmeister EP, Dao KD, Glowacki KA, Shin AY: The role of midcarpal arthroscopy in the diagnosis of disorders of the wrist. J Hand Surg [Am]. 2001; 26:407-414.

19. Culp RW, Osterman AL, Kaufmann RA: Wrist arthroscopy: operative procedures. In Green DP, ed: Operative Hand Surgery. New York: Elsevier, 2005.

20. Chen AC, Chan YS, Yuan LJ, et al: Arthroscopically assisted osteosynthesis of complex intra-articular fractures of the distal radius. J Trauma. 2002; 53:354-359.

21. Levy HJ, Glickel SZ: Arthroscopic assisted internal fixation of volar intra-articular wrist fractures. Arthroscopy. 1993; 9:122-131.

22. Melone CP: Articular fractures of the distal radius. Orthop Clin North Am. 1984; 15:217-236.

23. Geissler WB, Freeland AE, Savoie FH, et al: Intracarpal soft-tissue lesions associated with an intra-articular fracture of the distal end of the radius. J Bone Joint Surg Am. 1996; 78:357-365.

24. Hanker GJ: Radius fractures in the athlete. Clin Sports Med. 2001; 20:189-201.

25. Mathoulin C, Sbihi A, Panciera P: Interest in wrist arthroscopy for treatment of articular fractures of the distal radius: report of 27 cases. Chir Main. 2001; 20:342-350.

26. Shih JT, Lee HM, Hou YT, Tan CM: Arthroscopically-assisted reduction of intra-articular fractures and soft tissue management of distal radius. Hand Surg. 2001; 6:127-135.

27. Rose S, Frank J, Marzi I: Diagnostic and therapeutic significance of arthroscopy in distal radius fracture. Zentralbl Chir. 1999; 124:984-992.

28. Mayfield JK, Johnson RP, Kilcoyne RK: Carpal dislocations: pathomechanics and progressive perilunar instability. J Hand Surg [Am]. 1980; 5:226-241.

29. Weiss AP, Akelman E, Lambiase R: Comparison of the findings of triple-injection cinearthrography of the wrist with those of arthroscopy. J Bone Joint Surg [Am]. 1996; 78:348-356.

30. Cooney WP: Evaluation of chronic wrist pain by arthrography, arthroscopy, and arthrotomy. J Hand Surg [Am]. 1993; 18:815-822.

31. Walsh JJ, Berger RA, Cooney WP: Current status of scapholunate interosseous ligament injuries. J Am Acad Orthop Surg. 2002; 10:32-42.

32. Slade JF 3rd, Taksali S, Safanda J: Combined fractures of the scaphoid and distal radius: a revised treatment rationale using percutaneous and arthroscopic techniques. Hand Clin. 2005; 21:427-441.

Simultaneous Fractures of the Scaphoid and Distal Radius

21

Greg A. Merrell, MD and Joseph F. Slade III, MD

Although uncommon, simultaneous fractures of the distal radius and scaphoid can be challenging to treat. Once the decision has been made to surgically treat these injuries, the question arises on the order of treatment of these combined fractures. The goal of surgical treatment is rigid fixation. Once fixation is achieved in one fracture, the treatment of the second fracture risks disruption of fixation of the first fracture. If the scaphoid is fixed first, there is potential for screw pullout or loosening during the substantial forces applied during reduction of the distal radius. If the first fracture treated is the radius, reduction of the second fracture, that of the scaphoid, may result in a loss of reduction and a malunion in the radius. The purpose of this chapter is to present a tactical approach to the surgical treatment of these combined fractures, which results in rigid fixation of both fractures using arthroscopic and percutaneous techniques.

The incidence of combined injuries varies from 0.7% to 6.5% of all distal radius fractures.[1-4] The mechanism is a high-energy injury with rapid forced loading of an outstretched radial-deviated dorsiflexed wrist.[1,3,5,6] These injuries are often associated with a displaced and angulated scaphoid fracture.

The rare isolated stable nondisplaced scaphoid fracture and distal radius fracture might be safely managed with plaster immobilization for periods of 3 to 4 months. Unfortunately, this period of immobilization for the treatment of distal radius fractures, at best, results in delay in recovery of hand and wrist function and, at worst, permanent stiffness.[6,7]

A review of the relatively few published reports on combined scaphoid and distal radius fractures demonstrates that treatments have evolved over the past decade. Historical references site the primacy of addressing the distal radius fracture, but this predated the operative treatment of acute scaphoid fractures.[5,8,9] We now understand that both fractures must be adequately reduced and treated. The arthroscopic care of both distal radius and scaphoid fractures and the use of percutaneous techniques have permitted the rigid fixation of these fractures while preserving uninjured tissues.[10-13] This has allowed for the early recovery of hand function with minimal complications.

The techniques presented in this chapter will describe in a step-by-step manner the evaluation and fixation of a specific case to help provide clarity. This injury occurred in a 22-year-old right-handed skateboarder who had a fracture through an old scaphoid nonunion and a distal radius fracture (**Figs. 21-1 and 21-2**).

Indications

The typical patient who presents with these injuries is male in his 20s or 30s after a fall, motor vehicle accident, or sports injury. Any patient with combined fractures with displacement of either the scaphoid or distal radius greater than 1 mm would be an operative candidate. If the patient is going to benefit from operative intervention of one fracture and the other is nondisplaced, then stable fixation of the other fracture while in the operating room probably makes sense to allow for the earliest possible mobilization of the extremity. If both fractures are nondisplaced and the scaphoid fracture is mid to distal, one could make a case for either operative or nonoperative intervention depending on the specific circumstances of the patient (e.g., age, comorbidities, tolerance of a cast). Typically, these are treated within 2 weeks, although treatment after that date is not necessarily contraindicated.

Contraindications

Treatment of pediatric patients with nondisplaced fractures is relatively contraindicated because in these patients the scaphoid fracture will usually heal in a reasonable amount of time and there are not as many problems with joint stiffness. A common problem today with the treatment protocol of children is that many caregivers neglect to utilize a cast or limit casting in children, resulting in nonunions. It should be understood that adolescents have similar healing potential as adults and should be provided the same treatment as adults.

Overview of Surgical Technique

The treatment of combined fractures of the scaphoid and distal radius includes the arthroscopic-assisted/percutaneous reduction of both fractures and their rigid fixation. *The key to success is a three-step process:*

1. The percutaneous/arthroscopic reduction of the scaphoid fracture and provisional stabilization with a guidewire placed along its central axis
2. The reduction and rigid fixation of the distal radius fracture to permit early motion
3. The fixation of the scaphoid fracture by the percutaneous implantation of a cannulated headless compression screw along the central scaphoid axis

This surgical staging permits reduction of both fractures without compromising the final rigid fixation of either fracture. Arthroscopy is used to confirm fracture reduction and identify occult injuries.

Setup

Equipment includes a headless cannulated compression screw for scaphoid fixation to permit percutaneous fixation and some type of distal radius fixation system that can provide rigid fixation with the least complications. We prefer screws of standard size for scaphoid fractures of the middle third, because the larger core

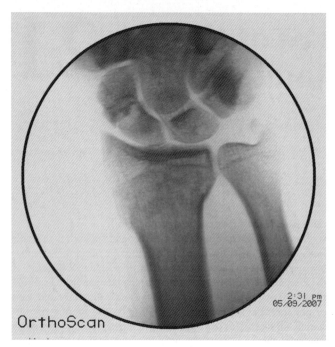

FIGURE 21-1 Anteroposterior radiograph demonstrating distal radius fracture and a combined scaphoid nonunion with a new fracture at the distal edge of the nonunion site. Sequential images of the technique for fixation of this injury form the basis for discussion of this chapter. The patient is a 19-year-old skateboarder.

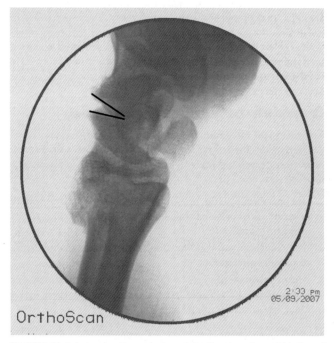

FIGURE 21-2 Lateral radiograph demonstrating dorsal comminution of the distal radius fracture and a flexion deformity of the scaphoid.

shaft increases the ability to resist lateral displacement forces.[14] Mini-fluoroscopy permits real-time imaging during surgery. Although standard fluoroscopy units can be used, they are cumbersome and emit a significant amount of radiation. Additional equipment includes 0.045-inch and 0.062-inch double-cut Kirschner wires (K-wires), a wire driver, and a small joint arthroscopy setup, including a traction system.

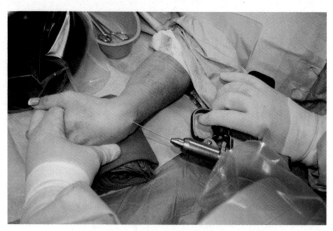

FIGURE 21-3 Driving the central axis wire.

Surgical Technique

Imaging

The patient is placed supine, with the upper extremity extended on a hand table in a neutral position with a roll under the ulnar side of the wrist. A fluoroscopic survey of the wrist and carpus is performed to evaluate the personality of the fractures, including the direction of displacement, the presence and degree of comminution, and associated ligamentous injuries. Radiographic views of the distal radius, to account for the palmar tilt and ulnar inclination, are useful in evaluating fracture displacement of the articular surface. Longitudinal traction is then applied to the wrist, and a second fluoroscopic survey is conducted through a 90-degree arc. This helps determine the reduction achieved by ligamentotaxis and whether there is any remaining displacement.

Scaphoid Fracture Reduction and Dorsal Guidewire Placement along the Scaphoid Central Axis

The wrist is in an ulnarly deviated position extended on the arm table with a mini-fluoroscopy unit placed horizontal on the arm table and perpendicular to the wrist. The starting position for the guidewire is the proximal scaphoid pole at the 3-4 arthroscopic portal (**Fig. 21-3**). This dorsal approach permits easy access to the central scaphoid axis because the base of the scaphoid is covered only by soft tissue. The distal scaphoid is covered by the trapezium and obstructs direct line of sight, making central axis wire placement difficult. With the wrist supported by a roll and mini-fluoroscopy perpendicular to the wrist, a guidewire is placed at the proximal scaphoid pole and driven dorsally along the central axis of the scaphoid passing through the trapezium. The wrist is maintained in a flexed position to avoid bending the guidewire. As the wire is advanced, its position in two planes is confirmed using fluoroscopy (**Fig. 21-4**). The wire is advanced from a dorsal to volar position until the dorsal trailing end of the wire clears the radiocarpal joint, permitting full extension of the wrist. The volar end of the wire exits from the radial base of the thumb, which is a safe zone devoid of tendons and neurovascular structures. Once the dorsal trailing end of the guidewire has been buried into the proximal scaphoid pole, the wrist can be extended for imaging to

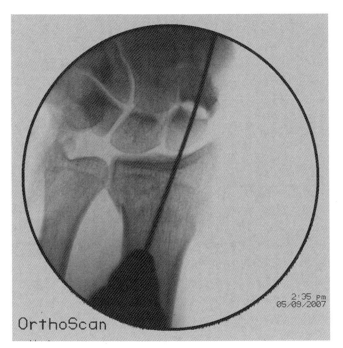

FIGURE 21-4 Central axis wire in correct position on the anteroposterior view.

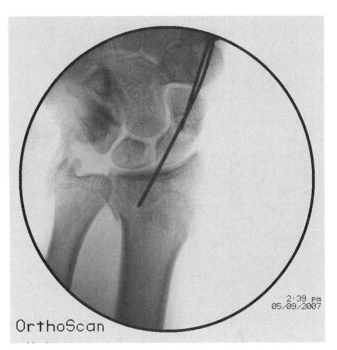

FIGURE 21-6 A second antirotation wire is placed.

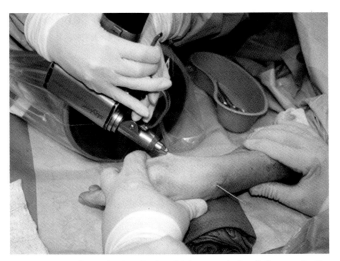

FIGURE 21-5 Central axis wire is withdrawn volarly all the way to the fracture site to allow reduction of the fracture. Wire placement in a displaced fracture is crucial in the distal fragment but initially less important in the proximal fragment until reduction is performed.

confirm scaphoid fracture alignment and correct positioning of the guidewire.

If the scaphoid is displaced, the proximal pole is ignored and the guidewire is placed through the distal scaphoid fragment along its central axis and withdrawn volarly beyond the fracture site (**Fig. 21-5**). A second antirotation wire is usually added, particularly in less stable displaced fractures (**Fig. 21-6**).

Often the lunate sits in a dorsiflexed intercalated segment instability (DISI) position. This is corrected by hyperflexing the wrist and driving a 0.062-inch wire from the distal radius into the lunate to capture the lunate in a corrected position (**Fig. 21-7**). This also helps stabilize the proximal pole of the scaphoid, assisting with the reduction. The scaphoid fracture is reduced percuta-

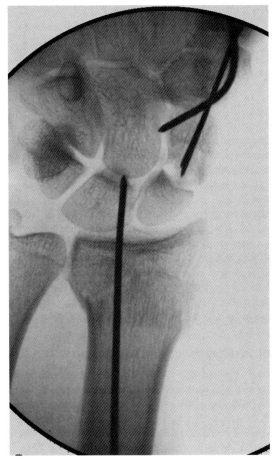

FIGURE 21-7 The wrist is hyperflexed to correct the lunate DISI position, and a 0.062-inch wire is driven from radius to lunate to hold this position. A joystick is also placed in the distal scaphoid.

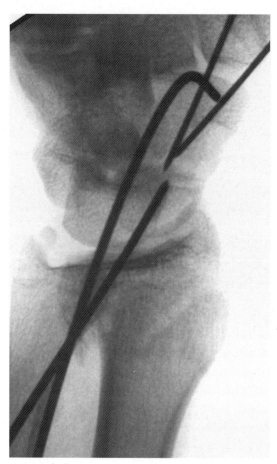

FIGURE 21-8 The joystick is used to extend the distal pole of the scaphoid while the two axis wires are driven retrograde to capture the reduction.

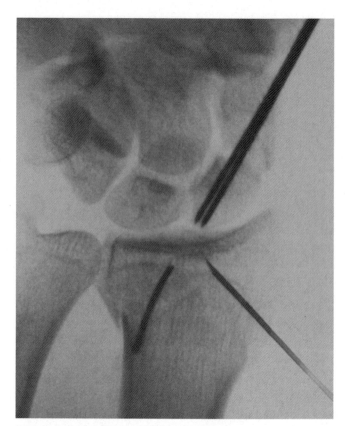

FIGURE 21-9 The distal radius fracture is reduced percutaneously with the use of Kapandji-type joystick K-wires.

neously using dorsally placed 0.062-inch K-wires as joysticks in each fracture fragment. When the dorsal joysticks are brought together, the flexion deformity of the scaphoid is corrected. This is best confirmed on lateral fluoroscopy (**Fig. 21-8**). The previously placed distal wires are driven retrograde to capture the reduction.

With acute fractures, there is usually no loss of volar cortex because the volar scaphoid fails in tension in a hyperextension injury. Older or impacted displaced fractures may require the direct introduction of a small hemostat at the fracture site to achieve reduction. The hemostat is introduced through a midcarpal or an accessory portal. Once reduction is achieved, the previously placed wire in the distal fragment is driven from its volar position into the proximal fragment to capture and secure reduction.

Distal Radius Fracture Reduction

Once the scaphoid fracture is reduced and provisionally stabilized, attention is turned to the distal radius fracture. Again, like the scaphoid, the distal radius is percutaneously reduced using mini-fluoroscopy, 19-gauge needles to locate the fracture site, a small curved hemostat placed percutaneously to achieve reduction, and K-wires to provide provisional fixation (**Fig. 21-9**). Depending on the fracture type and stability, the patient's needs and desires, and, finally, the surgeon's skill and experience, an appropriate wrist fracture system is selected. As a rule, the sim-

plest system that achieves rigid fixation and permits early recovery of hand function with the least complication is the best. Our goals should be restoration of a congruent joint surface and of the native metaphyseal cortical architecture. It has been the senior author's experience that every patient sustains two injuries. The first is his or her misfortune, and the second is our treatment. If we can limit the second injury by avoiding any additional injury to the uninjured structures, the patient often has fewer complications and a quicker recovery of hand function. The use of fluoroscopy and arthroscopy permits the use of percutaneous techniques, which limits these secondary injuries but still facilitates our ultimate goals of fracture reduction and rigid fixation. The wrist is placed in a neutral position perpendicular to a mini-fluoroscopy unit with the ulna supported by a towel roll. Imaging locates the fractures, and 19-gauge needles are placed dorsally, identifying the fracture site. Limited stab incisions are made, and a small curved hemostat is introduced into the fracture site. The distal fracture fragment is leveraged into a reduced position and a percutaneous 0.062-inch K-wire is placed to provide provisional fixation. Both the radial height and dorsal tilt should be restored. If an intra-articular fracture is detected on imaging, than this fracture is reduced and secured first, using the just-described techniques.

Arthroscopy and Soft Tissue Injuries

After fluoroscopy confirms fracture reduction of the scaphoid and the radius, arthroscopy can be used as a valuable tool to provide direct confirmation of articular fracture reduction of both the scaphoid and the radius.[10-12,15]

Longitudinal traction is applied through all fingers to allow for safe entry of the small joint arthroscope and instruments. With the use of mini-fluoroscopy, the midcarpal and radiocarpal portals are located and 19-gauge needles are used to mark these portal sites. After a small longitudinal incision is made, a small hemostat is used to dissect bluntly the soft tissue down to the joint capsule. A blunt trocar is used to enter the joint. An angled, 2.7-mm 30-degree small joint arthroscope is placed in the radial, midcarpal portal to confirm scaphoid fracture reduction.

The arthroscope is then placed in the radiocarpal joint through the 3-4 portal. The integrity of the scapholunate and lunotrique-tral interosseous ligaments is assessed from both the radiocarpal and midcarpal joints. These joints are explored with a probe. Partial tears can be treated with simple débridement. Complete carpal ligament disruptions require an open ligament repair using bone anchors and provisional fixation with K-wires or headless screws.

With the use of arthroscopy and imaging, the distal articular surface can now be directly examined for incongruencies. If displacement is detected, joystick K-wires are placed percutaneously into the fracture fragments. A small curved hemostat is introduced through a small stab incision into the fracture site to elevate the displaced fragment, and the joysticks are then used to align the fragments and capture the reduction. Once the fracture reduction is accomplished, multiple K-wires provide fracture stabilization. This effectively transforms an intra-articular fracture into an extra-articular fracture.

Rigid Fixation of the Distal Radius

The fracture system selected should provide rigid fixation of the distal radius and permit early recovery of hand function. Rigid fixation of unstable fractures can be provided by headless screws for radial styloid fractures (standard size Acutrak II Headless Screws; Acumed, Inc., Beaverton, OR), an internal medullary rod for extra-articular and some intra-articular fractures (Micronail; Wright Medical, Arlington, TN), and plating for complex or severely comminuted fractures (Medartis, Acumed, Depuy/Hand Innovations, Stryker, Trimed, Synthes, Wright Medical). Volar locked plating takes advantage of the stiff volar radial cortex to achieve rigid fixation.

Intramedullary rods are inserted just dorsal to the radial styloid between the first and second dorsal compartment (**Fig. 21-10**). The largest nail is inserted close to the radial cortex, and distal locking screws are used to provide secure distal radius fixation. Next, proximal locking screws are placed percutaneously into the intramedullary nail, completing fixation (**Fig. 21-11**).

Volar plates are commonly inserted through a modified Henry approach. The wrist is placed over a towel roll and approached through an incision centered over the flexor carpi radialis tendon. The tendon is exposed and retracted, and the tendon floor sheath is incised. Care is taken to protect the radial artery radially and the median nerve ulnarly. The flexor pollicis longus muscle origin is identified, protected, and retracted, exposing the pronator quadratus over the volar distal radius. The pronator quadratus is incised in an L shape off the radial and distal radius, with care taken to protect the volar radial carpal ligaments. A Cobb elevator is used to elevate the muscle ulnarly, exposing the fracture site. The brachioradialis tendon insertion on the radial styloid is identified and Z-plastied. The floor of the first dorsal extensor compartment is identified and incised. This exposure is often sufficient to expose the fracture site. If complete reduction has not been achieved, then K-wires are partially withdrawn and an anatomical reduction of the fracture is obtained. Early malunions and intra-articular fractures require greater exposure. In these cases, the

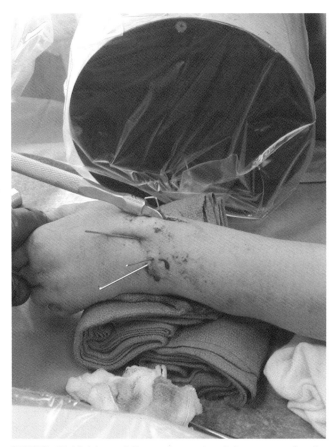

FIGURE 21-10 Intramedullary reamer placed to prepare for the Micronail.

dorsal periosteum of the distal radius is incised, fracture callus is excised, and the proximal radius may be delivered from the wound to assist in bone grafting and fracture reduction. The volar plate is secured to the radius proximal to the fracture site, and the distal radius is molded to the volar plate and secured with locking screws. Care is taken to position the plate to capture unstable distal volar fracture fragments. Distal screws are placed, being mindful to prevent both intra-articular penetration of screws and to keep them unicortical to prevent extensor ruptures. Careful assessment with live fluoroscopy is best to confirm proper screw position. Additional bone graft is applied radially as needed. The brachioradialis tendon is repaired in a lengthened position. The pronator quadratus is advanced, providing plate coverage to the radial styloid, and secured to the brachioradialis tendon.

Scaphoid Length and Screw Size

After distal radius fixation, the scaphoid fracture can now be rigidly fixed. In the case presented here, an added wrinkle is the need to percutaneously curet and bone graft the nonunion. One K-wire is withdrawn from the distal part of the scaphoid and the cannula for a Jam-Sheedy bone biopsy needle is placed up the reamed path for the screw to the nonunion site (**Fig. 21-12**). Cores of bone graft previously harvested from either the hip, distal radius, or tibial tubercle are passed through the cannula and deposited into the fracture site with the use of an obturator (**Fig. 21-13**). The nonunion site has now been filled with graft, and the K-wire is advanced back across the fracture site (**Fig. 21-14**).

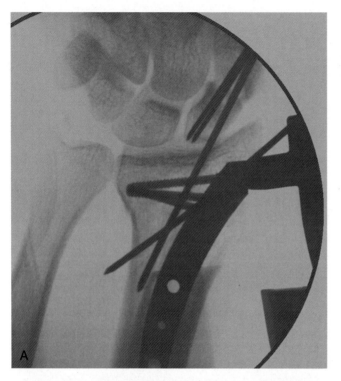

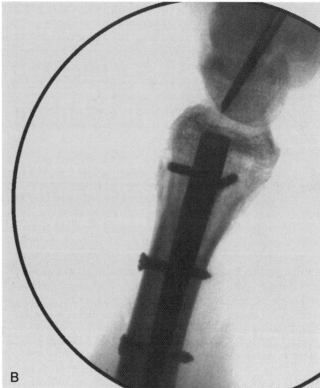

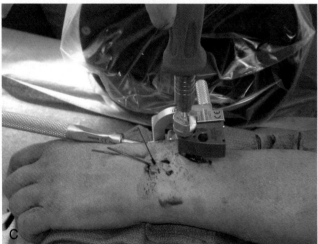

FIGURE 21-11 Anteroposterior (**A**) and lateral (**B**) radiographs of the Micronail. **C,** Clinical photo of the Micronail being placed.

The scaphoid length must now be determined.[15] The guidewire is adjusted until the distal end is in contact with the distal cortex of the scaphoid. A second wire of equal length is placed at the tip of the cortex of the proximal pole. The difference in length between these two wires is the exact length of the scaphoid.

The most common complication of percutaneous screw implantation is implantation of a screw that is too long. In our experience, to avoid this complication, the screw selected should provide for 2 mm of clearance between the screw's end and the scaphoid cortex. The screw length should be 4 mm shorter than the scaphoid length. This permits the complete implantation of a headless compression screw in bone without exposure.

Once the length of the screw has been determined, the appropriate width must be selected. Biomechanical studies suggest that the widest screws provide the strongest fixation.[14] One concern about introducing larger screws dorsally is the consequences of

the resulting cartilage defect, but these defects have been shown to heal over with cartilage in time without degenerative changes.[16]

With extremely small proximal pole fractures or avulsions there is a possible risk of fragmentation with implantation of a large screw. Under these circumstances, a smaller screw is inserted to decrease the risk of fracture fragmentation but a second headless screw or 0.062-inch K-wire should be placed from the scaphoid to the capitate temporarily locking the midcarpal joint and deflecting a strong torque force that is transferred along the long axis of the scaphoid. These strong forces can result in screw pullout and nonunion.

Screw Implantation

Headless compression screws are implanted dorsally for scaphoid fractures of the proximal pole and implanted volarly for distal pole

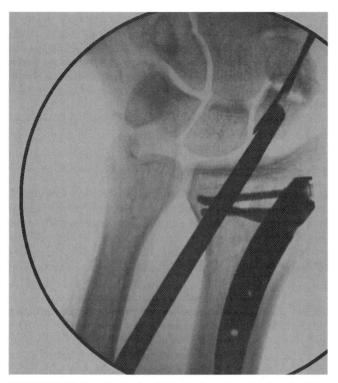

FIGURE 21-12 One K-wire is withdrawn from the distal part of the scaphoid and the cannula for a Jam-Sheedy needle is placed up the reamed path for the screw to the nonunion site.

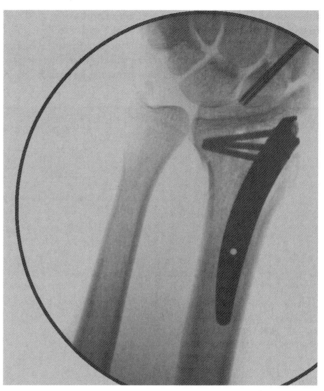

FIGURE 21-14 The nonunion site has now been filled with graft, and the K-wire is advanced back across the fracture site.

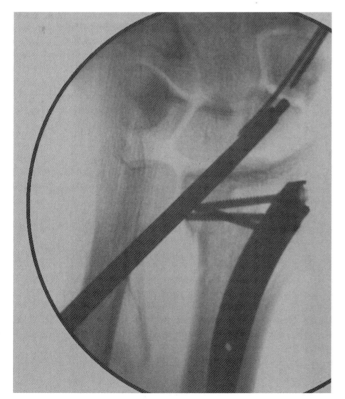

FIGURE 21-13 Cores of bone graft previously harvested from either the hip, distal radius, or tibial tubercle are passed through the cannula and deposited into the fracture site with the use of an obturator. The nonunion site had previously been curetted percutaneously.

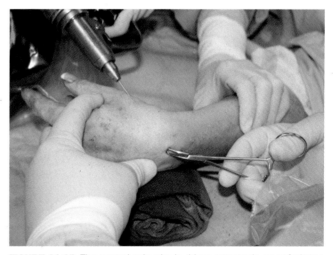

FIGURE 21-15 The central axis wire is driven retrograde as soft tissue is cleared. The wire is left out on both dorsal and volar sides to prevent shearing or allow wire removal if it does shear during screw placement.

fractures, because this permits maximum fracture compression.[15] Fractures of the waist may be fixed from a dorsal or volar approach as long as the screw is implanted along the central scaphoid axis. Blunt dissection along the guidewire exposes a tract to the dorsal wrist capsule and scaphoid base. Before drilling, the guidewire should be advanced so that both ends are exposed equally (**Fig. 21-15**). This will permit the wire from becoming dislodged during reaming. The scaphoid is prepared by hand drilling the scaphoid cortex with a cannulated hand drill. This allows the implantation of a headless compression screw completely within the scaphoid. The screw is advanced under fluoroscopic guidance to within 1 to 2 mm of the opposite cortex with excellent compression (**Fig. 21-16**). If the screw is advanced to the distal cortex, attempts to advance the screw farther will displace or penetrate the distal fragment. With unstable fractures, a joystick is left in

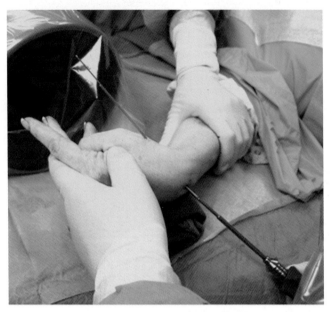

FIGURE 21-16 The screw is placed while keeping the wrist flexed to prevent bending of the guidewire.

the distal scaphoid fragment for screw implantation. As the screw is implanted, a counterforce is exerted through the joystick, compressing both fracture fragments and ensuring rigid fixation.

After screw placement, the guidewire is removed and wrist fluoroscopy confirms screw position, fracture reduction, and rigid fixation. Arthroscopy can also confirm reduction and complete seating of the screw.

Occasionally, as in the case presented, the unstable nature of the fracture requires additional fixation (screw and supplemental K-wires or two screws) (**Fig. 21-17**).

Postoperative Care

Postoperative care is directed at recovery of hand function. A bulky hand dressing is applied, and elevation of the limb is enforced to control early swelling. A digital exercise program is initiated immediately. Commercially available cooling pads are valuable in helping to control pain. If significant swelling is present intraoperatively, consideration is given to the release of the median nerve in the carpal tunnel. The control of postoperative pain is critical for the successful recovery of hand function.

At the first office visit, the surgical dressing is removed and a volar splint is applied. A vigorous hand and wrist therapy program is initiated to recover a full arc of motion of the digits and forearm. Patients with fractures of the scaphoid waist are started on an immediate wrist range-of-motion protocol. Patients with proximal pole fractures are protected for 6 weeks before the initiation of therapy. All patients are started on an immediate strengthening program. The purpose of this is to axially load the fracture site now secured with an intramedullary screw to stimulate healing.

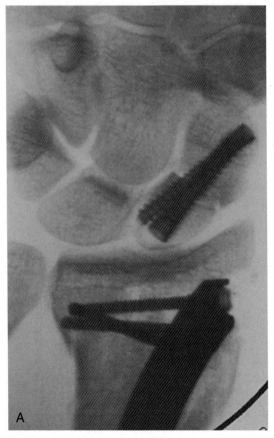
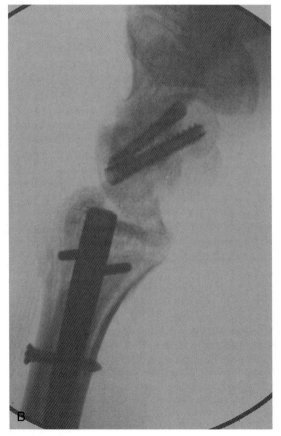

FIGURE 21-17 Given the unstable nature of the fracture, two screws are placed in the scaphoid, one dorsal to volar and one volar to dorsal. Anteroposterior (**A**) and lateral (**B**) radiographs show the final reduction and fixation.

Adjustments to this protocol are made to take into account any concerns for suboptimal fixation or bone quality. Heavy lifting and contact sports are restricted until the patient's arm is no longer tender and computed tomography (CT) confirms healing by bridging callus.

Authors' Case Results

The case presented here healed at 7 weeks based on both clinical evaluation and bridging bone on CT scan. Careful percutaneous technique permits fast recovery with limited morbidity. **Figures 21-18 through 21-22** demonstrate this patient's postoperative radiographs and his functional recovery.

We reviewed scaphoid fractures treated with percutaneous repair by one of us (JFSIII) on the Yale Hand Service between 1998 and 2002. Eight ipsilateral fractures of the scaphoid and distal radius were identified in adults. The average age was 30 years (range: 18 to 58 years), and there was a bimodal distribution, with the men having an average age of 22 years and the women having an average age of 49 years. The injuries were three of the right scaphoid and five of the left scaphoid. Six of the eight patients were male. In these cases the injury involved a fall from a substantial height, a motor vehicle accident, or, in one case, a skateboard accident. The two female patients were injured in falls.

All scaphoid fractures were displaced greater than 1 mm. Seven of the scaphoid fractures were located at the waist, and one involved the proximal pole of scaphoid. One scaphoid fracture involved a fresh fracture through and distal to a preexisting nonunion. An additional carpal fracture was identified on arthroscopic

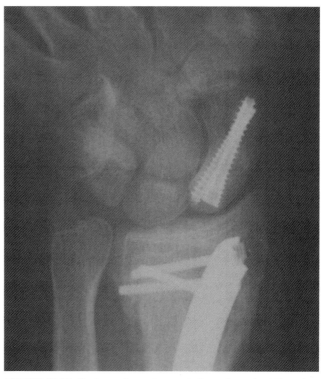

FIGURE 21-19 Postoperative anteroposterior radiograph at 7 weeks.

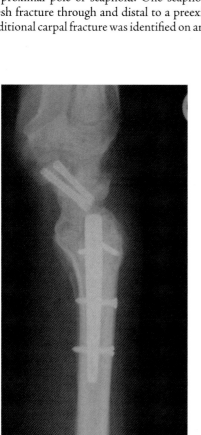

FIGURE 21-18 Postoperative lateral radiograph at 7 weeks.

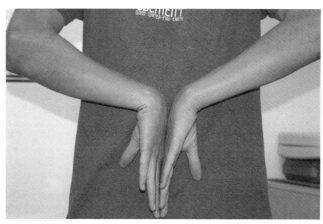

FIGURE 21-20 Wrist flexion at 7 weeks.

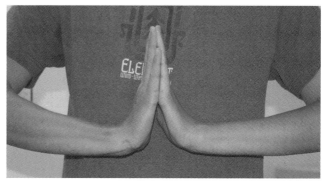

FIGURE 21-21 Wrist extension at 7 weeks.

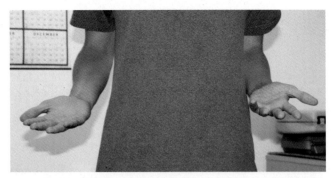

FIGURE 21-22 Supination at 7 weeks.

examination that involved a coronal split of the lunate (and was also percutaneously repaired). The distal radius fractures included two displaced radial styloid fractures and one volar shearing fracture. The remaining distal radius fractures were a "Colles" type fractures with dorsal comminution, and two fractures were intra-articular.

All fractures were operatively treated within 2 weeks of injury. All scaphoid fractures were treated with arthroscopic-assisted reduction and dorsal percutaneous fixation with a standard Acutrak screw, which is a headless cannulated compression screw. All radius fractures were treated with arthroscopic-assisted fracture reduction and rigid fixation. This was accomplished using percutaneous screws and/or open repair, with either a dorsal or volar plate system or a Micronail. No external fixation was used, and allograft was used in all radius fractures requiring bone grafting for structural support.

Average follow-up was 24 months (range: 6 to 42 months). All scaphoid fractures healed and demonstrated complete bridging bone on CT at an average of 14 weeks (range: 7 to 16 weeks). No scaphoid developed avascular necrosis by CT scan. All radius fractures clinically and radiographically healed within 6 weeks. At final follow-up, all radii had maintained height within 2 mm of the opposite normal wrist and at least neutral volar tilt. All intra-articular fractures maintained a congruent surface without displacement or gapping. Radial styloid fractures were treated with a percutaneous headless cannulated compression screw and healed without displacement.

The patients' wrist motion at follow-up averaged 65 degrees of extension, 50 degrees of flexion, 15 degrees of radial deviation, 26 degrees of ulnar deviation, 75 degrees of pronation, and 60 degrees of supination. The grip strength averaged 90 lb for the injured hand and 110 lb in the opposite hand.

There was one complication: a rupture of the extensor pollicis longus tendon, which was the result of a radial styloid and dorsal plate. The plate was removed at the time of tendon rupture, which occurred at 6 months after surgery. The tendon was repaired with a tendon graft/splint, and the patient went on to make a full recovery in manual labor.

Discussion

Simultaneous fractures of the distal radius and ipsilateral scaphoid represent a relatively small subset of upper extremity injuries. The choice of treatment for the distal radius or scaphoid fracture may significantly impact successful healing of the other fracture.

Published reports of these combined injuries are sparse but reflect a change in our treatment protocols over the past decade.

This transformation appears to have paralleled our evolving understanding of scaphoid fractures themselves.

Because of the relative infrequency of this injury combination, the actual incidence is difficult to determine with precision; reports vary from 0.7% to 6.5% of all distal radius fractures.[3] In 1983, Osterman and associates noted that concurrent distal radius fractures and scaphoid fractures constituted 1.9% of all distal radius fractures treated at their institution.[2] This number differs significantly from that of Vukov and colleagues, who reviewed 650 patients with fractures of the distal radius and noted that concomitant scaphoid fractures occurred in 4% of patients.[17] Because of the conflicting reports, Hove and coworkers attempted to specifically address this question. They performed a prospective 3-year study in which they enrolled all distal radius fractures and scaphoid fractures seen at their institution. During that time, they treated 2330 adults with distal radius fractures and 390 adults with scaphoid fractures. They noted only 12 combined injuries—0.05% of all distal radius fractures and 3% of all scaphoid fractures were combined injuries.[1]

Much of the early literature addressing these combined injuries focused on defining the "primary fracture," usually that of the distal radius. Treatment algorithms focused on the primary fracture. Smith and associates expressed concern that traction placed across the wrist in the reduction of the distal radius leads to displacement of the scaphoid.[5] They retrospectively reviewed nine patients with concurrent distal radius and scaphoid fractures and concluded that the reduction maneuvers used for the displaced distal radius fractures had no adverse affect on scaphoid healing. Although they used pins and plaster in their series, they advocated the use of external fixation placed across the wrist.[5]

Proubasta and Lluch presented two patients with displaced intra-articular fractures of the distal radius and nondisplaced scaphoid fractures who were treated by closed reduction and external fixation. They noted dorsal comminution of the distal radius and suggested that placing the wrist in a flexed position would adversely affect healing of the scaphoid. Their solution was to hold the wrist in neutral with an external fixator. They reported that both distal radius and scaphoid fractures healed uneventfully in this fashion.[8]

Tountas and Waddell suggested that treatment is dictated by the radius fracture alone. In their series all scaphoid injuries were typically nondisplaced stable fractures and treatment of radius fracture took precedence.[3] These observations were based on the mistaken belief that standard radiographs could confirm scaphoid healing at 12 weeks.

Richards and colleagues expressed renewed concern about placing traction across a carpus that contained a scaphoid fracture[9] and presented two patients who had combined scaphoid and distal radius fractures. In both cases the scaphoid was treated with Herbert screw internal fixation, prior to placing traction across the wrist, to avoid distraction across the scaphoid fracture.

Trumble and coworkers recognized that the closed treatment of the scaphoid often requires extended periods of immobilization and expressed concern that this would adversely affect the outcome of the distal radial fracture.[6] They also recognized that placing traction across the wrist would create a distraction force across the scaphoid and cautioned that this may decrease union rates. They recommended internal fixation of the scaphoid before reducing or fixing the radius with distractive forces, but forces required to reduce the radius fracture after scaphoid fixation could lead to scaphoid fracture displacement or reduction in compression at the fracture site. Because the most significant forces used in scaphoid fracture fixation appear to be the reduction and alignment of the fracture and the percutaneous screw fixation, it seems logical to divide these maneuvers to address reduction of the distal radius. This ensures rigid fixation of both fractures. These observations are supported by our small clinical series, which permitted the initiation of an immediate rehabilitation program without loss of reduction or motion at either fracture site.

REFERENCES

1. Hove LM: Simultaneous scaphoid and distal radius fractures. J Hand Surg [Br]. 1994; 19:384-387.

2. Osterman AL, Bora FW, Dalinka MK: Simultaneous fractures of the distal radius and scaphoid injuries. Presented before the American Academy of Orthopaedic Surgeons, Anaheim, CA, 1983.

3. Tountas AA, Waddell JP: Simultaneous fractures of the distal radius and scaphoid. J Orthop Trauma. 1987; 1:312-317.

4. Tumilty JA, Squire DS: Unrecognized chondral penetration by a Herbert screw in the scaphoid. J Hand Surg [Am]. 1996; 21:66-68.

5. Smith T, Keeve JP, Bertin KC, Mann RJ: Simultaneous fractures of the distal radius and scaphoid. J Trauma. 1988; 28:676-679.

6. Trumble TE, Schmitt SR, Vedder NB: Factors affecting functional outcome of displaced intra-articular distal radius fractures. J Hand Surg [Am]. 1994; 19:325-340.

7. Trumble TE, Clarke T, Kreder HJ: Non-union of the scaphoid: treatment with cannulated screws compared with treatment with Herbert screws. J Bone Joint Surg Am. 1996; 78:1829-1837.

8. Proubasta IR, Lluch A: Concomitant fractures of the scaphoid and distal radius: treatment by external fixation: a report of two cases. J Bone Joint Surg Am. 1991; 73:938-940.

9. Richards RR, Ghose T, McBroom RJ: Ipsilateral fractures of the distal radius and scaphoid treated by Herbert screw and external skeletal fixation. Clin Orthop. 1992; 282:219-221.

10. Doi K, Hattori Y, Otsuka K, et al: Intra-articular fractures of the distal aspect of the radius: arthroscopically assisted reduction compared with open reduction and internal fixation. J Bone Joint Surg Am. 1999; 81:1093-1110.

11. Geissler WB, Freeland AE: Arthroscopically assisted reduction of intraarticular distal radial fractures. Clin Orthop. 1996; 327:125-134.

12. Geissler WB, Freeland AE: Intercarpal soft-tissue lesions associated with an intra-articular fracture of the distal end of the radius. J Bone Joint Surg Am. 1996; 78:257-265.

13. Slade JF 3rd, Grauer JN, Mahoney JD: Arthroscopic reduction and percutaneous fixation of scaphoid fractures with a novel dorsal technique. Orthop Clin North Am. 2001; 32:247-261.

14. Toby EB, Butler TE, McCormack TJ, et al: A comparison of fixation screws for the scaphoid during application of cyclic bending loads. J Bone Joint Surg Am. 1997; 79:1190-1197.

15. Slade JF 3rd, Gutow AP, Geissler WB: Percutaneous internal fixation of scaphoid fractures via an arthroscopically assisted dorsal approach. J Bone Joint Surg Am. 2002; 84(Suppl 2): 21-36.

16. Slade JF 3rd, Moore AE: Dorsal percutaneous fixation of stable, unstable, and displaced scaphoid fractures and selected non-unions. Atlas of the Hand Clinics: Scaphoid Injuries. 2003; 8:1-18.

17. Vukov V, Ristic K, Stevanovic M, et al: Simultaneous fractures of the distal end of the radius and the scaphoid bone. J Orthop Trauma. 1988; 2:120-123.

Galeazzi Fracture-Dislocations

22

David E. Ruchelsman, MD, Keith B. Raskin, MD, and Michael E. Rettig, MD

Galeazzi fracture-dislocations are defined by fracture of the middle to distal third of the radial diaphysis with simultaneous traumatic disruption of the distal radioulnar joint (DRUJ), resulting in either dorsal or ulnar subluxation/dislocation of the ulnar head from within the sigmoid notch. Although first described by Cooper in 1882,[1,2] this complex forearm fracture-dislocation has been credited to Galeazzi,[3] who in 1934 reported a series of 18 patients with this injury pattern. Mikic[1] proposed that both-bone forearm fractures with concomitant DRUJ dislocation be considered within the spectrum of the classic Galeazzi fracture-dislocation because similar principles of management are applied.

Several early series demonstrated uniformly poor results with nonoperative management, and, as a result, the Galeazzi fracture-dislocation has been referred to as a "fracture of necessity." Hughston[4] reported that nonoperative treatment of the classic Galeazzi lesion resulted in unsatisfactory results in 92% (35 of 38) of patients. Mikic[1] reported an 80% failure rate with conservative management in 86 adults with Galeazzi fracture-dislocations due to both inability to control progressive displacement of the radius fracture as well as recurrent subluxation or dislocation of the DRUJ despite cast immobilization. Mikic postulated that rupture of the triangular fibrocartilage complex (TFCC) was the primary cause of redislocations and the poor results observed. Other early series reported similar disappointing results with closed reduction and immobilization.[2,5]

With advances in surgical techniques to achieve osteosynthesis and soft tissue reconstruction, open reduction and internal fixation (ORIF) has become the standard of care to optimize outcomes after forearm fractures associated with DRUJ disruption. Operative management has yielded satisfactory results in more than 80% of adult patients with these injuries.[6-9]

Regional Anatomy and Biomechanics

Stability of the forearm, and specifically the DRUJ, is dependent on the presence of dynamic (musculotendinous) and passive (ligamentous) soft tissue stabilizers and, to a lesser extent, osseous anatomy. Bony congruity between the ulnar head and sigmoid notch of the radius contributes only approximately 20% of total DRUJ stability. In the transverse plane, the sigmoid notch is shallow relative to the ulna seat and the radii of their articular seats are disparate; thus, appositional contact is small.[10,11] As a result, motion at the DRUJ is predominantly translational—a combination of sliding and rotation. However, its axis of motion remains adjacent to the center of the ulnar head.

Tolat and associates[11] analyzed the osseous characteristics of the sigmoid notch and ulnar head in 50 cadaveric specimens in the coronal and transverse planes with multiple articular surface-based measurements. Three midcoronal DRUJ articular types

(types I to III) were confirmed: type I DRUJ (55%)—apposing joint surfaces are parallel to the long axis of the radius and ulna; type II DRUJ (33%)—oblique apposing surfaces at the sigmoid and ulnar articular seats; and type III DRUJ (12%)—"reverse oblique" joint orientation with the DRUJ angular apex formed proximal to the DRUJ. In addition, four axial plane anatomical variants of the sigmoid notch were also noted and included flat face (42%), ski slope (14%), C-type (30%), and S-type (14%) notches. Furthermore, an extra-articular palmar osteocartilaginous lip was found in 80% of specimens and was found to serve as a consistent point of attachment for the volar radioulnar ligament and volar DRUJ capsule. When the TFCC is sectioned in the laboratory or incompetent in the clinical setting, this palmar lip serves as a buttress to palmar dislocation of the ulnar head and, thus, acts as a supplemental stabilizer to the interosseous membrane (IOM). This buttress effect is lost when there is a longitudinal tear in the interosseous membrane or fracture of the palmar rim (i.e., sigmoid notch fracture).

The soft tissue anatomy about the DRUJ is well defined,[12] and its stabilizers include the pronator quadratus, ulnocarpal ligaments, extensor carpi ulnaris subsheath, dorsal and volar radioulnar ligaments, IOM, and DRUJ capsule. The TFCC is considered the primary stabilizer of the DRUJ, and the IOM is a secondary restraint. The ulnar styloid projects 2 to 6 mm and is the site of attachment for the superficial (distal) limbs of the radioulnar ligaments and the extensor carpi ulnaris subsheath. The deep (proximal) fibers of the distal radioulnar ligaments and the ulnocapitate ligament insert into the fovea at the styloid base. Gofton and colleagues[13] found that the radioulnar ligaments and the triangular fibrocartilage maintain DRUJ kinematics with simulated active forearm motion when more proximal soft tissue stabilizers (i.e., pronator quadratus, IOM, extensor carpi ulnaris subsheath, ulnar collateral ligament) are sacrificed. Furthermore, the radioulnar ligaments may play a greater stabilizing role in DRUJ stability in patients with flat sigmoid notches.[11]

The IOM has multiple biomechanical functions: it helps to transmit force from the radius to the ulna, acts to prevent excessive supination, serves as an aponeurosis for insertions of the deep flexors and extensors, and resists radius and ulna diastasis. The complexity of the IOM structure has been studied by several groups.[14-16] In a cadaveric study, Hotchkiss and associates[14] defined a central band of ligamentous tissue that contributed 71% of the longitudinal stiffness of the IOM after radial head excision. Injury to this region may represent the pathoanatomy responsible for proximal migration of the radius after radial head excision. Skahen and coworkers[16] found that the IOM was consistently organized into a central band, one to five accessory bands, a dorsal proximal interosseous band, and membranous portions. Fibers from the central band originate from the radius and run in a distal-ulnar direction at a 20-degree angle to the long axis of the ulna. Peak strain occurs in the central band during pronation, the assumed position of the forearm when a Galeazzi fracture-dislocation is sustained. Other authors[17,18] have demonstrated that the IOM also serves as a coronal (transverse) and sagittal (dorsal-volar) plane stabilizer of the DRUJ, in addition to its described role as a longitudinal restraint. Analyses by Watanabe and colleagues[18] suggest that it is a specific injury to the distal portion of the IOM (distal to the central band) that confers increased dorsal-volar instability at the DRUJ throughout a range of forearm rotation when the TFCC and distal radioulnar ligaments are incompetent; when the midportion of the IOM (including the central band) is sectioned together with the distal IOM, the DRUJ becomes unconstrained. Similarly, in a cadaveric biomechanical model, Gofton and coworkers[13] demonstrated that the IOM was essential in the maintenance of DRUJ kinematics when distal soft tissue stabilizers are sacrificed (i.e., radioulnar ligaments and triangular fibrocartilage).

True Galeazzi fracture-dislocations have not been reproduced in an ex vivo biomechanical model.[19-21] As a result, although these injuries are assumed to occur in definable stages, the failure sequence of the regional soft tissue restraints after fracture of the radius has not been elucidated. However, the contributions of the TFCC and IOM to the biomechanics of the Galeazzi fracture-dislocation have been studied. Moore and associates,[20] in a cadaveric model, produced artificial Galeazzi fractures composed of transverse, uncomminuted radial metadiaphyseal fractures created with a Gigli saw at the distal insertion of the pronator teres followed by sequential sectioning of the TFCC and IOM. Moore and associates[20] and Schneiderman and coworkers[15] independently demonstrated that radial shortening greater than 10 mm required complete disruption of both the TFCC as well as the

IOM. Intermediate shortening occurred with isolated sectioning of the TFCC or IOM, respectively. The dorsal carpal retinaculum and ulnar collateral ligaments of the wrist were not found to be significant soft tissue constraints.

Classification

Galeazzi fracture-dislocations are relatively rare injuries, constituting 3% to 7%[22] of all forearm fractures. In a retrospective review, Ring and colleagues[23] reported that the incidence of isolated radial diaphyseal fractures without DRUJ involvement is greater than that of the true Galeazzi fracture-dislocations. Of the 36 radial shaft fractures, only 9 (25%) occurred in conjunction with DRUJ disruption, whereas 27 (75%) radial diaphyseal fractures occurred in isolation and had no evidence of DRUJ dysfunction at latest follow-up. If both-bone forearm fractures with DRUJ dislocation are included, the incidence is higher. In Mikic's series of 125 patients with Galeazzi fracture-dislocations,[1] 20% of cases included fractures of both the radius and ulna.

Dameron[24] originally subdivided Galeazzi fracture-dislocations into the ulna-volar type (ulna volar to the radiocarpal complex) and the ulna-dorsal type (ulna dorsal to the radiocarpal complex). In a retrospective review of 40 operatively treated Galeazzi fracture-dislocations, Rettig and Raskin[8] introduced a classification scheme for these injuries with prognostic value with regard to the probability of intraoperative DRUJ instability after ORIF of the radial shaft fracture. Two patterns of fracture-dislocation were identified based on the distance of the radial shaft fracture from the midarticular surface of the distal radius. In 12 of 22 (55%) type I fractures, occurring within the distal third of the radial shaft and within 7.5 cm of the midarticular surface (**Fig. 22-1**), operative stabilization of the DRUJ was required with percutaneous Kirschner wire (K-wire) fixation secondary to persis-

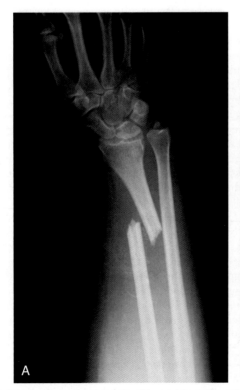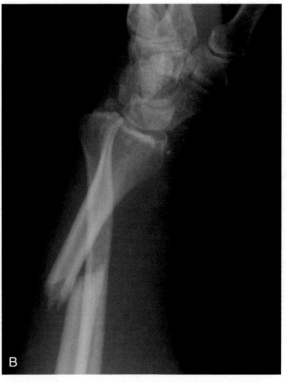

FIGURE 22-1 Preoperative posteroanterior (**A**) and lateral (**B**) radiographs reveal a fracture of the radial shaft within 7.5 cm of the midarticular surface of the distal radius—type I injury. DRUJ disruption as well as ulnar styloid fracture is appreciated.

tent DRUJ instability after ORIF of the radial shaft fracture. Three of these 12 patients underwent concomitant open repair of the TFCC because the DRUJ was found to be irreducible. In contrast, only 1 of 18 (6%) patients with a type II injury, within the middle third of the radial shaft and more than 7.5 cm from the

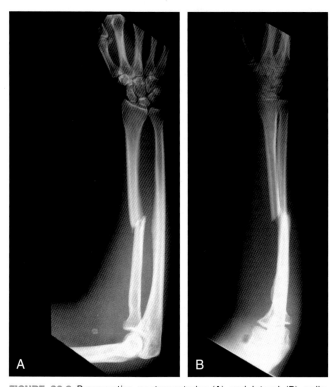

FIGURE 22-2 Preoperative posteroanterior (**A**) and lateral (**B**) radiographs demonstrating a short oblique fracture of the radial shaft more than 7.5 cm from the midarticular surface of the distal radius—type II injury.

midarticular surface of the distal radius (**Fig. 22-2**), required percutaneous fixation of an unstable DRUJ ($P < .001$).

The mechanism of injury includes a high-velocity direct impact with axial loading of an outstretched arm. Axial loading of the forearm combined with hyperpronation of the forearm is the most common mechanism and causes dorsal dislocation of the DRUJ[1]; conversely, hypersupination leads to volar dislocation of the ulnar head from the sigmoid notch. We have postulated that for distal radial shaft fractures (type I injuries) within 7.5 cm of the midarticular surface, a high-impact hyperextension mechanism results in a direct continuum of complete injuries through the TFCC and IOM, which predisposes the DRUJ to residual instability and dorsal subluxation despite anatomical radial shaft fracture fixation[8] (**Fig. 22-3A**). With fractures through the middle third of the radial shaft (type II injuries) an indirect pronation force is incurred with incomplete disruption to the regional stabilizing soft tissue structures (see **Fig. 22-3B**). This may account for the high likelihood of DRUJ and ulnar head stability within the sigmoid notch after fixation of more proximally located radial shaft fractures. However, a significant relationship between the magnitude of initial radial shortening and DRUJ stability was not identified. In a retrospective review of 36 patients with radial shaft fractures treated with plate and screw fixation, Ring and coworkers[23] observed a similar trend toward DRUJ stability with proximal and middle third fractures in accord with our findings. In this series, 5 of 8 distal third fractures were associated with DRUJ instability, whereas only 4 of 28 proximal/middle third radius fractures had DRUJ involvement.

Indications and Contraindications

ORIF of radial shaft fractures in the skeletally mature patient is indicated. The DRUJ is treated based on the clinical and radiographic examination after fixation of the radial shaft fracture. Nonoperative management of acute closed Galeazzi fracture-dislocations, in general, results in an unacceptable clinical result.

FIGURE 22-3 **A,** Posteroanterior radiograph demonstrating a type I fracture in the distal third of the radial shaft within 7.5 cm of the midarticular surface of the distal radius resulting from a high-impact hyperextension injury. **B,** Posteroanterior radiograph demonstrating a type II fracture in the middle third of the radial shaft more than 7.5 cm from the midarticular surface of the distal radius resulting from an indirect pronation force. Arrows represent an axial load force in *A* and a hyperpronation force in *B*.

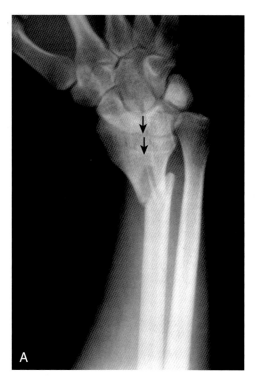

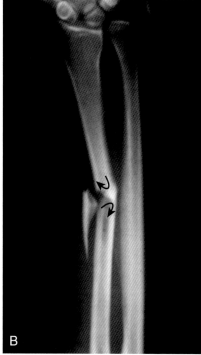

The timing of surgery is dependent on the soft tissue status and clinical condition of the patient. Contraindications to early ORIF include severe, high-grade open fractures with soft tissue loss and gross contamination. Jones[25] reported good or excellent results in 66% (12/18) of patients with grade III open forearm fractures treated with a protocol of immediate extensive primary débridement, open reduction and dynamic compression plate fixation, and serial re-débridements at 24- to 48-hour intervals until wound status allowed for soft tissue reconstruction. Duncan and coworkers[26] found statistically significant differences in the rate of satisfactory outcomes between grade I, II, and IIIA open forearm fractures and those seen in grade IIIB and IIIC injuries when immediate (<24 hours) ORIF was performed. Patients with grade IIIB and IIIC open forearm fractures may be managed with initial external fixation, serial débridements, and meticulous wound care, followed by delayed internal fixation. Bone grafting should be planned for open fractures with extensive comminution and/or segmental defects at a minimum of 6 weeks from the time a closed soft tissue envelope is obtained. Multisystem trauma or multiple medical comorbidities are clinical scenarios in which early ORIF may also be contraindicated.

Initial Evaluation and Management

Physical examination demonstrates forearm deformity. Prominence of the ulnar head may be present, especially with dorsal DRUJ dislocation, and significant skin tenting may be present. Deforming forces of the radial shaft fracture include the pronator quadratus insertion on the volar surface of the distal fragment, the brachioradialis, and the extrinsic thumb abductor and extensors.[4] A thorough neurovascular examination of the upper extremity should be performed and the status of the forearm compartments should be documented. Circumferential inspection of the skin is also performed to identify an open injury. Given the magnitude of energy required to produce this injury, a thorough secondary survey should be performed to rule out any additional musculoskeletal injuries. Prerequisite radiographs include those of the ipsilateral elbow, forearm, and wrist. Radiographic markers of DRUJ disruption are assessed and include fracture through the fovea of the ulnar styloid, DRUJ widening on the anteroposterior view, more than 5 mm of radial shortening, and dorsal subluxation/dislocation of the DRUJ on a true lateral view of the wrist. The importance of radiographic imaging of the ipsilateral elbow and wrist is highlighted by numerous reports of the presence of coincident ipsilateral upper extremity trauma.[9,23,27-32] In a series by Ring and coworkers,[23] 10 of 36 radial diaphyseal fractures were sustained together with ipsilateral upper extremity trauma, including diaphyseal humerus fracture (2), proximal humerus fracture (1), elbow dislocation (1), and scaphoid fracture (1). Strehle and Gerber[9] identified additional upper extremity fractures in 21% of their cases. Contralateral wrist radiographs may be obtained if radiographs are equivocal on the injured side. Although advanced imaging modalities are available,[33-35] they are rarely obtained preoperatively for true Galeazzi fracture-dislocations. Fester and colleagues[36] have recommended the use of both ultrasonography and magnetic resonance imaging when there is clinical suspicion of injury to the IOM because both modalities have impressive testing characteristics (sensitivity, specificity, and positive and negative predictive values).

In the emergency department and with appropriate pain control or sedation, restoration of gross alignment and radial length may be attempted utilizing digital traction applied through finger traps. A well-padded long-arm plaster splint is applied, and the forearm is splinted in supination if the DRUJ is clinically reducible. The patient may require admission for observation and serial neurovascular checks if there is concern for compartment swelling.

Surgical Technique

The patient is positioned supine on the operating room table. The involved upper extremity is positioned in supination on a standard armboard. A nonsterile tourniquet is applied to the upper arm area. After adequate anesthetic has been achieved (usually with regional anesthesia), the entire upper extremity is prepped and draped in a standard manner. Consideration should be given to preparing the ipsilateral iliac crest for harvesting of autogenous bone graft if preoperative radiographs reveal comminution at the radial shaft fracture site. The contralateral DRUJ should be examined preoperatively for intraoperative comparison to the injured wrist.

A volar (Henry) approach to the radial shaft is performed utilizing the flexor carpi radialis/radial artery interval. After retraction of the flexor carpi radialis tendon, the subtendinous space of Parona is developed to expose the pronator quadratus. Traumatic disruption of the pronator quadratus sustained with the injury may be appreciated. The distal extent of the exposure—the radiocarpal joint—is marked by the origin of the extrinsic volar wrist ligaments and fully identified after elevation of the pronator quadratus from the metaphysis of the radius. The pronator quadratus is progressively subperiosteally elevated in a distal-to-proximal as well as radial-to-ulnar fashion. Exposure of the sigmoid notch is possible with this approach and may be helpful if a concomitant comminuted ulnar head fracture is present. The proximal limit of the exposure is dictated by the location of the radial shaft fracture. More proximal exposure of the radial shaft fracture may require release of the flexor pollicis longus origin and pronator teres insertion.

Alternatively, a dorsal (Thompson) approach to the proximal radius may be performed for type II fractures. The interval between the extensor carpi radialis brevis and extensor digitorum communis is developed. The posterior interosseous nerve is then identified and protected as it emerges from the supinator, which is then elevated in a subperiosteal fashion toward its origin. If distal exposure is needed, the abductor pollicis longus and extensor pollicis brevis are reflected subperiosteally. After fracture reduction, dorsal plate fixation is performed.

The fracture site is identified and the extent of comminution is evaluated. Fracture site débridement is performed. Manual reduction of the radial shaft fracture is performed, and provisional reduction is maintained with bone reduction clamps. A 3.5-mm AO dynamic compression plate or low-contact dynamic compression plate may be applied to the volar surface and temporarily held with bone reduction clamps. Locked plating techniques may be utilized if there is significant comminution and/or osteoporosis. If the radial shaft fracture is located at the metadiaphyseal junction or within the distal radius metaphysis, consideration may be given to the use of a long volar fixed-angle plate and screw construct. Plate length, anatomical reduction, and restoration of radial length and bow are each evaluated and confirmed with intraoperative fluoroscopy. The chosen implant is then secured to the radial shaft with fully threaded cortical screws and the bone reduction clamps are then removed. Certain fracture patterns may be amendable to supplemental small or mini-fragment cortical lag screws to achieve interfragmentary compression (i.e., butterfly fragments) (**Fig. 22-4**).

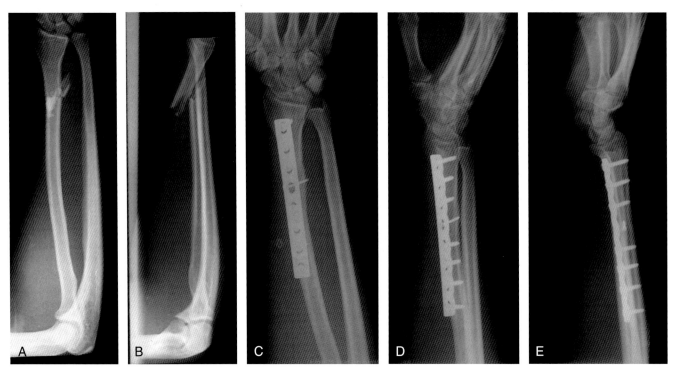

FIGURE 22-4 Preoperative posteroanterior (**A**) and lateral (**B**) forearm radiographs are consistent with a type I Galeazzi fracture-dislocation. Postoperative posteroanterior (**C**), oblique (**D**), and lateral (**E**) radiographs demonstrate anatomical reduction after volar plate fixation of the radius fracture. Lag screw fixation of the butterfly fragment was performed outside the plate construct.

The location and extent of comminution and cortical bone loss are noted on fluoroscopy. Release of the radial septum from the dorsoradial aspect of the radial shaft affords access for bone grafting of the fracture site, often eliminating the need to perform a separate dorsal incision. Cortical fragments devoid of soft tissue attachments should be removed because they represent a potential nidus for infection. Options for bone graft are multiple and include autogenous iliac crest and the ipsilateral distal radius, as well as a host of osteoconductive and/or osteoinductive commercially available products.

After anatomical reduction and fixation of the radial shaft fracture, the DRUJ is evaluated clinically with the forearm in supination for both stability and reducibility. Because it is possible to force the DRUJ into a reduced position despite soft tissue or bone interposition, accurate lateral radiographs without undue force are evaluated. Dorsally directed manual stress is applied to the DRUJ in an attempt to dorsally translate the ulnar head out from the sigmoid notch. If the DRUJ is stable to stress, an above-elbow splint is applied with the forearm in supination (**Fig. 22-5**). In Galeazzi fracture-dislocations without associated fracture of the ulna styloid, the triangular ligament is disrupted. Cast immobilization in supination allows for reapproximation and healing of the triangular ligament at the site of avulsion to ensure long-term DRUJ stability.

If the ulnar head is unstable but reducible within the sigmoid notch in supination and there is no associated basilar ulnar styloid avulsion fracture fragment, then percutaneous transfixion of the DRUJ is performed. With the forearm in supination and the ulnar head held reduced within the sigmoid notch, two 0.062-inch (1.6 mm) K-wires are percutaneously placed from the ulna through the radius transversely approximately 1 cm proximal to the sigmoid notch to stabilize the DRUJ in supination (**Fig. 22-**

6). The surgeon should be suspicious for and predict residual DRUJ instability after ORIF of the radial shaft fracture in type I injury patterns.[8]

Open reduction of the DRUJ may be necessary if the ulnar head remains unstable and irreducible after reduction and internal fixation of the radial shaft fracture. Soft tissue interposition usually prevents anatomical reduction of the ulnar head into the sigmoid notch. Several regional soft tissue structures have been implicated as blocks to DRUJ reduction in Galeazzi fracture-dislocations. Interposition of the extensor retinaculum, DRUJ capsule, extensor carpi ulnaris, extensor digitorum communis to the ring and little fingers, and the extensor digiti minimi have been separately reported[37-43] as causes of an irreducible DRUJ in these complex injuries.

For open reduction of the DRUJ, a dorsal approach to the distal ulna between the fifth and sixth extensor compartments is utilized. The dorsal sensory branch of the ulnar nerve is protected. The extensor retinaculum is elevated from the dorsal DRUJ capsule. A dorsal DRUJ capsulotomy is then completed. However, a traumatic capsulotomy may be present and the ulna head may be buttonholed through the dorsal capsule with dorsal DRUJ dislocations. The DRUJ is inspected for loose bodies and traumatic chondromalacia and then débrided. The TFCC is evaluated. In all three cases of type I injuries requiring open reduction of the DRUJ in our series,[8] the triangular fibrocartilage was observed avulsed from its insertion into the base of the ulnar styloid (Palmer class 1B)[44] and interposed within the DRUJ. In these cases, the insertion site was prepared for reattachment through drill holes (one patient) or bone suture-anchors (two patients).

Ulnar styloid repair may supplement soft tissue repair/reconstruction and is indicated if a displaced, large ulnar styloid

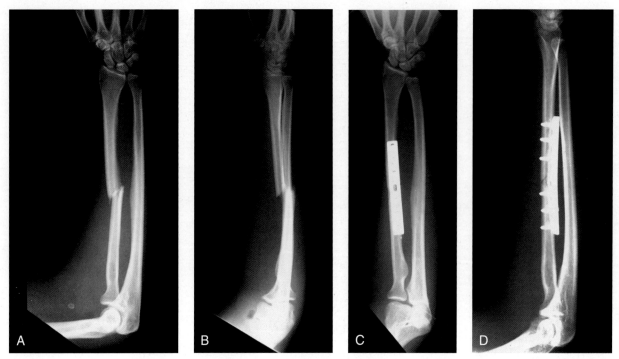

FIGURE 22-5 Preoperative posteroanterior (**A**) and lateral (**B**) forearm radiographs demonstrating a type II Galeazzi fracture-dislocation. A cortical butterfly fragment is seen. **C** and **D**, Postoperative radiographs demonstrate restoration of radial bow and length. ORIF was performed through a dorsal approach. Supplemental DRUJ fixation was not required.

fracture through its base is present. With a displaced ulnar styloid fracture through the fovea, the DRUJ can be unstable as the TFCC is attached to this fragment. Ulnar styloid fractures can be repaired with a 24- or 26-gauge stainless steel figure-of-eight tension band construct or K-wires. Of the nine Galeazzi fracture-dislocations presented by Ring and coworkers,[23] four were associated with displaced fractures through the base of the ulna styloid and underwent ORIF of the ulna styloid. Kikuchi and Nakamura[45] reported a case of a Galeazzi fracture-dislocation with an irreducible DRUJ secondary to entrapment of an avulsion fracture of the ulna fovea with its preserved attachments to the dorsal portion of the triangular ligament. After reattachment of the foveal fragment to its donor site and K-wire fixation of the ulnar styloid, DRUJ stability was achieved.

Salvage procedures for severe distal ulna fractures sustained with a Galeazzi injury include the Darrach procedure with subperiosteal distal ulnar head excision just proximal to the sigmoid notch with extensor carpi ulnaris tenodesis, the Bowers hemi-resection-interpositional arthroplasty, or some modification of these techniques. In the acute setting, selection of a salvage procedure is dependent on patient-specific characteristics.

Before wound closure, final orthogonal fluoroscopic images are obtained to confirm anatomical reduction of the radial shaft, distal ulna, and DRUJ. The pronator quadratus is positioned over the volar plate and may be reattached along its distal and radial border if it has been elevated as a continuous sleeve and the bony trauma has not disrupted it too extensively. The subcutaneous and skin layers are closed. If a dorsal approach to the distal ulna and DRUJ was utilized, the dorsal capsule is imbricated and the extensor retinaculum repaired. A sterile dressing is applied. A well-padded plaster long-arm splint in supination is applied.

At the initial postoperative office visit, the long-arm plaster splint is changed to an above-elbow cast with the forearm in

supination for 6 weeks. The transverse K-wires are removed at 6 weeks. At this time, progressive physical therapy is initiated.

Complications

Complications after operative treatment of Galeazzi fracture-dislocations are not uncommon, and several authors have reported a complication rate of 32% to 39%.[9,22] Complications include nonunion, malunion, infection, refracture after hardware removal, and persistent DRUJ pain and instability.

Symptomatic post-traumatic DRUJ instability may be due to ligamentous incompetence, bony deformity, or both. Clinical manifestations include pain and limited forearm rotation. The efficacy of conservative management of DRUJ instability with functional bracing is unclear, but bracing has been shown to reduce translational motion at the DRUJ experimentally in a cadaveric study.[46] The role of arthroscopic TFCC repair in the setting of chronic DRUJ instability is evolving. In the absence of DRUJ arthritis and significant incongruity, various ligamentous reconstructive procedures of the DRUJ may be considered when the TFCC is irreparable. Ulnar shortening may be considered for symptomatic ulnocarpal impaction and early DRUJ arthritis. Several salvage procedures are available, including the Darrach resection in the low-demand patient, the Sauvé-Kapandji procedure, hemi-resection arthroplasty, and implant arthroplasty. Procedure selection is dependent on individual patient characteristics, radiographic findings, and surgeon preference.

Results of Treatment

With advances in techniques for achieving rigid osteosynthesis and soft tissue reconstruction, ORIF has become the standard of care to optimize outcomes after forearm fractures associated with DRUJ disruption. Although the literature is limited to a relatively small number of retrospective reviews with modest cohort sizes,

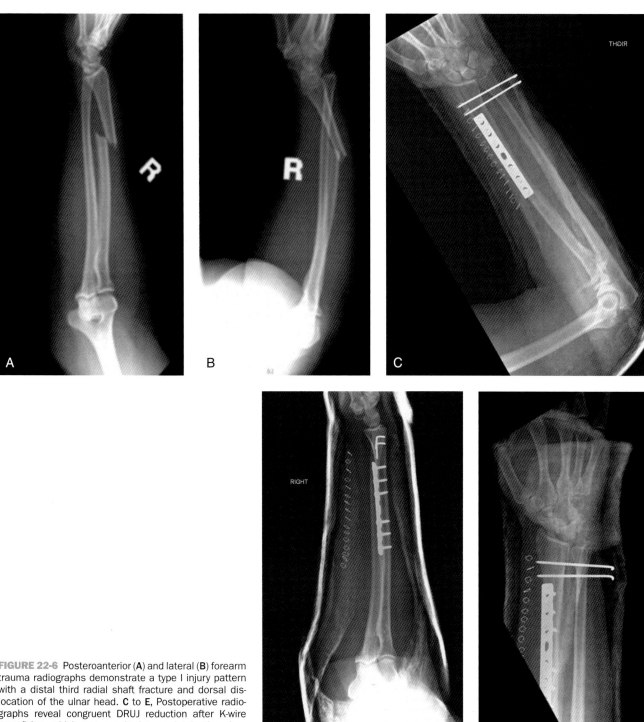

FIGURE 22-6 Posteroanterior (**A**) and lateral (**B**) forearm trauma radiographs demonstrate a type I injury pattern with a distal third radial shaft fracture and dorsal dislocation of the ulnar head. **C** to **E**, Postoperative radiographs reveal congruent DRUJ reduction after K-wire transfixion, which was required to maintain the ulnar head reduced within the sigmoid notch after radial shaft fracture fixation.

the data strongly indicate that operative management[6-9] yields results superior to those after closed treatment.[1,2,4,5]

We have previously reported excellent clinical results according to Mikic's criteria[1] in 38 of 40 patients with acute closed Galeazzi fracture-dislocations who were treated with a uniform surgical algorithm.[8] Only 2 patients had a poor result, and both had sustained a type I fracture-dislocation. Both subsequently required DRUJ reconstruction at an average of 9 months after the initial injury because of pain and limited supination. At 1-year follow-up, Mohan and associates[7] obtained good results in 80% (40/50) of cases treated with ORIF. Two patients subsequently underwent excision of the ulnar head secondary to limited supination and pronation. When anatomical alignment of the radius is achieved and congruent reduction of the DRUJ is maintained, full DRUJ function can be expected.[9] Kraus and Horne[47] reported a satisfactory outcome according to Hughston's criteria in 25 of 27 (93%) patients at 32 months postoperatively.

Conclusion

Galeazzi fracture-dislocations represent high-energy injuries involving the distal radial meta-diaphyseal region and the soft tissue stabilizers of the DRUJ, the TFCC, and the IOM. A high index of suspicion must be maintained for DRUJ disruption, especially with more distally located radial shaft fractures. Anatomical reduction and fixation of the radius does not reliably ensure stability of the DRUJ in every case. After fixation of the radial shaft fracture, DRUJ stability must be evaluated clinically and radiographically. Type I injuries represent a more severe soft tissue injury pattern to the regional stabilizers, which predisposes the DRUJ to residual instability and subluxation despite anatomical radial shaft fracture fixation. In contrast, DRUJ stability is more commonly found after fracture fixation of type II injuries. This may be due to incomplete soft tissue disruption and/or force transmission along the more substantial midportion of the IOM. Although percutaneous transfixion of the DRUJ is often possible, a low threshold for open reduction of the DRUJ and soft tissue or styloid repair should be maintained when an anatomical reduction is unobtainable with closed techniques. Anatomical fixation of the radial shaft fracture, thorough intraoperative assessment of DRUJ stability, and maintenance of a congruent reduction of the ulnar head within the sigmoid notch optimize the probability of uncomplicated fracture union and excellent functional results. Painful persistent, chronic DRUJ instability is a challenging clinical problem and may require a salvage procedure of the distal ulna.

REFERENCES

1. Mikic ZD: Galeazzi fracture-dislocations. J Bone Joint Surg Am. 1975; 57:1071-1080.
2. Reckling FW, Cordell LD: Unstable fracture-dislocations of the forearm: the Monteggia and Galeazzi lesions. Arch Surg. 1968; 96:999-1007.
3. Galeazzi R: Di una particolae sindrome traumatica dello scheletro dell'avambraccio. Atti Mem Soc Lomb Chir. 1934; 2:12.
4. Hughston JC: Fracture of the distal radial shaft; mistakes in management. J Bone Joint Surg Am. 1957; 39:249-264.
5. Wong PC: Galeazzi fracture-dislocations in Singapore 1960-1964: incidence and results of treatment. Singapore Med J. 1967; 8:186-193.
6. Macule Beneyto F, Arandes Renu JM, Ferreres Claramunt A, Ramon Soler R: Treatment of Galeazzi fracture-dislocations. J Trauma. 1994; 36:352-355.
7. Mohan K, Gupta AK, Sharma J, et al: Internal fixation in 50 cases of Galeazzi fracture. Acta Orthop Scand. 1988; 59:318-320.
8. Rettig ME, Raskin KB: Galeazzi fracture-dislocation: a new treatment-oriented classification. J Hand Surg [Am]. 2001; 26:228-235.
9. Strehle J, Gerber C: Distal radioulnar joint function after Galeazzi fracture-dislocations treated by open reduction and internal plate fixation. Clin Orthop Relat Res. 1993; 293:240-245.
10. Ekenstam F, Hagert CG: Anatomical studies on the geometry and stability of the distal radioulnar joint. Scand J Plast Reconstr Surg. 1985; 19:17-25.
11. Tolat AR, Stanley JK, Trail IA: A cadaveric study of the anatomy and stability of the distal radioulnar joint in the coronal and transverse planes. J Hand Surg [Br]. 1996; 21:587-594.
12. Palmer AK, Werner FW: The triangular fibrocartilage complex of the wrist—anatomy and function. J Hand Surg [Am]. 1981; 6:153-162.
13. Gofton WT, Gordon KD, Dunning CE, et al: Soft-tissue stabilizers of the distal radioulnar joint: an in vitro kinematic study. J Hand Surg [Am]. 2004; 29:423-431.
14. Hotchkiss RN, An KN, Sowa DT, et al: An anatomic and mechanical study of the interosseous membrane of the forearm: pathomechanics of proximal migration of the radius. J Hand Surg [Am]. 1989; 14:256-261.
15. Schneiderman G, Meldrum RD, Bloebaum RD, et al: The interosseous membrane of the forearm: structure and its role in Galeazzi fractures. J Trauma. 1993; 35:879-885.
16. Skahen JR 3rd, Palmer AK, Werner FW, Fortino MD: The interosseous membrane of the forearm: anatomy and function. J Hand Surg [Am]. 1997; 22:981-985.
17. Pfaeffle HJ, Fischer KJ, Manson TT, et al: Role of the forearm interosseous ligament: is it more than just longitudinal load transfer? J Hand Surg [Am]. 2000; 25:683-688.
18. Watanabe H, Berger RA, Berglund LJ, et al: Contribution of the interosseous membrane to distal radioulnar joint constraint. J Hand Surg [Am]. 2005; 30:1164-1171.
19. McGinley JC, Hopgood BC, Gaughan JP, et al: Forearm and elbow injury: the influence of rotational position. J Bone Joint Surg Am. 2003; 85:2403-2409.
20. Moore TM, Lester DK, Sarmiento A: The stabilizing effect of soft-tissue constraints in artificial Galeazzi fractures. Clin Orthop Relat Res. 1985; 194:189-194.
21. Snook GA, Chrisman OD, Wilson TC, Wietsma RD: Subluxation of the distal radioulnar joint by hyperpronation. J Bone Joint Surg Am. 1969; 51:1315.
22. Moore TM, Klein JP, Patzakis MJ, Harvey JP Jr: Results of compression-plating of closed Galeazzi fractures. J Bone Joint Surg Am. 1985; 67:1015-1021.
23. Ring D, Rhim R, Carpenter C, Jupiter JB: Isolated radial shaft fractures are more common than Galeazzi fractures. J Hand Surg [Am]. 2006; 31:17-21.

24. Dameron TBJ: Traumatic dislocation of the distal radioulnar joint. Clin Orthop Relat Res. 1972; 83:55-63.

25. Jones JA: Immediate internal fixation of high-energy open forearm fractures. J Orthop Trauma. 1991; 5:272-279.

26. Duncan R, Geissler W, Freeland AE, Savoie FH: Immediate internal fixation of open fractures of the diaphysis of the forearm. J Orthop Trauma. 1992; 6:25-31.

27. Clare DJ, Corley FG, Wirth MA: Ipsilateral combination Monteggia and Galeazzi injuries in an adult patient: a case report. J Orthop Trauma. 2002; 16:130-134.

28. Jones TR, Bond CD, Shin AY: Open Galeazzi fracture with concomitant radial head dislocation. Am J Orthop. 2001; 30:417-420.

29. Khurana JS, Kattapuran SV, Becker S, Mayo-Smith W: Galeazzi injury with an associated fracture of the radial head. Clin Orthop Relat Res. 1988; 234:70-71.

30. Sarup S, Bryant PA: Ipsilateral humeral shaft and Galeazzi fractures with a posterolateral dislocation of the elbow: a variant of the "floating dislocated elbow." J Trauma. 1997; 43:349-352.

31. Shiboi R, Kobayashi M, Wantanabe Y, Matsushita T: Elbow dislocation combined with ipsilateral Galeazzi fracture. J Orthop Sci. 2005; 10:540-542.

32. Stahl S, Freiman S: Simultaneous scaphoid and Galeazzi fractures. Hand Surg. 1999; 4:185-188.

33. Failla JM, Jacobson J, van Holsbeeck M: Ultrasound diagnosis and surgical pathology of the torn interosseous membrane in forearm fractures/dislocations. J Hand Surg [Am]. 1999; 24:257-266.

34. Matsuoka J, Beppu M, Nakajima H, Aoki H: Ultrasonography for the interosseous membrane of the forearm. Hand Surg. 2003; 8:227-235.

35. McGinley JC, Roach N, Hopgood BC, et al: Forearm interosseous membrane trauma: MRI diagnostic criteria and injury patterns. Skeletal Radiol. 2006; 35:275-281.

36. Fester EW, Murray PM, Sanders TG, et al: The efficacy of magnetic resonance imaging and ultrasound in detecting disruptions of the forearm interosseous membrane: a cadaver study. J Hand Surg [Am]. 2002; 27:418-424.

37. Alexander AH, Lichtman DM: Irreducible distal radioulnar joint occurring in a Galeazzi fracture-case report. J Hand Surg. 1981; 6:258-261.

38. Biyani A, Bhan S: Dual extensor tendon entrapment in Galeazzi fracture-dislocation: a case report. J Trauma. 1989; 29:1295-1297.

39. Borens O, Chebab EL, Roberts MM, Helfet DL: Bilateral Galeazzi fracture-dislocations. Am J Orthop. 2006; 35:369-372.

40. Cetti NE: An unusual cause of blocked reduction of the Galeazzi injury. Injury. 1977; 9:59-61.

41. Hanel DP, Scheid DK: Irreducible fracture-dislocation of the distal radioulnar joint secondary to entrapment of the extensor carpi ulnaris tendon. Clin Orthop Relat Res. 1988; 234:56-60.

42. Itoh Y, Horiuchi Y, Takahashi M, et al: Extensor tendon involvement in Smith's and Galeazzi fractures. J Hand Surg [Am]. 1987; 12:535-540.

43. Jenkins NH, Mintowt-Czyz WJ, Fairclough JA: Irreducible dislocation of the distal radioulnar joint. Injury. 1987; 18:40-43.

44. Palmer AK: Triangular fibrocartilage complex lesions: a classification. J Hand Surg [Am]. 1989; 14:594-606.

45. Kikuchi Y, Nakamura T: Irreducible Galeazzi fracture-dislocation due to an avulsion fracture of the fovea of the ulna. J Hand Surg [Br]. 1999; 24:379-381.

46. Millard GM, Budoff JE, Paravic V, Noble PC: Functional bracing for distal radioulnar joint instability. J Hand Surg [Am]. 2002; 27:972-977.

47. Kraus B, Horne G: Galeazzi fractures. J Trauma. 1985; 25:1093-1095.

Use of Bone Graft Substitutes and Bioactive Materials in Treatment of Distal Radius Fractures

23

Brian J. Hartigan, MD and Richard L. Makowiec, MD

The goals of treating distal radius fractures include anatomical reduction, stable fixation to allow early movement, reliable and rapid osteosynthesis, and restoration of pain-free function. Bone healing can be delayed by the presence of large metaphyseal defects or voids that are often seen in distal radius fractures. These defects, as well as segmental defects or osteoporotic bone, are amenable to bone grafting. Autologous bone graft has been frequently used in the treatment of distal radius fractures to aid in healing in those cases. Over the past several years there has been significant interest in the development of biomaterials that can augment fracture healing to preclude the need for autologous graft.

Medically, there has been increasing interest in restoring alignment through minimal incisions and with less invasive fracture fixation. The increased number of fractures related to aging and osteoporosis has contributed to this trend. Goals of limited invasive surgery include earlier mobilization and earlier return to function. Currently available bone graft substitutes for the distal radius can help achieve these goals by restoring structural integrity with limited morbidity and possibly by achieving more rapid healing of bone.

Economically, the high market value of these products has created a stimulus for their development.[1] As such, physicians may now choose from several products that are now commercially available. Unfortunately, there is currently little consensus on the indications for use of bone graft substitutes and a paucity of comparative studies between products. Rigorous comparison of the commercially available bone graft substitutes has proved difficult because of their diversity and the lack of standardized assays. Furthermore, comparable clinical studies have not been performed.[2] The U.S. government has contributed to this confusion as regulatory control of the different types of products, even similar products, has fallen under different agencies within the Food and Drug Administration.[3] This review will cover the indications and currently available materials for use as bone replacements in the treatment of distal radius fractures.

Bone Graft Properties

An ideal bone graft possesses four important properties: (1) osteogenic cells, which are naturally occurring cells with the potential to differentiate into bone forming cells; (2) osteoinductive factors, which are proteins, including growth factors, that stimulate and signal new bone growth; (3) osteoconductive matrix providing a scaffold for new bone growth; and (4) structural integrity.[4] Both cancellous and cortical autogenous bone graft possess the first three properties. Although cortical grafts are able to provide structural integrity, they are less osteogenic and osteo-

inductive when compared with cancellous grafts. Iliac crest autologus graft has long been the gold standard of bone grafts.

Alternatives to autogenous graft, or bone graft substitutes, are judged by their ability to provide aspects of these four components. Substitutes now available include allograft bone, demineralized bone matrix (DBM), synthetic ceramic mineral substitutes, and recombinant bone morphogenetic proteins BMP-7 and BMP-2.[1] Unfortunately, comparison of one substitute with another or with autogenous graft is difficult. Each substitute is made of unique materials and participates in healing in different ways. Additionally, there are no standardized assays specific for osteoinduction and osteoconduction in humans, making it impossible to accurately quantify their role in bone healing.

Indications

The distal radius has been the center of attention for the development of many of the bone graft substitutes because it is a common area to fracture with a relative lack of associated confounding variables.[5] The indications for the use of bone grafts or graft substitutes in the treatment of distal radius fractures, however, have not been clearly defined. Additionally, although autogenous graft has been proved to be beneficial,[6-9] there is no clear consensus with regard to bone graft substitutes.

The goal of treatment is to restore alignment of the radius and provide stability with minimal compromise of hand function.[10] This can be accomplished with either a cast, external fixator, or a variety of internal fixation techniques, depending on the fracture pattern, degree of displacement, stability of the fracture, patient age, and physical demands. Fracture healing is typically not a problem, because the fracture involves metaphyseal bone with ample vascularity.[11] However, comminuted fractures or fractures in osteoporotic bone often result in cortical comminution and metaphyseal defects, which if left unsupported can lead to collapse of the distal fragments and loss of alignment. Additionally, osteopenic or osteoporotic bone can limit fixation and result in loss of reduction after internal fixation. In either case, healing will typically occur but may result in a shortened or malaligned radius, which can produce pain, stiffness, and loss of strength.[12,13] It is in these osteoporotic or comminuted fractures that bone graft substitutes provide structural support or act as a scaffold for new bone formation and are particularly desirable.

The use of autogenous bone graft has been shown to be advantageous to support metaphyseal defects after distal radius fractures.[6-9] In addition to providing structural support, autogenous graft can accelerate and augment bone healing due to the presence of growth factors and viable osteoblasts. However, use of autogenous bone graft has been associated with donor site morbidity,

241

including infection, blood loss, and pain, as well as increased surgical time, hospital stay, and cost.[14] These potential disadvantages have helped lead to the development of numerous bone graft substitutes.

The decision to use graft or graft substitute should be based on the particular injury, with emphasis on fracture pattern, stability, comminution, soft tissue injury, as well as patient factors. Another consideration should be the type of fixation employed and whether the bone graft substitute is expected to provide structural stability. None of the available graft substitutes is ideal for all situations. A structural and osteoconductive material may be considered to augment fixation in the treatment of fractures with metaphyseal or diaphyseal defects or significant cortical comminution. An osteoinductive material may be used in fractures with potential impaired healing. These include local factors such as those extending into the diaphysis or those with extensive soft tissue disruption and host factors such as diabetes, smoking, or poor nutritional status. Further study regarding growth factors may expand the indications to include even the simple fractures in an effort to accelerate healing. It is also worthwhile to note that many of the modern fixed-angle implants impart rigid support of the distal end of the radius and that the use of bone graft or bone graft substitutes with these implants may be superfluous.

Graft Substitutes

There are several graft substitutes available for orthopaedic use in the United States. These include allograft, demineralized allograft bone matrix, mineral derived graft, composite graft, calcium sulfate, injectable cement, bioactive glass, and growth factors. These substitutes vary with regard to their osteoconductive properties, osteoinductive properties, structural strength, and rate of disappearance (**Table 23-1**).

Allograft

An allograft is tissue harvested from one individual and implanted into another individual of the same species. Allograft bone is harvested from human cadavers and is available as fresh, frozen, or freeze-dried preparations. Although fresh grafts are available,

they are not routinely used, owing to their antigenicity and potential for disease transmission. Most allografts are either frozen or freeze-dried. The method of preparation affects their performance, with frozen grafts maintaining greater strength but also greater infection and rejection potential compared with freeze-dried preparations. In both preparations the osteoprogenitor cells are killed while maintaining osteoinductive and osteoconductive properties as well as partial structural integrity. The host incorporates allograft bone by a process known as "creeping substitution," in which resorption and new bone formation occur at the graft-host interface.

Allograft is available in various forms, sizes, and shapes, depending on the individual need. Corticocancellous graft can be used to reconstruct larger defects or in cases where significant structural support is needed. Cancellous graft is better for smaller defects, especially in metaphyseal areas, and is particularly useful for the distal radius.[15] It can be used to augment autograft, or it can be mixed with autograft in order to introduce osteoprogenitor cells.

The disadvantages of allograft include its variable quality and potential for disease transmission. There have been several documented cases of bacterial infections transmitted by allografts and even a documented case of human immunodeficiency virus transmission.[1] When compared with autograft, other disadvantages include lack of osteogenic cells, fewer osteoinductive factors, and less structural integrity. Still, in a recent prospective and randomized study, no significant differences regarding fracture union or outcomes were noted when comparing allograft cancellous chips and autologous iliac crest bone grafting.[16]

Demineralized Bone Matrix

DBM is allograft bone that has been demineralized and processed by chemical and/or radiation treatment, leaving collagen as well as bone morphogenetic proteins and growth factors. It has been shown to be osteoinductive in an animal model and is therefore thought to maintain the presence of growth factors despite processing.[17] However, the potential for osteoinduction is variable, even among individual batches of the same product.

TABLE 23-1 Types of Graft Substitutes for Orthopaedic Use in the United States

Material	Osteogenic Cells	Osteoinductive Factors	Osteoconductive Matrix	Structural Integrity
Autogenous: cortical	+	+	+	+
Autogenous: cancellous	+	+	+	−
Allograft	−	+	+	±
Demineralized bone matrix	−	±	+	−
Mineral (ceramics/coralline)	−	−	+	−
Composites	−	±	+	−
Calcium sulfate	−	−	+	−
Cement	−	−	+	±
Bioglass	−	−	+	−
Growth factors	−	+	±	−

+, Present; −, absent; ±, variable.

DBM is available from several manufacturers, differing in its form and carrier. Forms available include those that can be injected or molded. Various carrier agents have also been used, including saline, glycerol, gelatin, polymers, hyaluronic acid, and collagen. Despite significant debate regarding the best form and carrier, no consensus exists. There has been concern regarding glycerol toxicity in an animal model, although this has not been seen in humans.[18]

DBM is believed to have both osteoconductive and osteoinductive properties and therefore may be useful in those fractures with impaired healing. However, the indication for use in the majority of distal radius fractures is limited because healing is of little concern and there is a greater need for a more structural, osteoconductive graft material. The main disadvantages include the possibility of disease transmission and immunogenicity, relatively poor structural integrity, and potential concerns about certain carriers.

Minerals

Calcium phosphate mineral grafts are osteoconductive grafts that are composed of hydroxyapatite, tricalcium phosphate, or a combination of the two. Most of these grafts, other than coralline hydroxyapatite, are ceramics that are made by heating mineral salts to high temperatures in a process known as sintering. This process increases strength but reduces the resorption and remodeling of the material. There has been significant, but unsubstantiated, concern about the slow rate of radiographic disappearance when used clinically. The rate of resorption depends on the chemical composition as well as material factors such as the surface area and pore size. Tricalcium phosphates of greater pore size allow better resorption by allowing osteoclasts into the pores, but this renders them mechanically weaker. The ideal pore size is between 150 and 500 μm.[19] Newer materials have been developed with increased porosity to increase the rate of resorption. This rate of resorption may or may not correlate with remodeling, depending on the material and the environment.[1]

Coralline hydroxyapatite is produced by a thermochemical reaction between Pacific coral and ammonium phosphate. This process converts the majority of the coral's calcium carbonate into hydroxyapatite, which is more slowly desorbed. Technically, this is not a ceramic because it does not undergo sintering. The pores are interconnected similar to cancellous bone, allowing bone ingrowth. Newer products have been produced with calcium carbonate on the surface to improve bone ingrowth and potentially graft resorption. True osteoclastic resorption does not occur and the graft disappears slowly. Similar to the ceramics, there is minimal remodeling. It has been shown to be useful to augment fixation of distal radius fractures.[20]

Calcium phosphate mineral grafts function purely as an osteoconductive implant on which bone will grow. Osteoinduction may be introduced when grafting is combined with autogenous platelets from a special autotransfusion process. They may be used to fill defects, although structural fixation is also needed. As a group, these grafts are brittle with little tensile strength, limiting their use to nonloaded defects or defects in which the bending, shear, and torsional stresses are neutralized with internal or external fixation.[21] Other disadvantages include variable quality and slow resorption/remodeling.

Composites

Various composite grafts have been used to obtain the beneficial properties of the various materials. Some composites have combined DBM with cancellous allograft bone or mineral substitutes (calcium sulfate). These have come in various forms, and their indication for use remains unclear. These grafts are potentially osteoconductive and osteoinductive but also have the disadvantages associated with both materials.

An additional composite is made up of bovine collagen, hydroxyapatite, and tricalcium phosphate. This material is osteoconductive but can be used along with aspirated autogenous bone marrow to make it osteoinductive and potentially osteogenic. Because it provides no structural support, it appears to be useful in fractures that have been stabilized but contain bone defects. It has been shown to be a viable alternative to autogenous bone graft in the treatment of fractures, including those of the distal radius.[22,23]

Calcium Sulfate

Calcium sulfate, also known as plaster of Paris, has been used to fill bone defects for many years. It acts as an osteoconductive filler for bone defects, but, unlike ceramics, the rate of resorption is rapid, with some variation depending on the formulation, configuration, and amount of material used. It is available in various forms including pellets, blocks, and in an injectable paste. Resorption occurs by both dissolution and replacement by bone.[24] It is indicated to fill metaphyseal defects but requires supplemental fixation.

Cement

Injectable cements are made up of calcium phosphate and have the advantage of complete filling of defects. They are either injected or molded into a defect in a liquid or putty form and solidify within several minutes without generating significant heat. The solid form provides structural support with compressive strength that is greater than cancellous bone, although it poorly resists torsion or shear.[25]

Bone cements have been shown to remodel with cutting cones and osteoclastic activity, because they strongly resemble the mineral phase of bone due to the presence of dahllite.[25] Radiographic disappearance of the material by 30% to 60% has been seen at 1 year, with cortical remodeling preceding medullary remodeling.[26]

Several studies have evaluated the use of calcium phosphate cement in the treatment of distal radius fractures. An initial study demonstrated improved clinical outcome compared with casting alone.[27] A larger, multicenter, prospective study compared bone cement (with or without Kirschner wires [K-wires]) to controls treated with casting or external fixation (with or without K-wires).[26] This demonstrated earlier functional return in the cement group without loss of measured radiographic parameters. However, long-term outcomes were similar.

The advantage of structural integrity and remodeling of this osteoconductive material certainly makes it attractive for use in the distal radius. Disadvantages include lack of osteoinduction and weakness of the material in torsion and shear. Additionally, care must be exercised during injection, as the material may extrude and solidify in the surrounding soft tissues.

Bioactive Glass

Bioactive glasses are a combination of silica, calcium, and phosphate materials that form a bond between the graft and host tissue. The silica is rapidly broken down with the release of calcium and phosphate. This process may prove useful for the delivery of newly derived growth factors. These substitutes are osteoconductive but do not provide structural support.

Growth Factors

Inflammation is the earliest stage of fracture healing and begins as a result of the hematoma from fracture bleeding. Cells within this initial fibrin clot secrete growth factors, which regulate the early events of fracture healing. These factors stimulate and regulate bone formation. One of the main limitations of the majority of the currently available graft substitutes is the lack of this osteoinductive or osteogenic potential. This is currently the most intense area of research with regard to bone graft substitutes.[1]

Autogenous bone marrow has been used to fill this deficit. It can be used to augment many of the synthetic or allogenic substitutes to add osteoinductive factors as well as potentially osteogenic cells.[28] Typically harvested from the ilium with limited morbidity, it must be used immediately in order to maintain the viability of the existing cells. Marrow has been shown to contain both osteoprogenitor cells and growth factors.[29]

Platelet-rich plasma is another source of these factors. This is obtained from ultraconcentration of centrifuged blood and therefore is most often used when significant blood loss occurs during a surgical procedure, which is not common in fractures of the distal radius.

More recently, recombinant growth factors such as the bone morphogenetic proteins and synthetic peptides have been introduced, primarily for the augmentation of spinal fusion. The recombinant forms of BMP-7 (osteogenic protein-1 [OP1]; Stryker, Kalamazoo, MI) and BMP-2 (Infuse; Medtronic Sofamor Danek, Memphis, TN) have been approved for selected trauma indications.[30,31] These recombinant bone morphogenetic proteins are produced in hyperphysiological concentrations and therefore may have the potential to impart an immunological reaction. In addition, these proteins require an additional substitute to act as a carrier and to provide an osteoconductive matrix. Antibodies to these factors, and also the carriers, have been seen in humans, but it is unclear if this represents a clinical problem.[30] Newer techniques will certainly continue to develop and, along with genetic engineering, will most likely represent the future of bone graft substitution.

Summary

Although autogenous bone graft has been shown to be useful in the treatment of distal radius fractures, the role of bone graft substitutes and the optimal replacement material remain unclear. It is clear that orthobiologics will play an increasing role in fracture care and that there will be an increasing number of products from which to choose. Commercially available products (each with differing osteoconductive, osteoinductive, and structural properties) offer the treating surgeon many choices. Hand surgeons need to be cognizant of the indications for use of bone graft substitutes and choose the most appropriate to provide the structural support, gap filling, or bone healing stimulation that the situation warrants. Further comparative research will hopefully help clarify the indications and most appropriate material for a given fracture and clinical situation.

REFERENCES

1. Ladd AL, Pliam NB: Bone graft substitutes in the radius and upper limb. J Am Soc Surg Hand. 2003; 3(4):227-245.

2. Ladd AL, Pliam NB: The role of bone graft and alternatives in unstable distal radius fracture treatment. Orthop Clin North Am. 2001; 32(2):337-351.

3. Bauer TW, Smith ST: Bioactive materials in orthopaedic surgery: overview and regulatory considerations. Clin Orthop Relat Res. 2002; 395:11-22.

4. Gazdag AR, Lane JM, Glaser D, Forster RA: Alternatives to autogenous bone graft: efficacy and indications. J Am Acad Orthop Surg. 1995; 3:1-8.

5. Owen RA, Meltron LJ, Johnson KA, et al: Incidence of Colles' fracture in a North American community. Am J Public Health. 1982; 72:605-607.

6. Swigart CR, Wolfe SW: Limited incision open techniques for distal radius fracture management. Orthop Clin North Am. 2001; 32:317-327.

7. Axelrod T, Paley D, Green J, McMurtry RY: Limited open reduction of the lunate facet in comminuted intra-articular fractures of the distal radius. J Hand Surg [Am]. 1988; 13:372-377.

8. Axelrod TS, McMurtry RY: Open reduction and internal fixation of comminuted, intra-articular fractures of the distal radius. J Hand Surg [Am]. 1990; 15:1-11.

9. Seitz WH, Froimson AI, Leb R, Shapiro JD: Augmented external fixation of unstable distal radius fractures. J Hand Surg [Am]. 1991; 16:1010-1016.

10. Simic PM, Weiland AJ: Fractures of the distal aspect of the radius: changes in treatment over the past two decades. J Bone Joint Surg Am. 2003; 85(3):552-564.

11. Segalman KA, Clark GL: Un-united fractures of the distal radius: a report of 12 cases. J Hand Surg [Am]. 1998; 23:914-919.

12. Knirk JL, Jupiter JB: Intra-articular fractures of the distal end of the radius in young adults. J Bone Joint Surg Am. 1986; 68:647-659.

13. Jupiter JB: Current concepts review: fractures of the distal end of the radius. J Bone Joint Surg Am. 1991; 73:461-469.

14. Younger EM, Chapman MW: Morbidity at bone graft donor sites. J Orthop Trauma. 1989; 3:192-195.

15. Herrera M, Chapman CB, Roh M, et al: Treatment of unstable distal radius fractures with cancellous allograft and external fixation. J Hand Surg [Am]. 1999; 24:1269-1278.

16. Rajan GP, Fornaro J, Trentz O, Zellweger R: Cancellous allograft versus autologous bone grafting for repair of comminuted distal radius fractures: a prospective, randomized trial. J Trauma. 2006;60:1322-1329.

17. Urist MR, Silverman BF, Burning K, et al: The bone induction principle. Clin Orthop Relat Res. 1967; 53:243-283.

18. Bostrom MP, Yang X, Kennan M, et al: An unexpected outcome during testing of commercially available demineralized bone graft materials: how safe are the nonallograft components? Spine. 2001; 26:1425-1428.

19. Geissler WB: Bone graft substitutes in the upper extremity. Hand Clin. 2006; 22(3):329-339.

20. Wolfe SW, Pike L, Slade JF III, Katz LD: Augmentation of distal radius fracture fixation with coralline hydroxyapatite bone graft substitute. J Hand Surg. 1999; 24:816-827.

21. Bucholz RW: Nonallograft osteoconductive bone graft substitutes. Clin Orthop Relat Res. 2002; 395:44-52.

22. Chapman MW, Bucholz R, Cornell C: Treatment of acute fractures with a collagen-calcium phosphate graft material: a randomized clinical trial. J Bone Joint Surg. 1997; 79:495-502.

23. Scaglione PH, Buchman MT: Collagraft bone substitute in upper extremity fractures: a preliminary study. Surg Forum. 1997; 48:563-565.

24. Kelly CM, Wilkins RM, Gitelis S, et al: The use of surgical grade calcium sulfate as a bone graft substitute: results of a multicenter trial. Clin Orthop Relat Res. 2001; 382:342.

25. Constantz BR, Ison IC, Fulmer MT, et al: Skeletal repair by in situ formation of the mineral phase of bone. Science. 1995; 24:1796-1799.

26. Cassidy C, Jupiter JB, Cohen M, et al: Norian SRS cement compared with conventional fixation in distal radius fractures: a randomized study. J Bone Joint Surg Am. 2003; 85:2127-2137.

27. Jupiter JB, Winters S, Sigman S, et al: Repair of five distal radius fractures with an investigational cancellous bone cement: a preliminary report. J Orthop Trauma. 1997; 11:110-116.

28. Burwell RG: The function of bone marrow in the incorporation of a bone graft. Clin Orthop Relat Res. 1985; 200:125-141.

29. Muschler GF, Nitto H, Boehm CA, Easley KA: Age- and gender-related changes in the cellularity of human bone marrow and the prevalence of osteoblastic progenitors. J Orthop Res. 2001; 19:117-125.

30. Friedlaender GE, Perry CR, Cole JD, et al: Osteogenic protein-1 (bone morphogenetic protein-7) in the treatment of tibial nonunions. J Bone Joint Surg Am. 2001; 83 (Suppl 1):S151-S158.

31. Grovender M, Scimma C, Genant HK, et al: Recombinant human bone morphogenetic protein-2 for treatment of open tibial fractures: a prospective, controlled, randomized study of four hundred and fifty patients. J Bone Joint Surg Am. 2002; 84:2123-2134.

Complex Regional Pain Syndrome after Distal Radius Fractures

24

George D. Chloros, MD, Ethan R. Wiesler, MD, Anastasios Papadonikolakis, MD,
Zhongyu Li, MD, Beth P. Smith, PhD, and L. Andrew Koman, MD

Complex regional pain syndrome (CRPS) occurring after distal radius fractures is a significant comorbid event. Symptoms and signs include delayed healing, pain, impaired recovery, persistent muscle stiffness, joint stiffness and contracture, severe cold sensitivity, and functional impairment. After trauma, persistent neuropathic pain of an inappropriate intensity with the absence of impending or ongoing tissue damage is defined as CRPS. In association with a distal radius fracture, CRPS may delay or prevent recovery (**Fig. 24-1**) and has a strong negative impact on health-related quality of life and function. In this chapter we will (1) provide a definition of CRPS, (2) detail clinical symptoms and signs to aid in the early recognition of this diagnosis, (3) provide an overview of treatment and referral that will improve outcomes, and (4) facilitate the practitioner's understanding of questions related to standard of care.

Definitions

Complex regional pain syndrome is a clinical entity—without a pathognomonic diagnostic test or marker—defined by regional pain, autonomic dysfunction, vasomotor changes or instability, atrophy (trophic), and functional impairment.

Synonyms for this syndrome include reflex sympathetic dystrophy, causalgia, and algodystrophy. CRPS type I includes pain, functional impairment, autonomic dysfunction, and dystrophic changes in the absence of an identifiable peripheral nerve lesion, injury, or irritation (traditionally reflex sympathetic dystrophy); CRPS type II is identical in the presence of an identifiable nerve lesion (traditionally causalgia).[1,2] CRPS type III expands the concept to include all extremity pain dysfunction and is not discussed (**Table 24-1**). CRPS type I or II may be sympathetically maintained (SMP) or sympathetically independent (SIP) based on relief or persistence of pain after sympatholytic intervention.[3,4] The SMP type may become SIP over time; this distinction recognizes the dynamic nature of dystrophic responses. In general, the SMP type has a better prognosis and different treatment approach.

Incidence and Prognosis

Fracture of the distal radius and ulna is one of the most common injuries producing CRPS.[5-10] Tight casts,[8] the presence of a nociceptive event such as compression of the median nerve, injury of the median or ulnar nerves, overdistraction, instability of the distal radioulnar joint (DRUJ), or ulnar fracture may contribute to CRPS after fractures of the distal radius.[11,12]

In prospective studies, CRPS type I or II is reported in 26% to 39% of patients,[5,8,10,13] whereas, in retrospective studies, incidences of less than 2% are reported.[14-20] This variation may be partly explained by the difference in study design, patient inclusion/exclusion criteria, and strictness of definition. CRPS after fracture of the distal radius is not linked statistically to patient age, sex, number of attempted fracture reductions, adequacy of reduction,[5] side affected, or time from fracture to reduction and immobilization.[13] Atkins and associates[5] found no relationship to the severity of the fracture, whereas Bickerstaff and Kanis found CRPS was more likely to occur in patients who have sustained severe fractures.[13]

Web Video

24-1

The importance of early recognition and management of CRPS cannot be overemphasized; this is the single most important predictor of functional recovery and pain relief.[9,21] However, delay in diagnosis of 6 to 26 weeks is common.[22] In general, for patients diagnosed within 1 year of onset, the overall prognosis is favorable in 80% of cases, whereas there is significant morbidity in 50% of patients for whom treatment is delayed for more than 1 year.[23] Unfortunately, the prognosis of CRPS occurring after fracture of the distal radius varies from other entities and good outcomes are less common, with stiffness at 12 weeks correlating with residual CRPS at 10 years.[24]

Diagnosis and Evaluation

There is significant variation in the presentation of CRPS. The classic dystrophic progression from the acute phase (<3 months) to the dystrophic phase (3 to 6 months) to the chronic phase (>6 months) occurs infrequently; therefore, staging CRPS by the number of months is often inappropriate.[23] In this chapter we discuss the use of objective instruments and tests that serve to stage CRPS physiologically and functionally.

Symptoms and Signs

Pain

CRPS does not exist in the absence of pain; however, different patients may have variable perceptions of pain, including allodynia, hyperalgesia, hyperesthesia or hypoesthesia, and hyperpathia. Pain descriptions also vary ("burning," "throbbing," "pressing," "cutting," "searing," "shooting," or "aching"). If present, nociceptive foci, including peripheral nerve lesions and mechanical derangements, must be identified. The nociceptive trigger may not be identified until the SMP is managed and the dystrophic manifestations are treated. An objective and reproducible analysis of pain symptoms is accomplished by the use of standardized and/or validated instruments,[25] including the visual analog scale (VAS),[26,27] the pain portion of the Rand Corporation Short Form 36 (SF-36),[28] the McGill Short Form Pain Questionnaire,[29] and/or self-administered questionnaires designed to assess upper

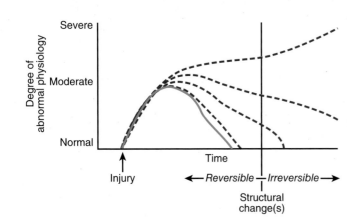

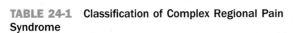

FIGURE 24-1 Abnormal physiology is a normal, expected process after injury. However, its persistence beyond normal time frames is abnormal and may result in permanent structural or functional damage within the extremity, the central nervous system, or both. *(From Koman LA, ed: Bowman Gray Orthopaedic Manual. Winston-Salem, NC: Orthopaedic Press, 1996.)*

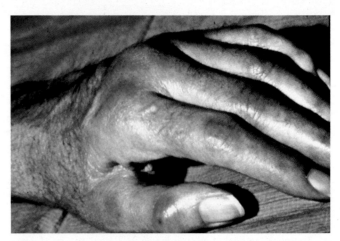

FIGURE 24-2 Hand of a CRPS patient with autonomic dysfunction and trophic changes. Note the metacarpophalangeal joints are extended or slightly flexed as are the proximal interphalangeal joints. *(From Koman LA, ed: Bowman Gray Orthopaedic Manual. Winston-Salem, NC: Orthopaedic Press, 1996.)*

TABLE 24-1 Classification of Complex Regional Pain Syndrome

CRPS Type	Traditional Designation	Features
Type I	Reflex sympathetic dystrophy	Pain, functional deficit, autonomic signs of dysfunction, dystrophic changes with absence of any identifiable clinical peripheral nerve lesion/injury
Type II	Causalgia	Pain, functional deficit, autonomic signs of dysfunction, dystrophic changes in the presence of an identifiable peripheral nerve injury
Type III	Other pain dysfunction etiologies	Pain of myofascial origin

Reproduced with permission from Koman LA, ed: Bowman Gray Orthopaedic Manual. Winston-Salem, NC: Orthopaedic Press, 2007.

extremity symptoms/function.[30,31] Cold intolerance, or pain on exposure to cold, may be analyzed by using the McCabe Cold Sensitivity Severity Scale.[32]

Trophic Changes

Upper extremity signs of CRPS include muscle and joint stiffness, edema, osteopenia, atrophy of the hair and nails, hypertrophy of skin, difficulty in fine finger manipulation, fixed posturing, and arthrofibrosis (**Fig. 24-2**). In 30% of cases, skin, hair, and/or nail changes may be apparent within 10 days of onset.[33] Osteopenia is common and involves both cortical and cancellous bone (**Fig. 24-3**).[6]

Autonomic Dysfunction

Eighty percent of CRPS patients report a medical history of symptoms of autonomic dysfunction.[34] Affected extremities may

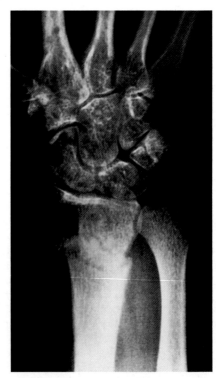

FIGURE 24-3 Plain radiograph showing diffuse osteopenia in a patient with CRPS after fracture of the distal radius and ulna (fracture line visible). Also note the juxtacortical demineralization, subchondral erosions, and cysts. *(From Koman LA, ed: Bowman Gray Orthopaedic Manual. Winston-Salem, NC: Orthopaedic Press, 1996.)*

either be "hot" or "cold." Sweating abnormalities (excessive or anhidrosis), vasomotor changes (redness or bluish discoloration of the extremity), and temperature (heat or cold) sensitivity/intolerance are the most common manifestations of autonomic dysfunction. During the painful stages of CRPS, autonomic dysfunction may be reported in up to 98% of patients.[25,35,36]

Diagnostic Testing

Evaluation of Pain

Although algometers,[37] dolorimeters,[38] computer-assisted stimuli,[39] or thermal pain thresholds may be used to quantify pain,[40] mechanical testing using Von Frey or Semmes-Weinstein monofilaments provides objective assessment of the quantity of pain and is a practical office procedure.[23]

Plain Radiographs

In approximately 80% of patients, regional osteopenia is evident on plain radiographs.[5,38] These changes are visible only if there is significant demineralization, which may not be apparent until after a long period from onset of symptoms.[41] The features of classic Sudeck's atrophy include diffuse osteopenia with juxtacortical demineralization and subchondral erosions or cysts (see Fig. 24-3).[23]

Bone Scintigraphy

Three-phase technetium-99m bone scintigraphy (TPBS) (**Fig. 24-4**) has a significant role in the diagnosis of CRPS.[36,42-45] The diagnostic accuracy of phase III of TPBS may equal that of the three-phase scan.[43] TPBS has a high specificity but poor sensitivity.[29,36,42,46] It provides objective support for the clinical diagnosis of CRPS, in combination with the other tests, but has no prognostic significance[25] or any value in determining the appropriate management approach.[21,36,47,48] The classic positive TPBS demonstrates increased periarticular uptake throughout the distal extremity.

Evaluation of Autonomic Control

Total digital blood flow equals the sum of the thermoregulatory flow (normally, 80% to 95%), and nutritional flow (normally, 5% to 20%).[23] In CRPS, inappropriate control of arteriovenous shunting leads to ischemia and deprivation of nutritional

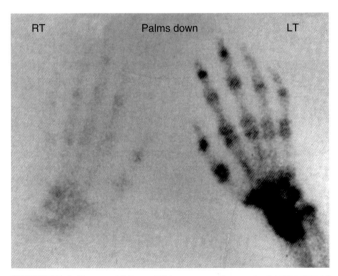

flow,[25,35,49,50] which is the common denominator in either a "warm, swollen" hand with high total flow or a "cold, stiff" hand with low total flow (**Fig. 24-5**). These components may be assessed by measurements of the digital temperatures, laser Doppler fluxmetry (LDF), vital capillaroscopy, laser Doppler perfusion imaging (LDPI), and isolated cold stress testing (ICST).[25,36,49,51-58] These measurements provide objective reproducible data, measure the effect of intervention, and guide treatment.[25,59-61] Sweat function may be evaluated quantitatively, and combined with the measurements of ICST, provides objective evidence of autonomic function.[9,25,62] Relief after sympatholytic intervention defines SMP.[3,4] SMP may be diagnosed by nerve blocks of the stellate ganglion (most common), epidural space, brachial plexus, or peripheral nerves using short-acting or intermediate-acting local anesthetics.[9] Stellate blocks are effective in only 70% to 75% of cases[2]; therefore, it is essential to confirm the sympatholysis by obtaining indirect evidence (i.e., Horner's syndrome, nasal congestion, and/or facial anhidrosis) or by direct evidence (i.e., increase in temperature (3°C), venous engorgement of the hand veins, dry skin, changes in skin color, and characteristic laser Doppler changes).[2,29,63] Thermography provides a large quantity of data and allows comparison with the contralateral extremity[64]; repeated measurements associated with stress over time are reproducible and correlate with symptoms.[65] However, higher temperatures measured by thermography do not correlate with skin surface flow in CRPS.[50] The use of a physiological stressor increases the predictive and diagnostic value of thermography.[29,66]

Management

General Principles

The two major pathophysiological stages associated with CRPS are (1) the "hot swollen" stage—increased total flow with decreased nutritional flow, and (2) the "cold stiff" stage—decreased total flow with decreased nutritional flow (**Table 24-2, Fig. 24-5**).[67]

Furthermore, after initial treatment, the response to sympatholytic intervention will classify the patient as having either SMP or SIP.[3,68,69] SMP more frequently occurs than SIP and has a more favorable prognosis.

Management of CRPS, based on physiological staging, addresses the pathophysiology, and its goals are (1) to control

TABLE 24-2 The Two States of Microvascular Perfusion Associated with Complex Regional Pain Syndrome

	Hot, Swollen	**Cold, Stiff**
Symptoms	• Increased total flow • Decreased nutritional flow	• Decreased total flow • Decreased nutritional flow
Signs	• Edema • Increased sweating	Atrophic
Pain	• With hyperalgesia • Without hyperalgesia	Hyperalgesia
	• With cold intolerance • Without cold tolerance	Cold

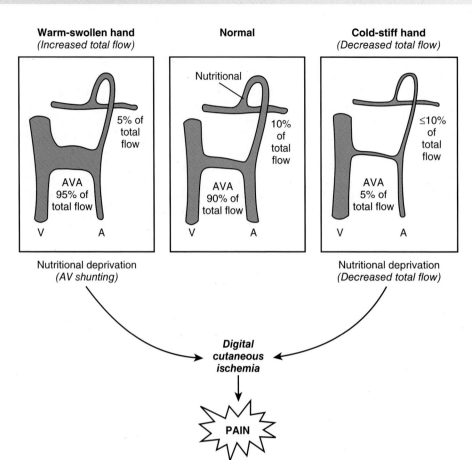

Warm-swollen hand
(Increased total flow)

Normal

Cold-stiff hand
(Decreased total flow)

Nutritional deprivation
(AV shunting)

Nutritional deprivation
(Decreased total flow)

Digital cutaneous ischemia

PAIN

FIGURE 24-5 The common underlying mechanism of CRPS is deprivation of nutritional flow and resulting pain via abnormal arteriovenous (AV) control through arteriovenous anastomoses (AVA). This is true in either a warm, swollen hand with increased total flow or a cold, stiff hand with decreased total flow. *(From Koman LA, ed: Bowman Gray Orthopaedic Manual. Winston-Salem, NC: Orthopaedic Press, 1996.)*

pain, (2) to identify a "trigger" (nociceptive focus) and correct it, (3) to manage the patient based on the response to treatment, and (4) to manage any extremity deformities.

Hand Therapy and Adaptive Modalities

The benefits of hand therapy in the management of CRPS are well established.[21,70,71] Hand therapy should address the entire limb; adhesive capsulitis to the shoulder may occur insidiously, and restoration of motion of the shoulder, elbow, and fingers is critical. Therapy should include active and passive range of motion, stress-loading activities,[71] transcutaneous electrical nerve stimulation (TENS), desensitization techniques, and/or sensory re-education. Besides TENS, adaptive modalities include contrast baths, continuous passive motion, intermittent positive pressure with pneumatic pumps, and hydrotherapy.[72-74]

Medications

Oral Medications

A myriad of oral medications with sympatholytic mechanisms are available; none is labeled by the U.S. Food and Drug Administration (FDA) for CRPS patients. Because they have no direct sympatholytic effect and are habit forming, narcotics are not ideal for CRPS; however, antidepressants, anticonvulsants, membrane stabilizers, adrenergic agents, calcium channel blockers, and neuromuscular blocking agents are beneficial. First-line drugs most frequently used include amitriptyline, phenytoin, carbamazepine, gabapentin, pregabalin, clonidine, nifedipine, and amlodipine (**Table 24-3**). Antidepressants may provide analgesia and modulate sympathetic hyperactivity in the peripheral and central

nervous systems.[4,75-77] One antidepressant may prove efficacious in one patient and not in another; thus, drug selection should be individualized. Often, the combination of two drugs belonging in different categories may be useful. For example, a tricyclic antidepressant combined with a selective serotonin reuptake inhibitor may be synergistic. Anticonvulsants have an incompletely delineated mechanism of action, including membrane stabilization. They are effective in the management of CRPS. Adrenergic agents include α_1 antagonists, α_2 antagonists, combined α_1 and α_2 antagonists, and α_2 agonists.[69,78,79] In patients with edema and hyperalgesia, administration of an α_2 agonist, such as clonidine (Catapres), in three divided doses or as a continuous transcutaneous patch, may result in improvement.[78,79] Calcium channel blockers often decrease pain, increase nutritional perfusion, and diminish abnormal arteriovenous shunting and have documented efficacy in CRPS.[25,80,81] The most commonly used calcium channel blockers are nifedipine (Adalat, Procardia) and amlodipine (Norvasc). Corticosteroids have multiple mechanisms of action, including membrane stabilization; they relieve dystrophic pain effectively in selected patients.[82-84] A high starting dose (e.g., 60 mg of prednisone) is rapidly tapered over 5 to 10 days.[84] Long-term low dosing has also been employed.[82,83] Currently, the use of corticosteroids is controversial because of their potential side effects, complications, and questionable benefit.

Parenteral Medications

Parenteral options include neuromuscular blocking agents, intravenous infusates, ganglion-blocking agents, continuous peripheral blocks with lidocaine, and intrathecal medications.

TABLE 24-3 Drugs Frequently Used in Complex Regional Pain Syndrome

Drug	Class	Mechanism of Action	Dosage (range)	Common Side Effects
Amitriptyline (Elavil, Endep)	Tricyclic antidepressant	Blocks reuptake of amines: serotonin, norepinephrine	25-75 mg (50-300 mg)	Anticholinergic effects, seizures, orthostatic hypotension, conduction abnormalities
Phenytoin (Dilantin)	Anticonvulsant	Membrane stabilization	100 mg tid (up to 400 mg/day)	*GI:* nausea, vomiting, constipation, hepatitis, liver damage *Hematologic:* thrombocytopenia, leukopenia, neutropenia *CNS:* nystagmus, ataxia, dizziness, convulsion *Other:* rashes *Contraindications:* liver disease, pregnancy
Carbamazepine (Tegretol)	Anticonvulsant	Blocks sodium influx across cell membranes	100 mg bid (1200 mg/day)	*GI:* nausea, vomiting, jaundice, hepatocellular, cholestatic *Hematologic:* aplastic anemia, agranulocytosis, thrombocytopenia *CNS:* dizziness, drowsiness, ataxia *Other:* rashes, epidermal necrolysis, congestive heart failure *Contraindications:* bone marrow depression, simultaneous MAO inhibitors
Gabapentin (Neurontin)	Anticonvulsant	Unknown, assumed to be GABA related	600-800 tid (2400 mg/day)	*GI:* anorexia, flatulence *Hematologic:* purpura *CNS:* somnolence, dizziness, ataxia *Other:* fatigue, hypertension Care must be taken with renal disease patients.
Pregabalin (Lyrica)	Anticonvulsant	Unknown, assumed to be GABA related	100 mg PO tid Starting dose: 50 mg PO tid; increase to 300 mg/day over 7 days; Max: 300 mg/day; to discontinue, taper over 7 days	Dizziness, somnolence, dry mouth, asthenia, blurred vision, edema, weight gain, confused thinking
Clonidine (Catapres)	Adrenergic agent	α_2 Agonist	Topical, intrathecal, or oral: 1 mg/hr patch weekly 1 mg tid initially	Dry mouth, sedation, contact dermatitis (transdermal system)
Nifedipine (Adalat, Procardia)	Calcium channel blocker	Blockade of calcium channel on vascular smooth muscle cell	10-30 mg PO tid or 30-90 mg qid sustained	Headache, flushing, dizziness, peripheral edema, postural hypotension
Amlodipine (Norvasc)	Calcium channel blocker	Blockade of calcium channel on vascular smooth muscle cell	2.5-5 mg/day	Edema, headache, fatigue, and dizziness; postural hypotension

Reproduced with permission from Koman LA, ed: Bowman Gray Orthopaedic Manual. Winston-Salem, NC: Orthopaedic Press, 2007.

Neuromuscular blocking agents such as botulinum toxins A and B result in relief of muscle spasm, dystonia, and skin hypersensitivity and have also been utilized in the management of pain.[85] However, their mechanism of action in CRPS is unknown. Intravenous regional infusion, once the mainstay of most treatment regimens, is used less frequently. The use of intravenous corticosteroids, guanethidine, lidocaine, and bretylium tosylate (Bretylol) has been described.[23,86] However, controlled studies do not support efficacy, and bretylium tosylate, which was the only

drug labeled by the FDA for chronic pain, has been discontinued from the U.S. market. In CRPS patients requiring reconstructive procedures, or mobilization of stiff joints by manipulation under anesthesia, bretylium or corticosteroids have been used in conjunction with regional anesthesia.[87]

Epidural administration of corticosteroids and clonidine may be used with success in selected patients.[88,89] A single block or a series of blocks of the stellate ganglion, brachial plexus, or spinal cord/nerve roots may be beneficial.[23] Continuous infusion of local anesthetic over the area of the stellate ganglion or paravertebral ganglia, along the brachial plexus, or within the epidural space has been effective in controlling chronic sympathetic pain[90,91] and is our modality of choice. Successful treatment occurs in 50% to 70% of patients.[91,92]

Sympathectomy, Implantable Devices, and Surgery

Sympathectomy

Chemical sympathectomy effects pain relief in selected patients without complete transection of the nerves; alternatively, sympathectomy may be accomplished using phenol or radiofrequency ablation. Both procedures result in reversible axonotmesis followed by recovery in 3 to 6 months. In contrast, surgical transection, which is irreversible, effects short-term benefit with delayed (6 to 9 weeks) upregulation of receptors; thus, we recommend the former.

Implantable Devices: Peripheral Nerve Stimulators, Spinal Cord Stimulators

Placement of an implantable electrical stimulator in the gray matter, dorsal column, spinal cord, and peripheral nerves is possible to control pain.[93-96] Spinal cord stimulation for CRPS provided successful pain relief for 50% of patients previously refractory to treatment[97]; however, these devices relieve pain without improving function.[98]

Management of the Nociceptive Focus

Neural nociceptive foci may include neuromas, neuromas-in-continuity, or compression neuropathies (e.g., median nerve at the carpal tunnel—the most frequent after distal radius fractures). Mechanical nociceptive foci include DRUJ or triangular fibrocartilage complex problems, joint subluxations or dislocations, and cartilage flaps in the wrist or metacarpal areas. After maximal conservative management has eliminated confounding factors due to the dystrophic process, clinical evaluation will confirm the suspicion of a neural nociceptive focus. Surgical correction of the neural or mechanical nociceptive foci should be performed only after maximal pharmacological intervention.[9,23]

The following general principles refer to a complete nerve transection or to a neuroma-in-continuity. A tension-free nerve repair site may be accomplished by using a graft. Adhesions between the skin and nerve may be managed using a "Z" plasty, local flaps, or distant flaps. Modification of the neural bed using autologous fat, rotational muscle flaps, pedicled muscle or fascial flaps, free muscle transfer, or autologous or allograft venous wraps is indicated in cases of excessive scarring or adhesion development (**Fig. 24-6**).[99-102] Internal neurolysis should be minimized so that

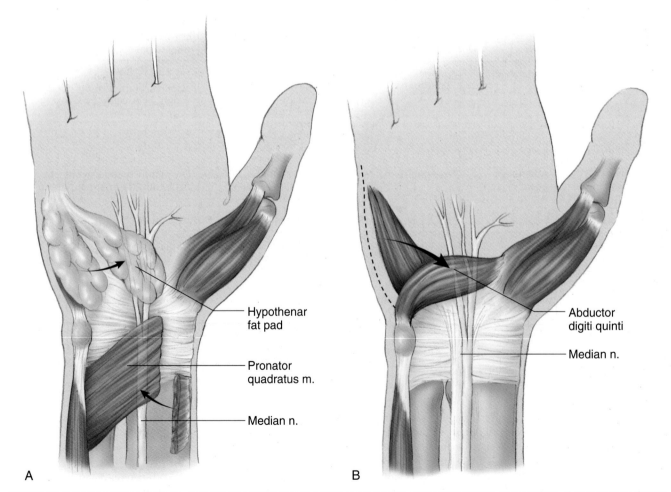

Hypothenar fat pad

Pronator quadratus m.

Median n.

Abductor digiti quinti

Median n.

A

B

FIGURE 24-6 Options for modifying the environment surrounding an injured median nerve at the wrist include transposition of pedicled hypothenar fat, the pronator quadratus muscle, or the abductor digiti quinti muscle. *(From Koman LA, ed: Bowman Gray Orthopaedic Manual. Winston-Salem, NC: Orthopaedic Press, 1996.)*

TABLE 24-4 Treatment of a "Hot Swollen" Complex Regional Pain Syndrome

Modality	Effect	Action	Example
Immobilization with splints or casts	Decrease pain Prevent progression to contracture Avoid tight casts		
Compressive dressings and elevation of the limb	Decrease edema Avoid tight dressing		
Hand therapy	Decrease pain Helps prevent arthrofibrosis/contracture	Active ROM (esp. proximal interphalangeal joints) Isometric exercises if active ROM causes too much pain Minimize passive ROM	
Stress loading activities	Decrease pain/edema		
Cryotherapy and TENS	Decrease pain/edema		
Contrast baths	Decrease pain		
NSAIDs	Decrease non-neuropathic pain Control edema	Important to control pain related to ongoing cell and tissue damage. Little effect on the neuropathic sympathetically maintained form of CRPS.	
Narcotics	Decrease non-neuropathic pain		
Calcium channel blockers	Decrease edema and increase nutritional flow Help to prevent arthrofibrosis	Increase nutritional flow (by diminishing the increased shunting via arteriovenous anastomoses)	Amlodipine (Norvasc) 2.5-5 mg/day PO, Nifedipine (Adalat, Procardia) 10-30 mg tid or 30-90 mg qid sustained
Corticosteroids	Decrease inflammation		10 mg/day PO
Tricyclic antidepressants	Decrease pain Sympatholytic action		Amitriptyline (Elavil), 25-75 mg tid
Selective serotonin reuptake inhibitors			Fluoxetine (Prozac), 20-80 mg/day
Anticonvulsants			Gabapentin (Neurontin), 600-800 mg tid
Adrenergic agent	Improves edema and hyperalgesia	Presynaptic α_2 agonist	Clonidine (Catapres), 1-mg/hr patch, weekly or 1 mg PO tid initially
Continuous autonomic blockade of the stellate ganglion	Decreases pain and sympathetic nervous system influence		

ROM, range of motion; TENS, transcutaneous electrical nerve stimulation.
Reproduced with permission from Koman LA, ed: Bowman Gray Orthopaedic Manual. Winston-Salem, NC: Orthopaedic Press, 2007.

further damage to the nerve is avoided. Appropriate hemostasis should control hematoma formation. Adequate postoperative care is essential to avoid a postoperative dystrophic flare and should include pharmacological interventions and hand therapy, including early active and passive range of motion. The use of nonocclusive dressings is proposed.

In the treatment of a nerve compression, careful evaluation is important. If symptoms are confirmed and warrant surgical intervention, nerve conduction studies should be considered. The nerve should be released, and if the neural bed is compromised it should be modified (see Fig. 24-6). Adequate postoperative care should be provided to prevent the recurrence of a dystrophic flare; it may include continuous blocks and/or oral medications.

Overview of Focused Approach

Early recognition and treatment of CRPS is the mainstay of management.[9,21] Pain, swelling, and/or vasomotor changes that are out of proportion to the traumatic or surgical event or are significantly prolonged should raise a high index of suspicion. The diagnosis of CRPS is clinical, supported by imaging modalities and evaluation of autonomic function. Physiological staging serves as the basis of treatment. A "multidisciplinary" management approach is recommended, and the team leader is determined by the circumstances of the pain process. As a general rule, "simple" modalities and drugs (oral medication and therapy) should be used first before progressing to more complex modalities (e.g., autonomic blocks). Treatment should be individualized and altered based on the patient's specific symptoms and his or her response to treatment. The goals of management are (1) to control the symptoms of pain, inflammation, and edema; (2) to improve nutritional flow; (3) to identify the presence of a nociceptive focus (if available); and (4) to prevent and/or manage deformity. The management of three possible clinical situations will be discussed.

Hot, Swollen Extremity

Cast or splint immobilization is used to decrease pain and prevent the development of contractures (**Table 24-4**). To decrease edema, the limb should be elevated above heart level and compressive dressings applied. Tight casts/dressings should be avoided. Early hand therapy is important and includes passive and active range of motion (ROM); it will prevent the development of arthrofibrosis, particularly in the proximal interphalangeal joints. Isometric muscle exercises may be used if active ROM is too painful; passive ROM should be minimal. Light activity or active motion is not enough, and a self-controlled, home program of stress loading activities may be helpful.[71] Contrast baths (alternate hot and cold therapy) are useful. Adaptive modalities, including TENS may be beneficial.[74,103] Nonsteroidal anti-inflammatory drugs (NSAIDs) may be helpful in controlling pain and inflammation. Narcotics may be used for pain due to ongoing cell and tissue damage caused by the initial trauma but have minimal effect on the SMP component of CRPS. By contrast, calcium channel blockers, antidepressants, anticonvulsants, corticosteroids, and membrane stabilizers all exhibit direct or indirect sympatholytic effects. Calcium channel blockers (e.g., amlodipine, nifedipine) increase nutritional flow and prevent the development of deformity. Antidepressants (e.g., tricyclics [amitriptyline] or selective serotonin reuptake inhibitors [fluoxetine]) act at the amine pump level to decrease pain. Anticonvulsants (e.g., gabapentin) decrease pain and sympathetic tone. Corticosteroids limit inflammatory effects. Typically, an early use of a tricyclic antidepressant (e.g., amitriptyline) in combination with an anticonvulsant (e.g., gabapentin) is advised for a patient with a hot, swollen hand. If the patient is not responding well to treatment, continuous autonomic blockade of the stellate ganglion or the use of intravenous bretylium may be attempted. After favorable response to the blocks, hand therapy as described previously should be continued. If there is no response to sympatholytic intervention, or there is no response whereas there was one previously, the patient is classified as having SIP. The treatment of SIP is complex and includes specialized modalities, and its discussion is beyond the scope of this chapter.

Cold, Stiff Extremity, No Significant Contracture

The use of the just discussed modalities for the "hot, swollen extremity" is advocated. Especially in this case, calcium channel blockers (e.g., amlodipine) combined with a tricyclic antidepressant (e.g., amitriptyline) may increase nutritional flow signifi-

cantly. The use of TENS may also increase nutritional flow by inhibition of the smaller nociceptive fibers. The application of a clonidine (an α^2 adrenergic agonist) patch in a dose of 0.1 to 0.2 mg may provide dramatic relief.

Management of Established Contracture

Common contractures that are associated with CRPS include those of the metacarpophalangeal joints in extension and those of the proximal interphalangeal joints in flexion or extension. Restriction of shoulder, elbow, and wrist ROM may be present. Although early symptom management may prevent the development of contractures, arthrofibrosis may still develop. Surgery to release contractures should be performed after maximal nonoperative treatment. Demonstration of the ability to control SMP by sympatholytics is recommended before surgical intervention. A nerve block or general anesthesia is used during this procedure; postoperative pain may be managed by a continuous epidural or nerve block. Surgery is indicated when health-related quality of life and function of the patient are compromised, for example in the presence of persistent contractures that prevent normal function of the hand and interfere with the performance of daily activities. After surgery for release of the metacarpophalangeal joint contractures, the patient's final range of motion will be 80% to 90% of the intraoperative range of motion. However, for the proximal interphalangeal joints, this range of motion is far less maintained postoperatively. Therefore, it should be made clear to patients that any surgical procedure that is performed is a salvage procedure aimed at providing a gross improvement of the function of their hands and that full restoration of hand function is not a realistic goal.

Summary

CRPS is a challenge both to recognize early and to treat. The diagnosis is clinical supported by imaging modalities and evaluation of autonomic nervous system function. Management, based on physiological staging, is individualized and will depend on the patient's response to treatment. Correcting the pathophysiology, alleviating symptoms, and preventing deformity are the mainstays of management.

REFERENCES

1. Merskey H, Bogduk N, eds: Classification of Chronic Pain: Descriptions of Chronic Pain Syndromes and Definitions of Pain Terms Prepared by the Task Force on Taxonomy of the International Association for the Study of Pain. 2nd ed. Seattle, WA: IASP Press, 1994.

2. Stanton-Hicks M, Janig W, Hassenbusch S, et al: Reflex sympathetic dystrophy: changing concepts and taxonomy. Pain. 1995; 63:127-133.

3. Amadio PC, Mackinnon S, Merritt W, et al: Reflex sympathetic dystrophy syndrome: consensus report of an ad hoc committee of the American Association for Hand Surgery on the definition of reflex sympathetic dystrophy syndrome. Plast Reconstr Surg. 1991; 87:371-375.

4. Czop C, Smith TL, Koman LA: The pharmacologic approach to the painful hand. Hand Clin. 1996; 12:633-642.

5. Atkins RM, Duckworth T, Kanis JA: Features of algodystrophy after Colles' fracture. J Bone Joint Surg Br. 1990; 72:105-110.

6. Bickerstaff DR, Charlesworth D, Kanis JA: Changes in cortical and trabecular bone in algodystrophy. Br J Rheumatol. 1993; 32:46-51.

7. Fernandez D, Jupiter J: Fractures of the Distal Radius: A Practical Approach to Management. New York: Springer-Verlag, 1996.

8. Field J, Protheroe DL, Atkins RM: Algodystrophy after Colles fractures is associated with secondary tightness of casts. J Bone Joint Surg Br. 1994; 76:901-905.

9. Koman LA, Smith TL, Smith BP, Pollock DC: Reflex sympathetic and other dystrophies. In Peimer CA, ed. Surgery of the Hand and Upper Extremity. New York: McGraw-Hill, 1996; 2295-2312.

10. Laulan J, Bismuth JP, Sicre G, Garaud P: The different types of algodystrophy after fracture of the distal radius. J Hand Surg [Br]. 1999; 22(4):441-447.

11. Herron M, Faraj A, Craigen MA: Dorsal plating for displaced intra-articular fractures of the distal radius. Injury. 2003; 34(7):497-502.

12. Sennwald GR, Della SD: Unstable distal radial fractures treated by external fixation: an analytical review. Scand J Plast Reconstr Surg Hand Surg. 2002; 36:226-230.

13. Bickerstaff DR, Kanis JA: Algodystrophy: an under-recognized complication of minor trauma. Br J Rheumatol. 1994; 33:240-248.

14. Frykman G: Fractures of the distal radius including sequelae—shoulder-hand-finger syndrome, disturbance in the distal radio-ulnar joint and impairment of nerve function. Acta Orthop Scand. 1967; 108:4-152.

15. Green JT, Gay FH: Colles' fracture—residual disability. Am J Surg. 1956; 91:636-641.

16. Lidstrom A: Fractures of the distal end of the radius: a clinical and statistical study of end results. Acta Orthop Scand. 1959; 30:1-118.

17. Pool C: Colles' fracture: a prospective study of treatment. J Bone Joint Surg Br. 1973; 55:540-544.

18. Bacorn RW, Kurtzke JF: Colles' fracture: a study of two thousand cases from the New York State Workmen's Compensation Board. J Bone Joint Surg Am. 1953; 35:643-658.

19. Plewes LW: Sudeck's atrophy in the hand. J Bone Joint Surg Br. 1956; 38:195-203.

20. Stewart HD, Innes AR, Burke FD: The hand complications of Colles' fractures. J Hand Surg [Br]. 1985; 10:103-106.

21. Koman LA, Poehling GG: Reflex sympathetic dystrophy. In Gelberman R, ed: Operative Nerve Repair and Reconstruction. Philadelphia: JB Lippincott, 1990; 1497-1524.

22. Li Z, Smith BP, Smith TL, Koman LA: Diagnosis and management of complex regional pain syndrome complicating upper extremity recovery. J Hand Ther. 2005; 18:270-276.

23. Koman LA, Poehling GG, Smith TL: Complex regional pain syndrome: reflex sympathetic dystrophy and causalgia. In: Green's Operative Hand Surgery. 4th ed. New York: Churchill Livingstone, 1999; 636-666.

24. Field J, Warwick D, Bannister GC: Features of algodystrophy ten years after Colles' fracture. J Hand Surg [Br]. 1992; 17:318-320.

25. Koman LA, Smith BP, Smith TL: Stress testing in the evaluation of upper extremity perfusion. Hand Clin. 1993; 1:59-83.

26. Davidoff G, Morey K, Amann M, Stamps J: Pain measurement in reflex sympathetic dystrophy syndrome. Pain. 1988; 32:27-34.

27. Huskisson E: Measurement of pain. Lancet. 1974; 1127-1131.

28. Ware JE Jr, Sherbourne CD: The MOS 36-item short-form health survey (SF0-36): I. Conceptual framework and item selection. Med Care. 1992; 30:473-481.

29. Koman LA, Smith TL, Poehling GG, Smith BP: Reflex sympathetic dystrophy. Curr Opin Orthop. 1993; 4(IV): 85-88.

30. Levine D, Simmons B, Koris M, et al: A self-administered questionnaire for the assessment of severity of symptoms and functional status in carpal tunnel syndrome. J Bone Joint Surg Am. 1993; 75:1585-1592.

31. McConnell S, Beaton DE, Bombardier C: The DASH Outcome Measure User's Manual. Toronto, Canada: Institute for Work & Health, 1999.

32. McCabe SJ, Mizgala C, Glickman L: The measurement of cold sensitivity of the hand. J Hand Surg [Am]. 1991; 16: 1037-1040.

33. Baron R, Maier C: Reflex sympathetic dystrophy: skin blood flow, sympathetic vasoconstrictor reflexes and pain before and after surgical sympathectomy. Pain. 1996; 67:317-326.

34. Cooke ED, Ward C: Vicious circles in reflex sympathetic dystrophy—a hypothesis: discussion paper. J R Soc Med. 1990; 83:96-99.

35. Kurvers HAJ, Jacobs M, Beuk R, et al: Reflex sympathetic dystrophy: evolution of microcirculatory disturbances in time. Pain. 1995; 60:333-340.

36. Pollock FE Jr, Koman LA, Smith BP, Poehling GG: Patterns of microvascular response associated with reflex sympathetic dystrophy of the hand and wrist. J Hand Surg [Am]. 1993; 18(5):847-852.

37. Bryan AS, Klenerman L, Bowsher D: The diagnosis of reflex sympathetic dystrophy using an algometer. J Bone Joint Surg Br. 1991; 73:644-646.

38. Atkins RM, Duckworth T, Kanis JA: Algodystrophy following Colles' fracture. J Hand Surg [Br]. 1989; 14:161-164.

39. Liu S, Kopacz D, Carpenter R: Quantitative assessment of differential sensory nerve block after lidocaine spinal anesthesia. Anesthesiology. 1995; (1):60-63.

40. Gracely R, Price D, Roberts W, Bennett G: Quantitative sensory testing in patients with complex regional pain syndrome (CRPS) I and II. In Janig W, Stanton-Hicks M, eds: Reflex Sympathetic Dystrophy: A Reappraisal, Progress in Pain Research and Management. Seattle: IASP Press, 1996; 151-170.

41. Arriagada M, Arinoviche R: X-ray bone densitometry in the diagnosis and followup of reflex sympathetic dystrophy syndrome. J Rheumatol. 1994; 21(3):498-500.

42. Davidoff G, Werner R, Cremer S, et al: Predictive value of the three-phase technetium bone scan in diagnosis of reflex sympathetic dystrophy syndrome. Arch Phys Med Rehabil. 1989; 70:135-137.

43. Mackinnon SE, Holder LE: The use of three-phase radionuclide bone scanning in the diagnosis of reflex sympathetic dystrophy. J Hand Surg [Am]. 1984; 9:556-563.

44. Steinert H, Nickel O, Hahn K: Three-phase bone scanning in reflex sympathetic dystrophy. In Stanton-Hicks M, Janig W, Boas RA, eds: Reflex Sympathetic Dystrophy: Current Management of Pain. Boston: Kluwer Academic Publishers, 1990; 177-185.

45. Zyluk A: The usefulness of quantitative evaluation of three-phase scintigraphy in the diagnosis of post-traumatic reflex sympathetic dystrophy. J Hand Surg [Br]. 1999; 24(1):16-21.

46. Kozin F, Soin J, Ryan L, et al: Bone scintigraphy in the reflex sympathetic dystrophy syndrome. Radiology. 1981; 138:437-443.

47. Hoffman J, Phillips W, Blum M, et al: Effect of sympathetic block demonstrated by triple-phase bone scan. J Hand Surg [Am]. 1993; 18(5):860-864.

48. Koman LA, Barden A, Smith BP, et al: Reflex sympathetic dystrophy in an adolescent. Foot Ankle. 1993; 5:273-277.

49. Irazuzta J, Berde C, Sethna N: Laser Doppler measurements of skin blood flow before, during, and after lumbar sympathetic blockade in children and young adults with reflex sympathetic dystrophy syndrome. J Clin Monit. 1992; 8(1):16-19.

50. Matsumura H, Jimbo Y, Watanabe K: Haemodynamic changes in early phase reflex sympathetic dystrophy. Scand J Plast Reconstr Hand Surg. 1996; 30:133-138.

51. Bej M, Schwartzman R: Abnormalities of cutaneous blood flow regulation in patients with reflex sympathetic dystrophy as measured by laser Doppler fluxmetry. Arch Neurol. 1991; 48:912-915.

52. Fagrell B: Vital capillaroscopy. Angiology. 1974; 23:284-298.

53. Fagrell B: Microcirculation of the Skin. 2nd ed. Orlando, FL: Academic Press, 1984.

54. Fagrell B: Skin preparations: advantages and disadvantages. In Baker CH, Nastuk WL, eds: Microcirculatory Technology. Orlando, FL: Academic Press, 1986; 19-42.

55. Fagrell B: Clinical studies of skin microcirculation. Klin Wochenschr. 1986; 64:943-992.

56. Fagrell B: Microcirculatory methods for evaluating the effect of vasoactive drugs in clinical practice. Acta Pharmacol Toxicol. 1986; 59:103-107.

57. Ide J, Yamaga M, Kitamura T, Takagi K: Quantitative evaluation of sympathetic nervous system dysfunction in patients with reflex sympathetic dystrophy. J Hand Surg [Br]. 1997; 22(1):102-106.

58. Ostergren J, Rosen L, Fagrell B, Stranden E: Skin microvascular circulation in the sympathetic dystrophies evaluated by videophotometric capillaroscopy and laser Doppler fluxmetry. Int J Microcirc Clin Exp. 1988; 7(3):289.

59. Cooke ED, Glick EN, Bowcock SA, et al: Reflex sympathetic dystrophy (algoneurodystrophy): temperature studies in the upper limb. Br J Rheumatol. 1989; 28:399-403.

60. Fagius J, Karhuvaara S, Sundlof G: The cold pressor test: effects on sympathetic nerve activity in human muscle and skin nerve fascicles. Acta Physiol Scand. 1989; 137:325-334.

61. Koman LA, Nunley J, Goldner J, et al: Isolated cold stress testing in the assessment of symptoms in the upper extremity: preliminary communication. J Hand Surg. 1984; 3:305-313.

62. Low PA, Caskey P, Tuck R, et al: Quantitative sudomotor axon reflex test in normal and neuropathic subjects. Ann Neurol. 1983; 14:573-580.

63. Malmqvist ELA, Bengtsson M, Sorensen J: Efficacy of stellate ganglion block: a clinical study with bupivacaine. Reg Anesth. 1992; 17:340-347.

64. Ecker A: Contact thermography in diagnosis of reflex sympathetic dystrophy: a new look at pathogenesis. Thermology. 1985; 1:106-109.

65. Sherman RA, Barja RH, Bruno GM: Thermographic correlates of chronic pain: analysis of 125 patients incorporating evaluations by a blind panel. Arch Phys Med Rehabil. 1987; 68:273-279.

66. Gulevich SJ, Conwell TD, Lane J, et al: Stress infrared telethermography is useful in the diagnosis of complex regional pain syndrome, type I (formerly reflex sympathetic dystrophy). Clin J Pain. 1997; 13:50-59.

67. Koman LA, Smith TL, Smith BP, Li Z: The painful hand. Hand Clin. 1996; 12(4):757-764.

68. Raja SN, Meyer RA, Campbell JN: Peripheral mechanism of somatic pain. Anesthesiology. 1988; 68:571-590.

69. Raja SN, Davis KD, Campbell JN: The adrenergic pharmacology of sympathetically-maintained pain. J Reconstr Microsurg. 1992; 8:63-69.

70. Haines BL: Rehabilitation of the painful upper extremity. Hand Clin. 1996; 12(4):801-816.

71. Watson HK, Carlson L: Treatment of reflex sympathetic dystrophy of the hand with an active "stress loading" program. J Hand Surg [Am]. 1987; 12(5):779-785.

72. Abram SE: Increased sympathetic tone associated with transcutaneous electrical stimulation. Anesthesiology. 1976; 45:575-577.

73. Long DM: Electrical stimulation for relief of pain from chronic nerve injury. J Neurosurg. 1973; 39:718-722.

74. Richlin DM, Carron H, Rowlingson JC, et al: Reflex sympathetic dystrophy: successful treatment by transcutaneous nerve stimulation. J Pediatr. 1978; 93:84-85.

75. Magni G: The use of antidepressants in the treatment of chronic pain. Drugs. 1991; 42(5):730-748.

76. Monks R: Psychotropic drugs. In Wall P, Melzack R, eds: The Textbook of Pain. 3rd ed. Edinburgh: Churchill Livingstone, 1994.

77. Watson CPN: Antidepressant drugs as adjuvant analgesics. J Pain Symptom Manage. 1994; 9(6):392-405.

78. Davis KD, Treede RD, Raja SN, et al: Topical application of clonidine relieves hyperalgesia in patients with sympathetically maintained pain. Pain. 1991; 47:309-317.

79. Kohn M, Chaprnka C, Caskey W, Ghignone M: Evaluation of transdermal clonidine in the treatment of reflex sympathetic dystrophy. ASSH Meeting, Toronto, Canada, September 27, 1990.

80. Raja SN, Turnquist JL, Meleka S, Campbell JN: Monitoring adequacy of alpha-adrenoceptor blockade following

systemic phentolamine administration. Pain. 1996; 64: 197-204.

81. Warfield C: Principles and practice of pain management. In Warfield C, ed: Principles and Practice of Pain Management. New York: MacGraw-Hill, 1993.

82. Christensen K, Jensen E, Noer I: The reflex dystrophy syndrome response to treatment with systemic corticosteroids. Acta Chir Scand. 1982; 148:653-655.

83. Glick EN: Reflex dystrophy (algoneurodystrophy): results of treatment by corticosteroids. Rheumatol Rehabil. 1973; 12:84-88.

84. Kozin F, Ryan L, Soin J, Wortmann R: The reflex sympathetic dystrophy syndrome (RSDS): III. Scintigraphic studies, further evidence for the therapeutic efficacy of systemic corticosteroids and proposed diagnostic criteria. Am J Med. 1981; 70:23-30.

85. Argoff CE: The use of botulinum toxins for chronic pain and headaches. Curr Treat Options Neurol. 2003; 5(6): 483-492.

86. Ford SR, Forrest WH, Eltherington L: The treatment of reflex sympathetic dystrophy with intravenous regional bretylium. Anesthesiology. 1988; 68:137-140.

87. Duncan K, Lewis R, Racz G, Nordyke M: Treatment of upper extremity reflex sympathetic dystrophy with joint stiffness using sympatholytic Bier blocks and manipulation. Orthopedics. 1988; 11(6):883-886.

88. Dirksen R, Rutgers MJ, Coolen JMW: Cervical epidural steroids in reflex sympathetic dystrophy. Anesthesiology. 1987; 66:71-73.

89. Rauck RL, Eisenach J, Jackson K, et al: Epidural clonidine treatment for refractory reflex sympathetic dystrophy. Anesthesiology. 1993; 79(6):1163-1169.

90. Betcher A, Bean G: Continuous procaine block of paravertebral sympathetic ganglions. JAMA. 1953; 151(4): 288-292.

91. Linson MA, Leffert R, Todd D: The treatment of upper extremity reflex sympathetic dystrophy with prolonged continuous stellate ganglion blockade. J Hand Surg. 1983; 8:153-159.

92. Byas-Smith M: Management of acute exacerbations of chronic pain syndromes. In Sinatra RS, ed: Acute Pain. St. Louis: Mosby-Yearbook, 1992; 432-443.

93. Ballantine HT: Treatment of intractable psychiatric illness and chronic pain by sterotactic cingulotomy. In Schmidek H, Sweet W, eds: Operative Neurosurgical Techniques: Indications, Methods, and Results. New York: Grune & Stratton, 1988; 1069-1075.

94. Hosobuchi Y: Subcortical electrical stimulation for control of intractable pain in humans. J Neurosurg. 1986; 64: 543-553.

95. Kumar K, Nath R, Wyant G: Treatment of chronic pain by epidural spinal cord stimulation: a 10-year experience. J Neurosurg. 1991; 75:402-407.

96. Young RF, Chambi VI: Pain relief by electrical stimulation of the periaqueductal and periventricular gray matter. J Neurosurg. 1987; 66:364-371.

97. Kemler MA, Schouten HJ, Gracely RH: Diagnosing sensory abnormalities with either normal values or values from contralateral skin: comparison of two approaches in complex regional pain syndrome I. Anesthesiology. 2000; 93(3):718-727.

98. Kemler MA, Barendse GA, van Kleef M, et al: Spinal cord stimulation in patients with chronic reflex sympathetic dystrophy. N Engl J Med. 2000; 343(9):618-624.

99. Jones NF: Treatment of chronic pain by "wrapping" intact nerves with pedicle and free flaps. Hand Clin. 1996; 12(4):765-772.

100. Koman LA, Ruch DS, Smith BP, et al: Reflex sympathetic dystrophy after wrist surgery. In Levin L, ed: Problems in Plastic and Reconstructive Surgery. Philadelphia: JB Lippincott, 1992; 300-322.

101. Masear VR, Colgin S: The treatment of epineural scarring with allograft vein wrapping. Hand Clin. 1996; 12(4): 773-779.

102. Sotereanos DG, Giannakopoulos PN, Mitsionis GI, et al: Vein-graft wrapping for the treatment of recurrent compression of the median nerve. Microsurgery. 1995; 16:752-756.

103. Melzack R: Prolonged relief of pain by brief, intense transcutaneous somatic stimulation. Pain. 1975; 1:357-373.

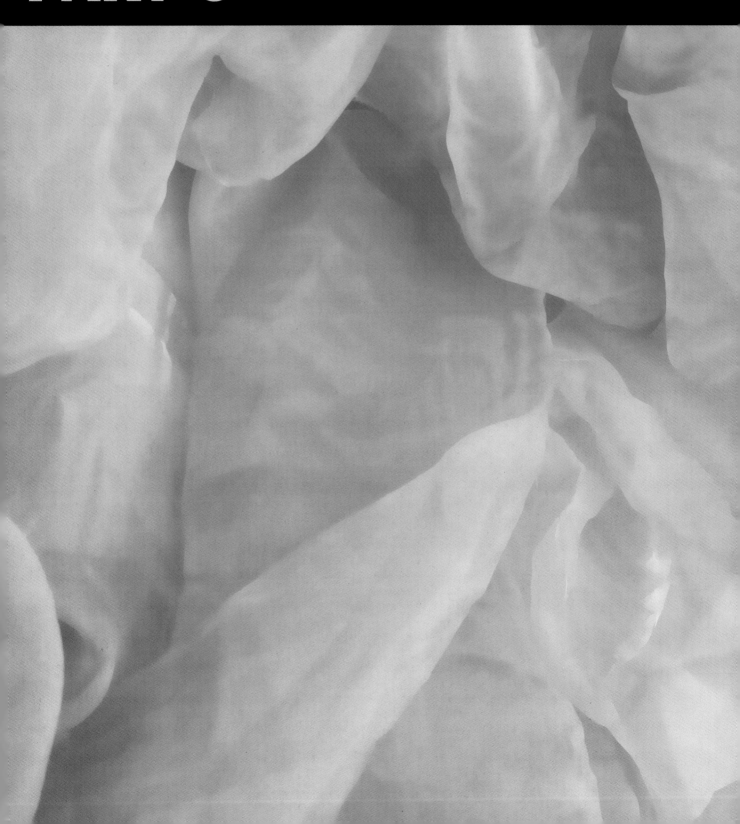

PART 6 THE ULNAR SIDE

Stability of the Distal Radioulnar Joint

25

William B. Kleinman, MD

The longitudinal axis of forearm pronation/supination passes through the center of the radial head proximally and through the foveal sulcus at the lateral base of the ulnar styloid distally. Af Ekenstam and Hagert[1] defined the pole of the distal ulna as that portion adjacent to the triangular fibrocartilage (TFC) that is covered by hyaline cartilage and responsible for absorption of load transferred to the forearm from the medial carpus, through the articular disc of the TFC onto the ulna. The fovea is the recess lying between hyaline cartilage of the ulnar pole and the ulnar styloid. This fossa is richly vascularized; it serves as a point of insertion of the major distal radioulnar joint (DRUJ), stabilizing the ligamentous components of the TFC.

Advances in Understanding of Anatomy and Biomechanics of the Distal Radioulnar Joint

Research published particularly over the past 30 years now gives us a clear understanding of how the anatomical position of the fovea and the deep components of the TFC are critical to the rotational and translational stability of the DRUJ. Anatomical works by Bednar and associates, in 1991,[2] and Thiru-Pathi and colleagues, in 1986,[3] independently demonstrate the rich vascularity within the ulnar fovea. These authors also described the source of vascular nutrition of all peripheral tissues of the TFC, both dorsal and palmar. Their two landmark papers also describe the avascular, central articular disc of the TFC, nourished by synovial fluid from both the DRUJ and the ulnocarpal joint.

At the ginglymus ulnotrochlear joint of the elbow, the ulna participates only in forearm flexion and extension; it does not rotate. Forearm pronation/supination involves rotation of the radiocarpal unit (with the attached hand) around a rotationally fixed and stable ulna. The complex architecture of the ulnotrochlear articular surfaces and the collateral ligament stabilizers of the elbow allow the ulna to move as a hinge only, without a rotational component. The longitudinal axis around which rotation takes place can be visualized in **Figure 25-1**. The anatomy of the sigmoid notch of the radius, the seat of the ulna (which articulates with the notch), and the guiding, checkrein potential of the components of the TFC allow 90 degrees of forearm supination (at which point the two forearm bones are essentially parallel, and the interosseous space the widest) to 90 degrees of pronation, at which point the radius has rotated across the anterior surface of the fixed ulna (**Fig. 25-2**). The principal axis* of load bearing at

the DRUJ tracks obliquely across the sigmoid notch as the radiocarpal unit pronates/supinates around the fixed ulna (**Fig. 25-3**). The tracking line is from distal/dorsal in pronation to proximal/palmar in supination.

In the human bipedal condition, with flexed elbows at the side (prepared for work), the radiocarpal unit rests "on top" of the ulnar seat, with gravity pulling the hand and its load toward the ground (**Fig. 25-4**). This so-called zero-rotation position of the forearm has been nicely described by Palmer.[4] In this position—the most common for human forearm function—a significant joint reaction force (JRF) can develop between the sigmoid notch of the radius and the rotationally fixed ulnar seat (see Fig. 25-4). Usually, radiographs of the carpus are viewed with the fingers toward the ceiling. Students of hand surgery learn that it is easier to develop three-dimensional thinking about the anatomy of the wrist and the distal end of the ulna if (1) their patients are clinically examined with their elbows on the examining table and their fingers toward the ceiling; (2) if radiographs are viewed with the fingers toward the ceiling; and (3) if arthroscopy of the wrist is performed with the fingers toward the ceiling.

I have reoriented **Figure 25-4**, however, to allow the reader an appreciation of the "zero-rotation" position of the *working* forearm, with the radial and ulnar styloids at their widest anatomical separation and the forearm in neutral rotation (0 degrees of pronation/supination). In this position, the principal axis of load bearing at the DRUJ passes through the center of the sigmoid notch and the center of the seat of the ulna. In zero rotation, the various radioulnar ligament components of the TFC are under the least amount of tension.[1,5]

The structural presence and health of articular surface cartilage on the ulnar seat (as well as the sigmoid notch) are critical in providing a painless mechanical fulcrum for all radioulnar load-bearing activity. In a state of equilibrium (no forearm motion), all moments around a fixed fulcrum (i.e., the seat of the ulna) *must be equal* (**Fig. 25-5**). The loaded hand (F) times the length of the loaded hand from the fulcrum provided by the seat of the ulna (L) must be equal to the moment ($F' \times L'$) on the proximal side of the fulcrum:

$$F \times L = F' \times L'$$

where F' is the stability provided at the radiocapitellar joint by the annular ligament encircling the radial head and L' is the entire length of the forearm. Because $F \times L = F' \times L'$, the relatively long forearm makes the requirement for proximal radius stability by the annular ligament (F') relatively small, regardless of the load in the hand.

---

*The *principal axis* is an engineering term used to define an imaginary point at the center of an infinite number of cluster points between two loaded surfaces, in contact with each other.

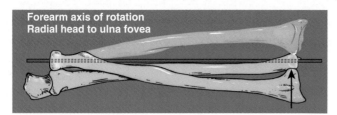

Forearm axis of rotation
Radial head to ulna fovea

FIGURE 25-1 The longitudinal axis of rotation of the forearm (*red bar*) passes through the head of the radius proximally and through the fovea of the ulna distally.

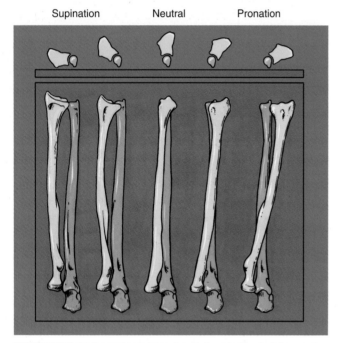

Supination　　Neutral　　Pronation

FIGURE 25-2 As the radius rotates from full supination to full pronation around a fixed ulna, the radiocarpal unit shortens relative to the ulna, resulting in ulnar-positive variance in the pronated position.

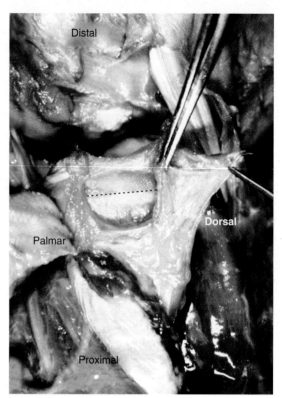

Distal

Dorsal

Palmar

Proximal

FIGURE 25-3 The principal axis of load-bearing tracks across the sigmoid notch from proximal/palmar in supination to distal/dorsal in pronation.

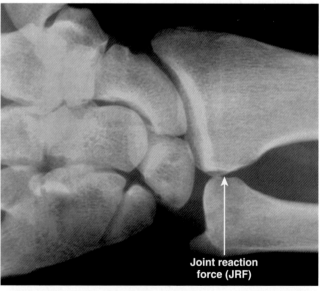

Joint reaction
force (JRF)

FIGURE 25-4 The seat of the ulna is the fulcrum for all DRUJ mechanics. Because most upper limb activities in the bipedal human occur with the radiocarpal unit "on top" of the ulnar seat, the joint reaction force (JRF) at the DRUJ can be enormous. The joint reaction force is proportional to the load in the hand, the force of all muscles acting to pull the radius and ulna together for stability, and the force of gravity acting on the hand/forearm unit.

The sum of *all* moments distal and proximal to this fulcrum equals the total load on the fulcrum (the ulnar seat) itself, defined as the joint reaction force (JRF) at the DRUJ (**Fig. 25-6**). Based on how much load is in the hand (F), and the size of the moment distal to the DRUJ, the reader begins to appreciate the potential magnitude of the JRF at the DRUJ and the importance of surface hyaline cartilage health at both the sigmoid notch and the ulnar seat for painless DRUJ function.

Using elegant cadaver dissections, in 1985 af Ekenstam and Hagert[1,6] demonstrated that the concave radius of curvature of the sigmoid notch is greater than that of the ulnar seat (**Fig. 25-7**). This incongruity of articular surfaces creates a geometrically nonconstrained articulation at the DRUJ, subject to translational dorsal and palmar instability of the sigmoid notch on the ulnar seat. Not only does the radiocarpal unit rotate around the fixed ulnar seat in pronation/supination, but the flatter surface of the sigmoid notch also has enough inherent instability through incongruous cartilage surfaces to allow *translation* of the notch palmarly or dorsally on the fixed ulna as the forearm *rotates* into pronation or supination, respectively. The DRUJ is *not* a ball-and-socket joint. **Figure 25-3** reveals the exposed cadaver sigmoid notch (the ulna has been dissected free and hinged palmarly out

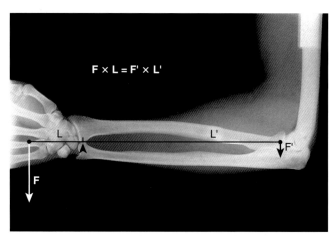

$$F \times L = F' \times L'$$

FIGURE 25-5 In equilibrium, the moments on the distal and proximal sides of the ulnar seat fulcrum must be equal. The load in the hand (F) times the distance of the load from the fulcrum (L) must be equal to the length of the forearm from the fulcrum (L') times the resistance to displacement provided by the annular ligament at the radial head (F').

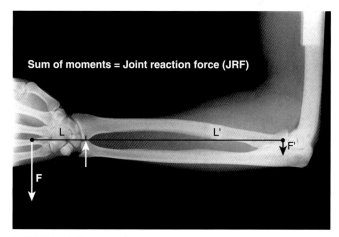

Sum of moments = Joint reaction force (JRF)

FIGURE 25-6 The sum of the moments on the distal and proximal sides of the fulcrum equals the joint reaction force (JRF) at the DRUJ.

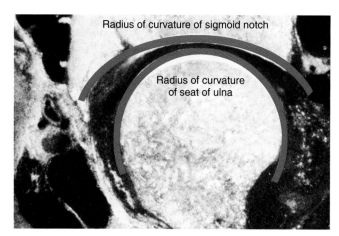

Radius of curvature of sigmoid notch

Radius of curvature of seat of ulna

FIGURE 25-7 Transverse section through the DRUJ. The radius of curvature of the sigmoid notch is greater than the radius of curvature of the seat of the ulna, leading to an inherent instability of the DRUJ through an arc of pronation/supination. Rotation of the forearm around a longitudinal axis of rotation (see Fig. 25-1) is manifest at the DRUJ by rotation and translation of the sigmoid notch against the ulnar seat. *(From Af Ekenstam F, Hagert CG: Anatomical studies on the geometry and stability of the distal radioulnar joint. Scand J Plast Reconstr Surg. 1985; 19:17-25.)*

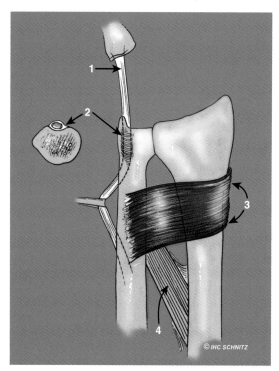

FIGURE 25-8 Extrinsic stabilizers of the inherently unstable DRUJ include (1) the tendon of the extensor carpi ulnaris; (2) the sixth dorsal compartment subsheath; (3) the superficial and deep heads of the pronator quadratus; and (4) the interosseous ligament of the forearm. Even considered all together, the extrinsic DRUJ stabilizers are fairly ineffective in physiologically maintaining DRUJ stability through the arc of pronation/supination under load.

of the notch to the reader's left), showing the oblique tracking line of the principal axis of forearm load bearing through a full pronation/supination arc at the DRUJ (see earlier). Because rotation of the radius across the ulna from supination to pronation results in relative ulnar-positive variance[4] at the end arc of forearm pronation, the tracking line of the principal axis of load bearing across the sigmoid notch must—by definition—be oblique. It tracks from slightly more proximal at the palmar edge of the notch in full supination to slightly more distal at the dorsal edge of the notch in full pronation.

Stability of the DRUJ

With inherently unstable, nonconstrained articular surfaces, anatomical stability of the DRUJ is achieved through *extrinsic* extracapsular as well as *intrinsic* intracapsular structures. Extrinsic stability is provided principally by (1) dynamic tensioning of the extensor carpi ulnaris (ECU) as its tendon crosses the distal head of the ulna[7,8]; (2) the semi-rigid sixth dorsal compartment itself, constraining the ECU tendon[7,8]; (3) dynamic support provided by the superficial and deep heads of the pronator quadratus[9]; and (4) the interosseous ligament of the mid forearm[10] (**Fig. 25-8**).

The extrinsic DRUJ stabilizers are of secondary importance compared with the more biomechanically effective intrinsic radioulnar components of the TFC.[1,2,6] Dorsal and palmar radioulnar TFC fibers arise from the medial border of the distal radius and insert on the ulna at two separate and distinct sites: (1) the fovea at the

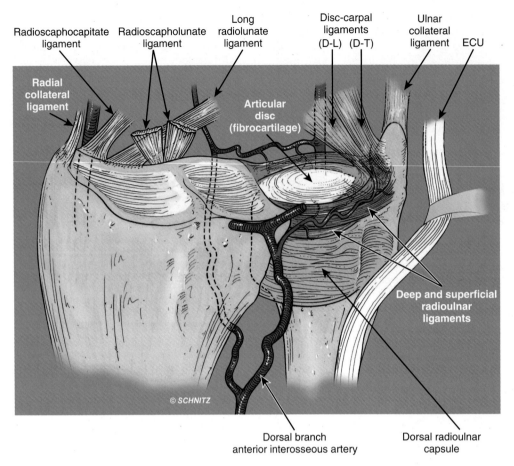

Radioscaphocapitate ligament   Radioscapholunate ligament   Long radiolunate ligament   Disc-carpal ligaments (D-L) (D-T)   Ulnar collateral ligament   ECU

Radial collateral ligament

Articular disc (fibrocartilage)

Deep and superficial radioulnar ligaments

© SCHNITZ

Dorsal branch anterior interosseous artery   Dorsal radioulnar capsule

FIGURE 25-9 The prime intrinsic stabilizer of the DRUJ is the triangular fibrocartilage (TFC). The TFC complex consists of superficial (*green*) and deep (*blue*) radioulnar fibers, the two disc-carpal ligaments (disc-lunate and disc-triquetral), and the central articular disc (*white*). The articular disc is responsible for transferring load from the medial carpus to the pole of the distal ulna. The vascularized, peripheral radioulnar ligaments (*green and blue*) are nourished by dorsal and palmar branches of the posterior interosseous artery and are responsible for guiding the radiocarpal unit around the seat of the ulna. ECU, extensor carpi ulnaris.

base of the ulnar styloid and (2) the ulnar styloid itself. **Figure 25-9** emphasizes the well-vascularized nature of the dorsal and palmar radioulnar ligaments. **Figure 25-10** illustrates the critical and clinically significant difference between the angle of attack of the dorsal and palmar *superficial* radioulnar fibers inserting on the ulnar styloid and the *deep* fibers inserting onto the fovea. Well-vascularized, longitudinally oriented connective tissue fibers of the TFC anchor the radius to the ulna along both its dorsal and palmar margins. The blood supply to both these areas of the periphery of the TFC is through branches of the posterior interosseous artery (see Fig. 25-9).[2,3] These vessels course along the dorsal and palmar radioulnar ligaments penetrating and nourishing the dorsal 20% and palmar 20% of the TFC.[2,3] Between these two sets of DRUJ checkreins, the articular disc is nourished by synovial fluid washing from the ulnocarpal joint distally and the DRUJ proximally. The articular disc is primarily responsible for load transmission from the medial carpus to the forearm, particularly with the hand-forearm unit in ulnar deviation. In neutral deviation of the hand-forearm unit, the principal axis of load transmission passes from the hand, through the head of the capitate, then the scapholunate ligament, and finally onto the articular surface of the distal radius at the interfossal ridge, which separates the elliptical (scaphoid-bearing) and spherical (lunate-bearing) fossae of the distal radius (see Figs. 25-10 and 25-11). Af Ekenstam and colleagues[6] have demonstrated in the laboratory that, in neutral position of the wrist, 84% of hand load is transferred to the radius and only 16% is transferred through the central articular disc of the TFC. With ulnar deviation of the hand-forearm unit (**Figs. 25-12 and 25-13**), the principal axis of load bearing

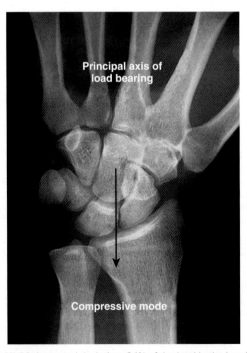

Principal axis of load bearing

Compressive mode

FIGURE 25-10 In neutral deviation, 84% of the load in the hand passes to the forearm through the radius, with the principal axis of load bearing passing through the scapholunate ligament and onto the interfossal ridge of the distal radius. Only 16% of the entire load transferred from the hand to the forearm is borne by the articular disc of the TFC in neutral deviation.

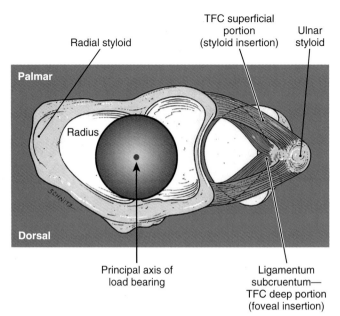

FIGURE 25-11 The deep radioulnar fibers of the TFC (dorsal and palmar) originate at the dorsal and palmar edges of the medial border of the distal radius and insert onto the fovea of the ulna (*blue fibers*, referred to as the ligamentum subcruentum). Their obtuse angle of attack makes them particularly effective in guiding the radius around the ulna through a functional arc of pronation/supination. In compressive mode, with the hand-forearm unit in neutral deviation, the principal axis of load bearing passes through the scapholunate ligament onto the articular surface of the distal radius.

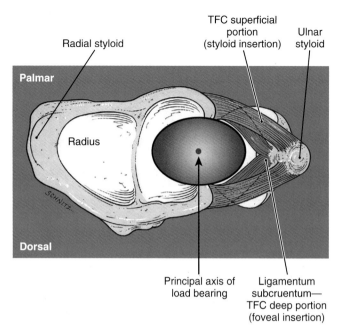

FIGURE 25-13 Deep fibers of the TFC (ligamentum subcruentum) insert onto the ulnar fovea at an obtuse angle of attack (*blue*). Superficial radioulnar fibers (*green*) insert onto the ulnar styloid and have little function in controlling forearm rotation at the DRUJ. As the principal axis of load bearing shifts onto the TFC in ulnar deviation, the articular disc is supported by the superficial palmar and dorsal (*green*) radioulnar ligaments, attaching directly to the bony ulnar styloid.

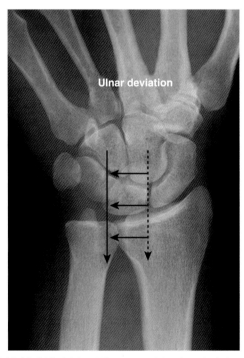

FIGURE 25-12 With the hand/forearm unit in ulnar deviation, the principal axis of load transfer is shifted medially onto the articular disc of the TFC, away from the distal radius. The principal axis now passes through the triquetrohamate joint onto the pole of the distal ulna.

shifts medially, placing more load on the articular disc and the pole of the distal ulna, rather than on the interfossal ridge of the distal radius when the hand-forearm unit is in neutral deviation.

How the TFC Components Guide the Radiocarpal Unit around a Fixed Ulna: The Significance of Rotation and Translation

The dorsal and palmar radioulnar ligaments consist of superficial components inserting directly onto the ulnar styloid and deep components inserting significantly more laterally, into the fovea adjacent to the articular surface of the pole of the distal ulna (**Fig. 25-14**). These two components of the TFC are distinct in both their anatomy and function. Scrutiny of Figure 25-14 reveals that fibers of the superficial component form an *acute* angle as they converge on the ulnar styloid from the medial radius. This narrow angle of attack gives the superficial TFC a poor mechanical advantage for guiding the radiocarpal unit through an arc of pronation/supination. The deep components of the TFC (arising along the medial border of the distal radius, but inserting into the fovea), however, form an *obtuse* angle of attack, which is much more mechanically advantageous in stabilizing rotation of the radius around the fixed ulna (see Fig. 25-14). The deep components of the TFC have been referred to by wrist investigators as the ligamentum subcruentum. In his landmark 1975 article on the "Articular Disc of the Hand," Kauer[11] gives credit to Henle[12] and Fick[13] for describing a vascularized fissure between the superficial and deep components of the TFC, which they called the "ligamentum subcruentum" but technically was not a ligament at all. More recently, however, the term "ligamentum subcruentum" has come to represent the deep fibers of the TFC (inserting into the fovea) and is now used commonly by many wrist investigators as interchangeable with the term "deep TFC radioulnar ligaments."

Figures 25-11 and 25-13 schematically represent the superficial radioulnar ligaments (green) and the deep ligamentum subcruentum (blue) in transverse section through the ulnocarpal joint. The distinct differences in fiber orientation and mechanical advantage of the deep radioulnar ligaments in controlling forearm rotation are apparent. It might be easier, however, to understand the relative difference in the effectiveness of the superficial and deep radioulnar ligaments of the TFC in controlling physiological forearm rotation and translation using an analogy of a team of

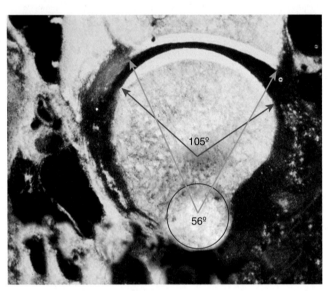

FIGURE 25-14 Stability of the DRUJ. The obtuse angle of attack of the ligamentum subcruentum (*blue*) from the medial radius to the fovea is much more mechanically advantageous in guiding the radius around the seat of the ulna through a full arc of pronation/supination. The superficial radioulnar ligaments (*green*) are much less effective in controlling distal radioulnar rotation and translation. *(From Af Ekenstam F, Hagert CG: Anatomical studies on the geometry and stability of the distal radioulnar joint. Scand J Plast Reconstr Surg. 1985; 19:17-25.)*

horses, a buckboard, and a driver (**Fig. 25-15**). The team of horses represents the radius; the seat of the buckboard is the fovea of the ulna. The buckboard driver holds the reins securely at the buckboard seat (the ulnar fovea). The angle of attack of the blue reins to the two outside horses of the team represents the angle of attack of the deep dorsal and palmar fibers of the ligamentum subcruentum from the radius (the team of horses) to the foveal sulcus of the ulna (the seated buckboard driver). Their orientation makes the angle of attack on the outside horses of the team much more effective in turning the team of horses (the radius) around the buckboard (the ulna). The narrower, acute angle of attack of the superficial TFC fibers is represented as green reins connecting the driver to the central horses of the team. This angle of attack is much less effective in controlling rotation of the team relative to the driver (see Fig. 25-15B). Like the diagrammatic obtuse blue fibers of the ligamentum subcruentum in **Figures 25-11 and 25-13**, the blue reins are much more effective in controlling the team of horses by virtue of their obtuse angle of attack on the two outside horses.

Af Ekenstam and Hagert first suggested in 1985[1] that the deep fibers of the TFC were the principal intrinsic stabilizers of the DRUJ. Although these investigators used cadaver dissections and experimental techniques that might be considered somewhat basic by today's standards, their conclusions were sound: in forearm supination the dorsal, deep fibers of the ligamentum subcruentum tighten significantly while the deep palmar fibers remain lax. This suggests a pulling, tethering mechanism for controlling stability during DRUJ rotation (**Fig. 25-16**). Conversely, these authors found that the palmar, deep fibers of the ligamentum subcruentum were the principal restraints against superphysiological palmar migration of the radiocarpal unit at the sigmoid notch in pronation (see Fig. 25-16).

In 1991, Schuind and associates,[5] from the Mayo Clinic Biomechanics Laboratory, refuting af Ekenstam and Hagert's 1985 work, suggested a totally different TFC function for controlling forearm stability. Using a sophisticated stereophotogrammatic technique with phosphorescent markers and computer analysis, the authors concluded that the dorsal fibers of the TFC tighten in pronation and the palmar fibers tighten in supination, conclusions opposite those published by af Ekenstam and Hagert 6 years earlier.

LIGAMENTUM SUBCRUENTUM

LIGAMENTUM SUBCRUENTUM
PLUS
TFC SUPERFICIAL PORTION

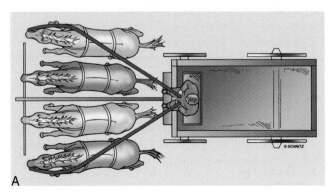
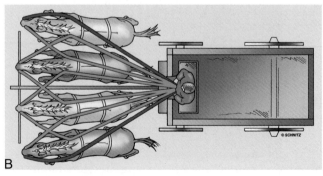

A   B

FIGURE 25-15 The TFC "buckboard" analogy. **A,** Outer reins from the driver seated on the buckboard (the ulna) to the outside horses of the team easily control the entire team because of their wide angle of attack from the seat of the buckboard to the horses. This wide angle represents the same effectiveness of the angle of attack of the deep ligamentum subcruentum of the TFC from the radius to the fovea of the ulna. **B,** A narrower angle of attack of green reins on the central horses of the team is much less effective in controlling the team. These more acutely angled reins represent the acutely angled and less-effective green-colored fibers of the TFC (superficial, and inserting onto the ulnar styloid).

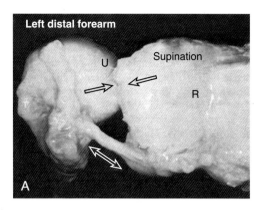

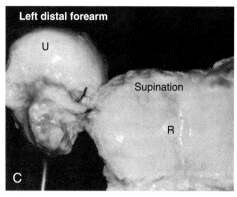

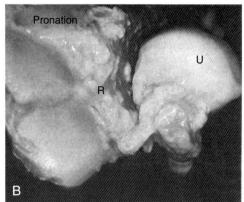

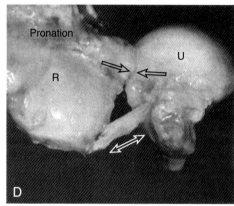

FIGURE 25-16 **A** and **B**, Cadaver photos illustrating palmar dislocation of the radius in pronation after division of the TFC palmar ligaments. **C** and **D**, Cadaver photos illustrating dorsal dislocation of the radius in supination after division of the TFC dorsal ligaments. *(From Af Ekenstam F, Hagert CG: Anatomical studies on the geometry and stability of the distal radioulnar joint. Scand J Plast Reconstr Surg. 1985; 19:17-25.)*

Controversy raged in the academic hand surgical world until 1994, when Hagert—carefully studying the conflicting conclusions from 1985 and 1991—recognized that both research groups were correct but that each was examining a different piece of the puzzle. In a small, but brilliant work published in 1994,[14] Hagert clarified the biomechanical effect of each component of the TFC for the first time. In this article he reasoned that his earlier 1985 publication studied only the deep components of the TFC—those inserting into the fovea of the ulna. This was a consequence of aggressive excision of the central articular disc for the 1985 study, which affected the integrity of the dorsal and palmar superficial TFC radioulnar ligaments. He also implied that the phosphorescent markers applied to the surface of the TFC by Schuind and associates[5] measured developing tension or tightening of the superficial radioulnar ligaments only, as these fibers enveloped the articular disc. The surface phosphorescent markers, however, did not consider the biomechanics of the radiofoveal deep fibers, with their much more mechanically effective angle of attack. Hagert clearly stated that in forearm pronation, the dorsal superficial fibers of the TFC must tighten for stability as do the deep palmar fibers of the ligamentum subcruentum. Conversely, in supination, the palmar superficial TFC radioulnar fibers (to the ulnar styloid) tighten as do the deep dorsal fibers of the ligamentum subcruentum, making both theories correct (**Fig. 25-17**).

Two critical anatomical factors are responsible for a more significant stabilizing effect of the ligamentum subcruentum on forearm rotation than the superficial radioulnar ligaments of the TFC: first, full forearm pronation allows the principal axis of load bearing at the DRUJ to track distally and dorsally along the sigmoid notch to a point where less than 10% of the dorsal notch is still in contact with the articular seat of the ulna.[1] In this position, most of the hyaline cartilage–covered distal end of the ulna has herniated against the dorsal DRUJ capsule,[15] out from under the confining cover of the dorsal superficial radioulnar fibers of the TFC that attach to the bony ulnar styloid. In maximum pronation, DRUJ stability is based almost entirely on the restraining, pulling action of the palmar, deep fibers of the ligamentum subcruentum, preventing superphysiological translation from occurring. Second, the obtuse angle of attack of these deep fibers (recall the analogy of the team of horses and the buckboard) is perfectly oriented to prevent DRUJ subluxation. More than any other intrinsic or extrinsic DRUJ-stabilizing components discussed earlier, these two anatomical considerations are responsible for DRUJ stability.

Conversely, in full supination (as the sigmoid notch migrates dorsally on the ulnar seat to less than 10% articular surface contact[1]) the superficial palmar TFC fibers become ineffective as the ulnar head rolls out beyond their effective confines, stretching the palmar DRUJ capsule.[15] At the same time, the dorsal ligamentum subcruentum tightens and its obtuse orientation becomes mechanically advantageous in restraining the radiocarpal unit from superphysiological dorsal migration on the seat of the ulna. The profound stabilizing importance of the ligamentum subcruentum relative to the superficial fibers of the TFC becomes quite clear.

Provocative Maneuvers for Determining the Health and Integrity of the Ligamentum Subcruentum: The Perpetual Role of Physical Diagnosis in Hand Surgery

Direct arthroscopy of the TFC through the ulnocarpal joint can, unfortunately, only provide information about the integrity and health of the superficial dorsal and palmar fibers of the TFC and

LEFT FOREARM

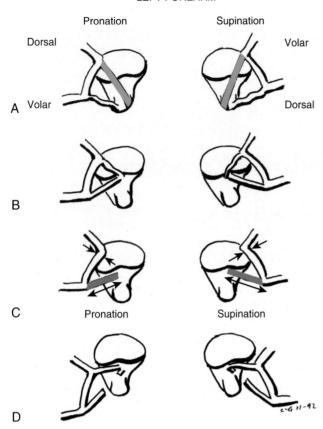

FIGURE 25-17 Reproduction of Hagert's 1994 work illustrating the effectiveness of the deep fibers of the TFC in controlling distal radioulnar rotation and the relative ineffectiveness of the superficial fibers. The critical factor is the angle of attack of the ligamentum subcruentum from the radius to the fovea of the ulna. *(From Hagert CG: Distal radius fracture and the distal radioulnar joint—anatomical considerations. Handchir Mikrochir Plast Chir. 1994; 26:22-26.)*

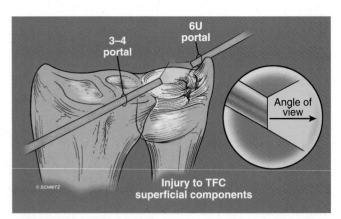

FIGURE 25-18 The ligamentum subcruentum (deep dorsal and palmar fiber of the TFC) cannot be visualized by ulnocarpal arthroscopy. Only injuries of the superficial radioulnar ligaments and articular disc can be seen.

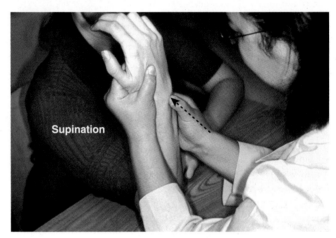

FIGURE 25-19 Stress-testing the dorsal, deep fibers of the ligamentum subcruentum for pain and/or mechanical instability (findings must be compared with those of the opposite, uninjured side).

the articular disc (**Fig. 25-18**). Ulnocarpal arthroscopy will not allow the surgeon visualization of the deeper ligamentum subcruentum unless the superficial TFC has been completely ruptured and retracted from its moorings on the bony ulnar styloid, or if a large, central degenerative hole has been worn through the articular disc.[16] The clinician can, however, examine the distal forearm for health and integrity of the dorsal *and* palmar components of the ligamentum subcruentum using precise provocative maneuvers and physical diagnostic techniques.

If we assume that in full forearm supination the dorsal radiofoveal fibers of the ligamentum subcruentum are under maximum tension (the palmar superficial fibers are also under tension, but less mechanically advantageous) and in full forearm pronation the palmar radiofoveal fibers of the ligamentum subcruentum are under maximum tension, then the dorsal and palmar components of the deep TFC can be stress-tested employing these two provocative maneuvers:

1. The examiner sits opposite the patient, with the patient's elbow on the examining table and his or her fingers toward the ceiling. The patient's forearm is rotated into full supination. In this position, the dorsal fibers of the ligamentum subcruentum will be under maximum tension. The examiner then pushes the distal ulna toward the patient while pulling the radiocarpal

unit toward himself or herself (**Fig. 25-19**). This maneuver introduces a superphysiological load into the DRUJ; it will be painless only if the dorsal fibers of the ligamentum subcruentum are healthy. If inflamed, or suffering from relatively minor injury, the two forearm bones will be grossly stable on stress-testing but the patient will experience considerable pain on loading the DRUJ beyond its physiological limits. If the deep dorsal fibers have been severely sprained and detached from the fovea, this maneuver will not only be painful but will also lead to superphysiological movement of the sigmoid notch off the seat of the ulna, resulting in subtle subluxation or even gross instability, depending on the magnitude of injury to the dorsal fibers of the ligamentum subcruentum.

2. **Figure 25-20** demonstrates the clinician stress-testing the deep palmar ligamentum subcruentum by applying a dorsally directed superphysiological load to the distal ulna (along the vector of the arrow), while supporting the forearm in full pronation. The hand/forearm unit is gently pulled toward the examiner while the examiner's thumb pushes the ulna toward the patient. If the deep palmar radioulnar portion of the TFC is either ruptured or attenuated, the sigmoid notch will translate beyond its normal end-arc relationship to the seat of the ulna, resulting in painful instability in full pronation.

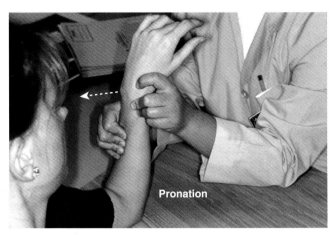

FIGURE 25-20 Stress-testing the palmar, deep fibers of the ligamentum subcruentum for pain and/or mechanical instability (findings must be compared with those of the opposite, uninjured side).

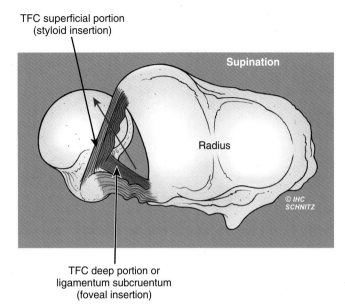

FIGURE 25-21 An illustration of tightening of the dorsal, deep fibers of the ligamentum subcruentum as the radius rotates and translates dorsally off the seat of the ulna in supination. The head of the ulna translates along the sigmoid notch and herniates out from under cover of tightening superficial palmar TFC fibers, rendering these (green) fibers ineffective in controlling DRUJ mechanics.

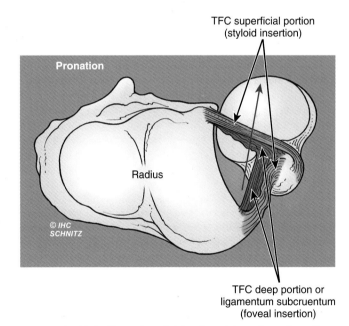

FIGURE 25-22 An illustration of tightening of the palmar, deep fibers of the ligamentum subcruentum as the radius rotates and translates palmarly off the seat of the ulna in pronation. The head of the ulna translates along the sigmoid notch and herniates out from under cover of tightening superficial dorsal TFC fibers, rendering these (green) fibers ineffective in controlling DRUJ mechanics.

Physical findings of pain and/or instability with these two provocative maneuvers must always be compared with findings of the opposite, uninjured extremity.

These physical diagnostic techniques are highly reliable. They are precise in detecting painful instability of the DRUJ, whether secondary to inflammatory arthropathy or trauma. The importance of provocative maneuvers that can isolate the deep TFC ligamentum subcruentum from the superficial radioulnar ligaments cannot be overstated, especially because no information about the condition of the ligamentum subcruentum can be gleaned from ulnocarpal arthroscopy (see Fig. 25-18). In full supination, essentially all load introduced by the examiner's hand stresses the dorsal ligamentum subcruentum (**Fig. 25-21**), as the seat of the ulna is translated along the sigmoid notch beyond the confines of the superficial palmar TFC fibers. In full pronation, introduction of a superphysiological load by the examiner's thumb against the distal ulna stress-tests the palmar ligamentum subcruentum, eliciting pain and/or instability in its pathological state (**Fig. 25-22**). Physical diagnosis of injury to the deep fibers of the TFC should be considered the "gold standard" in clinical evaluation of the TFC. Once the clinician understands the significance of TFC fiber orientation and can appreciate the importance of the critical angle of attack of the deep TFC fibers from the medial radius to the ulnar fovea, injuries to the TFC leading to either subtle or gross instability can be readily identified by careful physical examination.

A new generation of wrist coils has improved the diagnostic potential of magnetic resonance imaging (MRI) over the past 15 years. There are many published studies corroborating MRI findings at the distal end of the ulna by open surgical exploration; diagnostic accuracy has become much more reasonable in recent years. But MRI with or without gadolinium contrast should *not* be regarded as a substitute for a thorough physical examination of the DRUJ and the TFC, particularly through use of direct palpation of the periphery of the TFC and stress-testing techniques. The MR image in **Figure 25-23A** clearly shows integrity of the superficial radioulnar ligaments arising from the medial radius and inserting into the ulnar styloid; contrast agent is observed streaming around the pole of the distal ulna, across the fovea to the base of the styloid, suggesting complete avulsion of the ligamentum subcruentum (deep TFC fibers) from the foveal sulcus. This massive injury to the deep components of the

TFC resulted in painful dorsal and palmar translational instability at the DRUJ in this patient. Provocative stress-testing (described earlier) was clinically positive in both pronation and supination. **Figure 25-23B** demonstrates intraoperative findings of complete avulsion of the ligamentum subcruentum from the ulnar fovea. While possibly corroborating the clinician's physical findings, MRI should be considered only helpful in assessing the

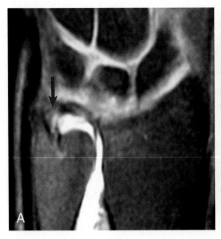 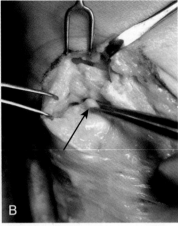

FIGURE 25-23 A and **B,** Improved wrist coils have made wrist MRI more useful in establishing a working diagnosis of a TFC injury. In this example, it appears that the superficial TFC components attaching directly to the bony ulnar styloid are still intact (*arrow*); however, contrast material streams across the ulnar pole and through the fovea, suggesting that the ligamentum subcruentum has been completely avulsed from the fovea. These MRI findings were confirmed at the time of surgery. The *arrow* on **B** points to the stump of the avulsed ligamentum subcruentum, deep in the ulnar fovea.

condition of a patient's TFC but not definitively diagnostic. The incidence of false-positive and false-negative MRI findings still remains very high today. MRI findings should always require clinical correlation by the examining physician.

Displaced Basilar Ulnar Styloid Fractures

With newfound understanding of the integral role played by the ligamentum subcruentum in DRUJ mechanics, more critical attention should be given to displaced basilar ulnar styloid fractures, so often occurring in association with fractures of the distal radius. Laboratory cadaver studies by Viegas and colleagues, in 1990,[17] demonstrate certain conditions necessary for traumatic ulnar styloid failure and displacement. Their results suggest that with certain losses of radius length, palmar tilt, and/or angle of inclination associated with distal radius fractures, enough tension could be placed on the ulnar styloid through the intact superficial radioulnar ligaments of the TFC that the bony styloid could be avulsed from its base as the fractured distal radius fragments displace. With the ulnar styloid (and TFC) intact, the authors could osteotomize the radius but achieve only the following in their laboratory: (1) radius shortening of 2 and 4 mm; (2) an angle of radius inclination of 10 degrees; and (3) a radius tilt of 0 degrees. However, if they first osteotomized the ulnar styloid through its base, the radius could be then shortened beyond 4 mm, the inclination could be reduced to at least 0 degrees, and a dorsal tilt of 15 degrees or 30 degrees could be achieved. The clinical implication of their work is clear: a distal radius fracture with metaphyseal collapse and shortening and/or dorsal tilt beyond the authors' experimental methods can result in either a concomitant displaced fracture of the ulnar styloid (an avulsion fracture via intact superficial TFC components inserting onto the bony ulnar styloid) or an avulsion or tear of the TFC superficial ligaments from the styloid itself, with the bone remaining intact.[18] In the clinical setting, one can readily appreciate that with displaced distal radius fractures, if the ulnar styloid has been avulsed at its base by the superficial TFC fibers that insert directly into the bony ulnar styloid, then—by definition—the deep fibers of the ligamentum subcruentum must also be avulsed and displaced from the fovea of the ulna, precisely the same distance as the ulnar styloid displacement from its bony base (**Fig. 25-24**). The potential effect of a ligamentum subcruentum injury of this nature on DRUJ stability, with or without concomitant avulsion of the ulnar

styloid through its base, should be obvious. The hand surgeon must exercise judgment in determining whether the degree of ulnar styloid displacement is sufficient to justify surgical open reduction and stabilization. By surgically anchoring the displaced basilar ulnar styloid fracture back to its bony base by open reduction and internal fixation (at the same time as any required anatomical open reduction and internal fixation of the displaced distal radius fracture), the surgeon essentially ensures that the concomitantly avulsed ligamentum subcruentum is most closely approximated to the fovea. Once healed, the DRUJ-stabilizing function of the deep radioulnar component of the TFC has been restored. After anatomical alignment of the bony ulnar styloid, the deep TFC fibers can be maintained in this position by immobilization with a long arm cast for 6 weeks (preventing forearm rotation), with or without adjunctive percutaneous 0.062-inch Kirschner wires (K-wires) through the ulna into the radius in "zero rotation." A more secure and predictable reattachment of the ligamentum subcruentum can be performed using bone-anchoring techniques directly to the foveal sulcus of the ulna (see later).

Consequences of Failing to Appreciate TFC Anatomy When Treating Displaced Distal Radius Fractures

An example of the consequences of failing to respect this type of disruption of anatomy—and potential disturbance of normal DRUJ biomechanics—is seen in **Figure 25-25A-C**. A 19-year-old female college student fell off her bicycle onto the outstretched dominant hand, incurring this grossly displaced, extra-articular distal radius fracture. The extent of shortening and dorsal angulation is clear (see Fig. 25-25A, B). Also readily seen is the significant displacement of the ulnar styloid, avulsed through its base by the intact superficial radioulnar components of the TFC. The patient was treated elsewhere by closed reduction of her distal radius fracture and cast immobilization until radius bony union (see **Fig. 25-25C**). She presented for a second opinion in my office 9 months after her initial treatment (see Fig. 25-25D), complaining of disabling pain at the distal end of the ulna, particularly with loaded pronation and supination. Physical examination revealed (1) subtle hypermobility at the sigmoid notch on stress-testing the ligamentum subcruentum using the provocative maneuvers described earlier (relative to the opposite side); (2) full pronation and supination; and (3) 65 degrees of wrist extension

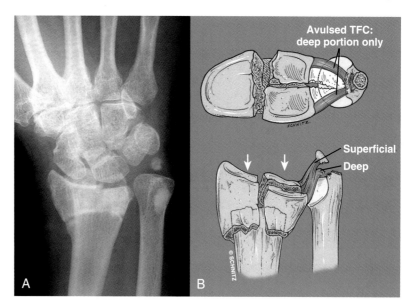

FIGURE 25-24 A and **B**, Basilar ulnar styloid fractures can be displaced in association with displaced distal radius fractures through tension on the intact superficial dorsal and palmar radioulnar ligaments (*green*). As the radius fracture fragments displace, the intact superficial radioulnar ligaments (*green*) can either rupture (see Palmer's[19] classification of traumatic TFC lesions) or remain intact, avulsing the entire styloid from its base (as in this example). If the superficial radioulnar ligaments (*green*) remain intact, as the styloid displaces from its base the deep fibers of the ligamentum subcruentum (*blue*) will be avulsed from their insertion at the ulnar fovea and displace the same distance as the initial displacement of the ulnar styloid. Figure **A**, Radiograph of the displaced radius and ulnar styloid fractures. **B**, Schematic representation of the tearing and separation of the critical ligamentum subcruentum (*blue*) as its foveal insertion fails.

and 75 degrees of wrist flexion. There was no tenderness on direct palpation of the ulnar styloid fracture nonunion. The "piano key" sign was negative. This traditional sign of micro-instability of the DRUJ is elicited by placing the seated patient with his or her palm flap on the examining table. The hypothenar eminence is forced firmly against the table by the patient, which causes a prominent and unstable distal ulna to relocate at the DRUJ. The action of the unstable ulna being forced up and down mimics the action of a piano key.

Radiographs of this young woman show a 6-mm, radially displaced malunion of the distal radius, with a 6-mm displacement of her ulnar styloid, avulsed through its bony base by the superficial dorsal and palmar radioulnar components of the TFC (see Fig. 25-25). The styloid is displaced from its base exactly the same distance as the lateral displacement of the distal radius fragment at the malunion site. The original displacement of the metaphyseal radius fracture at the time of injury impact pulled the ulnar styloid from its base by force-transmission through the intact superficial dorsal and palmar components of the TFC. As the bony styloid was avulsed from its base, the deep foveal attachments of the ligamentum subcruentum failed as well, destabilizing the DRUJ by loss of this critical anchor point. Failure by the first treating surgeon to anatomically reduce the distal radius not only resulted in a radius malunion and ulnar styloid nonunion (see Fig. 25-25) but also left the avulsed fibers of the deep ligamentum subcruentum adjacent to hyaline cartilage covering the distal ulnar pole. There was no potential whatsoever for the ligamentum subcruentum to heal to the fovea because of the magnitude of the initial fracture displacement.

In this patient, failure of the ligamentum subcruentum to heal properly to its anatomical insertion onto the ulnar fovea resulted in chronic, painful DRUJ instability under load.

The patient's 6-mm radius malunion not only shifted the ulnar styloid from its anatomical base but also left the ligamentum subcruentum displaced to a position from which it could not be reanchored to the fovea without corrective osteotomy of the radius. A dome osteotomy of the radius was performed (see Fig. 25-25E), allowing a 6-mm medial shift of the distal radius, along with the superficial radioulnar ligaments and articular disc, all still attached to the ulnar styloid. The restored anatomy of the radius allowed the ulnar styloid fibrous union to be taken down, reduced,

and anchored anatomically to its base using a tension-band wiring technique. With the ulnar styloid anatomically reduced, the deep fibers of the TFC could be restored to their anatomical insertion into the fovea. A bone anchor placed directly into the fovea (with an additional 2-0 Fiberwire added to the 2-0 Ethibond suture already attached) ensured an anatomical insertion of the deep fibers of the TFC. Fixation techniques for the radius dome osteotomy (four 0.062-inch K-wires in this case) are of secondary importance to understanding the profound importance of repairing the deep components of the TFC to the fovea in this patient. The critical concept was to shift the entire distal forearm unit medially, enabling anatomical restoration of the ligamentum subcruentum to the fovea and restoration of normal DRUJ mechanics. **Figure 25-25E** demonstrates the intraoperative technique of preparing the fovea for reattachment of the ligamentum subcruentum, installing the bone anchor (with additional 2-0 Fiberwire attached), and passing sutures through the TFC before pulling the deep fibers securely into the fovea. As seen in the postoperative radiograph (see Fig. 25-25E), two additional percutaneous 0.062-inch K-wires were passed through the distal ulna into the radius before tying the bone anchor sutures as tightly as possible. The K-wires maintain rigid stability of the DRUJ during the early postoperative healing process. All eight percutaneous K-wires seen in Figure 25-25E were removed 6 weeks after surgery. After rehabilitation the patient regained full, painless pronation/supination, with normal load-bearing capacity at the DRUJ. Her final radiograph is seen in **Figure 25-25J**.

Conclusions

By applying our newfound knowledge of TFC anatomy and biomechanics, and by using new physical examination techniques like the ones I introduced in this chapter, we are able to make much more precise diagnoses.

I am hopeful that the reader now understands why the works of af Ekenstam and Hagert in 1985, and Schuind and associates, in 1991, deemed so controversial then, should now be considered corroborative. Special credit should also go to Dr. Carl-Goran Hagert, who recognized the reasons for our misunderstandings in 1994 and provided a clear explanation of how the different components of the TFC work in conjunction with each other, in providing functional stability at the DRUJ. The superficial radio-

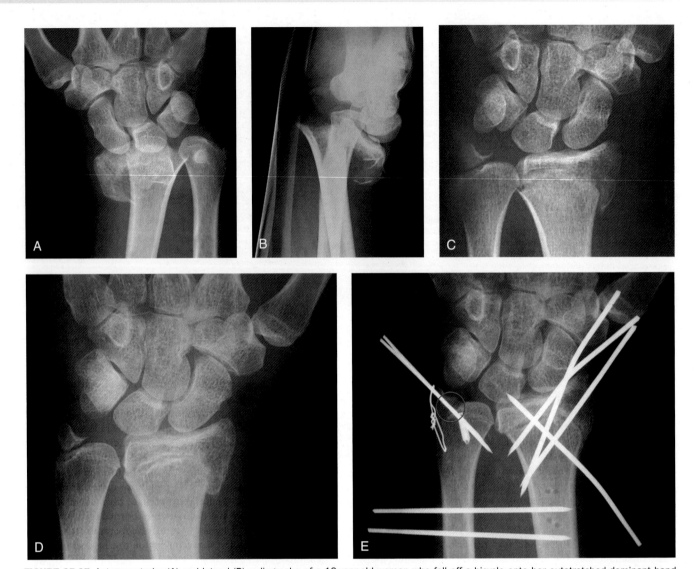

FIGURE 25-25 Anteroposterior (**A**) and lateral (**B**) radiographs of a 19-year-old woman who fell off a bicycle onto her outstretched dominant hand. The magnitude of radius shortening, dorsal angulation, and complete loss of inclination is readily seen. **C,** The patient was treated elsewhere by closed reduction and cast immobilization for 6 weeks. Anteroposterior radiograph out of plaster reveals lateral displacement of the distal radius fragment, with similar lateral displacement of the ulnar styloid through its base, avulsed by the intact superficial radioulnar ligaments of the TFC. **D,** Nine months after the initial injury, the radius is healed, the displaced ulnar styloid fracture nonunion is ankylosed and nontender, but the DRUJ is painful and unstable through a full arc of pronation/supination. Provocative maneuvers that stress the deep dorsal and deep palmar fibers of the ligamentum subcruentum were positive for pain and instability. **E,** Dome osteotomy of the radius malunion allowed a 6-mm medial shift of the distal radius fragment in this patient. The ulnar styloid could then be anatomically reduced at its base and held with tension-band wires. With the bony anatomy restored, the critical, deep radioulnar ligaments of the ligamentum subcruentum were now juxtaposed to the fovea (*red circle*) and could be securely reattached with a bone anchor. To eliminate any forearm rotation for 6 weeks, two 0.062-inch K-wires were introduced percutaneously through the distal shaft of the ulna into the radius.

ulnar components of the TFC maintain stability of the hypovascular articular disc for load transmission from the medial side of the carpus to the pole of the ulna. The clinical manifestation of chronic, superphysiological load on the superficial components of the TFC is progressive deterioration of the articular disc, the ulnar pole, and, eventually, the lunatotriquetral joint, referred to by Milch in 1941[16] as "ulnocarpal abutment syndrome" and classified by Palmer as progressive degenerative lesions of the TFC.[16] Deep peripheral tears of the TFC have an effect on DRUJ rotational stability that is quite different from the effects of central degenerative TFC tears classified by Palmer in 1989.

The deep components of the TFC (palmar and dorsal ligamentum subcruentum), with their obtuse and mechanically

advantageous angle of attack from the palmar and dorsal medial edges of the distal radius to the ulnar fovea, principally guide the radius around a fixed ulna through a full functional arc of pronation/supination. That the DRUJ can be destabilized by rupture of the deep fibers of the TFC alone, with the superficial radioulnar ligaments still intact, is now well recognized. In the past 3 years we have treated 10 patients at the Indiana Hand Center with intraoperative documentation of ligamentum subcruentum avulsion from the ulnar fovea but a normal ulnocarpal arthroscopic examination, with intact superficial radioulnar ligaments and articular disc. Recent improvements in contrast MRI have made our presumptive diagnoses more clear, but the value of preoperative physical diagnostic maneuvers cannot be overstated. Bone

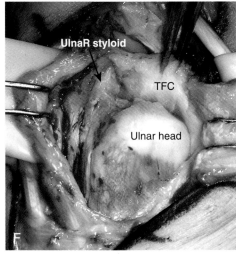

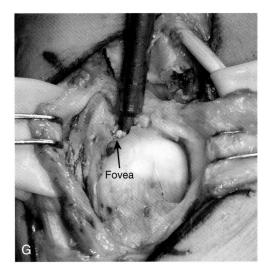

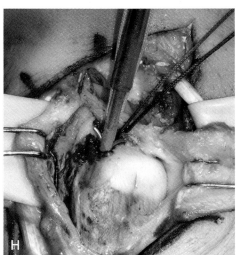

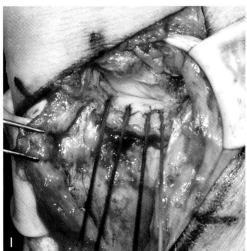

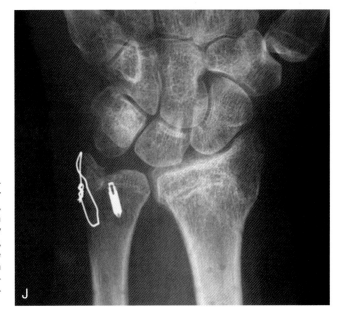

FIGURE 25-25, cont'd   **F** to **I,** A sequence of intra-operative steps used to prepare the ulnar fovea for a bone anchor. Once placed deeply into the fovea, the standard 2-0 suture material manufactured with the anchor can be reinforced by the surgeon by adding additional suture material to the anchor, giving a potential four-strand attachment of the avulsed, deep radioulnar fibers of the ligamentum subcruentum to bone. **J,** Long-term follow-up antero-posterior radiograph. The patient recovered full, pain-less pronation/supination under load.

anchoring of the avulsed ligamentum subcruentum to the ulnar fovea is now a regularly performed surgical procedure in our practice, in those cases in which provocative stress-testing of the ligamentum subcruentum has been positive. Certainly, the chronicity and magnitude of the patient's symptoms, as well as a failure of conservative management, are factors that enhance the indications for surgical intervention.

ACKNOWLEDGMENT

Special thanks to Mr. Gary Schnitz, my friend and colleague, who has provided all the partners of The Indiana Hand Center with some of the finest medical illustrations in all of academic hand surgery. His brilliant work is recognized throughout the hand surgery world. His drawings have helped an untold number of students of hand surgery more clearly understand our research, our clinical work, and our professional endeavors in general.

REFERENCES

1. Af Ekenstam F, Hagert CG: Anatomical studies on the geometry and stability of the distal radioulnar joint. Scand J Plast Reconstr Surg. 1985; 19:17-25.

2. Bednar MS, Arnoczky SP, Weiland AJ: The microvasculature of the triangular fibrocartilage complex: its clinical significance. J Hand Surg [Am]. 1991;16:1101-1105.

3. Thiru-Pathi RG, Ferlic DC, Clayton ML, McClure DC: Arterial anatomy of the triangular fibrocartilage of the wrist and its clinical significance. J Hand Surg [Am]. 1986; 11:258-263.

4. Palmer AK, Werner FW: Biomechanics of the distal radioulnar joint. Clin Orthop Relat Res. 1984; 187:26-35.

5. Schuind F, An KN, Berglund L, et al: The distal radioulnar ligaments: a biomechanical study. J Hand Surg [Am]. 1991; 16:1106-1114.

6. Af Ekenstam FW, Palmer AK, Glisson RR: The load on the radius and ulna in different positions of the wrist and forearm: a cadaver study. Acta Orthop Scand. 1984; 55:363-365.

7. Goldner JL, Hayes MG: Stabilization of the remaining ulna using one-half of the extensor carpi ulnaris tendon after resection of the distal ulna. Orthop Trans. 1979; 3:330-331.

8. Spinner M, Kaplan EB: Extensor carpi ulnaris: its relationship to stability of the distal radioulnar joint. Clin Orthop Relat Res. 1970; 68:124-128.

9. Ruby LK, Ferenz CC, Dell PC: The pronator quadratus interposition transfer: an adjunct to resection arthroplasty of the distal radioulnar joint. J Hand Surg [Am]. 1996; 21:60-65.

10. Hotchkiss RN, An KN, Sowa DT, et al: An anatomic and mechanical study of the interosseous membrane of the forearm: pathomechanics of the proximal migration of the radius. J Hand Surg [Am]. 1989; 14:256-261.

11. Kauer JMG: The articular disc of the hand. Acta Anat. 1975; 93:590-605.

12. Henle J: Handbuch der Bänderlehre des Menschen. Braunschweig: Friedrich Vieweg, 1856.

13. Fick RA: Handbuch der Anatomie und Mechanik der Gelenke unter Berucksichtigung der bewegenden Muskeln. Vol 1. Anatomie der Gelenke. Jena: Fischer, 1904.

14. Hagert CG: Distal radius fracture and the distal radioulnar joint—anatomical considerations. Handchir Mikrochir Plast Chir. 1994; 26:22-26.

15. Kleinman WB, Graham TJ: The distal radioulnar joint capsule: clinical anatomy and role in posttraumatic limitation of forearm rotation. J Hand Surg [Am]. 1998; 23:588-599.

16. Milch H: Cuff resection of the ulna for malunited Colles' fracture. J Bone Joint Surg. 1941; 23:311-313.

17. Viegas SF, Pogue DJ, Patterson RM, Peterson PD: Effects of radioulnar instability on the radiocarpal joint: a biomechanical study. J Hand Surg [Am]. 1990; 15:728-732.

18. Pogue DJ, Viegas SF, Patterson RM, et al: Effects of distal radius fracture malunion on wrist joint mechanics. J Hand Surg [Am]. 1990; 15:721-727.

19. Palmer AK: Triangular fibrocartilage complex lesions: a classification. J Hand Surg [Am]. 1989; 14:594-606.

Arthroscopic Treatment of Triangular Fibrocartilage Complex Injuries

26

John M. Bednar, MD and A. Lee Osterman, MD

The triangular fibrocartilage complex (TFCC) is a complex anatomical structure located at the ulnar side of the wrist. It has the important biomechanical function of providing stability to both the ulnar carpus and the distal radioulnar joint (DRUJ). Disorders of the TFCC are responsible for the ulnar-sided wrist symptoms of pain, weakness, and instability that affect function. The diagnosis and treatment of these injuries to the TFCC will restore stability, resulting in pain relief and a good prognosis for return of function.

Anatomy

The TFCC is a cartilaginous and ligamentous structure interposed between the ulnar carpus and the distal ulna (**Fig. 26-1**). It arises from the distal aspect of the sigmoid notch of the radius and inserts into the base of the ulnar styloid. The TFCC attaches to the ulnar carpus via the ulnocarpal ligament complex (ulnolunate, ulnotriquetral, and ulnar collateral ligaments).[1-3] The radioulnar ligaments stabilize the DRUJ, limiting rotational as well as axial migration.[4] The dorsal and volar radioulnar ligaments (**Fig. 26-2**) are fibrous thickenings within the substance of the TFCC. As a result of this anatomical configuration, they function as a unit rather than as independent ligaments. The central, horizontal portion of the TFCC is the thinnest portion, composed of interwoven obliquely oriented sheets of collagen fibers[5] for the resistance of multidirectional stress.

The vascularity of the TFCC has been carefully studied.[5-7] The TFCC receives its blood supply from the ulnar artery through its radiocarpal branches and the dorsal and palmar branches of the anterior interosseous artery (**Fig. 26-3**). These vessels supply the TFCC in a radial fashion. Histologic sections demonstrate that these vessels penetrate only the peripheral 10% to 40% of the TFCC. The central section and radial attachment is avascular (**Fig. 26-4**). This vascular anatomy supports the concept that peripheral injuries possess the ability to heal if injured and treated appropriately, whereas the tears of the central portion do not heal if sutured and are usually débrided.

Biomechanics

The TFCC has several important biomechanical functions. It transmits 20% of an axially applied load from the ulnar carpus to the distal ulna, it is the major stabilizer of the DRUJ, and it is a stabilizer of the ulnar carpus.[3,8-12]

The amount of the load transferred to the distal ulna varies with ulnar variance. A greater amount is transferred in ulnar-positive variance than ulnar-negative variance. This results in a corresponding decreased thickness of the central portion of the TFCC in ulnar-positive wrists.[10] In addition, there is a variable load placed on the TFCC with forearm rotation. Supination causes ulnar-negative variance owing to the proximal migration of the ulna. This is reversed with pronation as the ulna moves distally, causing it to become ulnar positive.[13] The ulnar head also moves within the sigmoid notch in a dorsal direction with pronation and volar with supination.[8] The dorsal and volar radioulnar ligaments that form the peripheral portion of the TFCC become tight with forearm rotation, serving as major stabilizers of the DRUJ, which control this translation during rotation.[9]

Mechanism of Injury

Traumatic injuries of the TFCC result from the application of an extension/pronation force to the axially loaded wrist or by a distraction force to the ulnar aspect of the wrist.[1,14] This will most commonly occur with a fall on the outstretched hand. The lesions are more common with ulnar-positive and ulnar-neutral patients and are commonly found in those patients being treated for fractures of the distal radius.

Several authors have examined the incidence of intracarpal soft tissue injuries associated with distal radial fractures. Geissler and coworkers[15] studied 60 patients, finding a TFCC injury in 26 (43%). In Lindau and colleagues' series of 51 patients,[16] a TFCC injury was found in 43 (84%): 24 had a peripheral tear, 10 had a central perforation, and 9 had a combined central and peripheral tear. Richards and associates in their series of 118 patients[17] reported a TFCC injury in 35% of the patients with intra-articular fractures and 53% of those with extra-articular fractures.

Classification

The classification system described by Palmer[1] is the most useful for describing TFCC injuries that are both traumatic and degenerative. Only traumatic lesions are discussed here.

Traumatic lesions are classified according to the location of the tear within the TFCC. The traumatic class has been designated by Palmer as class 1 with subclasses of A, B, C, and D assigned to anatomical lesions within the TFCC.

A class 1A lesion represents a tear in the horizontal or central portion of the TFCC (**Fig. 26-5A**). The tear is 2 to 3 mm medial to the radial attachment of the cartilage. It is usually oriented from dorsal to volar.

A class 1B lesion (see Fig. 26-5B) is an avulsion of the peripheral aspect of the TFCC from its insertion onto the distal ulna. This can occur either with a fracture of the ulnar styloid or as a pure avulsion from its bony attachment. This type of injury disrupts the stabilizing effect of the TFCC on the DRUJ, resulting in clinical instability.

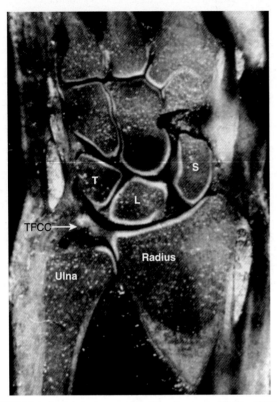

FIGURE 26-1 Anatomical coronal section demonstrating the TFCC and relation to the lunate (L), triquetrum (T), scaphoid (S), and distal ulna and radius. *(From Palmer AK, Werner FW: The triangular fibrocartilage complex of the wrist—anatomy and function. J Hand Surg. 1981; 6A:154.)*

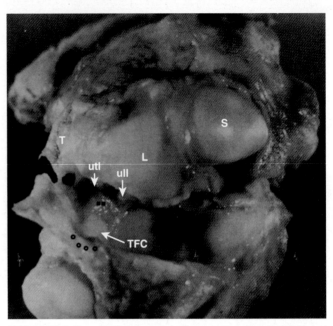

FIGURE 26-2 Dorsally disarticulated wrist demonstrating the TFCC and its volar ulnocarpal ligaments: ulnolunate ligament (ull), ulnotriquetral ligament (utl), and the dorsal radioulnar ligament (*four circles*). T, triquetrum; L, lunate; S, scaphoid. *(From Palmer AK: Triangular fibrocartilage complex lesions: a classification. J Hand Surg. 1989; 14A:595.)*

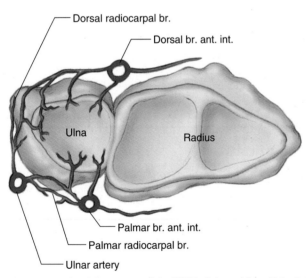

FIGURE 26-3 Arterial anatomy of the TFCC. *(Adapted from Thiru-Pathi RG, Ferlic DC, Clayton ML, et al: Arterial anatomy of the triangular fibrocartilage of the wrist and its surgical significance. J Hand Surg. 1986; 11A:261.)*

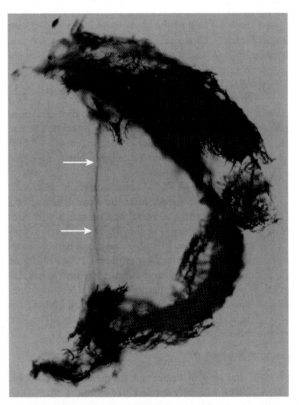

FIGURE 26-4 Axial view of the TFCC demonstrating the vascular supply to the periphery and avascular radial attachment (*arrows*). *(From Bednar MS, Arnoczky SP, Weiland AJ: The microvasculature of the triangular fibrocartilage complex: its clinical significance. J Hand Surg. 1991; 16A:1103.)*

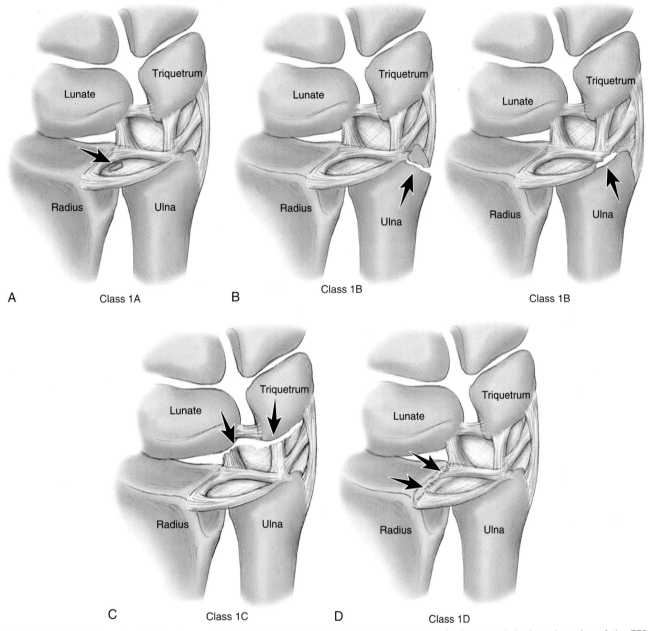

FIGURE 26-5 **A,** Palmer classification for acute TFCC injuries. Class 1A lesion involves a tear in the central, horizontal portion of the TFCC. **B,** Class 1B lesion is a tear of the TFCC from the distal ulna with or without an ulnar styloid fracture. **C,** Class 1C lesion is a tear of the TFCC distal attachment to the lunate and triquetrum through the ulnolunate and ulnotriquetral ligaments. **D,** Class 1D lesion is a detachment of the TFCC from its insertion onto the radius at the distal sigmoid notch. *(Adapted from Palmer AK: Triangular fibrocartilage complex lesions: a classification. J Hand Surg. 1989; 14A:601.)*

A class 1C lesion (see Fig. 26-5C) is an avulsion of the TFCC attachment to the ulnar carpus by disruption of the ulnocarpal ligaments. This lesion will result in ulnar carpal instability with volar translocation of the carpus.

A class 1D lesion (see Fig. 26-5D) is an avulsion of the TFCC from its radial attachment. Involvement of the dorsal and or volar radioulnar ligaments will result in instability of the DRUJ.

Diagnosis

Clinical symptoms consist of ulnar-sided wrist pain frequently with clicking and typically occur after a fall. The initial physical examination reveals swelling over the ulnar aspect of the wrist with inflammation of the tendon of the extensor carpi ulnaris. Point tenderness is present over the TFCC and distal ulna. Ulnar deviation and axial loading of the wrist (TFCC compression test) (**Fig. 26-6**) will elicit a painful response. A click is frequently present with forearm rotation. The DRUJ must be assessed for instability. Instability is best assessed with the forearm in neutral rotation, but it is also checked in full supination and full pronation. The examiner stabilizes the distal radius with one hand and applies a force to the distal ulna, moving it dorsal and volar in a search for increased motion or subluxation of the distal ulna relative to the radius compared with the opposite uninjured wrist. Significant instability would present as laxity of the distal ulna

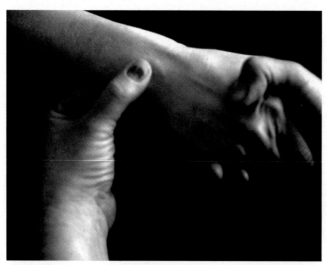

FIGURE 26-6 TFCC compression test: ulnar deviation and axial load applied to wrist produces a painful response.

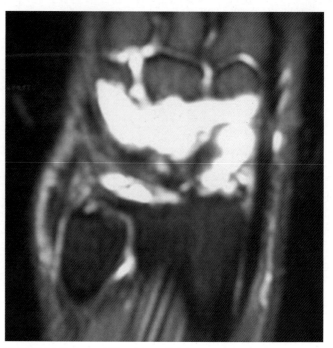

FIGURE 26-7 Coronal T2-weighted MR image of the wrist. High signal of the joint fluid outlines the low signal substance of the TFCC. Tears will show as high signal intensity within the TFCC periphery or central region.

with a positive "piano key" sign and dorsal prominence of the distal ulna. This would represent a significant tear or detachment of the dorsal or volar radioulnar ligaments.

TFCC injuries do not occur in isolation but are a component of a spectrum of injury to the ulnar side of the wrist.[18] The examiner must therefore evaluate all of the commonly injured structures on the ulnar side of the wrist. The lunatotriquetral joint must be assessed for instability due to a lunatotriquetral ligament tear. This would cause tenderness over the lunatotriquetral interval with a positive shuck test. The dorsal radial carpal ligament complex should be examined to determine if traumatic midcarpal instability is present.

The differential diagnosis for ulnar-sided wrist pain consistent with a TFCC tear would include extensor carpi ulnaris subluxation, lunatotriquetral ligament injury, triquetral avulsion fracture, pisotriquetral arthritis, ulnar artery thrombosis, neuritis of the dorsal ulnar sensory nerve, and ulnar neuropathy at Guyon's canal. It is a common finding that one or more of these diagnoses are present in addition to the TFCC injury.

Imaging

The diagnostic workup should include plain radiography to include a neutral rotation posteroanterior and a lateral view. This will allow assessment for fracture, ligament instability resulting in carpal malalignment, as well as determination of ulnar variance. The determination of ulnar variance is important in that it will influence treatment options. The DRUJ must also be examined radiographically to determine if subluxation, arthritis, or ulnar styloid abnormalities such as an acute or chronic nonunited fracture fragment are present.

Magnetic resonance imaging (MRI) is useful in the diagnosis of TFCC tears, especially the class 1A and D lesions.[19,20] T2-weighted MR images in the coronal plane are of the greatest diagnostic value (**Fig. 26-7**). The TFCC has a homogeneous low signal intensity. The synovial fluid of the joint appears as a bright image on T2-weighted images and will outline tears in the TFCC. The addition of a gadolinium arthrogram enhances the visualization of TFCC tears.

The series in the literature reviewing the sensitivity and specificity of MRI in diagnosing injuries of the TFCC show significant

variation in the reported results. Golimbu and coworkers[19] reported a 95% accuracy of MRI in the detection of TFCC tears. They studied 20 patients with the use of MRI. Fourteen of these patients had positive MR studies for TFCC pathology. These patients had surgical examination of the wrist confirming the TFCC pathologic process in 13 of the patients with a positive MRI. None of the patients with a negative MRI had a TFCC pathologic process found at the time of surgery. Schweitzer and associates[21] reported in 15 patients a sensitivity of 72%, specificity of 95%, and an accuracy of 89%. Zlatkin and colleagues[22] reported a sensitivity of 89%, specificity of 92%, and an accuracy of 90% in 23 patients. Potter and coworkers[23] reported a sensitivity of 100%, specificity of 90%, and an accuracy of 97% in 59 patients studied with a high-resolution magnet but they performed arthroscopy only in patients with a positive MRI and therefore could not determine how many patients with a clinical diagnosis of a TFCC injury but a negative MRI had a pathologic process of the TFCC.

Bednar and coworkers[24] reported on a series of 75 wrists in 70 patients with a diagnosis of TFCC injury based on clinical criteria. All patients had an MRI examination read by an experienced bone radiologist and then had wrist arthroscopy. The arthroscopic findings were correlated with the MRI and clinical examination. Seventy-one (95%) of the 75 wrists with a clinical diagnosis of TFCC pathology were confirmed to have a TFCC tear by arthroscopy. Thirty-four (48%) had a central tear, 33 (46%) had a peripheral tear, and 4 (6%) had both a central and a peripheral tear. Comparing the arthroscopic with the MRI findings produced 31 (44%) with positive arthroscopic findings and a positive MRI and 40 (56%) with positive arthroscopic findings but a negative MRI; and one of the four wrists with negative findings on arthroscopy had a positive MRI. Correlating TFCC tear type with MRI showed 34 central tears with 19 (56%) MRI positive, 33 peripheral tears with 11 (33%) MRI positive, and 4 central and peripheral tears with 1 (25%) MRI positive. This study produced an MRI sensitivity of 44% (sensitivity is the probability of a positive MRI when a TFCC lesion is present). The clinical examination sensitivity was 95%. If the patients are evaluated using the criteria employed by Potter, the Bednar and coworkers' study had 32 wrists with a positive MRI, of which 31 were positive by arthroscopy. The sensitivity for this subgroup of MRI-positive patients was 97%. The MRI specificity in the Bednar and coworkers' study was 75% (specificity is the probability of a negative MRI when a TFCC lesion is absent). The MRI correlated with arthroscopic findings in 45% of the wrists studied.

Joshy and colleagues[25] reported a series of 24 patients with a clinical suspicion of TFCC tear studied by direct MR arthrography and then wrist arthroscopy. They found the MR arthrography to have a sensitivity of 74%, specificity of 80%, and accuracy of 79% in detecting a full-thickness TFCC tear. They caution that negative results of MR arthrography in patients with clinical suspicion of TFCC tear should be interpreted with caution.

Conservative Treatment

The treatment of acute TFCC injuries is initially conservative by immobilization of the wrist and DRUJ. The patient must be examined carefully to look for instability of the DRUJ or radiocarpal joint. Routine radiographs should be obtained to detect a fracture or subluxation of the distal ulna. If the radiographs are negative and instability is not present, then immobilization for 4 to 6 weeks is recommended to allow healing of the TFCC disruption. A peripheral tear would be expected to heal if the torn edges are held in close contact, owing to the good vascularity of the periphery of the TFCC. Many central tears also become asymptomatic with immobilization even though there is no significant vascularity to the central portion. Mikic[26] examined the TFCC in 180 cadavers ranging in age from infant to 97 years old. He found no TFCC perforations in those wrists of individuals younger than 30 years of age. A linear progression of perforations with age was present over time such that all specimens in individuals over age 50 were found to have a TFCC perforation. This supports the concept that a defect in the central portion of the TFCC can occur without symptoms. It is those tears involving the ligamentous portion of the TFCC or those that heal with a flap of cartilage that impinges on the carpus or distal ulna that will clinically fail conservative treatment and require further treatment.

Surgical Treatment

Those patients who present acutely with instability by clinical and/or radiographic criteria should be treated by arthroscopic evaluation with TFCC and ligament repair.

Those patients who remain symptomatic after adequate immobilization should be subjected to further workup to include MR arthrography and be treated arthroscopically.

The specific treatment for each class 1 lesion is determined by the type of tear found arthroscopically.

Class 1A lesions are isolated stable central tears of the TFCC (**Fig. 26-8**). In patients with ulnar-neutral or ulnar-negative variance, who have failed conservative treatment, arthroscopic limited débridement of the central portion of the tear will give excellent relief of symptoms.[27] The biomechanical effect of excision of the central portion of the TFCC has been examined.[12,28,29] The excision of the central two thirds of the TFCC with maintenance of the dorsal and volar radioulnar ligaments as well as the ulnocarpal ligaments had no statistically significant effect on forearm axial

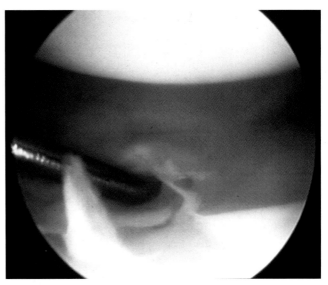

FIGURE 26-8 Arthroscopic view of a Palmer class 1A central tear.

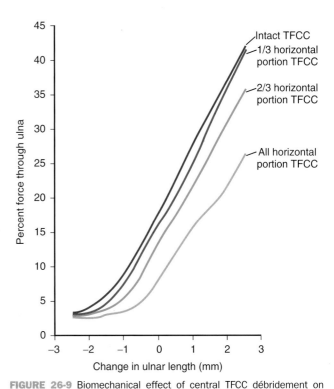

FIGURE 26-9 Biomechanical effect of central TFCC débridement on load transfer. (*Adapted from Palmer AK: The distal radioulnar joint: anatomy, biomechanics, and triangular fibrocartilage complex abnormalities. Hand Clin. 1987; 3:39.*)

load transmission (**Fig. 26-9**). The removal of more than two thirds will unload the ulnar column, shifting load to the distal radius and destabilizing the DRUJ.[12] Adams further emphasized that the peripheral 2 mm of the TFCC must be maintained during central débridement to not have a biomechanical effect on load transfer.[28]

Arthroscopic débridement is performed by insertion of the arthroscope through the 3-4 portal to visualize the tear and by insertion of a small punch and shaver through the 6R portal to trim the tear (**Fig. 26-10**). The dorsal ulnar portion of the TFCC

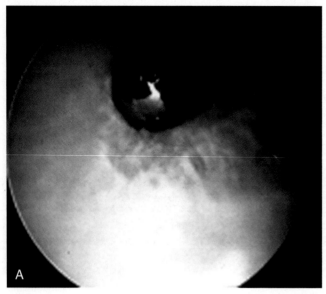
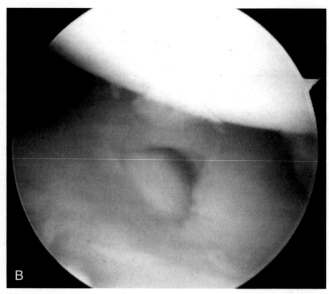

FIGURE 26-10 **A,** Arthroscopic débridement of a Palmer class 1A central tear. **B,** Débridement of the central one third of the TFCC produces a stable rim.

cannot be trimmed from the 6R portal using a punch. It can be trimmed using a small arthroscopic knife or the edge of an 18-gauge needle, raising a flap sufficient for the punch to trim. The alternative solution is to switch the scope to the 6R portal and use the punch through the 3-4 portal to accomplish the trimming of the ulnar portion of the tear.

Patients with central tears who are ulnar positive or who demonstrate chondromalacia may have degenerative lesions with an overlying acute tear. These lesions are best treated by limited débridement and ulnar recession by wafer resection or ulnar shortening osteotomy.

Class 1B lesions without an ulnar styloid fracture and a stable DRUJ can be immobilized for 4 weeks in a cast. If an ulnar styloid fracture is present, closed reduction should be attempted. If adequate reduction is achieved, then cast immobilization is sufficient. If the styloid remains displaced, then open reduction and internal fixation is required. The ulnar styloid fracture is best approached through the sixth compartment. The distal one third of the retinaculum is longitudinally divided. The extensor carpi ulnaris tendon is retracted, taking care not to disrupt the subsheath. The ulnar styloid fracture will be visible once the tendon is retracted. It can be mobilized by a longitudinal incision in the periosteum. The fracture is reduced by ulnar deviation and slight supination. Fixation is performed by either longitudinal Kirschner wire, screw, or tension band. If the ulnar styloid is comminuted and will not hold a fixation device, it should be excised and the TFCC attached to the ulna by a suture placed through drill holes in the ulna proximal to the fracture. The suture should be placed in the periphery of the TFCC under arthroscopic guidance to confirm proper placement of the suture and restoration of proper TFCC tension.

A peripheral avulsion of the TFCC should be ruled out in all patients treated for a distal radial fracture and treated in a manner similar to an isolated lesion.

Class 1B lesions that are present in the chronic stage of more than 3 months after injury require arthroscopic evaluation. A peripheral tear that involves the dorsal radioulnar ligament can easily be repaired by arthroscopic means. This is performed by a

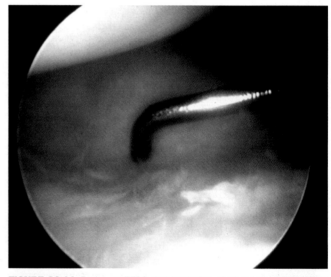

FIGURE 26-11 Probe on TFCC demonstrates absent trampoline effect indicating a peripheral TFCC detachment.

two-needle technique similar to that employed for the repair of a knee meniscus. Initial arthroscopic evaluation may not show a discrete tear of the TFCC periphery. A probe placed through the 6R portal will demonstrate loss of the normal trampoline effect of the TFCC, indicating a peripheral tear and loss of mechanical function (**Fig. 26-11**). Synovitis and thin scar will be seen along the periphery of the TFCC at the location of the tear. A shaver will easily débride the synovium and scar to demonstrate the tear (**Fig. 26-12**). Adhesions will be present between the undersurface of the TFCC and the distal ulna. These must be released and the TFC mobilized sufficiently to allow advancement to reattach it and to restore proper tension. Failure to adequately débride and mobilize the chronic TFCC tear will prevent an adequate repair. After débridement, two hollow needles are passed across the tear

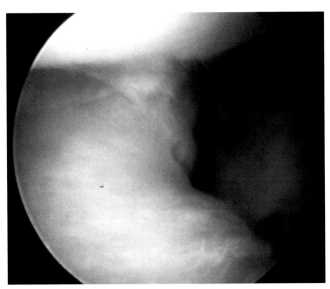

FIGURE 26-12 Arthroscopic view of a Palmer class 1B peripheral TFCC tear.

percutaneously under arthroscopic vision (**Fig. 26-13**). A wire loop is passed through one needle to retrieve a 2-0 PDS suture, which is passed through the other needle. This allows the passage of a horizontal mattress-type suture across the tear. We prefer a horizontal type of suture for TFCC repair. Many other authors have reported good results using multiple simple vertical sutures placed at the periphery of the TFCC. As the suture is drawn tight it approximates the tear and restores tension to the TFCC. The suture can be tied under the skin, over the dorsal wrist capsule, or out of the skin over a bolster. The patient is immobilized in a long arm cast for 4 to 6 weeks before restarting rotational motion and suture removal. Those patients with a nonunited ulnar styloid fragment and instability of the DRUJ due to the disruption of the TFCC require open reattachment of the styloid fragment or excision of the fragment and reattachment of the TFCC to the remaining proximal ulna.

Class 1C lesions involve a disruption of the ulnocarpal ligament complex (**Fig. 26-14**). Those tears that do not heal with immobilization require operative repair to stabilize the ulnar carpus. Peripheral tears that involve the volar radioulnar ligaments or the ulnocarpal ligament complex can be repaired arthroscopically with limited open exposure to retract the ulnar nerve and artery (**Fig. 26-15**). The success rate for open repair is 80% to 85% good and excellent results.[30,31]

Class 1D lesions involve the radial detachment of the TFCC from the sigmoid notch of the distal radius. The treatment of these lesions remains controversial. There appears to be no vascularity to this portion of the TFCC. Theoretically, a reattached cartilage would not heal at this repair site. Clinical experience with open repair of these tears, however, has been good.[31] This may be attributed to vascular ingrowth from the radial insertion site, which occurs with abrasion of the attachment site, stimulating the formation of new vessels. The tear needs to be assessed arthroscopically to determine its extent. If the radial tear includes disruption of one or both of the radioulnar ligaments, repair is required to prevent chronic instability of the DRUJ.

Short[32] has described an arthroscopic technique for repair of class 1D lesions. The arthroscope is placed in the 3-4 portal. A bur is placed through the 6R portal to roughen the radial attach-

ment of the TFCC. A 0.062-inch Kirschner wire is used to predrill two holes for the placement of the repair suture. The wires need to exit the radius on the radial side just volar to the first extensor compartment. An incision is made to retract the radial sensory nerve and the tendons of the first extensor compartment. A cannula is placed in the 6R portal through which a meniscal repair suture (suture with a long straight needle at each end) is passed through the radial aspect of the TFCC in a horizontal mattress fashion with each needle passing through the predrilled holes in the radius. The suture is tied over the radius.

The placement of the needles into the predrilled holes can be challenging because the holes are not visible by the scope in the 3-4 portal. Two 18-gauge spinal needles can be placed from the radial side of the radius through the bone until they can be seen in the joint at the attachment site for the TFCC. The needles provide a visible target for the meniscal repair suture needles. If the meniscal repair suture needles are not available, the 18-gauge needles can be passed directly through the radial attachment site of the TFCC. A 2-0 PDS suture is then passed from one 18-gauge needle to the other using a wire retrieval loop, the needles are removed, and the suture is tied over the radius.

Results

The results of arthroscopic repair of class 1B TFCC lesions are equivalent to those reported for open repair. Hermansdorfer and Kleinman[30] reported the results of open repair in 11 patients, with 8 of 11 having complete pain relief and grip strength return to 87% of normal. Cooney and colleagues[31] reported the results of open repair in 33 patients evaluated using the Mayo Modified Wrist Score. The average score was 83, with 11 excellent, 15 good, 6 fair, and 1 poor result. Bednar[33] reported the results of arthroscopic repair of a class 1B lesion in 40 wrists assessed by the Mayo Modified Wrist Score. The average score was 86, with 11 excellent, 22 good, 6 fair, and 1 poor result.

Trumble and associates[34] reported the results of arthroscopic repair in 24 wrists (9 1B, 2 1C, and 13 1D lesions). The average postoperative grip strength was 85%, with 89% excellent or good, 11% fair, and 0% poor results. Corso and coworkers[35] reported the results of a multicenter study evaluating 45 wrists from three institutions: 27 of the 45 wrists had other associated injuries (4 with distal radial fracture, 7 with scapholunate ligament injury, 9 with lunatotriquetral ligament injury, 2 with ulnocarpal ligament injury, and 2 with radiocarpal ligament injury). All TFCC injuries were repaired arthroscopically. The patients were evaluated by the Mayo Modified Wrist Score with 29 excellent, 12 good, 1 fair, and 3 poor results.

The treatment of class 1B TFCC tears in an ulnar-positive patient is determined by history and arthroscopic findings. If the patient reports an acute injury in a previously asymptomatic wrist and arthroscopic evaluation demonstrates an acute peripheral tear with no arthroscopic findings of ulnar abutment (chronic central tear, osteochondral lesion on the ulnar aspect of the lunate), then an arthroscopic repair of the TFCC is performed. Note that the long ulna will decrease the available working space in the joint between the TFCC and the carpus, which will increase the technical difficulty of passing the repair suture. Bednar[36] presented the results of arthroscopic repair of a class 1B lesion in an ulnar-positive wrist in 20 patients assessed by the Mayo Modified Wrist Score. The average score was 83, with 5 excellent, 9 good, 5 fair, and 1 poor result. The average grip strength was 73% of normal. If there is a history of ulnar abutment type symptom before acute tear and arthroscopic evaluation demonstrates evidence of ulnar

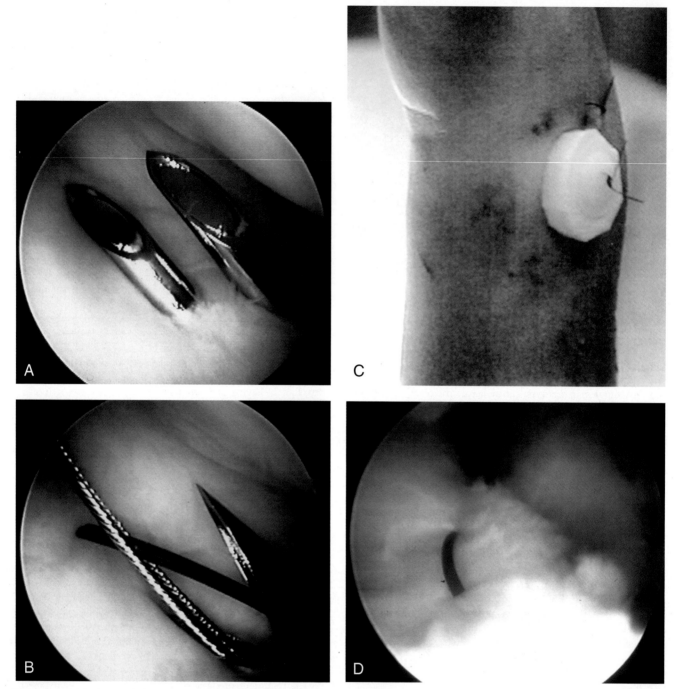

FIGURE 26-13 Arthroscopic repair of a Palmer class 1B peripheral TFCC tear. **A,** Two hollow needles passed across the tear. **B,** Wire loop in one needle used to pass 2-0 suture across tear. **C,** Suture tied over bolster. **D,** Suture approximates tear and restores tension to TFCC.

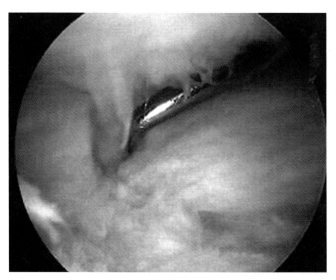

FIGURE 26-14 Arthroscopic view of a Palmer class 1C tear.

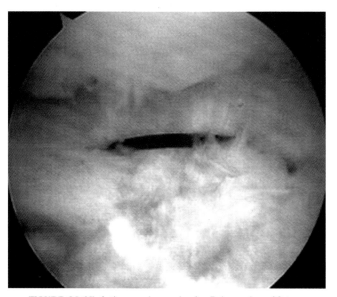

FIGURE 26-15 Arthroscopic repair of a Palmer class 1C tear.

abutment in addition to an acute TFCC injury, then, in addition to TFCC repair, ulnar shortening osteotomy is recommended. Trumble and associates[37] reported the results of arthroscopic TFCC repair with ulnar-shortening osteotomy in 21 patients (9 1B, 2 1C, 10 1D lesions) with 90% pain relief and grip strengths of 81% of normal.

Short[32] reported 79% excellent and good results in his series, with return of grip strength to 90% after an arthroscopic repair of a radial TFCC tear.

If the radial tear does not involve the radioulnar ligaments it is not destabilizing, and débridement of the central one to two thirds of the TFCC is recommended. Osterman[38] reported a series of 19 patients with radial TFCC tears. All tears were chronic, and no patient had instability of the DRUJ. Ten patients were treated with arthroscopic débridement and 9 with arthroscopic repair. Eighty percent of the débridement group and 67% of the repair group were asymptomatic at follow-up. The data suggested that débridement of the radial TFCC tear was equally effective to repair in the patients with no instability.

Summary

Injuries to the TFCC result in incapacitating ulnar-sided wrist pain in many patients who have sustained a pronation/extension injury to the wrist or a traction injury to the ulnar side of the wrist. Early diagnosis and immobilization in those patients with no instability of the carpus or DRUJ will result in the rapid resolution of symptoms and return to function in the majority of patients. Those patients with clinical instability should be acutely treated with arthroscopic evaluation and stabilization. Those patients with persistent symptoms despite adequate conservative treatment require further evaluation by MR arthrogram. A TFCC lesion repaired by arthroscopic treatment will result in 80% to 85% good to excellent results with relief of pain and return to work or sports activities without restriction.

REFERENCES

1. Palmer AK: Triangular fibrocartilage complex lesions: a classification. J Hand Surg [Am]. 1989; 14:594-606.
2. Palmer AK: Triangular fibrocartilage disorders: injury patterns and treatment. Arthroscopy. 1990; 6:125-132.
3. Palmer AK, Werner FW: The triangular fibrocartilage complex of the wrist—anatomy and function. J Hand Surg [Am]. 1981; 6:153-162.
4. Schuind F, An KN, Berglund L, et al: The distal radioulnar ligaments: a biomechanical study. J Hand Surg [Am]. 1991; 16:1106-1114.
5. Chidgey LK: Histologic anatomy of the triangular fibrocartilage. Hand Clin. 1991; (2):249-262.
6. Bednar MS, Arnoczky SP, Weiland AJ: The microvasculature of the triangular fibrocartilage complex: its clinical significance. J Hand Surg [Am]. 1991; 16:1101-1105.
7. Thiru-Pathi RG, Ferlic DC, Clayton ML, et al: Arterial anatomy of the triangular fibrocartilage of the wrist and its surgical significance. J Hand Surg [Am]. 1986; 11:258-263.
8. Ekenstein FW, Palmer AK, Glisson RR: The load on the radius and ulna in different positions of the wrist and forearm. Acta Orthop Scand. 1984; 55:363-365.
9. Palmer AK: The distal radioulnar joint. In Taleisnik J, ed: Hand Clinics—Management of Wrist Problems. Philadelphia: WB Saunders, 1987; 3:31-40.
10. Palmer AK, Glisson RR, Werner FW: Relationship between ulnar variance and TFCC thickness. J Hand Surg [Am]. 1984; 9:681-683.
11. Palmer AK, Werner FW: Biomechanics of the distal radioulnar joint. Clin Orthop Relat Res. 1984; 187:26-34.
12. Palmer AK, Werner FW, Glisson RR, et al: Partial excision of the triangular fibrocartilage complex. J Hand Surg [Am]. 1988; 13:391-394.
13. Palmer AK, Glisson RR, Werner FW: Ulnar variance determination. J Hand Surg [Am]. 1982; 7:376-379.
14. Coleman HM: Injuries of the articular disc at the wrist. J Bone Joint Surg Br. 1960; 42:552-559.
15. Geissler WB, Freeland AE, Savoie FH, et al: Intracarpal soft-tissue lesions associated with an intra-articular fracture of the distal end of the radius. J Bone Joint Surg Am. 1996; 78:357-365.
16. Lindau T, Adlercreutz C, Aspenberg P: Peripheral tears of

the triangular fibrocartilage complex cause distal radioulnar joint instability after distal radial fracture. J Hand Surg [Am]. 2000; 25:464-468.

17. Richards RS, Bennett JD, Roth JH, Milne K Jr: Arthroscopic diagnosis of intra-articular soft tissue injuries associated with distal radial fractures. J Hand Surg [Am]. 1997; 22(5):772-776.

18. Melone CP Jr, Nathan R: Traumatic disruption of the triangular fibrocartilage complex: pathoanatomy. Clin Orthop Relat Res. 1992; 275:65-73.

19. Golimbu CN, Firooznia H, Melone CP Jr, et al: Tears of the triangular fibrocartilage of the wrist: MR imaging. Radiology. 1989; 173:731-733.

20. Skahen JR, Palmer AK, Levinsohn EM, et al: Magnetic resonance imaging of the triangular fibrocartilage complex. J. Hand Surg [Am]. 1990; 15: 552-557.

21. Schweitzer ME, Brahme SK, Hodler J, et al: Chronic wrist pain: spin-echo and short tau inversion recovery MR imaging and conventional and MR arthrography. Radiology. 1992; 182:205-211.

22. Zlatkin MB, Chao PC, Osterman AL, et al: Chronic wrist pain: evaluation with high-resolution MR imaging. Radiology. 1989; 173:723-729.

23. Potter HG, Asnis-Ernberg L, Weiland AJ, et al: The utility of high-resolution magnetic resonance imaging in the evaluation of the triangular fibrocartilage complex of the wrist. J Bone Joint Surg [Am]. 1997; 79:1675-1684.

24. Bednar JM, Bos M, Giacobetti F: Comparison of the accuracy of clinical exam and MRI in diagnosing TFCC lesions. Presented before the 52nd annual meeting of the American Society for Surgery of the Hand, Denver, CO, September 11, 1997.

25. Joshy S, Lee K, Deshmukh SC: Accuracy of direct magnetic resonance arthrography in the diagnosis of triangular fibrocartilage complex tears of the wrist. Int Orthop. 2008; 32:251-253. Epub 2007; Jan 11.

26. Mikic ZD: Age changes in the triangular fibrocartilage of the wrist joint. J Anat. 1978; 126:367-384.

27. Osterman AL: Arthroscopic debridement of triangular fibrocartilage complex tears. Arthroscopy. 1990; 6(2):120-124.

28. Adams BD: Partial excision of the triangular fibrocartilage complex articular disk: a biomechanical study. J Hand Surg [Am]. 1993; 18:334-340.

29. Menon J, Wood VE, Schoene HR, et al: Isolated tears of the triangular fibrocartilage of the wrist: results of partial excision. J Hand Surg [Am]. 1984; 9:527-530.

30. Hermansdorfer JD, Kleinman WB: Management of chronic peripheral tears of the triangular fibrocartilage complex. J Hand Surg [Am]. 1991; 16:340-346.

31. Cooney WP, Linscheid RL, Dobyns JH: Triangular fibrocartilage tears. J Hand Surg [Am]. 1994; 19:143-154.

32. Short WH: Arthroscopic repair of radial-sided triangular fibrocartilage complex tears. J Am Soc Surg of the Hand. 2001; 1:258-266.

33. Bednar JM: Arthroscopic repair of peripheral tears of the triangular fibrocartilage complex. Presented before the American Academy of Orthopaedic Surgeons. Atlanta, GA, February 23, 1996.

34. Trumble TE, Gilbert M, Vedder N: Isolated tears of the triangular fibrocartilage: management by early arthroscopic repair. J Hand Surg [Am]. 1997; 22:57-65.

35. Corso SJ, Savoie FH, Geissler WB, et al: Arthroscopic repair of peripheral avulsions of the triangular fibrocartilage complex of the wrist: a multicenter study. Arthroscopy 1997; 13:78-84.

36. Bednar JM: Arthroscopic TFCC repair in the ulna positive wrist. Presented before the International Federation of the Society of Surgery of the Hand, Vancouver, BC, Canada, May 25, 1998.

37. Trumble TE, Gilbert M, Vedder N: Ulnar shortening combined with arthroscopic repairs in the delayed management of triangular fibrocartilage complex tears. J Hand Surg [Am]. 1997; 22:807-813.

38. Osterman AL: Radial triangular fibrocartilage tears: debride or repair? Presented at the ASSH/ASHT annual meeting, San Antonio, TX, September 23, 2005.

Anatomy and Biomechanics of Forearm Rotation

27

Michael Sauerbier, MD and Frank Unglaub, MD

Evolution

Pronation and supination are rotational motions that exist exclusively in the forearm. The mechanical bases for these movements are the existence of two forearm bones and the presence of two coupled trochoid joints—the proximal and distal radioulnar joints (PRUJ and DRUJ).[1] Two bones at the forearm are an inheritance from a remote ancestor, the icthyostega, a crossopterygian tetrapod that sprang up from the sea 300 million years ago, transforming its fins into members.[2] This unique ability to transfer rotational force to the grasping hand must have played a decisive role in the human evolution.[3] Two bones in comparison to one bone with one joint bring advantages—no tendon, nerve, and vessel twisting at the wrist with decreased function. Furthermore, only two bones at the forearm provide a wide range of motion but stable and light construction.[4]

The DRUJ and PRUJ together work as a single "forearm joint," resulting in pronation/supination. Hagert[5] compared the montages of the forearm with a ventral view of the leg. The proximal ulnar and distal radial segments create a unit similar to the tibia. The olecranon resembles the patella fused with the tuberosity of the tibia; the radial styloid resembles the medial malleolus at the ankle. The proximal radial and distal ulnar segments create a unit reminiscent of the fibula with the ulnar styloid resembling the lateral malleolus.

Anatomy
Distal Radioulnar Joint

The DRUJ consists of two parts: the radioulnar articulation and the ulnoligamentous articulation. The border between these two components is defined as the ulnar extension of a line along the subchondral bone of the distal radius. The articular surface of the distal radius toward the ulnar head is the sigmoid notch, and the corresponding surface of the ulnar head constitutes the seat of the joint.[6] The sigmoid notch is a shallow concave articular surface for the ulnar head; it is convex proximally and concave distally, where it meets the lunate facet on its medial surface.[7] The radius and ulna are constrained from proximal to distal by the annular ligament, interosseous membrane (IOM), and triangular fibrocartilage (TFC) (**Fig. 27-1**).[7] There is a variation in the relative lengths of the forearm bones, as measured at the wrist. By convention, an ulnar-neutral variance is one in which the distal cortical surface of the ulnar pole is level with the cortical surface of the most proximal aspect of the lunate fossa. This is measured perpendicular to the longitudinal axis of the forearm when the radiograph is taken with the forearm and wrist in neutral extension and neutral deviation and with the x-ray tube perpendicular to the plane of the radiocarpal joint.[7] An ulnar-negative variance

indicates an ulna that is shorter than the lunate fossa of the radius and an ulnar-positive variance indicates an ulna that is longer. Although most forearms are within 2 mm of a positive variance and 4 mm of a negative variance, pathological conditions are more prevalent at the extremes.[8] The shape of the ulnar head depends on the lengths of the ulna and radius. If the ulna is shorter than the radius (ulnar negative), the ulnar head is cone shaped. If the ulna and radius are similar in length, the ulnar head is cylindrical (ulnar neutral). If the ulna is longer than the radius (ulnar positive), the ulnar head is spherical (**Fig. 27-2**).[9,10]

Aside from the seat, the ulnar head articulates with the TFC.[7] The triangular fibrocartilage complex (TFCC) consists of the dorsal and palmar radioulnar ligaments, the meniscus homologue, and the articular disc. The dorsal radioulnar ligament attaches to the dorsal rim of the distal radius at the level of the sigmoid notch and courses obliquely ulnarly and anteriorly to insert with the palmar radioulnar ligament into the fovea of the ulnar head and the styloid process. The palmar radioulnar ligament attaches radially to the palmar rim of the distal radius at the level of the sigmoid notch and courses obliquely ulnarly and dorsally to attach with the dorsoulnar ligament to the fovea of the ulnar head and the ulnar styloid process (**Fig. 27-3**).[11]

Interosseous Membrane

The IOM is a quadrangular sheath that extends from the radius to the ulna, filling the interosseous space. It links both bones of the forearm and also separates the anterior and the posterior

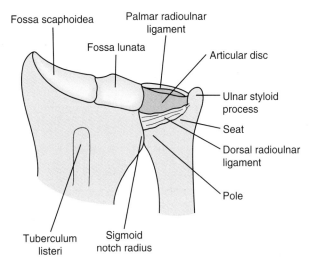

FIGURE 27-1 Distal radioulnar joint with its anatomical structures for stability.

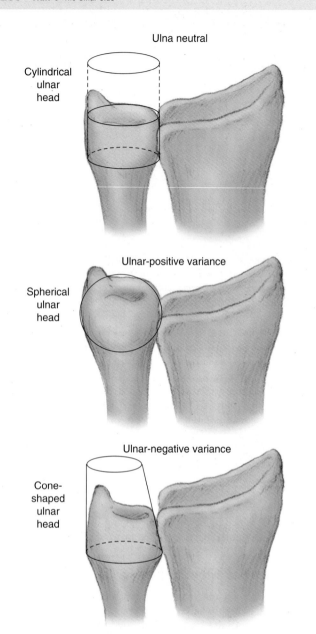

Ulna neutral

Cylindrical ulnar head

Ulnar-positive variance

Spherical ulnar head

Ulnar-negative variance

Cone-shaped ulnar head

FIGURE 27-2 Shaping of the ulnar head depends on the length of the bone and its different anatomical configurations.

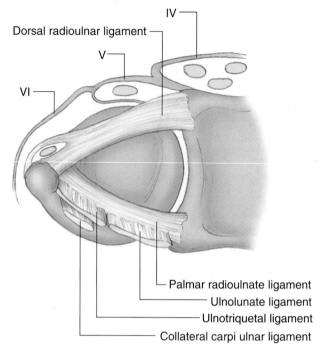

IV

Dorsal radioulnar ligament

V

VI

Palmar radioulnate ligament
Ulnolunate ligament
Ulnotriquetal ligament
Collateral carpi ulnar ligament

FIGURE 27-3 Different important ligaments for stabilization of the DRUJ.

compartments of the forearm. Proximally and distally the membrane is not continuous and is perforated by posterior and anterior interosseous vessels (**Fig. 27-4**).[1]

Fibers in the anterior plane run distally and obliquely from the medial border of the radius to the lateral border of the ulna. Three bundles are distinguished: the proximal descending fibers are almost horizontal, the intermediate descending fibers follow a short oblique direction, and the distal descending fibers have a long, oblique trajectory.[1] In the posterior plane, fibers run proximally and obliquely from the radius to the ulna. The proximal ascending bundle is short, oblique, and quite strong. It arises from the interosseous tubercle of the radius and ends at the proximal ulna. The distal ascending bundle is inconstant. Its direction is long oblique. It arises from the distal radius and reaches the proximal ulna.[1] Hotchkiss and coworkers studied the role of the IOM in preventing proximal migration of the radius. In their cadaver study, they found a discrete central band or thickening.[12] The

central band was responsible for 71% of the longitudinal stiffness of the forearm, whereas the TFCC was responsible for only 8%.

From the IOM of the forearm a tract extends to the dorsal capsule of the DRUJ. It originates from the radius 22 mm proximal to the distal dorsal corner of the sigmoid notch and inserts distally at the capsule of the DRUJ between the tendon sheaths of the extensor digiti minimi and extensor carpi ulnaris. The tract of the IOM is taut in pronation and loose in supination. It strengthens the dorsal capsule of the DRUJ, forming a sling that protects the ulnar head during pronation.[13]

Proximal Radioulnar Joint

The PRUJ is not a "hinge" but rather a ball-and-socket type of articulation.[5] The radial head has a 360-degree convex articulating surface. The head is ovoid rather than circular and is offset approximately 15 degrees from the longitudinal axis of the radius. Cartilage covers 240 degrees of the radial head, which articulates with the ulna at the PRUJ.

The stability of the PRUJ is excellent because the radial head is enclosed in a very strong osteoligamentous cavity that is made of the radial notch of the ulna and the annular ligament, which is a very resistant ligament (**Fig. 27-5**). There are rarely problems with the joint, except in fractures of the radial head.[4]

Biomechanics
Kinetics

The ulnar head moves in a rolling and sliding motion from the dorsal to the palmar rim of the sigmoid notch as the joint moves from pronation to supination.[7] From pronation to supination, the TFC is taut first dorsally and then palmarly in the same sequence.[7] The radius rotates around the ulnar head about a longitudinal axis that passes roughly through the center of the radial head at the PRUJ at the elbow to the fovea of the ulnar head at the level of the wrist (**Fig. 27-6**).[7] The axes of the two radioulnar joints must

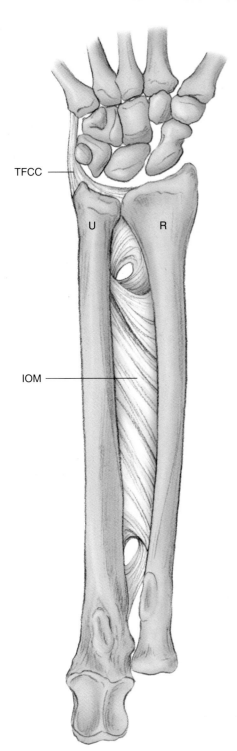

FIGURE 27-4 Forearm with important anatomical structures that contribute to the stability of the DRUJ. U, ulna; R, radius; TFCC, triangular fibrocartilage complex; IOM, interosseous membrane.

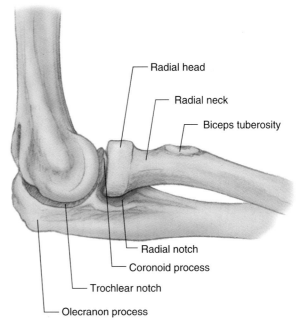

FIGURE 27-5 Proximal radioulnar joint with its anatomical structures for stability.

be aligned coaxially; if not, forearm rotation is blocked. Kapandji compared this situation with a door where two hinges of the door are not aligned; thus, the door cannot be opened.[4]

The ulnar variance depends on the length of both forearm bones (see earlier), as well as gripping and forearm rotation. The radius migrates proximally with forearm pronation, which increases ulnar variance.[14] Maximal ulnar variance is found when gripping with the forearm in pronation; minimal ulnar variance

occurs when the hand is relaxed and the forearm is in supination.[15] In the pronated position the radius becomes shorter than the ulna and the inferior aspect of the ulna head moves palmarward with regard to the lower rim of the radial sigmoid notch. When there is loss of radial height after a distal radius fracture, resulting in an ulnar-positive variance, pronation increases the impaction to the carpus, particularly the lunate and triquetrum.[4]

Rotation of the forearm allows the palm of the hand to be directed facing upward, medially, and downward while the elbow is flexed and anteriorly, medially, and posteriorly with an extended elbow. The total arc of rotation is close to 180 degrees. Rotation of the forearm associated with rotation of the shoulder allows for 270 degrees of rotation of the upper limb.[1] Because the seat of the ulna fills the sigmoid notch of the radius only in a sector of 90 to 135 degrees, increasing pronation and supination gradually diminishes the contact area. In maximal pronation or supination, the joint surfaces of the seat and sigmoid notch have a marginal contact of 2 to 3 mm.[6] Joint surface contact is optimal only in a neutral forearm position (**Fig. 27-7**).

The ulna and radius transmit loading forces to the elbow and wrist, respectively. Eighteen percent of the load that is transmitted through the wrist passes through the ulna and 82% passes through the radius.[16] With the elbow extended, 60% of the load is transmitted through the radius and 40% through the ulna.[1] The force transmission through the wrist was investigated by Schuind and associates, who found that the force transmission ratio at the radioulnocarpal joint was 55% through the radioscaphoid and 35% through the radiolunate joints. The remaining 10% of the load passed through the TFC.[17]

Stability is provided by the contour of the joints, the surrounding ligaments, and the crossing muscles.[18] However, the dominant structures stabilizing the DRUJ are the ligamentous components of the TFCC proper. The major constraint to dorsal translation of the distal ulna relative to the radius is the palmar radioulnar ligament. Palmar translation of the distal ulna relative to the

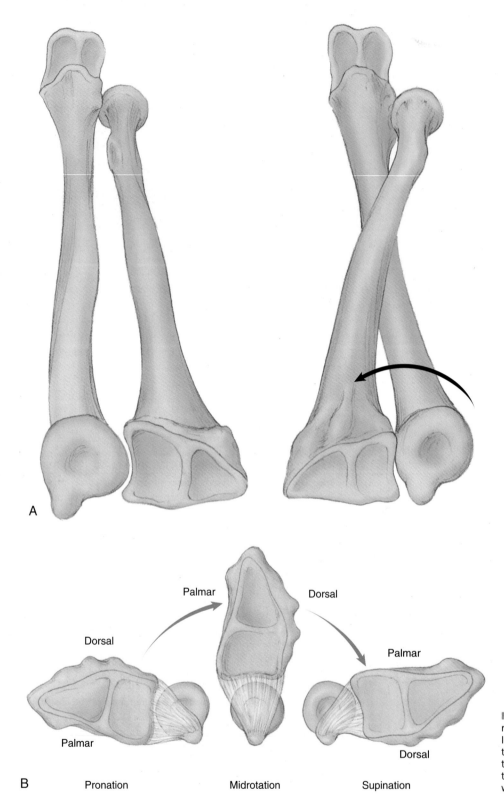

FIGURE 27-6 A and **B**, The radius rotates around the ulnar head about a longitudinal axis that passes roughly through the center of the radial head at the PRUJ at the elbow to the fovea of the ulnar head at the level of the wrist.

radius is constrained primarily by the dorsal radioulnar ligament, with secondary constraint provided by the palmar radioulnar ligament and IOM. In each position the IOM becomes the main stabilizing structure that prevents dislocation of the DRUJ.[5] Hotchkiss and colleagues reported that the IOM was most stiff in forearm supination and least stiff in pronation.[12] The trajectories of the collagen fibers that make up these two ligaments run

in a somewhat helical course from origin to insertion. They do not resist axial radial translation well. Schuind and associates examined the role of the TFCC in stabilizing the DRUJ in pronation and supination and in the transverse plane. They found that the palmar radioulnar ligament of the TFCC is taut in supination and the dorsal radioulnar ligament is taut in pronation. In full pronation, the palmar radioulnar ligament decreased to an average

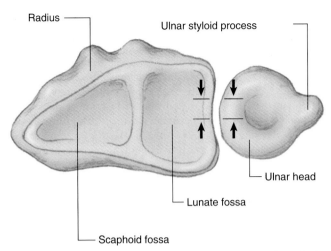

FIGURE 27-7 Contact area (*arrows*) between the radius and ulna in the DRUJ in neutral position. Joint surface contact is optimal only in neutral forearm position.

of 71% of its length in tension. In full supination, the dorsal radioulnar ligament decreased to an average of 90% of its length. Furthermore, they observed that in the transverse plane the TFCC was less stiff in neutral forearm rotation than in pronation and supination.[18] The ulnocarpal ligaments and extensor carpi ulnaris subsheath did not contribute significantly to DRUJ stability; however, approximately 20% of DRUJ constraint is provided by the articular contact of the radius and ulna.[19] Additionally, the extensor retinaculum does not play a part in stabilization of the DRUJ, but the tension of the extensor carpi ulnaris in its intact fibro-osseus tunnel does.[20]

Motor Muscles of Pronation and Supination

Four important major muscles provide active motion of the DRUJ: the pronator quadratus muscle and the pronator teres, innervated by the median nerve, pronate the forearm; and the biceps brachii, which is innervated by the musculocutaneus nerve,

and the supinator muscle, innervated by the radial nerve, provide supination (**Fig. 27-8**).[5] The supinator muscle originates from the lateral epicondyle of the humerus, supinator crest of the ulna, and radial collateral ligament and inserts at the lateral proximal radial shaft. The muscle acts by a mechanism of unrolling. It has been established that slow unresisted supination is brought about by the independent action of the supinator, whereas fast resisted and unresisted supination is assisted by the action of the biceps muscle.[21] The pronator quadratus muscle is shown to be the prime pronator for the forearm in all positions of elbow flexion and extension.[21] There are two distinct heads of the pronator quadratus: superficial and deep.[22] The superficial head takes origin from a short tendon on the dorsoulnar border of the ulna and inserts into a broad flat facet on the palmar surface of the radius. The deep head takes origin in a similar manner to the superficial head, but with a slightly less distinct tendon and from a slightly more palmar position of the ulna.[23] The pronator teres has two heads. The humeral head, which is larger and more superficial, arises immediately above the medial epicondyle of the humerus. The ulnar head is a thin fasciculus that arises from the medial side of the coronoid process of the ulna. The muscle passes obliquely across the forearm and ends in a flat tendon, which is inserted into a rough impression at the middle of the lateral surface of the radius, just below the insertion of the supinator. The pronator teres muscle is stronger in the flexed elbow than in the extended elbow. The flexor and extensor carpi ulnaris muscles may be responsible for initiating pronation from maximal supinated position.[24] Supination is accomplished through the action of the supinator muscle and the biceps at the proximal quarter of the forearm, whereas pronation is achieved through the actions of the pronator teres and pronator quadratus, which act distal to the midpoint of the forearm.[7] Supinatory torque is approximately 15% greater than pronatory torque.[25] The brachioradialis muscle is not usually a supinator, except when the forearm is in complete pronation (see Fig. 27-8). The S-shaped configuration of the radius around the axis of pronation/supination determines, anatomically, the sizes of the lever arms of the pronating/supinating muscles[5] (see Fig. 27-6).

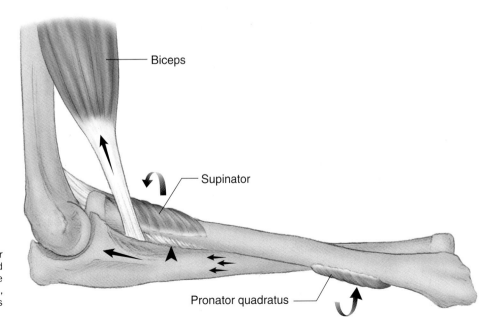

FIGURE 27-8 Important muscles for pronation/supination. The S-shaped configuration of the radius around the axis of pronation/supination determines, anatomically, the sizes of the lever arms of the pronating/supinating muscles.

Clinical Consequences

Dislocation/Subluxation

Clinically, the majority of dislocations involving the DRUJ are dorsal, where the distal ulna is dorsal to the radius. It has been believed that the combination of forearm pronation and wrist hyperextension predisposes to this injury pattern.[26-28] Instability of the distal ulna at the DRUJ can result from dislocations, radius and ulna fractures, malunions, and ligament injuries. Avulsion of the radioulnar ligaments from either the radial or ulnar origins results in increased mobility of the ulnar head on the radius, which may be detected by ballottement tests such as the "piano key sign" (**Fig. 27-9**). The unstable distal ulna most commonly presents with dorsal displacement of the ulnar head and a carpal supination deformity (see Fig. 27-9).[29]

Adams recently described true anatomical reconstruction of the distal radioulnar ligament for post-traumatic DRUJ instability (**Fig. 27-10**).[30,31] The DRUJ is stabilized by a tendon graft (e.g., palmaris longus tendon) for reconstruction of the palmar and dorsal radioulnar ligament.

Fractures

Traumatic subluxations and dislocations of the DRUJ can be isolated phenomena,[28,32] but they can also occur in association with fractures of the radius, ulna, or both. Distal radius fractures with concomitant DRUJ instability are more common than previ-

ously thought.[33] Recent studies have shown that the associated pathology in the DRUJ is a major contributor to long-term loss of motion and poor clinical outcomes after distal radius fractures.[34,35] Recent data, however, seem to indicate that it is not merely the presence of a styloid fracture that matters but the location of that fracture relative to the base and its amount of displacement that relates to the outcome.[36] Fracture at the base of the ulnar styloid and significant displacement of an ulnar styloid fracture were found to increase the risk of DRUJ instability. Significant displacement of an ulnar styloid is an indication for internal fixation (**Fig. 27-11**).

In the case of Galeazzi fracture-dislocation, there is a complex traumatic disruption of the DRUJ that is associated with an unstable radius fracture, commonly at the junction of the middle and distal thirds of the radial shaft. This injury represents nearly 7% of all fractures of the forearm.[37] The mechanism of injury is often a high-velocity direct impact with forceful forearm pronation.[38] This injury is often treated with open reduction and internal fixation of the radius fracture and open or pin fixation of the DRUJ and repair of the ligaments.

The Monteggia fracture consists of a fracture to the proximal third of the ulna with a concomitant dislocation of the radial head. The Galeazzi lesion is three times more common than the Monteggia pattern of injury. The most common mechanism for a Monteggia fracture-dislocation is a fall on an outstretched and hyperpronated hand, resulting in an ulnar shaft fracture and ante-

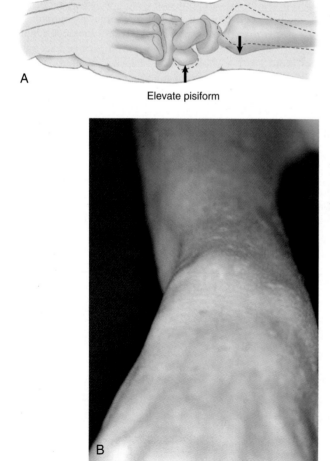

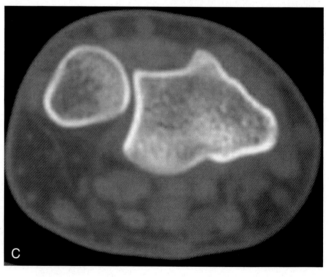

FIGURE 27-9 A, "Piano key" sign. **B,** Dorsal subluxation of the DRUJ. **C,** CT scan (axial view) of dorsal subluxation. *(Courtesy of Dr. Richard A. Berger, Mayo Clinic, Rochester, Minnesota)*

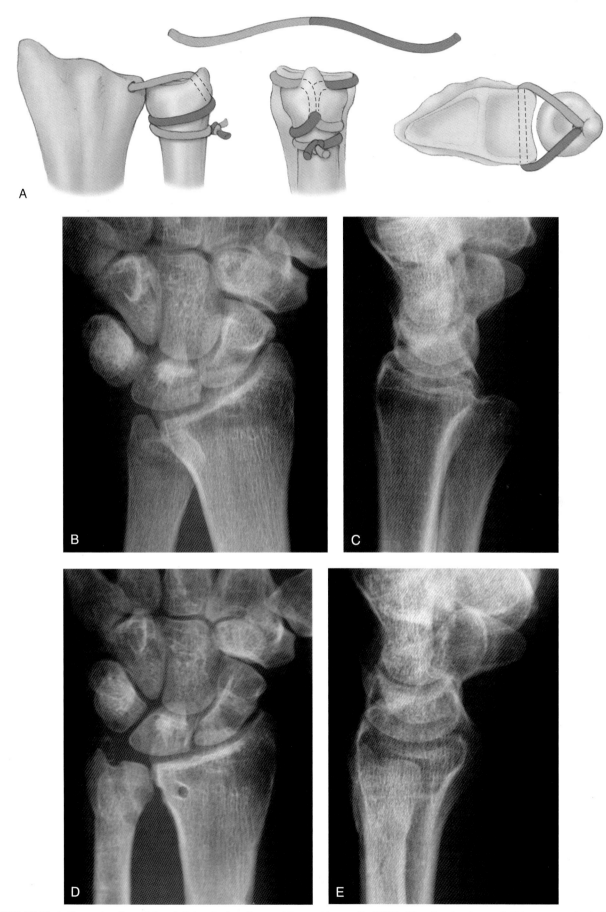

FIGURE 27-10 A, Reconstruction of the distal radioulnar ligament for post-traumatic DRUJ with a free tendon graft (Adams procedure). **B** and **C,** Radiographs showing DRUJ instability. **D** and **E,** Radiographs showing Adams procedure, with reconstruction with a palmaris longus tendon (see text).

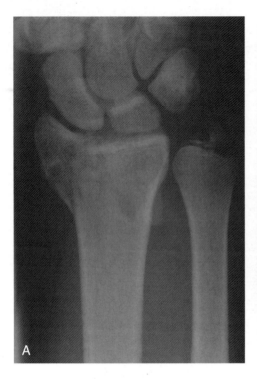

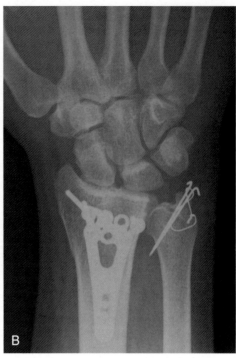

FIGURE 27-11 A, Radiograph of distal radius fracture with fracture at the base of the ulnar styloid. **B,** Fixation of the fracture. *(Courtesy of Hermann Krimmer, MD, Center for Hand Surgery, Ravensburg, Germany.)*

rior radial head dislocation.[39] Monteggia fracture-dislocations are usually considered a more severe injury in adults, who most often require open reduction and internal fixation.[40]

The longitudinal stability of the forearm can be altered in some high-energy radial head fractures, such as the Essex-Lopresti lesion.[41] In this lesion there is a comminuted radial head fracture. This injury is associated with a proximal migration of the radius in case of a dislocation of the DRUJ and the IOM is ruptured completely.[1] This type of accident is one of the worst case sce-

narios in forearm injuries. Radiographs of the elbow should be routinely performed when there is suspicion of PRUJ injury (**Fig. 27-12**).

To allow for longitudinal migration of the radius, the whole membrane must be disrupted, because one ascending and one descending group of fibers suffice to prevent these displacements.[1] If the IOM is intact, even with excision of the PRUJ and DRUJ, the radius maintains its longitudinal stability.[1] As mentioned earlier, the central band of the IOM is responsible for 71% of the

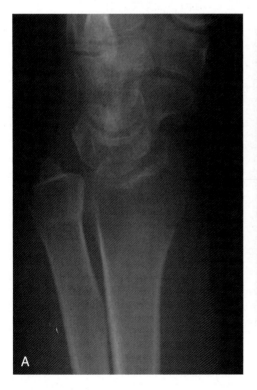

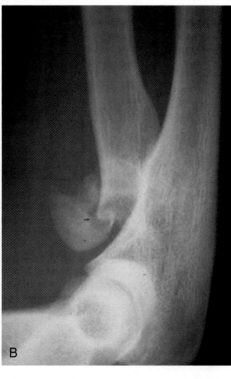

FIGURE 27-12 Essex-Lopresti injury. **A,** Radiograph shows dislocation of the DRUJ. **B,** Radial head fracture. *(Courtesy of Hermann Krimmer, MD, Center for Hand Surgery, Ravensburg, Germany.)*

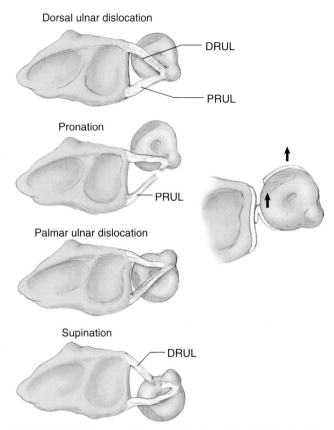

Dorsal ulnar dislocation

— DRUL

— PRUL

Pronation

— PRUL

Palmar ulnar dislocation

Supination

— DRUL

FIGURE 27-13 Palmar and dorsal dislocation of the DRUJ after injury. The majority of dislocations involving the DRUJ are dorsal, where the distal ulna is dorsal to the distal radius. DRUL, distal radioulnar ligament; PRUL, proximal radioulnar ligament.

longitudinal stiffness of the forearm, whereas the TFCC is responsible for 8%.[12] The stability of the DRUJ is minimally supported by bony architecture.[42]

The potential importance of dynamic stabilization of the DRUJ by the extensor carpi ulnaris and the pronator quadratus, especially the deep head, has been proposed and even recognized in some innovative surgical reconstruction procedures. The majority of dislocations involving the DRUJ are dorsal, where the distal ulna is dorsal to the distal radius. The radius of the curvature of the sigmoid notch is 4 to 7 mm larger than that of the ulnar head; and, consequently, pronation and supination are a combined rotation and sliding movement in the DRUJ.[6] In the DRUJ, stability supported by joint surface architecture is minimal and the ligament is therefore of particular importance for stability.[6]

With the forearm in neutral position the palmar and dorsal ligaments are relaxed.[6] If the palmar ligament is injured, the radius dislocates palmarly in pronation. In supination, the opposite occurs: the dorsal radioulnar ligament is taut (**Fig. 27-13**).[6]

Arthrosis

Arthrosis of the DRUJ is a common problem, often leading to substantial disability from pain, weakness, and instability. Such degenerative changes can result from mismatches in the length of the radius and ulna distally, traumatic disruptions of the soft tissues that stabilize the DRUJ, fractures involving the mutual articulating surfaces of the radius and ulna, or any combination thereof. Therefore, resection of one or both articular surfaces of the DRUJ is the treatment of choice. This can take several forms, such as resection of the entire ulnar head (Darrach procedure) (**Fig. 27-14**),[43] partial resection of the joint surfaces with or without interposition of connective soft tissue (**Fig. 27-15**).[44,45]

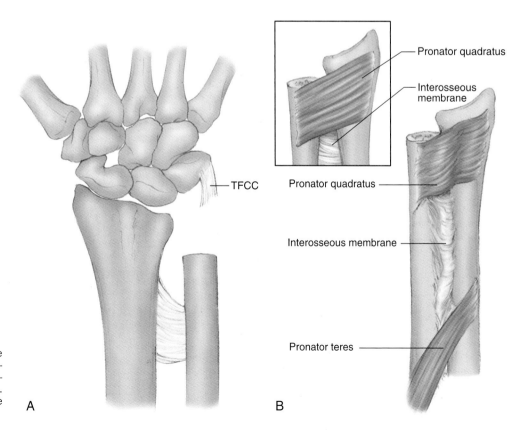

Pronator quadratus

Interosseous membrane

Pronator quadratus —

Interosseous membrane —

Pronator teres —

— TFCC

FIGURE 27-14 Resection of the distal ulna. **A,** The Darrach procedure. **B,** Typical radioulnar impingement after Darrach procedure. TFCC, triangular fibrocartilage complex.

A

B

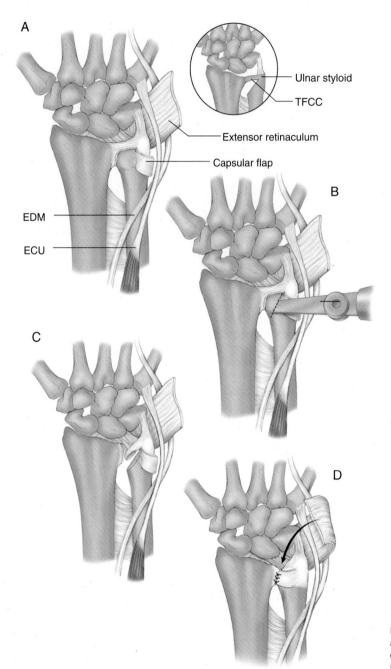

FIGURE 27-15 **A** to **D**, Ulnar head hemi-resection interposition arthroplasty (Bowers procedure). TFCC, triangular fibrocartilage complex; ECU, extensor carpi ulnaris; EDM, extensor digiti minimi.

or fusion of the distal radius and ulna with creation of a proximal pseudarthosis.[46] The results of a biomechanical investigation showed less instability of the hemi-resection arthroplasty in comparison with the Darrach procedure.[47]

In a recently performed biomechanical study, the implantation of an ulnar head endoprosthesis effectively restored the stability of the DRUJ by simulating the geometry of the ulnar head (**Fig. 27-16**).[48] There were significantly better results after the implantation of the prosthesis compared with the Darrach procedure. The interposition of the pronator quadratus muscle or tenodesis with the extensor and flexor carpi ulnaris tendons[49] did not reduce the radioulnar convergence created by resection of the distal ulna[50] and showed significantly worse results in comparison with the prosthesis implantation.[48] Neither of the two soft tissue stabilizations could prevent radioulnar impingement.[48] Implant

arthroplasty of the distal ulna combined with an adequate soft tissue repair is recommended to improve pain, function, and strength of the wrist and forearm to treat painful disorders of the DRUJ secondary to instability and arthrosis.[51]

Summary

The DRUJ, IOM, and PRUJ are essential for painless, powerful, and stable motions of the forearm. Forearm rotation, which occurs as the radius wraps around the ulna, guided by soft tissues at the wrist and elbow joint, also contributes to upper extremity mobility. Force transmission in the forearm is a complex interaction of the radius, ulna, IOM, and TFCC. An understanding of elbow, forearm, and wrist anatomy is crucial to the surgeon evaluating and treating complex forearm pathological processes.

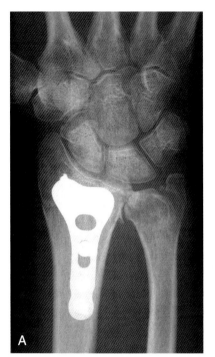
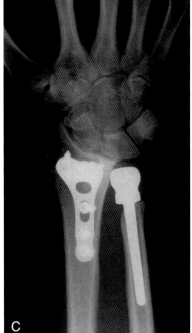
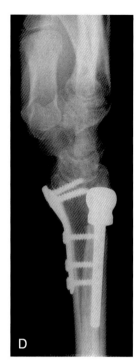

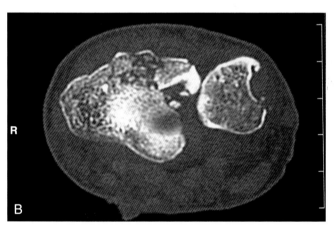

FIGURE 27-16 **A,** Radiograph of a 6-week-old distal radius fracture after open reduction and internal fixation with a palmar plate. **B,** CT scan (axial view) with destruction of the sigmoid notch of the radius. **C** and **D,** The distal ulna was replaced with an ulnar head prosthesis 6 weeks after injury.

REFERENCES

1. Poitevin LA: Anatomy and biomechanics of the interosseous membrane: its importance in the longitudinal stability of the forearm. Hand Clin. 2001; 1:97-110.

2. Kapandji AI: Why are there two bones in the forearm? Ann Chir. 1975; 29:463-470.

3. Lewis OJ: Evolutionary change in primate wrist and inferior radio-ulnar joints. Anat Rec. 1965; 151:275-285.

4. Kapandji A: Biomechanics of pronation and supination of the forearm. Hand Clin. 2001; 17:111-122.

5. Hagert CG: The distal radioulnar joint in relation to the whole forearm. Clin Orthop Relat Res. 1992; 275:56-64.

6. Ekenstam F: Anatomy of the distal radioulnar joint. Clin Orthop Relat Res. 1992; 275:14-18.

7. Linscheid R: Biomechanics of the distal radioulnar joint. Clin Orthop Relat Res. 1992; 275:46-55.

8. Czitrom AA, Dobyns JH, Linscheid RL: Ulnar variance in carpal instability. J Hand Surg [Am]. 1987; 2:205-208.

9. Forstner H: The distal radio-ulnar joint: morphologic aspects and surgical orthopedic consequences. Unfallchirurg. 1987; 11:512-517.

10. De Smet L: Ulnar variance: facts and fiction. Review article. Acta Orthop Belg. 1994; 1:1-9.

11. Berger RA: The anatomy of the ligaments of the wrist and distal radioulnar joints. Clin Orthop Relat Res. 2001; 383:32-40.

12. Hotchkiss RN, An KN, Sowa DT, et al: An anatomic and mechanical study of the interosseous membrane of the forearm: pathomechanics of proximal migration of the radius. J Hand Surg [Am]. 1989; 14:256-261.

13. Gabl M, Zimmermann R, Angermann P, et al: The interosseous membrane and its influence on the distal radioulnar joint: an anatomical investigation of the distal tract. J Hand Surg [Br]. 1998; 23:179-182.

14. Goodfellow JW, Bullough PG: The pattern of ageing of the articular cartilage of the elbow joint. J Bone Joint Surg Br. 1967; 49:175-181.

15. Jung JM, Baek GH, Kim JH, et al: Changes in ulnar variance in relation to forearm rotation and grip. J Bone Joint Surg Br. 2001; 83:1029-1033.

16. Palmer AK, Werner FW, Glisson RR, Murphy DJ: Partial excision of the triangular fibrocartilage complex. J Hand Surg [Am]. 1988; 3:391-394.

17. Schuind F, Cooney WP, Linscheid RL, et al: Force and pressure transmission through the normal wrist: a theoretical two-dimensional study in the posteroanterior plane. J Biomech. 1995; 28:587-601.

18. Schuind F, An KN, Berglund L, et al: The distal radioulnar ligaments: a biomechanical study. J Hand Surg [Am]. 1991; 6:1106-1114.

19. Stuart PR, Berger RA, Linscheid RL, An KN: The dorso-palmar stability of the distal radioulnar joint. J Hand Surg [Am]. 2000; 4:689-699.

20. Spinner M, Kaplan EB: Extensor carpi ulnaris: its relationship to the stability of the distal radio-ulnar joint. Clin Orthop Relat Res. 1970; 68:124-129.

21. Basmajian J, Deluca CJ. In Butler J, ed: Muscles Alive. Their Functions Revealed by Electromyography. Baltimore: Williams & Williams, 1985; 280-289.

22. Johnson RK, Shrewsbury MM: The pronator quadratus in motions and in stabilization of the radius and ulna at the distal radioulnar joint. J Hand Surg [Am]. 1976; 3:205-209.

23. Stuart PR: Pronator quadratus revisited. J Hand Surg [Br]. 1996; 21:714-722.

24. Haugstvedt JR, Berger RA, Berglund LJ: A mechanical study of the moment-forces of the supinators and pronators of the forearm. Acta Orthop Scand. 2001; 72:629-634.

25. Askew LJ, An KN, Morrey BF, Chao EYS: Isometric elbow strength in normal individuals. Clin Orthop Relat Res. 1987; 222:261-266.

26. Hui FC, Linscheid RL: Ulnotriquetral augmentation tenodesis: a reconstructive procedure for dorsal subluxation of the distal radioulnar joint. J Hand Surg [Am]. 1982; 3:230-236.

27. Buterbaugh GA, Palmer AK: Fractures and dislocations of the distal radioulnar joint. Hand Clin. 1988; 3:361-375.

28. Heiple KG, Freehafer AA: Isolated traumatic dislocation of the distal end of the ulna or distal radio-ulnar joint. J Bone Joint Surg Am. 1962; 44:1387-1394.

29. Bowers WH: Problems of the distal radioulnar joint. Adv Orthop Surg. 1984; 7:289-303.

30. Adams BD: Anatomic reconstruction of the distal radioulnar ligaments for DRUJ instability. Tech Hand Up Extrem Surg. 2000; 4:154-160.

31. Adams BD, Berger RA: An anatomic reconstruction of the distal radioulnar ligaments for posttraumatic distal radioulnar joint instability. J Hand Surg [Am]. 2002; 2:243-251.

32. Rainey RK, Pfautsch ML: Traumatic volar dislocation of the distal radioulnar joint. Orthopedics. 1985; 7:896-900.

33. Frykman GK: Fractures of the distal radius including sequelae of shoulder-hand-finger syndrome, disturbance in the distal radio-ulnar joint and impairment of nerve function: a clinical and experimental study. Acta Orthop Scand Suppl. 1967; 108: 7-153.

34. Cooney WP 3rd, Dobyns JH, Linscheid RL: Complications of Colles' fractures. J Bone Joint Surg Am. 1980; 62:613-619.

35. Stoffelen D, De Smet L, Broos P: The importance of the distal radioulnar joint in distal radial fractures. J Hand Surg [Br]. 1998; 23:507-511.

36. May MM, Lawton JN, Blazar PE: Ulnar styloid fractures associated with distal radius fractures: incidence and implications for distal radioulnar joint instability. J Hand Surg [Am]. 2002; 27:965-971.

37. Dameron TB: Traumatic dislocation of the distal radioulnar joint. Clin Orthop Relat Res. 1972; 83:55-63.

38. Mikic ZD: Galeazzi fracture-dislocations. J Bone Joint Surg Am. 1975; 57:1071-1080.

39. Boyd HB, Boals JC: The Monteggia lesion: a review of 159 cases. Clin Orthop Relat Res. 1969; 66:94-100.

40. Ring D, Jupiter JB: Current concepts review: fracture-dislocation of the elbow. J Bone Joint Surg. 1998; 80:566-580.

41. Essex-Lopresti P: Fractures of the radial head with distal radioulnar dislocation: report of two cases. J Bone Joint Surg Br. 1951; 33:244-247.

42. Ekenstam F, Hagert CG: Anatomical studies on the geometry and stability of the distal radio ulnar joint. Scand J Plast Reconstr Surg. 1985; 1:17-25.

43. Darrach W: Partial excision of lower shaft of ulna deformity following Colles fracture. Ann Surg. 1913; 57:764-765.

44. Bowers WH: Distal radioulnar joint arthroplasty: the hemiresection–interposition technique. J Hand Surg [Am]. 1985; 10:169-178.

45. Watson HK, Ryu JJ, Burgess RC: Matched distal ulnar resection. J Hand Surg [Am]. 1986; 11:812-817.

46. Kapandji IA: Opération de Kapandji-Sauvé: techniques et indications dans les affections non rhumatismales. Ann Chir Main. 1986; 5:181-193.

47. Sauerbier M, Fujita M, Hahn ME, et al: The dynamic radio-ulnar convergence of the Darrach procedure and the ulnar head hemiresection interposition arthroplasty: a biomechanical study. J Hand Surg [Br]. 2002; 4:307-316.

48. Sauerbier M, Hahn ME, Fujita M, et al: Dynamic radioulnar convergence after Darrach operation, soft tissue stabilizing operations of the distal ulna, and ulnar head prosthesis implantation—an experimental biomechanical study. Unfallchirurg. 2002; 8:688-698.

49. Breen TF, Jupiter JB: Extensor carpi ulnaris and flexor carpi ulnaris tenodesis of the unstable distal ulna. J Hand Surg [Am]. 1989; 4:612-617.

50. Sauerbier M, Berger RA, Fujita M, Hahn ME: Radioulnar convergence after distal ulnar resection: mechanical performance of two commonly used soft tissue stabilizing procedures. Acta Orthop Scand. 2003; 4:420-428.

51. Willis AA, Berger RA, Cooney WP 3rd: Arthroplasty of the distal radioulnar joint using a new ulnar head endoprosthesis: preliminary report. J Hand Surg [Am]. 2007; 32:177-189.

Ulnar Head and Styloid Fractures

28

Douglas A. Campbell, ChM

Fractures of the distal ulna have potentially important functional implications for the wrist. Fractures of the ulnar head can disrupt the congruency and/or stability of the distal radioulnar joint (DRUJ) and limit pain-free forearm rotation and hand positioning. Similarly, fractures of the ulnar styloid process, seen more frequently, can on occasion produce secondary instability of either the ulnocarpal joint or the DRUJ if left untreated. It is not necessary to actively treat all fractures of the distal ulna. Those situations in which treatment is necessary to restore function, limit complications, and provide an optimal outcome for these injuries are discussed in this chapter.

Anatomy and Functional Biomechanics

The meticulous histological analysis of the radioulnar ligaments by Nakamura and colleagues[1] reveals two predominant attachments to the distal ulna: the fovea and the base of the ulnar styloid process. The foveal attachment—just radial to the base of the ulnar styloid—is over a broad area and gives rise to near-vertical fibers. The styloid base attachment is over a smaller area, and its fibers are orientated horizontally. Both attachments are dense in Sharpey's fibers. The foveal and styloid base fibers coalesce and then divide to embrace the palmar and dorsal edges of the proximal portion of the articular disc.

Isolated sectioning studies of the ulnar insertions of these structures have shown that each part plays an equal role in stability *when no load is applied across the wrist*. One of the primary functions of the distal ulna, however, is as a weight-bearing joint (**Fig. 28-1**); and when these sectioning studies are repeated under load, the foveal attachment of the radioulnar ligament is found to contribute significantly greater stability to the DRUJ than the styloid attachment.[2] This view would be supported by the proximity of the fovea to the rotation axis of the forearm, making it more likely that this is the critical part of the radioulnar ligament's bony anchorage under dynamic conditions.

No direct bone/ligament connection has been identified over the styloid process from its midportion to the tip, although fibers do originate from the hyaline cartilage to coalesce with a somewhat lax sleevelike structure that some investigators refer to as the "ulnar collateral ligament."

Ulnar Head Fractures

Ulnar head fractures are rare, occurring in only 6% of all wrist fractures.[3] The frequency of each fracture configuration is shown in **Figure 28-2**. More recently, distal ulnar fractures have been classified according to the Comprehensive Classification of Fractures with an associated Q modifier (**Fig. 28-3**).[4]

The risk of disabling complications in this injury is unlikely to be DRUJ instability. The attachments of the triangular fibrocar-

tilage complex (TFCC) usually remain undisturbed. These articular fractures will give rise to the usual risks of this group of injuries. Coexistent fractures of the distal radius and ulna significantly increase the incidence of radial nonunion.[5] Indeed, this is the most likely circumstance in which the unusual complication of radial nonunion will be seen (**Fig. 28-4**). In spite of this knowledge, combined distal radius and ulna fractures continue to be managed by treating the radius alone.

Indications

Displaced or potentially unstable ulnar head fractures require accurate reduction and stabilization. These injuries should be recognized early and treated, ideally, within 7 days of injury.

Standard radiographs will provide most of the information about the fracture pattern (**Fig. 28-5**). Computed tomography (CT) may be necessary on occasion to fully evaluate the injury.

The advent of angularly stable small locking plates allows patients of all ages to be considered for internal fixation, irrespective of their bone quality.

Contraindications

There are no absolute contraindications to internal fixation of displaced ulnar head fractures except the multifragmentary injury pattern that is rendered unable to be reconstructed by virtue of fragment size.

Surgical Technique

General or regional anesthesia is required. Contrary to previous reports,[6] regional anesthesia is a safe and comfortable technique that can allow treatment on an outpatient basis.

The affected arm is placed on an arm table. The tip of the ulnar styloid is easier to expose when the forearm is placed in pronation. For this reason, the surgeon may choose to sit at the cranial edge of the arm table. If a distal radius fracture coexists, the surgeon will most likely choose to sit at the caudal edge of the arm table. It is therefore essential that the operating equipment (including mini-C-arm intensifier) is arranged in such a way that surgeon and assistant can move freely around the arm table during surgery.

An upper arm tourniquet is applied. The limb should be prepared and draped to the level of the tourniquet cuff. Intravenous prophylactic antibiotics are recommended immediately preoperatively.

A straight longitudinal incision along the course of the subcutaneous distal ulna is recommended. The dorsal sensory branch of the ulnar nerve lies immediately underneath the skin at the level of the ulnar neck. Extreme care must be taken to avoid this structure in the initial surgical approach.

The approach is deepened ulnar to the sixth extensor compartment to enable the stabilizing implant to be applied on the surface of the distal ulna between the tendons of the flexor carpi ulnaris and extensor carpi ulnaris. It is unusual to need to visualize the articular fragments directly, but in these rare instances a second approach can be made using the same skin incision but passing through the floor of the fifth extensor compartment. Retraction of the tendon of the extensor digiti minimi will allow direct inspection of any articular fragments.

Reduction of the fracture fragments is best performed indirectly using a small angularly stable implant. If reduction is

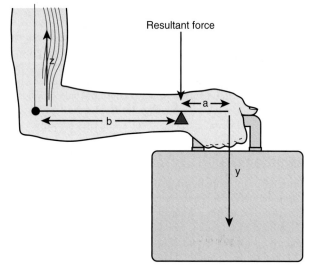

FIGURE 28-1 Force transmission through the DRUJ.

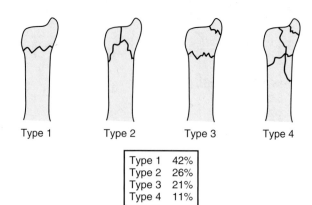

Type 1	42%
Type 2	26%
Type 3	21%
Type 4	11%

FIGURE 28-2 Incidence of ulnar head fractures.

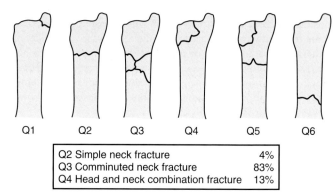

Q2 Simple neck fracture	4%
Q3 Comminuted neck fracture	83%
Q4 Head and neck combination fracture	13%

FIGURE 28-3 Incidence of distal ulnar fractures.

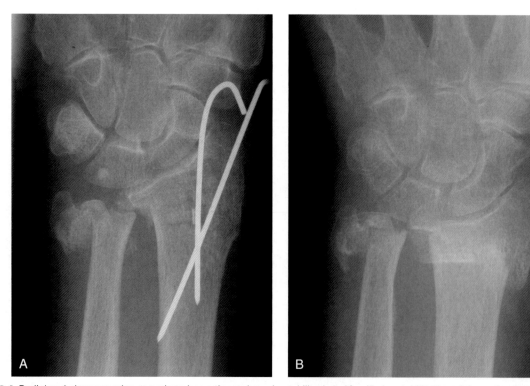

FIGURE 28-4 Radial and ulnar nonunion occurring when only one bone is stabilized. **A,** After K-wire stabilization of the radius fracture. **B,** Displaced nonunion after K-wire removal.

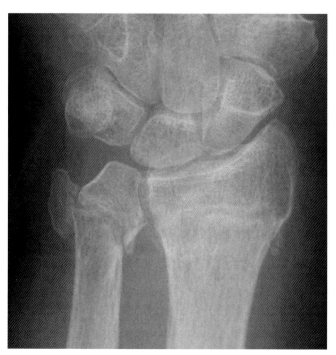

FIGURE 28-5 Plain radiograph clearly outlines articular fracture pattern.

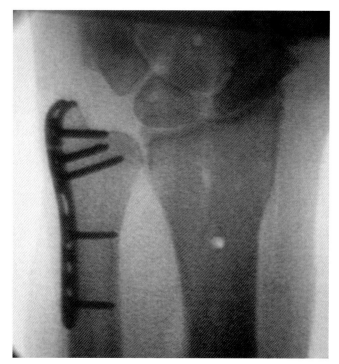

FIGURE 28-6 Use of a specially designed low-profile locking plate for a distal ulnar fracture.

attempted using pointed reduction forceps, the thin cortical bone of the ulnar head often fragments under load, leading to further comminution and possible failure.

The implant is best placed on the medial border of the ulna directly in line with the ulnar styloid. This acts as a buttress for the distal radius to be reduced onto (**Fig. 28-6**), in this case utilizing a specially designed implant for treating distal ulnar fractures.

Clinical testing of DRUJ stability will reveal if a coexistent unstable TFCC tear is present.

An above elbow cast or sugar tong splint is applied with the elbow flexed to 90 degrees and the forearm in neutral rotation. Early movement is begun depending on stability of fixation.

The skin overlying the distal ulna is thin. As a result, implants placed here are frequently palpable—and may give rise to discomfort. A low threshold for implant removal, once union is certain, is recommended.

Clinical Examples
Case 1
A 77-year-old woman presented after a fall with a painful and deformed wrist. The initial radiographs reveal a displaced articular fracture of the distal radius and a minimally displaced long oblique extra-articular fracture of the distal ulna (**Fig. 28-7A, B**). Initial treatment consisted of the application of a bridging external fixator. The surgeon clearly concentrated on the reduction of the distal radius fracture, but—in the absence of an intact ulnar buttress—displacement of the unstable ulnar fracture was inevitable (see **Fig. 28-7C, D**).

Attempts were then made to provide an ulnar buttress by stabilizing the distal ulnar fragment with a longitudinal Kirschner wire (K-wire). This method provided insufficient stability, and it was not possible to maintain a reduction.

Stabilization by open reduction and internal fixation (ORIF) using a 2.0-mm mini-condylar plate (Synthes) (see **Fig. 28-7E**) and a volar distal radius plate (Synthes) allowed early movement and an almost complete recovery of function 3 months after surgery.

Had the necessity for the distal ulna to act as a weight-bearing buttress been appreciated at an early stage, the ulnar fracture could have been treated by a much simpler method of stabilization such as multiple lag screws. An example of this method of treatment for a similar fracture is shown in **Figure 28-8**.

Case 2
A 20-year-old man was involved in a motor vehicle accident, sustaining multiple life-threatening injuries. His initial treatment concentrated on his major visceral trauma and unstable pelvic fracture. He sustained a displaced fracture of the distal radius and ulna (**Fig. 28-9A, B**) that was managed initially by a bridging external fixator (see **Fig. 28-9C, D**).

It was recognized 4 weeks after injury that the distal ulnar fracture had never been reduced and that the ulnar head lay in a palmar position.

ORIF of both fractures using a 2.0-mm mini-condylar plate (Synthes) and a dorsal distal radius plate (Synthes) (see **Fig. 28-9E**) allowed immediate rehabilitation and a return to full function.

The immediate requirement to treat life-threatening injuries resulted in early basic stabilization of the wrist fracture. Referral for definitive treatment of the radius and ulna fractures was delayed, although accurate anatomical stabilization was still possible. There had been no early attempt to reduce the distal ulna fracture, and this led to greater technical difficulty at the time of surgery.

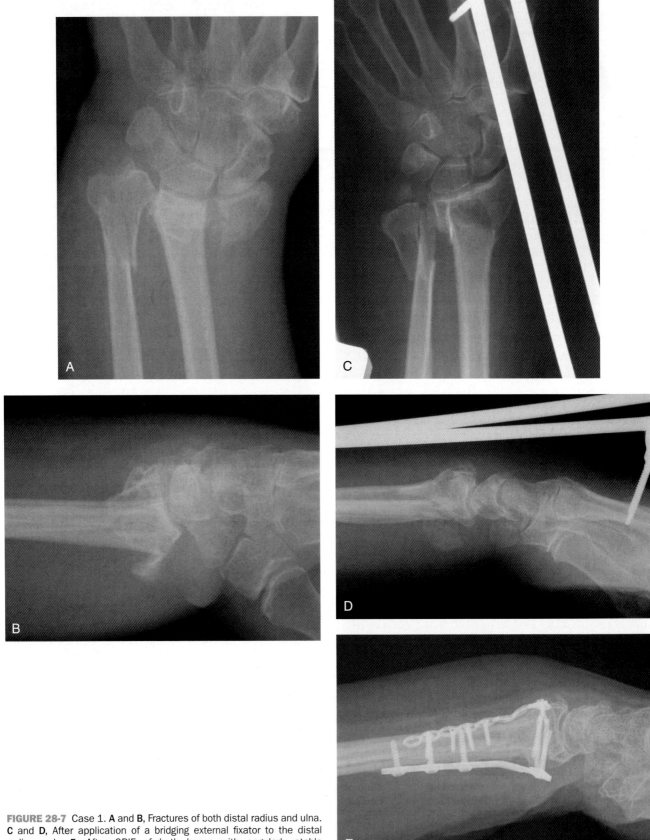

FIGURE 28-7 Case 1. **A** and **B,** Fractures of both distal radius and ulna. **C** and **D,** After application of a bridging external fixator to the distal radius only. **E,** After ORIF of both bones with angularly stable implants.

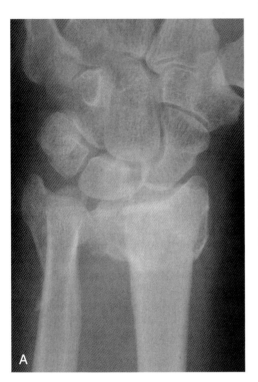

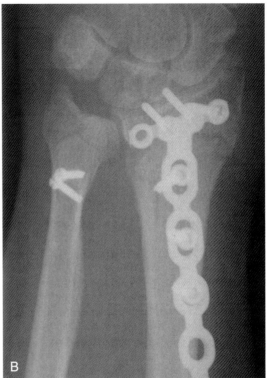

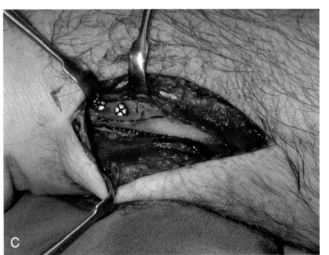

FIGURE 28-8 A and **B,** Ulnar fracture treated with two lag screws. **C,** Operative view.

Results

Reports of treatment of these unusual fractures are rare.

In 2004, we reported our series of 24 distal ulna fractures, associated with fractures of the distal radius, stabilized with a mini-condylar plate (Synthes).[4] The majority of cases (83%) were comminuted neck fractures. In a small number of isolated ulnar head fractures, simple lag screws were also used. An average range of rotation of 146 degrees (76 degrees of pronation, 70 degrees of supination) was achieved at an average of 26 months after surgery. The average flexion/extension arc was 102 degrees (50 degrees flexion, 52 degrees extension). Nonunion of the distal ulna was seen in only one case and was treated by revision grafting and plating and went on to uneventful union.

Ulnar Styloid Fractures

It is generally recognized that there are four distinct fracture configurations of the ulnar styloid process (**Fig. 28-10**).

The level of the styloid fracture is relevant to the risk of development of instability of the DRUJ. The basal oblique fracture is more likely to disturb the foveal attachment of the radioulnar ligament.

Incidence

All authors agree that more than 50% of distal radial fractures are accompanied by fractures of the ulnar styloid. In a study of 130 distal radius fractures,[7] 71 were noted to have a coexistent ulnar

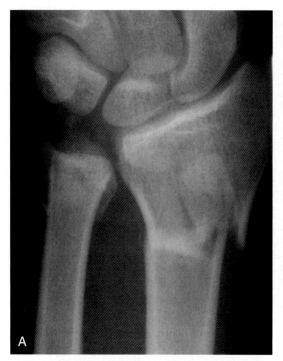

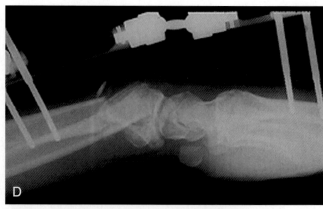

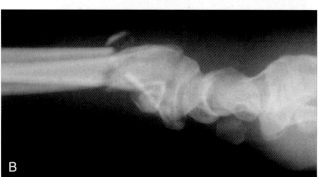

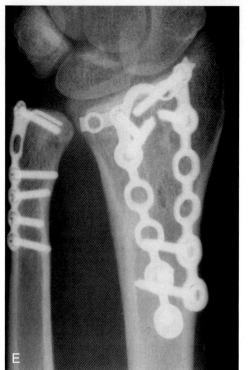

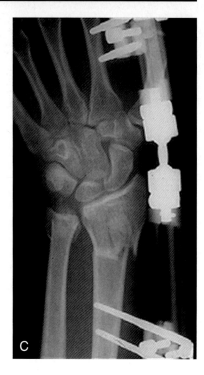

FIGURE 28-9 Case 2. **A** and **B,** Extra-articular fracture of distal radius with associated palmarly displaced ulnar head fracture. **C** and **D,** After initial stabilization with bridging external fixator to the distal radius only. **E,** After ORIF to stabilize both bones using angularly stable implants.

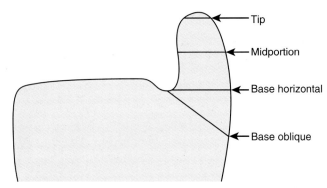

FIGURE 28-10 Fracture configurations of the ulnar styloid process.

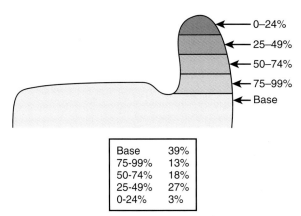

Base	39%
75-99%	13%
50-74%	18%
25-49%	27%
0-24%	3%

FIGURE 28-11 Incidence of site of ulnar styloid fractures.

styloid fracture (55%). Of these, 39% involved the base (**Fig. 28-11**).

Radiographic Prediction of DRUJ Instability

Instability of the DRUJ complicates a reported 3% to 37% of distal radius fractures,[8,9] yet fewer than 10% of distal radius fractures demand a surgical procedure on the distal ulna.[7,10] Instability relates to detachment of a significant portion of the TFCC—significant in either size or location. These situations arise either by a direct tear through a critical amount of the soft tissue component or by fracture through its bony anchorage.

Nakamura and colleagues[11] assessed the relevance of each of the four levels of ulnar styloid fracture on DRUJ stability in 10 cadaveric wrists and found no instability in styloid tip or midportion fractures but up to a 20% loss of stiffness (stability) in basal horizontal fractures. Basal oblique fractures, however, produced up to 70% loss of stiffness.

Wide displacement of any type of ulnar styloid fracture was also recognized as a significant risk for development of DRUJ instability—presumably because wide displacement would not be possible without a significant soft tissue tear (**Fig. 28-12**).

Indications

Ulnar styloid fractures only ever require stabilization when they are the cause (either partly or wholly) of DRUJ instability.

Assessment of DRUJ stability will therefore allow the surgeon to select which individual fractures require active treatment. Stability can only be assessed in the presence of an intact or stable reconstructed distal radius. In a wrist injury involving fractures to both distal radius and ulna, stable reconstruction of the radius must be achieved before judging DRUJ stability.

Passive anteroposterior glide of the distal ulna relative to the distal radius in positions of neutral rotation, full pronation, and full supination will provide this information. Assessment of the uninjured limb will give a guide to the normal laxity of the joint for any given individual.

If stabilization is deemed necessary, a choice of techniques is available. The fracture configuration will partly dictate the choices available. Fracture fragments of significant size (oblique and horizontal basal fractures) are suitable for bony reconstruction. More distal or comminuted fragments are suitable for reconstruction by soft tissue reattachment—ignoring the fracture fragments.

Contraindications

There are no contraindications to stabilization of the DRUJ. As noted earlier, small or comminuted fragments may preclude bony reconstruction, but soft tissue stabilization (by TFCC reattachment) should still be performed.

Surgical Technique

The surgical approach is identical to that described for stabilization of ulnar head fractures. However, the distal ulnar shaft need not routinely be exposed.

Soft tissue reattachment of the TFCC is not discussed in this chapter.

A number of different bony reconstruction techniques can be used.

Tension Band Wiring This technique is ideal if the fragments are of insufficient size to safely place a lag screw or if they are comminuted.

Two 1.0-mm K-wires are passed through the fragment, as nearly parallel as possible, to engage the far cortex. A thin-gauge stainless-steel prestretched wire loop is passed through a perpendicular drill hole in the distal ulnar shaft and looped around the K-wires before tightening. It is critical to attempt to reduce the prominence of both the K-wires and the wire loop, because the skin in this region is very thin.

Lag Screw This technique will provide excellent stability to the DRUJ and allow early movement but relies on extremely accurate placement of a small screw through an often tiny fragment of bone. The technical difficulties of this technique cannot be overemphasized. Should the drill for the gliding hole be introduced slightly off center, there is a substantial risk that the single piece of ulnar styloid will fragment, rendering this technique redundant. In these circumstances, tension band wiring should be used to secure the styloid fragments and restore stability. It is therefore recommended that an "inside out" technique of drilling the gliding hole in the distal fragment from the fracture surface out will provide the best opportunity for accurate placement of the lag screw.

The rehabilitation of these injuries is similar to that recommended for ulnar head fractures. The surgeon must be confident of the stability of fixation before allowing early movement.

External Fixation This unusual technique involves the application of an outrigger from the distal radius external fixator to the distal ulnar shaft, securing the forearm in supination. It is reported to produce improved results with fewer complications than standard tension band wiring.[12]

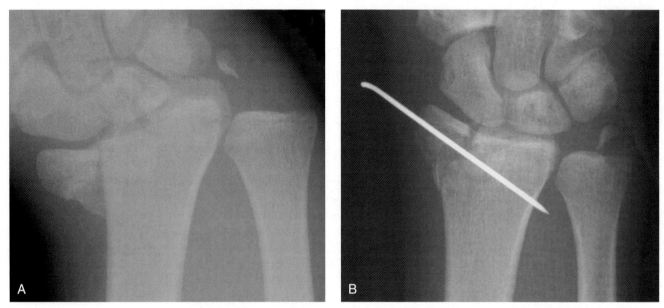

FIGURE 28-12 **A** and **B,** Radiographs at time of injury reveal true nature of styloid fragment displacement, which is not appreciated after reduction.

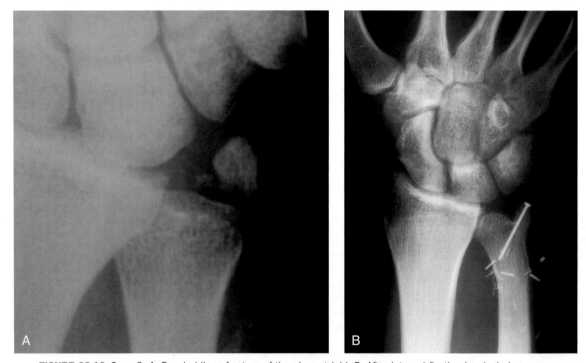

FIGURE 28-13 Case 3. **A,** Basal oblique fracture of the ulnar styloid. **B,** After internal fixation by single lag screw.

Clinical Examples

Case 3

A 35-year-old man was involved in a motor vehicle accident in which he was thrown from his vehicle. He sustained an open injury to the ulnar side of his right wrist (**Fig. 28-13A**). After appropriate wound débridement, the displaced ulnar styloid basal oblique fracture was reduced and secured with a single 1.5-mm lag screw (see **Fig. 28-13B**). After reconstruction of the soft tissue defect with a lateral arm free flap, the skeletal stability allowed early rehabilitation and return to full function.

This fragment was of sufficient size to accept a gliding hole drill diameter of 1.5 mm. Central placement of the drill hole reduced the risk of fragmentation.

Case 4

A 23-year-old male professional rugby player complained of pain and "clunking" in his wrist on impact after an injury sustained during play. Plain radiographs revealed a displaced basal oblique fracture of the ulnar styloid (**Fig. 28-14A**). There was a suspicion that this was not a totally new injury and that a fibrous union of

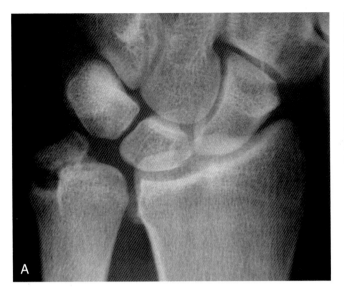

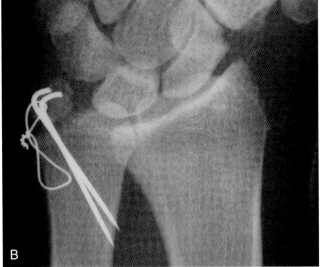

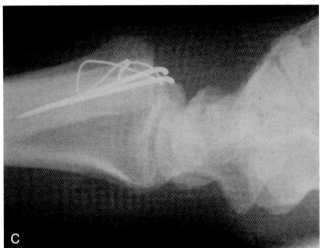

FIGURE 28-14 Case 4. **A**, Displaced basal oblique fracture of the ulnar styloid. **B** and **C**, Tension band wiring.

a previous fracture had been disrupted. Perifracture sclerosis was seen, suggesting a mature injury. The fracture was opened as described earlier and the fracture surfaces débrided to healthy cancellous bone. A tension band wiring was performed to stabilize the DRUJ and prevent further instability and "clunking" (see **Fig. 28-14B, C**), allowing a stable normal active range of motion.

The maturity of this injury and the need for débridement of the fracture surfaces meant that an accurate anatomical reduction with fragment interdigitation was not possible. Tension band wiring was selected as a technique more likely to provide a greater area of compression across the fracture site.

An alternative method of securing the tension band wire loop is shown (**Fig. 28-15**). This technique should be used with caution in the distal ulna because of the often uncomfortable prominence of the screw head through the skin.

Results

It remains the case that the presence of an ulnar styloid fracture represents a poor prognostic sign in wrist injuries.[13-17] The natural progression of this idea is to recommend regular operative stabilization of these injuries,[18] but this approach fails to differentiate between different styloid fracture patterns.

In contrast to an interventional approach, Tsukazaki and coworkers[19] examined 83 distal radius fractures to assess prognostic factors. In keeping with other descriptions on incidence, 44 cases (53%) had evidence of ulnar styloid injury. Again, no information was provided on the exact fracture configurations, yet only 19 fractures (43%) showed radiological evidence of union. There was no correlation between functional outcome, residual pain, and the presence or absence of an ulnar styloid fracture or nonunion. It is likely that the vast majority of these injuries were stable injuries of the DRUJ.

Few studies comment on the effects of fixation of ulnar styloid fractures.[20] No correlation between TFCC stabilization and outcome was found in a heterogenous group of Colles' fractures. Since these studies were published, the accuracy of classification has improved enormously. We now accept that the exact fracture configuration in both the radial and ulnar sides of each injury is the critical determinant in stability and, therefore, outcome.

Nonunion

As previously stated, there seems to be no correlation between ulnar styloid nonunion and functional outcome. Fractures of the tip of the ulnar styloid frequently fail to unite but appear to be

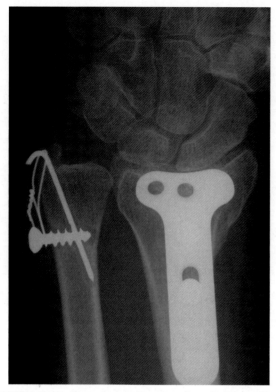

FIGURE 28-15 Alternative configuration of tension band wiring.

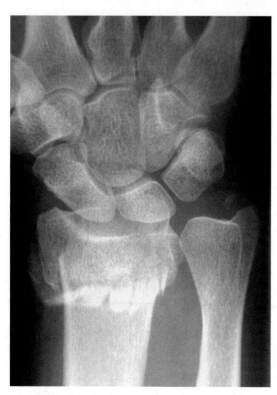

FIGURE 28-16 Avulsion of tip of ulnar styloid.

less of a clinical problem because they are unlikely to be associated with instability[17] (**Fig. 28-16**).

Ulnar styloid nonunion has been classified[21] into type 1 (with a stable DRUJ) and type 2 (with an unstable DRUJ). Those patients with symptomatic type 1 nonunion respond well to

simple excision of the ununited fragment, whereas those patients with symptomatic type 2 nonunion require formal reconstruction and TFCC reattachment.

Summary

Fractures of the distal part of the ulna can influence outcome dramatically. Appreciation of both their configuration and relationship to DRUJ congruency and stability is critical in reaching the correct treatment decision.

REFERENCES

1. Nakamura T, Takayama S, Horiuchi Y, Yabe Y: Origins and insertions of the triangular fibrocartilage complex: a histological study. J Hand Surg [Br]. 2001; 26; 446-454.

2. Haugstvedt JR, Berger RA, Nakamura T, et al: Relative contributions of the ulnar attachments of the triangular fibrocartilage complex to the dynamic stability of the distal radioulnar joint. J Hand Surg [Am]. 2006; 31; 445-451.

3. Biyani A, Simison AJM, Klenerman L: Fractures of the distal radius and ulna. J Hand Surg [Br]. 1995; 20; 357-364.

4. Ring D, McCarty LP, Campbell D, Jupiter JB: Condylar blade plate fixation of unstable fractures of the distal ulna associated with fracture of the distal radius. J Hand Surg [Am]. 2004; 29; 103-109.

5. McKee MD, Waddell JP, Yoo D, Richards RR: Nonunion of distal radial fractures associated with distal ulnar shaft fractures: a report of four cases. J Orthop Trauma. 1997; 11:49-53.

6. Kambouroglou G: Fractures of the distal ulna. In Giannoudis PV, Pape HC, eds: Orthopaedic Trauma Surgery. Cambridge, England: Cambridge University Press, 2006; 56-59.

7. May MM, Lawton JN, Blazar PE: Ulnar styloid fractures associated with distal radius fractures: incidence and implications for distal radioulnar joint instability. J Hand Surg [Am]. 2002; 27; 965-971.

8. Frykman G: Fractures of the distal radius including sequelae of shoulder-hand-finger syndrome, disturbance in the distal radioulnar joint and impairment of nerve function: a clinical and experimental study. Acta Orthop Scand Suppl. 1967; 108; 1-124.

9. Solgaard S: Function after distal radius fracture. Acta Orthop Scand. 1988; 59; 39-42.

10. Fernandez DL: Fractures of the distal radius: operative treatment. AAOS Instruct Course Lect. 1993; 42:73-88.

11. Nakamura T, Moy OJ, Peimer CA: Relationship between the ulnar styloid fracture and DRUJ instability. J Hand Surg [Br]. 2003; 28(Suppl 1):48.

12. Ruch DS, Lumsden BC, Papadonikolakis A: Distal radius fractures: a comparison of tension band wiring versus ulnar outrigger external fixation for the management of distal radioulnar instability. J Hand Surg [Am]. 2005; 30:969-977.

13. Knirk JL, Jupiter JB: Intraarticular fractures of the distal end of the radius in young adults. J Bone Joint Surg [Am]. 1986; 68:647-659.

14. De Bruijn HP: Functional treatment of Colles' fracture. Acta Orthop Scand Suppl. 1987; 223:1-95.

15. Roumen RMH, Hesp WLEM, Bruggink EDM: Unstable Colles fractures in elderly patients: a randomised trial of

external fixation for redisplacement. J Bone Joint Surg Br. 1991; 73:307-311.

16. Sanders RA, Keppel FL, Waldrop JI: External fixation of distal radius fractures: results and complications. J Hand Surg [Am]. 1991; 16:385-391.

17. Stoffelen D, De Smet L, Broos P: The importance of the distal radioulnar joint in distal radial fractures. J Hand Surg [Br]. 1998; 23:507-511.

18. Buterbaugh GA, Palmer AK: Fractures and dislocations of the distal radio-ulnar joint. Hand Clin. 1988; 4:361-375.

19. Tsukazaki T, Takagi K, Iwasaki K: Poor correlation between functional results and radiographic findings in Colles' fracture. J Hand Surg [Br]. 1993; 18:588-591.

20. Ekenstam F, Jakobsson OP, Wadin K: Repair of the triangular ligament in Colles' fracture: no effect in a prospective randomized study. Acta Orthop Scand. 1989; 60:393-396.

21. Hauck RM, Hershey PA, Shahen J, Palmer AK: Classification and treatment of ulnar styloid nonunion. J Hand Surg [Am]. 1996; 21:418-422.

Ligament Reconstruction/Sigmoid Notch Plasty for DRUJ Instability

29

Brian Adams, MD

The bony or ligamentous structures of the distal radioulnar joint (DRUJ) are often disrupted in association with a distal radius fracture, which is the most common cause for DRUJ instability. In some studies, up to 10% of patients with distal radius fractures had a DRUJ injury necessitating primary operative repair.[1] In addition, arthroscopy at the time of fracture identified the presence of triangular fibrocartilage complex (TFCC) injury in 43 of 51 patients examined by Lindau and colleagues.[2] The TFCC lesions were associated with DRUJ instability in 17 patients. Younger patients and those sustaining high-energy injuries are more likely to have DRUJ injuries in association with distal radius fractures.[2]

Failure to recognize and treat DRUJ disruption can contribute to a poor outcome. In particular, residual DRUJ instability after distal radius fracture is associated with worse objective and subjective outcome measures.[3] When treated acutely by either closed reduction or soft tissue or bony repair, most patients will not develop DRUJ instability. However, some patients with distal radius fractures will go on to develop chronic DRUJ instability owing to failure of the soft tissues to heal or to malunion of the radius or ulna (**Fig. 29-1**). Multiple techniques have been described to restore stability to the chronically unstable DRUJ. These techniques can be divided into three categories: (1) a direct radioulnar tether that is extrinsic to the joint, (2) an indirect radioulnar link through an ulnocarpal sling or tenodesis, or (3) reconstruction of the distal radioulnar ligaments.

Multiple biomechanical studies have shown that the dorsal and palmar radioulnar ligaments are key stabilizers of the DRUJ.[4,5] The radioulnar ligaments are condensations of fibers at the combined junctures of the triangular fibrocartilage articular disc, DRUJ capsule, and ulnocarpal capsule. As they pass toward the ulna, each ligament divides into superficial and deep fibers (**Fig. 29-2**). The superficial fibers insert on the ulnar styloid near its midportion. Disruption of the superficial fibers in the absence of other injury does not result in DRUJ instability. The deep radioulnar ligament fibers insert into the fovea on the ulnar head, which is a bony depression between the base of the styloid and the articular cartilage on the dome of the ulnar head. Disruption of these fibers can result in DRUJ instability.

Because of the importance of the dorsal and palmar radioulnar ligaments for DRUJ stability, reconstruction of these ligaments offers the best anatomical restoration of joint stability. The technique described in this chapter uses a tendon graft that nearly mimics the native ligaments. The two limbs of the tendon graft pass from the volar and dorsal margins of the sigmoid notch and converge to insert on the ulnar head at the fovea (**Fig. 29-3**). A recent biomechanical study by Gofton and coworkers[6] found that this radioulnar ligament reconstruction nearly restored the kine-matics of the unstable DRUJ, and it provided better joint stability than the nonanatomical reconstruction described by Fulkerson-Watson, which has been shown to provide the best stability among the radioulnar tether methods.

Reconstruction of the soft tissue DRUJ restraints, however, will be insufficient in the presence of a substantial osseous abnormality. The articular surfaces of the DRUJ are not congruent in the normal wrist. The sigmoid notch has a radius of curvature that is much larger than that of the ulnar head (**Fig. 29-4**). It is a combination of ligament tension and joint compression between the ulnar head and rims of the notch that provides joint stability. The dorsal and particularly the volar rims of the notch often have fibrocartilaginous extensions or labrums that augment its relatively flat surface, which improves joint congruency and capture and thus substantially increases DRUJ stability.[7] A developmentally flat notch or one that is deficient from injury poses greater risks to develop DRUJ instability and for the failure of a ligament reconstruction (**Fig. 29-5**). Sigmoid notch osteoplasty increases the prominence of the rim and improves joint stability.

Extra-articular deformity of the radius alone is sufficient to substantially impair DRUJ function. In cadaver studies, dorsal angulation of the distal radius or loss of radial inclination alters DRUJ mechanics and reduces forearm rotation.[8,9] Corrective osteotomy of the radius can be performed in conjunction with a radioulnar ligament reconstruction.

Indications

Distal radioulnar ligament reconstruction is indicated in patients with symptomatic chronic DRUJ instability. The instability may be unidirectional or bidirectional. Physical examination will show increased translation, which is typically greater with the forearm in neutral rotation. However, it is important to test passive translation in all forearm positions because palmar instability is best demonstrated with the forearm supinated. A painful clunk may occur with forearm rotation, especially if manual compression is applied during active motion. There is no specific age limit in adults, with the procedure having been performed in ages ranging from 16 to 45 years in the original reported series. There is also no specific time limit for the presence of instability as long as no other factors have developed to compromise the procedure. The procedure has successfully restored stability in patients who had their original injury 4 months to 30 years previously.

Computed tomography (CT) should be performed if there is any question regarding the competency of the sigmoid notch or the presence of arthritis. CT is performed on both wrists in equivalent neutral, pronation, and supination positions. The comparison between sides will help assess direction of instability and if the shape of the notch has been altered by injury. If the notch

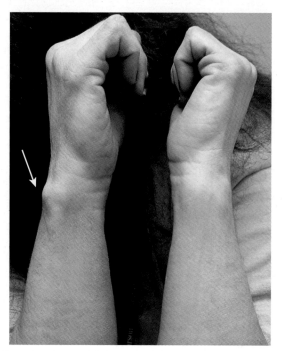

FIGURE 29-1 Chronic DRUJ instability after a distal radius fracture. *Arrow* points to the prominent ulnar head on the affected side.

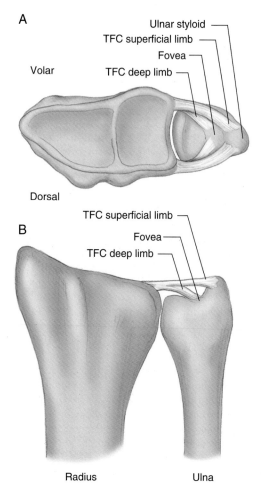

FIGURE 29-2 Volar and dorsal radioulnar ligaments each divide into superficial and deep limbs. Deep limbs insert into the ulnar fovea and are more important for DRUJ stability.

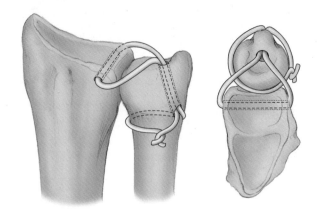

FIGURE 29-3 Final graft placement mimics the native insertion sites of the distal radioulnar ligaments.

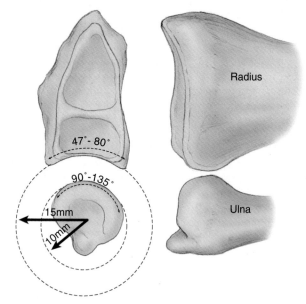

FIGURE 29-4 Radius of curvature of the sigmoid notch is greater than that of the ulnar head.

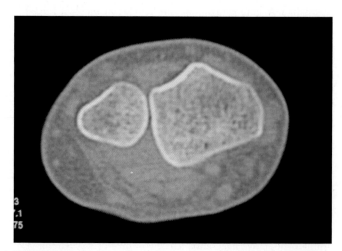

FIGURE 29-5 CT of a patient with symptomatic DRUJ instability shows a flat sigmoid notch with no substantial volar or dorsal rims. Ligamentous reconstruction alone in this patient would not be sufficient to restore stability; reconstruction was augmented with a volar sigmoid notch osteoplasty.

is developmentally flat or a rim has been traumatically damaged, a sigmoid notch osteoplasty at the time of ligamentous reconstruction may be necessary.

Contraindications

Because bony tunnels are made through the distal ulna and radius, the procedure is contraindicated in skeletally immature patients, owing to the risk of physeal injury. DRUJ reconstruction is contraindicated in patients with DRUJ arthritis and advanced ulnar impaction syndrome because the procedure is less likely to relieve pain despite improving joint stability.

Patients with generalized ligament laxity, particularly younger patients with bilateral DRUJ instability, are not good candidates because of the risk of recurrent instability over time.

Malunions of the distal radius or ulna, including acquired ulnar-positive variance, must be corrected either before or concomitant with the ligament reconstruction. A substantial incongruency of the sigmoid notch involving its central portion due to fracture malunion that is not indicated for corrective osteotomy is a relative contraindication due to the risk of arthritis.

Surgical Technique

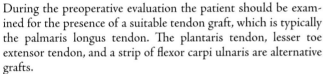

During the preoperative evaluation the patient should be examined for the presence of a suitable tendon graft, which is typically the palmaris longus tendon. The plantaris tendon, lesser toe extensor tendon, and a strip of flexor carpi ulnaris are alternative grafts.

The patient is positioned supine with the operative arm extended on a hand table. An upper arm tourniquet is applied. A 4-cm longitudinal skin incision is made over the interval between the fifth and sixth extensor compartments. The fifth compartment is entered, and the extensor digiti minimi is retracted. The DRUJ is identified by palpation. An L-shaped capsulotomy is made overlying the DRUJ. Its longitudinal limb extends along the dorsal rim of the sigmoid notch, stopping just short of the radiocarpal joint to preserve any remnant of the dorsal radioulnar ligament. The transverse limb extends ulnarward from the sigmoid notch, just proximal and parallel to the normal location of the dorsal radioulnar ligament (**Fig. 29-6**).

The capsular flap is reflected ulnarward, allowing inspection of the TFCC, ulnar head, and sigmoid notch. TFCC repair should be performed instead of ligament reconstruction if there is sufficient tissue. If the TFCC is insufficient for repair, one can proceed with ligamentous reconstruction.

The graft may be harvested at this point, and its diameter is assessed to plan for appropriate drill size to make the bony tunnels.

The periosteum is elevated from the dorsal distal radius adjacent to the sigmoid notch. A small back-cut along the dorsal rim of the distal radius may be necessary to provide sufficient elevation and retraction of the fourth extensor compartment. A guidewire for a 3.5-mm cannulated drill is driven from dorsal to volar through the distal radius several millimeters from the articular surfaces of the lunate fossa and sigmoid notch. The distance between the guidewire and the articular surfaces must be sufficient to allow a drill hole of sufficient size that will accommodate the graft. Guidewire position is confirmed with fluoroscopy. The cannulated drill is used over the guidewire with care not to drive the guidewire into the volar tissues. If necessary, the hole is enlarged with standard drill bits (**Fig. 29-7**).

When the surgical plan includes a corrective osteotomy for a distal radial malunion it is easier to create the radial tunnel before

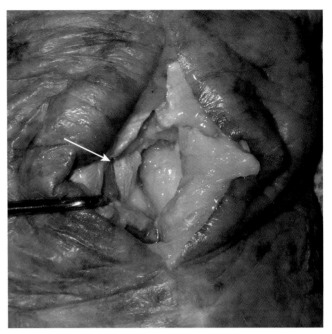

FIGURE 29-6 An L-shaped capsulotomy allows visualization of the sigmoid notch (*arrow*) and ulnar head.

making the osteotomy. Whether done before or after the osteotomy, the tunnel should be made parallel to the malaligned lunate fossa. Any osteotomies should be positioned and stabilized before graft tensioning.

The distal ulna tunnel extends between the fovea and the subcutaneous border of the ulnar neck just volar to the extensor carpi ulnaris tendon. If sufficient exposure cannot be obtained by flexing the wrist and retracting the TFCC remnant, the guidewire is inserted through the fovea to exit the ulnar neck. Alternatively, in patients with stiff wrist flexion or a large wrist, the guidewire can be passed more easily in the opposite direction, that is, from the ulnar neck to the fovea. Using this latter method, a 4- to 5-mm drill hole is first made in the ulnar neck at its subcutaneous border. A guidewire is inserted in the hole and driven through the fovea. Regardless of the direction of guidewire placement, the cannulated drill should be passed from proximal (ulnar neck) to distal (fovea) to prevent damage to the carpus. One should begin with a 3.5-mm cannulated drill bit and if necessary enlarge the tunnel with standard drill bits to accommodate both limbs of the graft (**Fig. 29-8**).

The volar opening of the radius tunnel is exposed through a 3- to 4-cm longitudinal incision extending proximally from the proximal wrist crease between the ulnar neurovascular bundle and finger flexor tendons. Careful dissection between the ulnar neurovascular bundle and finger flexors reveals the pronator quadratus and distal portion of the volar DRUJ capsule. A suture retriever is passed through to the radius tunnel from dorsal to volar. The retriever is used to pull one end of the graft from volar to dorsal through the radius. From dorsal to volar, a straight hemostat is passed just distal to the ulnar head and proximal to the residual TFCC. The volar DRUJ capsule is punctured, and the volar limb of the graft is grasped and pulled back into the dorsal wrist wound (**Fig. 29-9**). One should be careful not to entrap any nervous, vascular, or tendinous structures in the graft loop. Both ends of the tendon graft should now lie in the dorsal wrist exposure (**Fig. 29-10**).

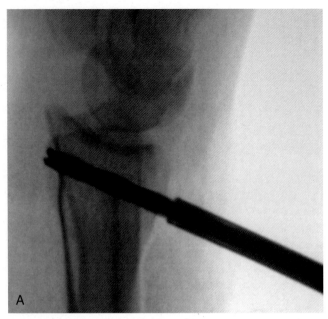

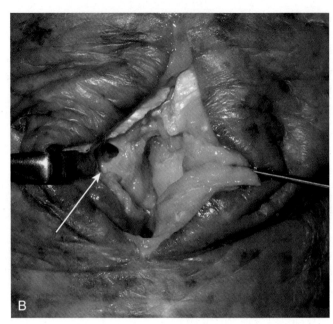

FIGURE 29-7 A, In this patient with a distal radius malunion, fluoroscopy is used to confirm guidewire and cannulated drill placement. Note that the drill hole is parallel to the distal radius articular surface. **B,** A distal radius drill hole (*arrow*) has been made several millimeters away from the articular surfaces of the sigmoid notch and lunate fossa.

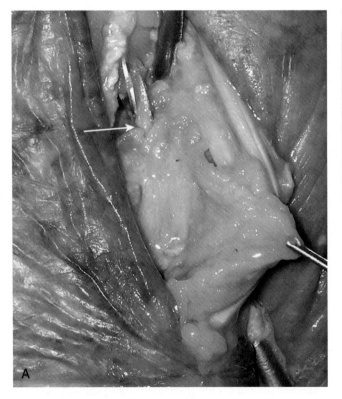

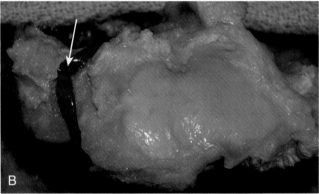

FIGURE 29-8 A, Cannulated drill passes over the guidewire from the ulnar neck to the fovea of the ulnar head. *Arrow* indicates the location of the fovea. **B,** After removal of the surrounding soft tissues, the red vessel loop can be seen exiting the fovea in the ulnar head.

The suture retriever is passed through the distal ulna tunnel from the neck to fovea, exiting in the dorsal wound. Both limbs of the tendon graft are pulled back through the ulna to exit at the ulnar neck (**Fig. 29-11**). A hemostat is passed ulnarward under the extensor carpi ulnaris sheath at the ulnar neck and used to pull one limb of the graft toward the radius (**Fig. 29-12**). From the dorsal exposure, a right-angled clamp is passed volarly around the ulnar neck to grasp the second graft limb and pull it back around the neck. Both limbs of the tendon graft should now be resting on the dorsal ulnar neck (**Fig. 29-13**).

The two graft limbs are pulled taut and tied in a half-hitch while the forearm is held in neutral rotation and manual pressure is applied to compress the DRUJ (**Fig. 29-14**). The half-hitch is secured with 3-0 nonabsorbable sutures (**Fig. 29-15**). The dorsal DRUJ capsule and the extensor retinaculum are closed in a single layer, with care to avoid the extensor tendons (see Fig. 29-20).

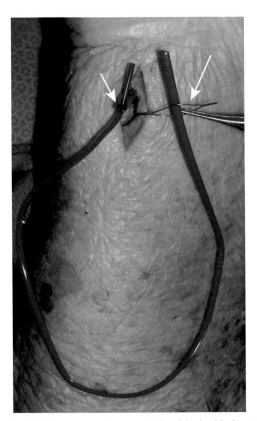

FIGURE 29-9 Suture passer is seen to the right in this image, while the tip of the hemostat is to the left. Hemostat grasps one end of the graft (*long arrow*) while the other graft end is placed in the suture retriever loop (*short arrow*). (A red vessel loop has been used instead of tendon graft in this cadaver specimen for illustrative purposes.)

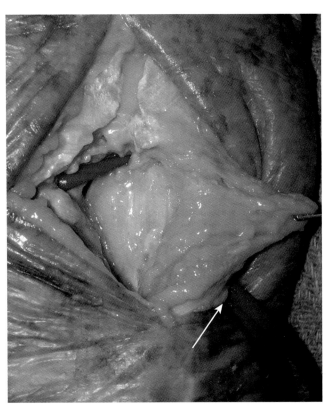

FIGURE 29-11 A suture retriever is used to pass both ends of the tendon graft through the distal ulna tunnel to exit at the ulnar neck (*arrow*).

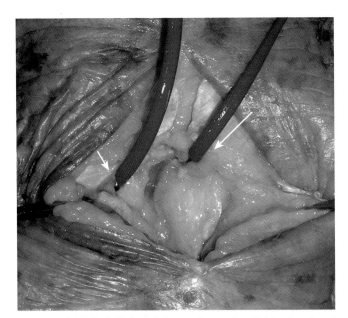

FIGURE 29-10 Both limbs of the tendon graft exit into the dorsal wound—one limb exiting through the distal radius tunnel (*short arrow*), and the second limb though the volar DRUJ capsule just distal to the ulnar head (*long arrow*).

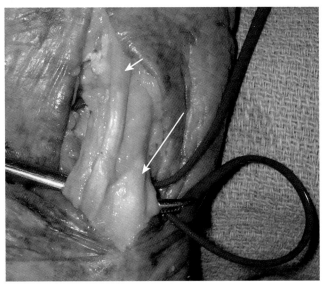

FIGURE 29-12 A hemostat pulls one end of the tendon graft over the dorsal ulnar neck and beneath the extensor carpi ulnaris sheath (*long arrow*). The *short arrow* indicates the location of the extensor digiti minimi tendon.

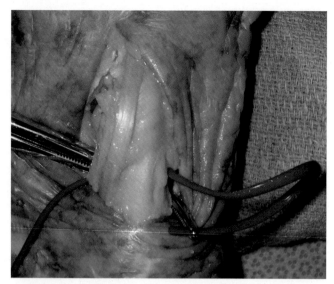

FIGURE 29-13 A right-angled clamp passes around the volar ulnar neck to retrieve the other end of the tendon graft.

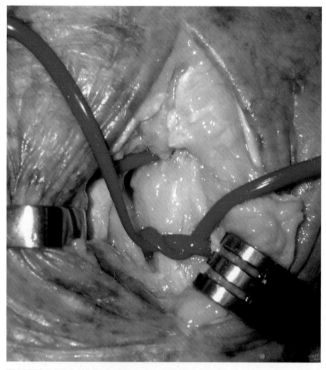

FIGURE 29-14 While holding the DRUJ reduced, the two ends of the graft are pulled taut and tied in a half-hitch over the ulnar neck. The ECU sheath is being retracted by the rake retractor (*right*).

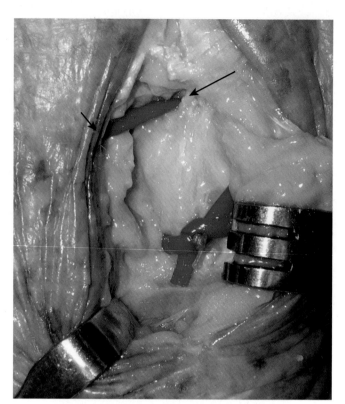

FIGURE 29-15 Final appearance of the graft from the dorsal wrist wound. The graft is seen exiting the radial drill hole (*short arrow*) and entering the fovea on the ulnar head (*long arrow*).

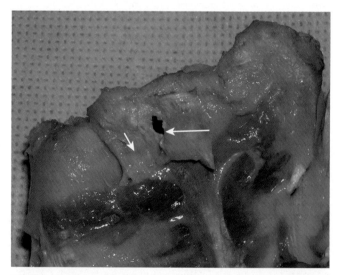

FIGURE 29-16 Bony surface of the radius adjacent to the volar rim of the DRUJ is exposed (*short arrow*) extending to the exit of the radial tunnel (*long arrow*).

The extensor digiti minimi tendon is left superficial over the DRUJ. A temporary large-diameter Kitschner wire (K-wire) may be placed across the DRUJ if desired but I very rarely do this.

The patient is placed in a long arm splint with the forearm in neutral to slight supination or pronation depending on the most stable position. At the first postoperative visit at 10 days, the patient is converted to a long arm cast extending to just above the elbow to control forearm rotation. Three weeks later the cast is changed to a short arm well-molded cast that partially limits forearm rotation for an additional 2 to 3 weeks.

The patient is then converted to a removable wrist brace to be used for an additional 2 more months as motion and strength are recovered. Therapy begins with active and gentle passive wrist flexion, extension, pronation, and supination. No limitations are placed on active motion, but only gentle passive motion should be used during the first month of therapy. Strengthening is started early, but high forces with the arm in full pronation and supination are avoided. At 4 months after the surgical procedure, more aggressive passive range of motion and strengthening exercises are added. No use of the hand for sports or other stress-

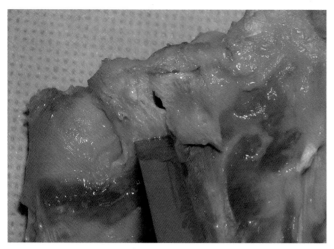

FIGURE 29-17 A small osteotome is used to make the proximal cut of the osteoplasty at the proximal margin of the sigmoid notch.

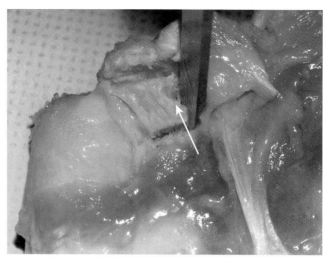

FIGURE 29-18 An osteotome is used to make the second transverse limb parallel to both the lunate fossa and the proximal osteotomy. The longitudinal cut of the osteotomy passes through the ulnar edge of the radial tunnel (arrow).

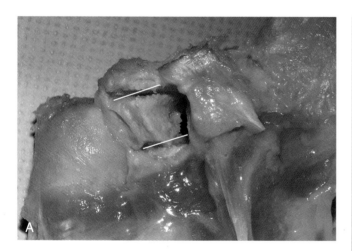

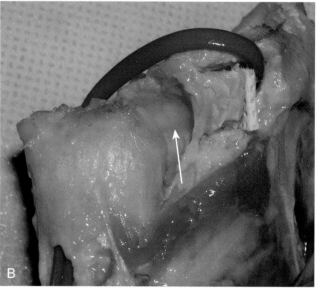

FIGURE 29-19 A, Osteotomy fragment is gently levered toward the ulnar head, which should bend but not break the articular cartilage and subchondral bone. The lines are adjacent to the proximal and distal osteotomy cuts. B, Oblique view of the wrist with the DRUJ distracted shows the intact articular cartilage of the sigmoid notch (arrow).

ful activities is allowed until at least the fourth month after surgery.

If the sigmoid notch is flat or deformed, then an osteoplasty may be performed at the same setting as the DRUJ ligament reconstruction. Sigmoid notch osteoplasty augments the volar or dorsal rim of the sigmoid notch to increase DRUJ stability. Wallwork and Bain[10] originally described the sigmoid notch osteoplasty for the volar rim, but the same technique may also be used to augment the dorsal rim.

The osteoplasty may be performed through the same volar or dorsal approach used for DRUJ ligament reconstruction. For the volar side, the periosteum is incised and raised 3 to 4 mm radial to the rim of the sigmoid notch (see Fig. 29-16). For the dorsal side, the previously incised capsule is raised in continuity with the adjacent periosteum. With the use of a small osteotome, a trans-

verse cut about 4 mm deep is made in the rim of the notch at its proximal edge (Fig. 29-17). A second parallel osteotomy is made 2 to 3 mm proximal to the radiocarpal joint. A longitudinal cut about 4 mm from the margin of the rim connects the two transverse limbs. If a simultaneous ligament reconstruction is part of the surgical plan, the radial drill hole is made first. The longitudinal limb of the osteotomy passes through the ulnar margin of the radial drill hole (Fig. 29-18). The osteotome is slowly advanced to the depth of the longitudinal cut (one-fourth to one-third the width of the radius) and used to gently lever the rim a few millimeters toward the ulna. The articular cartilage and subchondral bone are bent but not broken through. The gap is filled with bone graft harvested from the nearby distal radius (Fig. 29-19). The tendon graft should be passed through the distal radius drill hole but not tensioned before bone graft placement. Because the

---

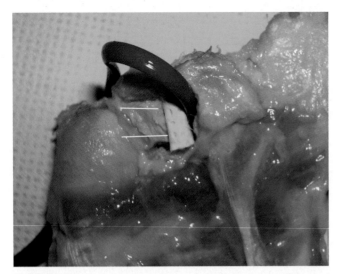

FIGURE 29-20 Tendon graft has been passed through the radial tunnel and into ulna tunnel. A small wedge of bone graft from the distal radius is wedged into the defect left by the osteotomy (*shown as a blue spacer*). Tension on the tendon graft secures the bone graft and the osteotomy position. The *lines* indicate the proximal and distal osteotomy cuts.

tendon graft will pass directly over the bone graft when tensioned in its final position, it will typically secure the bone graft, but sutures through the nearby periosteum can be added (**Fig. 29-20**).

The addition of a sigmoid notchplasty does not alter the postsurgical management except that the long arm immobilization is used for the first 6 weeks instead of 4 weeks; however, the time in the short arm cast can be reduced to 2 weeks.

Complications

Potential operative complications include injury to the dorsal cutaneous branch of the ulnar nerve or the ulnar neurovascular bundle during the exposures, and articular fractures when making the tunnels. Long-term potential complications include wrist stiffness, loss of forearm rotation, failure to relieve pain, and recurrent instability.

Results

The majority of patients treated with DRUJ ligament reconstruction will maintain near-full forearm rotation and have restored DRUJ stability and improved grip strength. This procedure successfully restored stability in 12 of 14 patients in Adams and Berger's original series,[11] and 9 of 14 patients had complete relief of pain at minimum 1 year follow-up. Patients averaged 72 degrees of pronation and 70 degrees of supination. One of the

patients with recurrent instability was later noted to have a deficient sigmoid notch volar rim, whereas the other had only ulnocarpal residual instability. A later follow-up with an additional 8 patients showed maintained stability in the first 12 successful procedures and good stability in the additional 8 patients.

Teoh and Yam reported similar results in their series of 9 patients treated with a slight variation of this technique. Seven of 9 patients had restored DRUJ stability and regained 90% of forearm rotation when compared with the normal side.[12]

REFERENCES

1. Geissler WB, Fernandez DL, Lamey DM: Distal radioulnar joint injuries associated with fractures of the distal radius. Clin Orthop Relat Res. 1996; 327:135-146.
2. Lindau T, Adlercreutz C, Aspenberg P: Peripheral tears of the triangular fibrocartilage complex cause distal radioulnar joint instability after distal radial fractures. J Hand Surg [Am]. 2000; 25:464-468.
3. Lindau T, Hagberg L, Adlercreutz C, et al: Distal radioulnar instability is an independent worsening factor in distal radial fractures. Clin Orthop Relat Res. 2000; 376:229-235.
4. Kihari H, Short WH, Werner FW, et al: The stabilizing mechanism of the distal radioulnar joint during pronation and supination. J Hand Surg [Am]. 1995; 20:930-936.
5. Ward LD, Ambrose CG, Masson MV, Levaro F: The role of the distal radioulnar ligaments, interosseous membrane, and joint capsule in distal radioulnar joint stability. J Hand Surg [Am]. 2000; 25:341-351.
6. Gofton WT, Gordon KD, Dunning CE, et al: Comparison of distal radioulnar joint reconstructions using an active joint motion simulator. J Hand Surg [Am]. 2005; 30:733-742.
7. Tolat AR, Stanley JK, Trail IA: A cadaveric study of the anatomy and stability of the distal radioulnar joint in the coronal and transverse planes. J Hand Surg [Br]. 1996; 21:587-594.
8. Adams BD: Effects of radial deformity on distal radioulnar joint mechanics. J Hand Surg [Am]. 1993; 18:492-498.
9. Kihari H, Palmer AK, Werner FW, et al: The effect of dorsally angulated distal radius fractures on distal radioulnar joint congruency and forearm rotation. J Hand Surg [Am]. 1996; 21:40-47.
10. Wallwork NA, Bain GI: Sigmoid notch osteoplasty for chronic volar instability of the distal radioulnar joint: a case report. J Hand Surg [Am]. 2001; 26:454-459.
11. Adams BD, Berger RA: An anatomic reconstruction of the distal radioulnar ligaments for posttraumatic distal radioulnar joint instability. J Hand Surg [Am]. 2002; 27:243-251.
12. Teoh LC, Yam AKT: Anatomic reconstruction of the distal radioulnar ligaments: long-term results. J Hand Surg [Br]. 2005; 30:185-193.

Dorsal Capsuloplasty in Volar Subluxation of the Distal Radius

30

A. Richard Koch, MD and Tijmen de Jong, MD

Instability of the distal radioulnar joint (DRUJ) may be responsible for reduced hand and wrist function from loss of strength and chronic pain on the ulnar side of the wrist. As Bowers noted in 1991, this condition was believed to be rare but became more and more diagnosed and therefore the subject of much discussion and investigation.[1] At this time, Bowers' observation is still of current interest.

The ulna is the stable unit of the forearm, supporting the radius and the hand and allowing controlled movement of the radius along its axis and the DRUJ. The bony anatomy of the DRUJ, however, adds very little to stability. A variety of other structures are responsible for stability of the DRUJ. It is currently assumed that these comprise the pronator quadratus, ulnocarpal ligament, extensor carpi ulnaris subsheath, dorsal radioulnar ligament, volar radioulnar ligament, interosseous membrane, the bony anatomy (sigmoid notch), and the DRUJ capsule.[2-10]

The soft tissues, together with normal articular cartilage surfaces of the lower end of the ulna and the medial articular facet of the distal radius, ensure a smooth and complete forearm in pronation/supination.[1,11] This specific movement is provided not only by rotation from the radius about the ulna but can also only be executed when there is a variable degree of dorsopalmar translation.[12,13]

Garcia-Elias described in his article on soft tissue anatomy and relationships about the distal ulna that the radius in supination rotates and translates dorsally about the stable ulna, whereas in pronation it rotates and translates palmarly.[14] As a result, there is a great variance in joint surface contact of the DRUJ between the sigmoid notch of the distal radius and the articulating surface of the ulnar head. In the neutral forearm position the surface contact is maximal (about 60%). In all other forearm positions there is joint surface contact until it is lost almost completely (less than 10%).[15]

A stable DRUJ allows rotation, axial motion, as well as translational movement in the dorsopalmar plane. All these movements are based on the osseous contours around the joint, supported by a complex of surrounding soft tissues, which Bowers[1] calls the major retaining ligaments. The triangular fibrocartilage complex (TFCC) is considered the major retaining ligament of the DRUJ, with two ligament subsets, the dorsal and volar marginal ligaments (DML-TFC, VML-TFC). These thickenings on the dorsal and volar margins of the central part of the TFCC on the triangular fibrocartilage proper are also referred to as the dorsal and volar radioulnar ligaments.[16] There is experimental evidence[6,17,18] suggesting that both palmar and dorsal distal radioulnar ligaments need to be intact to maintain complete

stability of the joint throughout the whole range of forearm rotation. The relative contribution of each ligament in stabilizing the DRUJ during pronation/supination remains, however, contradictory.[6,7,13,17,19]

Post-traumatic rupturing, laxity, or attenuation of the suspending soft tissues around the DRUJ may lead to DRUJ instability and cause chronic ulnar wrist pain, with decreased grip strength and a reduced sensation of wrist stability, affecting many activities of daily life. The inability of normal wrist function and subsequent pain may finally result in full work incapacitation.

Most of the current treatment options regarding instability of the DRUJ refer to reconstruction of the TFCC. A great variety of techniques have been published. Adams and Berger have classified these techniques into three categories[20]: (1) a direct radioulnar tether that is extrinsic to the joint,[21] (2) an indirect radioulnar link through an ulnocarpal sling or tenodesis,[22] and (3) reconstruction of the distal radioulnar ligaments.[16,23]

In their article, Adams and Berger describe their own technique for reconstruction of both dorsal and palmar radioulnar ligaments, because they believe that gross instability of the DRUJ requires disruption of both ligaments. Reconstruction of both ligaments would therefore be the optimal surgical treatment for post-traumatic, chronic DRUJ instability. For this purpose they use a tendon graft (usually the palmaris longus), which is passed through drill holes in the distal radius and ulna.[20]

In this chapter we describe the history and fate of 20 of our patients with only limited instability of the DRUJ. The basic cause for instability is a post-traumatic attenuation of the dorsal capsule, which we consider an extension of the dorsal marginal ligament. This instability permits a volar subluxation of the distal radius, resulting in chronic ulnar wrist pain.

Reefing of the dorsal capsule and thereby tightening the DML is our therapy of choice. This surgical approach is a result of a fortuitous observation during arthroscopy and open surgery in a patient with typical complaints of a painful DRUJ instability. As a routine, we perform an arthroscopy to improve our diagnostic differentiation. One of the most striking features during this examination was a clear laxity of the TFCC exclusively in the dorsal part. During the subsequent operation (see later), we observed a notable surplus of soft tissues over the ulnar head just proximal to the DML, becoming most evident when reducing the volar subluxation of the radius with the ulna. This tissue was not only found to be in continuation with the ligamentous part of the TFCC (DML) but also appeared surprisingly strong and sufficient for capsuloplasty.

The Authors' Experience

Patient Selection

The course of 20 consecutive patient treatments during the period from 2003 until 2005 was analyzed retrospectively. Charts were reviewed for preoperative history and physical findings. Fifteen of the patients were female,[14] and 5 were men. Of this group, 4 patients were excluded. One patient could not be traced for follow-up, 1 patient developed a pain syndrome (although on the radial side of the wrist), and 2 patients were excluded because of the severity of their TFCC degeneration, which became apparent during operation. Nevertheless we attempted a reefing of the DML, which later proved insufficient. In these 2 patients an ulnar shortening was performed in a second operation.

Therefore, 16 patients were included in the study, with an average age of 26 years (range: 9 to 56 years). In 10 patients the dominant wrist was involved. The mean duration of symptoms before first contact in our clinic was 31 months (12 to 108 months). The average follow-up was 12 months (5 to 23 months). All of these patients except 2 had a history of wrist trauma, of whom 6 suffered fractures of the distal radius or scaphoid. They were all treated with closed reduction and casting. None had previous surgery for DRUJ instability.

Physical Findings

We observed that patients suffering from painful DRUJ instability usually presented with painful rotation and ulnar deviation, often in combination with a painful click sensed over the dorsal aspect of the DRUJ while making rotational movements. Most patients complained of a reduced grip strength and periodic sensations of sudden wrist instability, provoked by rotational movements during (heavy) lifting.

In most of the patients, swelling around the ulnar side of the wrist could be observed. Sometimes, the ulnar head, however, was more prominent on the affected side. Subluxation of the extensor carpi ulnaris tendon in the sixth extensor sheet could be excluded. Rotation of the forearm was usually not restricted. Extreme supination was sometimes painful. Flexion and extension were symmetrical on both sides. A painful joint click in active and passive forearm rotation was present in seven patients.

In all patients an increased anteroposterior translation of the DRUJ was found, with passive manipulation, compared with the uninvolved wrist. When performing this maneuver, we ask the patient to lay the flexed elbow on a table with the hand pointing to the ceiling. Bringing the forearm in neutral position with the thumb pointing to the nose, the patient is asked to hold the wrist in full relaxation. Thus, we compare the translation of both wrists in neutral, supination, and pronation to evaluate the severity of instability. With the arm in the same position, we also perform the ulnar compression test. With the wrist in ulnar deviation, force is executed, thus compressing the ulnar side of the proximal row of the carpus against the TFCC. In only three patients, the ulnar compression pain was positive.

All patients had tenderness around the distal ulna, which varied from just distal and palmar of the ulnar styloid, dorsal to the distal edge of the ulnar head, or over the DRUJ.

Imaging

As a routine we obtain posteroanterior and true lateral plain radiographs in radial as well as in ulnar deviation. The lateral radiographs had our interest for objectivation of an altered prominence of the ulnar head, which was the case in six patients.

No wrists showed a widening of the joint in the posteroanterior radiograph. There were no signs of earlier trauma to the ulnar styloid process. The joint surfaces of the DRUJ and distal ulna showed no signs of earlier trauma or arthrosis. Before referral to our clinic, arthrography or magnetic resonance imaging (MRI) was performed in two patients. MRI showed a peripheral lesion of the TFCC, and arthrography demonstrated a central leak. Computed tomography was not performed.

Arthroscopy

Every patient in this series was subjected to wrist arthroscopy. A constant finding of the TFCC was observed in those patients who were suspected of having an instability of the DRUJ region. With the scope through the 3-4 portal and the probe via the RU portal, we obtained a clear view of the TFCC. When testing the tension of the TFCC with the probe, it often showed a normal movement (trampoline effect) of the central part of the TFCC; however, there was laxity in the area of the dorsal radioulnar ligament of the TFCC when compressing and pulling it with the curved probe. We often found an excess of fibrous tissue in this area, which was sometimes accompanied by a localized synovitis. To obtain a better view on the dorsal TFCC area we performed an arthroscopic synovectomy, but we have never seen clear tears in that area.

During arthroscopy of the ulnar side of the wrist, other pathological processes were excluded, especially lateral and medial tears of the TFCC.

We consider a combination of dorsal laxity of the TFCC and localized fibrous hypertrophy or synovitis highly suggestive of a DRUJ instability caused by attenuation of the fibrous tissues in the area of the DML.

Indications

Dorsal capsuloplasty in volar subluxation of the distal radius should be reserved for patients without significant TFCC disruption or central degeneration.

Our primary diagnostic parameters in patients selected for this reefing procedure are based on the specific history, physical examination, radiographs, and arthroscopy. Trauma is most often the primary cause for DRUJ instability. Increased volar-dorsal translation is apparent, with compression pain over the DML and DRUJ. Ulnar compression pain is normally absent.

Contraindications

On plain radiographs, styloid process pseudarthrosis and widening of the DRUJ should be excluded, because we believe that this technique is not appropriate for lateral or medial tears of the TFCC.

Other contraindications would include a nonreconstructable TFCC, ulnar head osteoarthritis, sigmoid notch incongruity, rheumatoid arthritis, and patients using systemic corticosteroids.

Surgical Technique

All our patients were operated on as outpatients under regional (axillary block) or general anesthesia with a pneumatic tourniquet around the upper arm to operate under bloodless conditions. The arm is laid on a hand table with the elbow extended and the forearm in pronation. To expose the ulnar head and DRUJ, we make an L-shaped (hockey stick) skin incision of about 5 cm along the sixth extensor sheet area from proximal to distal, curving 5 mm distal to the ulnar styloid to the dorsal aspect of the wrist,

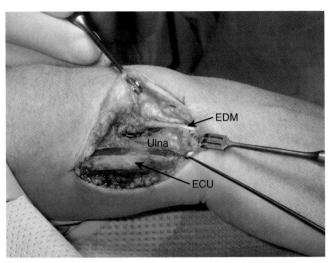

FIGURE 30-1 The ulnar head is exposed after skin incision and opening of the fifth and sixth extensor sheet. ECU, extensor carpi ulnaris; EDM, extensor digiti minimi.

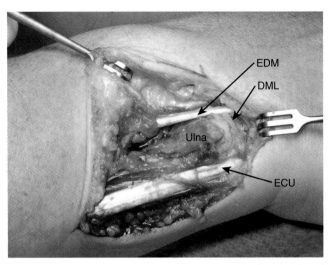

FIGURE 30-3 Opening the dorsal capsule just proximal to the dorsal marginal ligament (DML), exposing the ulnar head. EDM, extensor digiti minimi; ECU, extensor carpi ulnaris.

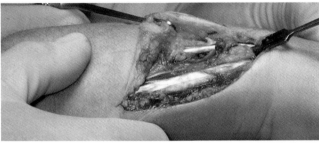

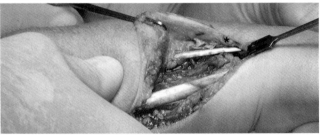

FIGURE 30-2 Wrinkling of dorsal capsular tissue (*asterisk*) when depressing the ulna.

and ending just radial to the fifth extensor sheet. To prevent the formation of a painful neuroma it is important to protect the sensory branches of the ulnar nerve, running from volar to dorsal especially in the distal part of the incision. We free the skin from the extensor retinaculum along the fifth and sixth tendon sheets and open them in the same manner as the skin, with a curved incision. The floor of the sixth extensor sheath, however, is preserved. To expose the DRUJ capsule, the extensor carpi ulnaris (ECU) and extensor digiti quinti (EDQ) tendons are retracted radially and ulnarward, respectively (**Fig. 30-1**).

With the wrist still in pronation, the ulnar head can be depressed in a volar direction, that is, correcting the DRUJ instability. In this manner, soft tissue wrinkling is observed around the distal and dorsal aspect of the ulnar head, just proximal to the DML of the TFCC (**Fig. 30-2**).

This wrinkling surplus of capsular tissue, which is surprisingly strong, is considered the elongated or attenuated DML. A few millimeters proximal to the DML an incision is made to create a

small flap, which is freed from the distal ulnar head but is left connected to the DML. By lifting this flap, the dorsal aspect of the ulnar head and DRUJ are exposed and can be inspected for cartilage condition (**Fig. 30-3**). A Mitchell trimmer can be inserted and moved between the TFCC and the ulnar head to feel if there are any adhesions that can be released. We then make an incision just distal to the radioulnar ligament to open the ulnocarpal joint for inspection of the triquetrum, the lunate, and the lunotriquetral ligament, as well as the TFCC. In case of TFCC lesions or signs of ulnocarpal abutment, a wafer procedure may be performed simultaneously.

We then start with the final part of the operation—reefing of the DML. After flexing the patient's elbow, the assistant holds the patient's wrist in a neutral position with the forearm in a 0-degree position with the thumb pointing toward the patient's nose. For better visibility and comfort, the surgeon will move to the "lower side" of the arm table. In **Figure 30-4**, note that the DML is now clearly demonstrated. With the forearm in this neutral position, the ulnar head is only slightly compressed volarly and the DML is brought over the dorsal capsule (**Fig. 30-5**). We then attach the dorsal portion of the DML with just slight tension to the periosteum of the ulnar head with usually no more than four separate PDS 4-0 stitches (**Fig. 30-6**). The site of fixation is thus more proximal to the point of original insertion of the DML, but it should never be too tight, in order to prevent a permanent reduction of supination (**Fig. 30-7**). Transfixion wires through the DRUJ are not used. It is important to maintain the wrist in a neutral position, until the final plaster is applied. The tourniquet is released, and hemostasis is obtained. The fifth and sixth extensor sheaths are closed with resorbable sutures, and the skin is closed with a subcuticular running suture. The site of the incision is covered with a nonadhesive gauze pad, fluffy dressings are applied around the hand and wrist, and a long forearm plaster splint is applied with the elbow flexed and the forearm in neutral position.

Rehabilitation

After 2 weeks the splint is replaced by a circular upper arm cast, for another 4 to 5 weeks. The duration of immobilization is 6 to

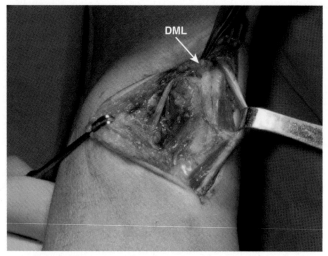

FIGURE 30-4 Dorsal marginal ligament (DML) held in forceps.

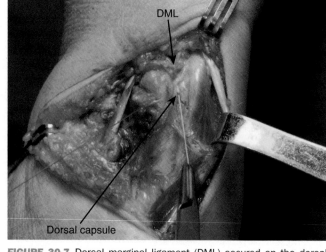

FIGURE 30-7 Dorsal marginal ligament (DML) secured on the dorsal capsule, however under no or little tension.

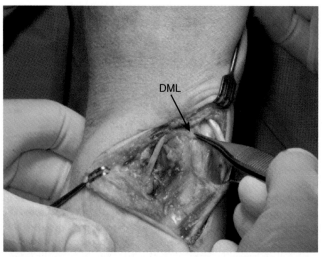

FIGURE 30-5 With forearm in neutral position, advancing the dorsal marginal ligament (DML) over the ulnar head.

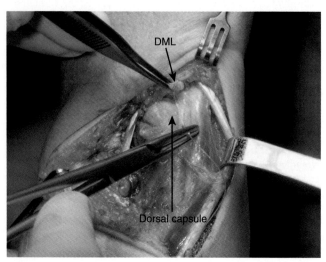

FIGURE 30-6 Inserting a stitch in the dorsal marginal ligament (DML).

7 weeks, depending on the quality of the capsular (DML) tissue.

After removal of the cast, patients are encouraged to start moving their wrist, with the assistance of a hand therapist, encouraging restoration of strength and movement. In general, recovery of supination consumes most of the time, but after 2 to 3 months normal rotation of the wrist can be anticipated. Restoration of flexion and extension is usually faster. Recovery of elbow flexion and extension does not require intensive assistance from the hand therapist. Gradual increase in lifting and impact loading is permitted in the course of the therapy. We believe that after 4 months of recovery, the wrist and hand can be used under all conditions, except for extreme loading during heavy work or sports, for which patients are advised to carry a mobile support cast for use around the wrist until 6 months after surgery.

Results

Twenty consecutive patients with DRUJ instability were studied retrospectively after DML reefing for dorsal radioulnar ligament attenuation, with a mean follow-up of 12 months. Four patients were excluded. Two were lost to follow up, and 1 patient suffered from an unrelated pain syndrome on the radial side of the wrist. One patient was found to have unforeseen severe TFCC degeneration, which proved unfit for DML reefing.

We observed no intraoperative or postoperative complications, except transient paresthesias on the ulnar side of the hand, which disappeared within a few weeks. The wound healing was uneventful (**Fig. 30-8**).

In all of the 16 patients, reefing of the DML resulted in a clinically stable DRUJ, although minor differences of translational movement between both wrists could be observed in all patients. To obtain objective values for the functional outcome, we measured the total range of motion on the operated wrist compared with the contralateral side (91%), grip strength (78%), and pain according to the visual analog scale.[3] When extrapolating these figures to the Mayo Modified Wrist Score combining motion, pain, grip strength, and functional status, the postoperative result score was 85 (excellent: 90-100 points; good: 80-90; fair: 70-80; poor: less than 65). Mean flexion of the operated side versus the contralateral side was 81 versus 86 degrees; extension: 67 versus

76 degrees; pronation: 85 versus 91 degrees; supination: 76 versus 87 degrees; radial deviation: 23 versus 29 degrees; and ulnar deviation: 27 versus 34 degrees.

Discussion

Bowers defines *instability* as an abnormal path of articular contact occurring during or at the end of the arc of motion attempted. This abnormal path or end point is permitted by alterations in

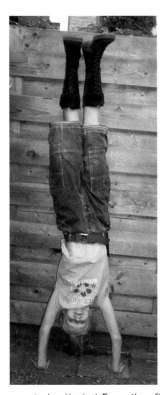

FIGURE 30-8 Our youngest patient at 5 months after surgery demonstrating her functional result.

joint surface or by deficiencies in the ligaments that retain the surfaces of the joint or both. DRUJ stability relies mainly on the strength of the supporting soft tissues.[1,15] The DML is one of these reinforcing structures, which we use for the dorsal capsuloplasty of the distal ulna.

The advantage of this technique is that it is technically easy and there is limited dissection, which may be helpful in reducing the chance of postoperative limitation of joint motion due to fibrosis. The basic mechanical aim is correcting the volar subluxation of the distal radius. Reefing the DML promotes lifting of the radius along the vertical axis of the sigmoid notch in a dorsal direction and thereby restoring the normal relationship between the radius and ulna in the DRUJ (**Fig. 30-9**). The vector used for repair is exclusively volar-dorsal and not ulnoradial, which differentiates this from a repair of a peripheral lesion of the TFCC. Another advantage is the use of vascularized, vital tissue instead of a free tendon graft. These grafts may lengthen in time as a result of structure loss of the collagen fibers, with subsequent recurrence of instability. Because the reefing is confined exclusively to the area of the DML, and is done under no tension, the risk of fibrosis and secondary impairment of motion is limited.

Arthroscopy remains our main diagnostic tool in patient selection. It is considered an investigational tool with a high sensitivity and specificity, especially in the diagnosis of lesions of the TFCC.[24-26] We believe that clearly visualizing the quality of the tissues along with the ability to test the mechanical quality of the TFCC tissue is of greatest importance in the surgical decision-making. A focal increase in the laxity of the dorsal TFCC is highly suggestive of this type of DRUJ instability.

Previous studies have indicated that the TFCC must rupture for a DRUJ dislocation to occur.[6,12,17] In our selected patients we could not detect a rupture of the TFCC during arthroscopy or operation. We believe the instability is caused by attenuation of the fibrous extension of the DML. Wong and coworkers have described a technique for treatment of a specific type of DRUJ instability that they find also on the dorsal side.[27] It consists of a duplication capsulorrhaphy of the dorsal capsular structures of

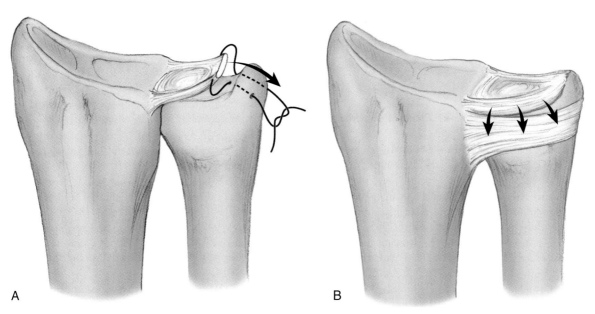

A   B

FIGURE 30-9 The vector of force is not radioulnar but volar-dorsal.

the DRUJ in a transverse way. Their series is small (only six patients, but with fairly good results). We use essentially the same fibrous tissues as Wong and coworkers, but we consider the capsule an integral part of the DML, with no relation to the floor of the fifth and sixth extensor sheets. Wong and coworkers' reefing technique is in a transverse direction, whereas we consider a reefing (or plication) from distal to proximal to be more sound biomechanically in the treatment of a volar-dorsal DRUJ instability. As in our series, no significant TFCC injury could be identified even though typically radioulnar joint laxity usually indicates disruption of soft tissue structures of the DRUJ. Laxity or attenuation of the dorsal extension of the DML seems to explain the volar subluxation of the distal radius and not a lesion of the TFCC itself, which remains inconsistent with earlier reports.[10]

When during surgery unexpected TFCC lesions or signs of ulnocarpal abutment became visible, we have simultaneously performed a wafer procedure[28] in four patients. Some authors prefer a shaft osteotomy for a partial ulnar head resection because the latter may result in scarring between the graft and the exposed bony surface.[20] With our technique this sequela is less probable, because we add no other tissue. Indeed in these four cases, which were otherwise not included in our study, no functional loss was observed in relation to scar formation.

An alternative for open surgical repair is arthroscopic suturing of tears of the TFCC, which is now commonly performed. Surgeons in favor of this technique claim a lower risk of neurovascular damage, reduced postoperative pain, and faster rehabilitation. These lesions are mainly ulnar- and radial-sided lesions.[29-34] Arthroscopic reefing of the dorsal extension of the DML seems, for the present, not feasible.

Dorsal capsuloplasty in volar subluxation of the distal radius should be reserved for patients without significant volar and dorsal TFCC disruption. For those selected patients with chronic dorsal instability, our technique has some advantages. It is simple without extensive soft tissue dissection. No drill holes for the passage of tendon grafts are needed, thus avoiding the risk of causing iatrogenic fracture, especially of the ulnar styloid. The tissue for reconstruction is strong and vascularized, reinforcing the DRUJ with a vector that runs from volar to dorsal.

Our results seem promising. Comparison with results of other series is difficult because they concern reconstructions of the peripheral tears of the TFCC. The only study on this specific type of instability[27] includes only six patients but describes favorable results comparable with ours.

REFERENCES

1. Bowers WH: Instability of the distal radioulnar articulation. Hand Clin. 1991; 7:311-327.
2. Kauer TMC, Landsmeer JMF: Functional anatomy of the wrist. In Tubiana R, ed: The Hand. Philadelphia: WB Saunders, 1981.
3. Ishii S, Palmer AK, Werner FW, et al: An anatomic study of the ligamentous structure of the triangular fibrocartilage complex. J Hand Surg [Am]. 1998; 23:977-985.
4. Johnson RK, Shrewsbury MM: The pronator quadratus in motion and in stabilization of the radius and ulna at the distal radioulnar joint. J Hand Surg. 1976; 1:205-209.
5. Spinner M, Kaplan EB: Extensor carpi ulnaris: its relationship to the stability of the distal radio-ulnar joint. Clin Orthop Relat Res. 1970; 68:124-129.
6. Kihara H, Short WH, Werner FW, et al: The stabilizing mechanism of the distal radioulnar joint during pronation and supination. J Hand Surg [Am]. 1995; 20:930-936.
7. Schuind F, An KN, Berglund L, et al: The distal radioulnar ligaments: a biomechanical study. J Hand Surg [Am]. 1991; 16:1106-1114.
8. Ward LD, Ambrose CG, Masson MV, Levaro F: The role of the distal radioulnar ligaments, interosseous membrane and joint capsule in distal radioulnar joint stability. J Hand Surg [Am]. 2000; 25:341-351.
9. Tolat AR, Stanley JK, Trail IA: A cadaveric study of the anatomy and stability of the distal radioulnar joint in the coronal and transverse planes. J Hand Surg [Br]. 1996; 21:587-594.
10. Watanabe H, Berger RA, Berglund LJ, et al: Contribution of the interosseous membrane to distal radioulnar joint constraint. J Hand Surg [Am]. 2005; 30:1164-1171.
11. af Ekenstam FW, Hagert CG: Anatomical studies on the geometry and stability of the distal radioulnar joint. Scand J Plast Reconstr Surg. 1985; 19:17.
12. Palmer AK, Werner FW: Biomechanics of the distal radioulnar joint. Clin Orthop Relat Res. 1984; 187:26-35.
13. Hagert CG: The distal radioulnar joint. Hand Clin. 1987; 3:41.
14. Garcia-Elias M: Soft-tissue anatomy and relationships about the distal ulna. Hand Clin. 1998; 14:165-176.
15. af Ekenstam FW: Osseous anatomy and articular relationships about the distal ulna. Hand Clin. 1998; 14:161-164.
16. Scheker LR, Belliappa PP, Acosta R, German DS: Reconstruction of the dorsal ligament of the triangular fibrocartilage complex: a biomechanical study. J Hand Surg [Br]. 1994; 19:310-318.
17. Stuart PR, Berger RA, Lindscheid RL, An KN: The dorsopalmar stability of the distal radioulnar joint. J Hand Surg [Am]. 2000; 25:689-699.
18. Pirela-Cruz MA, Goll SR, Klug M, Windler D: Stress computed tomography analysis of the distal radioulnar joint: a diagnostic tool for determining translational motion. J Hand Surg [Am]. 1991; 16:75-81.
19. Adams BD, Holley KA: Strains in the articular disk of the triangular fibrocartilage complex: a biomechanical study. J Hand Surg [Am]. 1993; 18:919-925.
20. Adams BD, Berger RA: An anatomic reconstruction of the distal radioulnar ligaments for posttraumatic distal radioulnar joint instability. J Hand Surg [Am]. 2002; 27:243-251.
21. Fulkerson JP, Watson HK: Congenital anterior subluxation of the distal ulna: a case report. Clin Orthop Relat Res. 1978; 131:179-182.
22. Breen TF, Jupiter JB: Extensor carpi ulnaris and flexor carpi ulnaris of the unstable distal ulna. J Hand Surg [Am]. 1989; 14:612-617.
23. Bowers WH: The distal radioulnar joint. In Green DP, Hotchkiss RN, Peterson WC, eds: Green's Operative Hand Surgery. 4th ed. Philadelphia: Churchill Livingstone, 1999; 986-1014.
24. Cooney W: Evaluation of chronic wrist pain by arthrography, arthroscopy and arthrotomy. J Hand Surg [Am]. 1993; 18:815-822.

25. Johnstone D, Thorogood S, Smith W, Scott T: A comparison of magnetic resonance imaging and arthroscopy in the investigation of chronic wrist pain. J Hand Surg [Br]. 1997; 22: 714-718.

26. Pederzini L, Luchetti R, Soragni O, et al: Evaluation of the triangular fibrocartilage complex tears by arthroscopy, arthrography and magnetic resonance imaging. Arthroscopy. 1992; 6:191-197.

27. Wong KH, Yip TH, Wu WC: Distal radioulnar joint distal instability treated with dorsal capsular reconstruction. Hand Surg. 2004; 9:55-61.

28. Feldon P, Terrono AL, Belsky MR: Wafer distal ulna resection for triangular fibrocartilage tears and/or ulna impaction syndrome. J Hand Surg [Am]. 1992; 17:731-773.

29. Corso SJ, Savoie FH, Geissler WB, et al: Arthroscopic repair of peripheral avulsion of the triangular fibrocartilage complex of the wrist: a multicenter study. Arthroscopy. 1997; 13: 78-84.

30. Haugstvedt JR, Husby T: Results of repair of peripheral tears in the triangular complex using an arthroscopic suture technique. Scand J Plast Reconstr Surg Hand Surg. 1999; 33:439-447.

31. Chou CH, Lee TS: Peripheral tears of the triangular fibrocartilage complex: results of primary repair. Int Orthop. 2001; 25:392-395.

32. Trumble T, Gilbert M, Vedder N: Isolated tears of the triangular fibrocartilage: management by early arthroscopic repair. J Hand Surg [Am]. 1997; 22:57-65.

33. Cober SR, Trumble TE: Arthroscopic repair of triangular fibrocartilage complex. Orthop Clin North Am. 2001; 30:279-294.

34. Miwa H, Hashizume H, Fujiwara K, et al: Arthroscopic surgery for traumatic triangular fibrocartilage complex injury. J Orthop Sci. 2004; 9:354-359.

Essex-Lopresti Fractures

31

Kathryne J. Stabile, MD and Matthew M. Tomaino, MD

Injury Pattern and Biomechanics

When a fall on an outstretched hand leads to a comminuted radial head fracture, longitudinal radioulnar dissociation (LRUD) may result if the forearm interosseous ligament (IOL) tears as well. This is often referred to as the Essex-Lopresti lesion. This injury pattern was initially described by Curr and Coe in 1946,[1] but Essex-Lopresti illustrated the importance of diagnosing longitudinal radioulnar instability.[2] Fracture of the radial head, disruption of the central third of the IOL, historically referred to as the interosseous membrane,[3-7] and injury to the distal radioulnar joint (DRUJ), contribute to loss of forearm stability. In LRUD, lack of forearm stability leads to loss of forearm rotation, decreased wrist extension, ulnar wrist pain, and elbow pain.[3-7] Understanding normal forearm biomechanics facilitates treatment of this challenging clinical problem.

The biomechanics of the forearm axis are best explained in terms of load transfer and stability. With use of the hand, and forceful grip, forces are transferred through the wrist to the elbow via the forearm IOL. Abnormal load transfer may result in pain secondary to abnormally high joint contact stresses at the elbow and ulnocarpal joints. As the forearm is loaded axially in compression, the IOL is loaded in tension. The IOL functions not only to transfer load from the radius to the ulna but also to pull the radius and ulna together at the proximal and distal radioulnar joints (**Fig. 31-1**).[8-12] Numerous studies have shown that the IOL and the triangular fibrocartilage complex (TFCC) help to provide stability to the DRUJ.[13-17]

Diagnosis

With a high-energy axial load applied to the forearm through the wrist, the radial head can fracture. With enough energy, the IOL and DRUJ can also be disrupted. Injury to the IOL and DRUJ can be easily overlooked if attention is focused on the radial head fracture alone.[18] After a few weeks, patients with LRUD can present with ulnar-sided wrist pain, loss of forearm rotation, and elbow pain. Physical examination will show painful rotation and ulnar deviation, forearm swelling, and lateral elbow tenderness.

Minimal radial shortening of up to 2 mm may be expected with a simple fracture of the radial head.[19,20] However, greater than 2 mm of radial shortening and radial head comminution are strongly suggestive of LRUD (**Fig. 31-2**).[21]

Edwards and Jupiter[22] proposed a classification system for the Essex-Lopresti type radial head fractures:

Type I—radial head fractures with minimal comminution amenable to open reduction and internal fixation

Type II—comminuted radial head fractures requiring excision and radial head replacement

Type III—chronic cases with irreducible proximal radial migration

Patients presenting with a comminuted radial head may present acutely with symptomatic LRUD, but they also have the potential to develop late LRUD. Although patients with LRUD may present acutely with wrist pain and forearm swelling, this is typically not the case. Forearm and wrist films should be obtained along with elbow films. Magnetic resonance imaging and ultrasonography have also proved useful in imaging IOL tears.[23-27] Radius stability can be assessed intraoperatively by applying axial load to the radius ("shuck" test). Proximal migration of the radius in late LRUD may be frank or occult. In frank cases, LRUD is seen on plain radiographs. In occult cases, power grip and axial stress views may elicit ulnar-positive variance.[28,29] Proximal migration of the radius may be fixed or reducible; distinguishing this can help guide treatment. If frank, dynamic fluoroscopic evaluation utilizing finger traps can illustrate if the deformity is reducible, then ulnar-positive variance may be "reduced" to ulnar-neutral variance. In the occult case, ulnar-positive variance is, by definition, dynamic.

Current Treatment and Surgical Technique

Traditionally, treatment approaches have focused on restoring a normal radioulnar relationship, which means restoring radial length. This has been accomplished by repair or replacement of the radial head and pinning of the radius to the ulna at the level of the DRUJ after restoration of length—to allow the IOL, TFCC attachment, and DRUJ capsule to heal. In the acute setting, the radius can usually be reduced; that is, proximal migration of the radius is not fixed and can be corrected by radial head open reduction and internal fixation (ORIF) or arthroplasty. In the late setting, however, proximal migration of the radius may be a fixed deformity requiring ulnar shortening at the wrist or use of a distraction device such as an Ilizarov frame to restore radioulnar length.

When the IOL is torn, the radial head is essential for maintaining longitudinal stability. If ORIF is not possible, radial head arthroplasty functions to share the load at the elbow and prevent proximal migration of the radius. Although Silastic radial heads have been used in the past, nonmetallic implants have been shown to collapse over time and may cause synovitis.[16,30-33] Metallic prostheses are stiffer than Silastic ones and are more effective in preventing proximal migration of the radius.[34-37] However, long-term clinical results of metallic radial heads in cases of LRUD are still lacking in the literature. There may be complications due to implant loosening and dislocation and elbow stiffness and capitellar wear from oversizing the implant.

Modular radial heads offer a more anatomical design. Grewal and associates recently reported favorable short-term clinical results at 2 years with modular radial head replacement for comminuted radial head fractures.[37] Even though this study lacked a control group, the authors found no evidence of overstuffing and 81% did not have arthritic changes. However, the outcomes of modular radial heads in patients with Essex-Lopresti fracture-dislocations in particular remain to be seen.

Treatment of Acute LRUD

The overall goal of treatment is to restore load sharing between the radius and ulna and prevent long-term proximal migration of the radius. The structures that require attention include the radial head, the TFCC, and the IOL. The radial head should be preserved if ORIF is possible. However, comminution of the radial head may prevent repair. Therefore, restoring radial length

will require metallic radial head arthroplasty (**Fig. 31-3**). In addition, pinning of the DRUJ for 4 weeks is recommended to allow the TFCC and DRUJ capsule to heal. Furthermore, because failure of this acute treatment strategy has significant consequences, and as the technique of open foveal reattachment of the torn TFCC has been refined, we advise a more aggressive approach to address the wrist after radial head replacement and restoration of the normal radioulnar relationship—open TFCC repair plus DRUJ pinning. This will ensure as precise a restoration of normal anatomy at the wrist as possible.

Little clinical data exist to support a clear role for reconstruction of the IOL acutely; and although suture repair of the IOL has been suggested, there are no data to suggest this is any better than just allowing the IOL to scar in once a normal radioulnar relationship has been restored. Biomechanical data suggest, however, that the IOL is necessary to unload the radial head. Acute reconstruction, in that light, may be a defensible strategy once the technical aspects of the procedure are refined.

Indications

Radial head repair or replacement is essential when addressing an acute Essex-Lopresti lesion. A number of modular head systems are available. It is important to preserve the lateral collateral ligament and to size the implant appropriately to avoid overstuffing the joint. This usually means that the proximal extent of any implant will line up with the coronoid process on a lateral radiographic view but not more proximally.

Contraindications

Silastic radial heads and radial head allografts are contraindicated. Any decision to salvage the radial head fracture must be based on feasibility of repair. Metallic radial head arthroplasty is probably

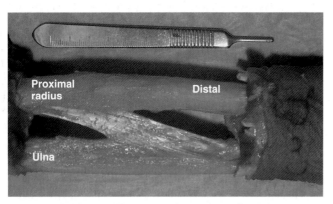

FIGURE 31-1 The forearm interosseous ligament.

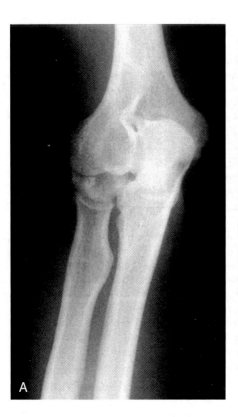

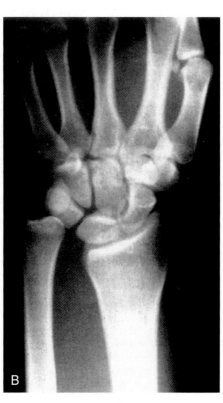

FIGURE 31-2 Anteroposterior radiographs of the elbow (**A**) and wrist (**B**) in a case of acute LRUD.

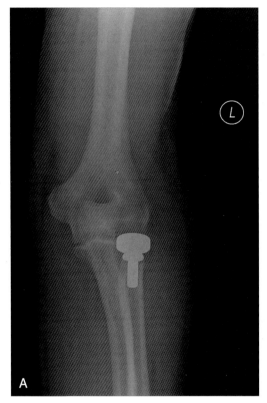
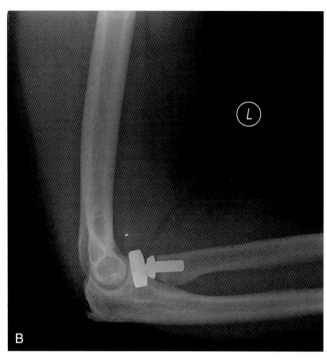

FIGURE 31-3 Anteroposterior (**A**) and lateral (**B**) radiographs after radial head replacement.

the better option when comminution exists such that rigid fixation and articular reconstruction are not possible.

Surgical Approach

The Kaplan approach is used at the elbow for radial head repair or arthroplasty. The deeper interval is between the extensor carpi radialis longus and the extensor digitorum communis. Open repair with a direct reattachment of the TFCC to the fovea is recommended to ensure optimal restoration of DRUJ stability. Suture anchors may be used in conjunction with temporary radioulnar pinning. The surgical approach is between the fifth and sixth extensor compartments.

Complications

Complications include stiffness from overstuffing the elbow joint. In addition, ulnar impaction syndrome and DRUJ arthritis, as well as radiocapitellar degeneration, may develop from proximal migration of the radius despite radial head arthroplasty and TFCC repair. This is the very rationale for IOL reconstruction in the acute setting, but most surgeons are probably well advised to evaluate postoperative outcome after the strategy mentioned earlier before reconstructing the IOL at the outset. This may change as IOL reconstruction techniques evolve and outcomes are reported.

Treatment of Late LRUD

When LRUD is unrecognized, hence untreated, restoration of radial length may not be possible. Characterizing proximal migration of the radius as fixed or reducible is critical to the

decision-making in such "chronic" cases.[38] Traction films with finger traps may be helpful. Fundamentally, intraoperative assessment relies on whether the proximal radius can be "pushed distally" when grasped with a towel clamp. In such cases, radial head replacement is recommended. Treatment recommendations for the reducible DRUJ are the same as for the acute case. However, if the radius cannot be pushed distally, and the DRUJ reduced, ulnar shortening osteotomy or use of an Ilizarov fixator (in a staged procedure) should be used to obtain ulnar-neutral variance. As experience with metallic ulnar head replacement increases, ulnar head arthroplasty may have a role when DRUJ arthritis exists. Although ulnar impaction, DRUJ arthritis, or an irreducible DRUJ may have been treated with distal ulna resection in low-demand wrists, this should not be performed in these types of cases. Grip strength will be compromised because of radioulnar impingement, and load transfer between the hand and elbow will be even more compromised. Indeed, understanding that transverse force vectors exist at the wrist and that the forearm unit functions with the IOL to unload the proximal radius mandates that neither the distal ulna nor the radial head is ever simply resected.

Although IOL reconstruction is still considered experimental, late cases of LRUD may represent the most compelling indication for such a strategy—to improve load sharing between the radius and ulna and reduce loads on the radial head implant.[39,40]

If capitellar wear has developed in chronic cases of untreated LRUD, capitellar resurfacing may be an option at the same time that radial head replacement is performed. Little data exist to support this innovative strategy, but uniarthroplasty (Small Bone Innovations, Inc., New York, NY) may hold promise in the future for such cases (**Fig. 31-4**).

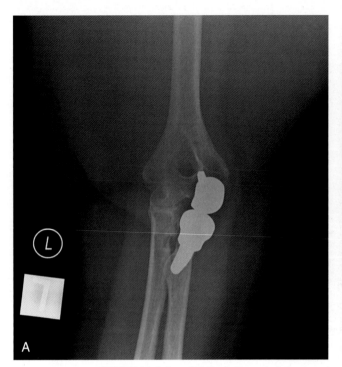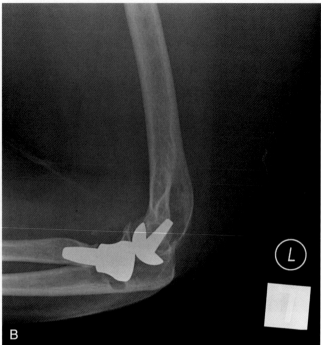

FIGURE 31-4 **A** and **B**, Capitellar resurfacing may have a role when radiocapitellar arthritis has developed.

IOL Reconstruction

In evaluating treatment of the Essex-Lopresti fracture-dislocation, a strategy that includes IOL reconstruction as well as radial head replacement and TFCC repair may be most attractive because historical options described earlier have provided inconsistent and, too frequently, inadequate results.[3,6,39-46] Because IOL reconstruction is still considered experimental, it is not typically recommended. However, reconstruction of the IOL is feasible and likely efficacious based on anatomical and biomechanical studies.

The goal of IOL reconstruction is to restore anatomical load transfer without limiting forearm rotation. Chandler and associates and Forster and coworkers have suggested that tendon graft be placed at an angle of 20 to 24 degrees to the long axis of the ulna.[47,48] Chandler and associates also found that the IOL inserts on the radius at a point 57% proximal to the distal radius and 34% proximal to the distal ulna.[48] These findings correlate well with those of Skahen and associates[49] and Fujita.[50] Despite agreement regarding where the IOL footprint is, however, there remains debate on the graft type, placement, and reconstruction technique. Grafts such as hamstring tendons or patellar tendon have similar material properties to the IOL.[46,51,52] However, these grafts pose issues with donor site morbidity.[53-57] Graft stiffness of the palmaris longus and single-bundle flexor carpi radialis have been shown to be significantly different from the intact IOL.[43,52] There is some clinical and basic science experience with the patellar tendon graft using a dorsal onlay technique described by Ruch and associates.[46] However, this reconstruction is nonanatomical and graft length may dictate graft placement.[43-46] Long-term clinical outcomes remain to be seen with the patellar tendon graft and onlay technique. Other authors have investigated IOL reconstruction techniques in the laboratory by placing the graft in line with the axis of rotation Ulnar, but, again, this is nonanatomical and remains a cadaveric experiment.[58,59]

In our laboratory we have investigated IOL reconstruction using a flexor carpi radialis graft placed anatomically in the footprint of the IOL on the radius and ulna. We found that an anatomical single-bundle graft restored approximately 76% of the load transferred through the intact IOL. We also found that an anatomical double-bundle graft was able to restore normal forearm load transfer to that of the intact IOL.[39,40] As favorable experience with tendon allograft for such procedures as elbow MCL and LCL reconstruction has grown, we have found that the potential morbidity of autograft use can be safely eliminated. This allows the selection of a lengthy graft such as the tibialis anterior as an alternative to the flexor carpi radialis autograft. Our proposed technique utilizes an anatomical single-bundle technique; this is expected to restore load transfer to approximately 75% of normal (**Fig. 31-5**). Tibialis anterior tendon graft can be anchored at the radius and ulna with biotenodesis screws (Arthrex, Naples, FL). As experience develops, a double-bundle reconstruction may become feasible, with the added benefit that biomechanical data suggest restoration of normal load transfer.

Indications

The indications for IOL reconstruction are unclear at this time but probably should include chronic cases for which intraoperative evidence of LRUD exists and for which radial head arthroplasty is planned. Regardless of whether a distal ulna procedure is required, IOL reconstruction will unload the proximal radius and diminish, if not prevent, the risk of subsequent radiocapitellar arthritis.

Contraindications

Contraindications revolve around how likely pain relief and functional restoration are with this approach as compared with

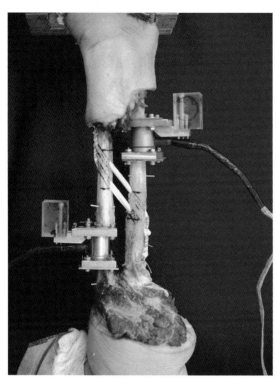

FIGURE 31-5 Proposed anatomical IOL reconstruction.

creation of a one-bone forearm. In other words, if concern exists over the amount of distal and proximal radioulnar degeneration and if little forearm rotation exists, salvage alone may be advisable.

Results

We have no results to report at this time because our recommendations for surgical technique are based solely on biomechanical and anatomical studies. However, Osterman and associates[45] treated 16 patients for chronic LRUD injuries with ulnar-shortening osteotomy and bone-ligament-bone reconstruction using a patellar tendon graft. The initial diagnoses were radial head fracture, radial head fracture with posterior dislocation, Monteggia fracture, radial head fracture with distal radius fracture, and Essex-Lopresti fracture. Interosseous ligament instability was identified an average of 10 months after radial head excision (range: 2 months to 12 years), with 75% of patients presenting within 2 years. The average ulnar variance was 3 mm (range: 2 to 5 mm) on standard posteroanterior radiographs. Other pathological processes included lunate impaction (4 patients), DRUJ arthritis (2 patients), and mild elbow arthritis (5 patients).

All patients received an ulnar-shortening osteotomy, and through the same incision a bone-ligament-bone autograft was anchored to the ulna. Through a plane beneath the extensors, the graft was tunneled and fixed to the radius at an acute angle. Grafts were tensioned in neutral to 20 degrees of supination. Concomitant procedures included radial head excision (1 patient), removal of radial head prosthesis (2 patients), wrist arthroscopy (3 patients), DRUJ resection (1 patient), Sauvé-Kapandji procedure (1 patient), and carpal tunnel release (1 patient).

Outcomes at an average of 78 months demonstrated that no patient was worse in terms of pain or function than before the surgery. Fifteen of 16 patients had improved wrist pain, 2 had

worse elbow arthritis radiographically, no patient had radiocapitellar impingement, and 4 patients had knee aches with weather change. No patient needed secondary surgery to address forearm instability. Grip strength improved from 59% to 86% of the unaffected limb. Ten of the 14 patients who were employed before their injury returned to their regular work duties, whereas 3 of 14 required job modification. Initial postoperative ulnar variance was −2 mm (range: −4 mm to +1 mm) and on follow-up averaged −1.5 mm (range −3 mm to +1 mm). Complications included one ulnar nonunion, one ulnar delayed union, 1 patient with extensor tendon adhesions, and 4 patients with knee aches.

Salvage

The ultimate solution for failed treatment of LRUD remains the creation of a one-bone forearm. This is considered, by some, the most reliable solution.[4,60,61] However, this procedure sacrifices function for pain relief.

REFERENCES

1. Curr JF, Coe WA: Dislocation of the inferior radio-ulnar joint. Br J Surg. 1946; 34:74.
2. Essex-Lopresti P: Fractures of the radial head with distal radio-ulna dislocation. J Bone Joint Surg Br. 1951; 33:244-247.
3. Hotchkiss RN: Fractures of the radial head and related instability and contracture of the forearm. Instr Course Lect. 1998; 47:173-177.
4. Hotchkiss RN: Injuries to the interosseous ligament of the forearm. Hand Clin. 1994; 10:391-398.
5. Mikic ZD, Vukadinovic SM: Late results in fractures of the radial head treated by excision. Clin Orthop Relat Res. 1983; 220-228.
6. Skahen JR 3rd, Palmer AK, Werner FW, Fortino MD: Reconstruction of the interosseous membrane of the forearm in cadavers. J Hand Surg [Am]. 1997; 22:986-994.
7. Sowa DT, Hotchkiss RN, Weiland AJ: Symptomatic proximal translation of the radius following radial head resection. Clin Orthop Relat Res. 1995; 106-113.
8. Halls AA, Travill A: Transmission of pressures across the elbow joint. Anat Rec. 1960; 150:243-248.
9. Pfaeffle HJ, Fischer KJ, Manson TT, et al: Role of the forearm interosseous ligament: is it more than just longitudinal load transfer? J Hand Surg [Am]. 2000; 25:683-688.
10. Palmer AK, Glisson RR, Werner FW: Relationship between ulnar variance and triangular fibrocartilage complex thickness. J Hand Surg [Am]. 1984; 9:681-682.
11. Markolf KL, Lamey D, Yang S, et al: Radioulnar load-sharing in the forearm: a study in cadavera. J Bone Joint Surg Am. 1998; 80:879-888.
12. Birkbeck DP, Failla JM, Hoshaw SJ, et al: The interosseous membrane affects load distribution in the forearm. J Hand Surg [Am]. 1997; 22:975-980.
13. Kleinman WB, Graham TJ: The distal radioulnar joint capsule: clinical anatomy and role in posttraumatic limitation of forearm rotation. J Hand Surg [Am]. 1998; 23:588-599.
14. Stuart PR, Berger RA, Linscheid RL, An KN: The dorso-palmar stability of the distal radioulnar joint. J Hand Surg [Am]. 2000; 25:689-699.

15. Ward LD, Ambrose CG, Masson MV, Levaro F: The role of the distal radioulnar ligaments, interosseous membrane, and joint capsule in distal radioulnar joint stability. J Hand Surg [Am]. 2000; 25:341-351.

16. Hotchkiss RN, An KN, Sowa DT, et al: An anatomic and mechanical study of the interosseous membrane of the forearm: pathomechanics of proximal migration of the radius. J Hand Surg [Am]. 1989; 14:256-261.

17. Rabinowitz RS, Light TR, Havey RM, et al: The role of the interosseous membrane and triangular fibrocartilage complex in forearm stability. J Hand Surg [Am]. 1994; 19:385-393.

18. Jungbluth P, Frangen TM, Arens S, et al: The undiagnosed Essex-Lopresti injury. J Bone Joint Surg Br. 2006; 88:1629-1633.

19. Morrey BF, Chao EY, Hui FC: Biomechanical study of the elbow following excision of the radial head. J Bone Joint Surg Am. 1979; 61:368.

20. Stephen IB: Excision of the radial head for closed fracture. Acta Orthop Scand. 1981; 52:409-412.

21. Davidson PA, Moseley JB Jr, Tullos HS: Radial head fracture: a potentially complex injury. Clin Orthop Relat Res. 1993; 224-230.

22. Edwards GS Jr, Jupiter JB: Radial head fractures with acute distal radioulnar dislocation. Essex-Lopresti revisited. Clin Orthop Relat Res. 1988; 61-69.

23. Failla JM, Jacobson J, van Holsbeeck M: Ultrasound diagnosis and surgical pathology of the torn interosseous membrane in forearm fractures/dislocations. J Hand Surg [Am]. 1999; 24:257-266.

24. Nakamura T, Yabe Y, Horiuchi Y: In vivo MR studies of dynamic changes in the interosseous membrane of the forearm during rotation. J Hand Surg [Br]. 1999; 24:245-248.

25. Starch DW, Dabezies EJ: Magnetic resonance imaging of the interosseous membrane of the forearm. J Bone Joint Surg Am. 2001; 83:235-238.

26. Wallace AL, Walsh WR, van Rooijen M, et al: The interosseous membrane in radio-ulnar dissociation. J Bone Joint Surg Br. 1997; 79:422-427.

27. Soubeyrand M, Lafont C, Oberlin C, et al: The "muscular hernia sign": an original ultrasonographic sign to detect lesions of the forearm's interosseous membrane. Surg Radiol Anat. 2006; 28:372-378.

28. Tomaino MM: The importance of the pronated grip x-ray view in evaluating ulnar variance. J Hand Surg [Am]. 2000; 25:352-357.

29. Shen J, Papadonikolakis A, Garrett JP, et al: Ulnar-positive variance as a predictor of distal radioulnar joint ligament disruption. J Hand Surg [Am]. 2005; 30:1172-1177.

30. Gordon M, Bullough PG: Synovial and osseous inflammation in failed silicone-rubber prostheses. J Bone Joint Surg Am. 1982; 64:574-580.

31. Morrey BF, Askew L, Chao EY: Silastic prosthetic replacement for the radial head. J Bone Joint Surg Am. 1981; 63:454-458.

32. Vanderwilde RS, Morrey BF, Melberg MW, Vinh TN: Inflammatory arthritis after failure of silicone rubber replacement of the radial head. J Bone Joint Surg [Br]. 1994; 76:78-81.

33. Worsing RA Jr, Engber WD, Lange TA: Reactive synovitis from particulate silastic. J Bone Joint Surg Am. 1982; 64:581-585.

34. Judet T, Massin P, Bayeh PJ: Radial head prosthesis with floating cup in recent and old injuries of the elbow: preliminary results. Rev Chir Orthop Rep Appareil Moteur. 1994; 80:123-130.

35. Knight DJ, Rymaszewski LA, Amis AA, Miller JH: Primary replacement of the fractured radial head with a metal prosthesis. J Bone Joint Surg Br. 1993; 75:572-576.

36. Popovic N, Gillet P, Rodriguez A, Lemaire R: Fracture of the radial head with associated elbow dislocation: results of treatment using a floating radial head prosthesis. J Orthop Trauma. 2000; 14:171-177.

37. Grewal R, MacDermid JC, Faber KJ, et al: Comminuted radial head fractures treated with a modular metallic radial head arthroplasty: study of outcomes. J Bone Joint Surg Am. 2006; 88:2192-2200.

38. Smith AM, Urbanosky LR, Castle JA, et al: Radius pull test: predictor of longitudinal forearm instability. J Bone Joint Surg Am. 2002; 84:1970-1976.

39. Pfaeffle HJ, Stabile KJ, Li ZM, Tomaino MM: Reconstruction of the interosseous ligament unloads metallic radial head arthroplasty and the distal ulna in cadavers. J Hand Surg [Am]. 2006; 31:269-278.

40. Pfaeffle HJ, Stabile KJ, Li ZM, Tomaino MM: Reconstruction of the interosseous ligament restores normal forearm compressive load transfer in cadavers. J Hand Surg [Am]. 2005; 30:319-325.

41. Harrington IJ, Sekyi-Otu A, Barrington TW, et al: The functional outcome with metallic radial head implants in the treatment of unstable elbow fractures: a long-term review. J Trauma. 2001; 50:46-52.

42. Sellman DC, Seitz WH Jr, Postak PD, Greenwald AS: Reconstructive strategies for radioulnar dissociation: a biomechanical study. J Orthop Trauma. 1995; 9:516-522.

43. Tejwani SG, Markolf KL, Benhaim P: Graft reconstruction of the interosseous membrane in conjunction with metallic radial head replacement: a cadaveric study. J Hand Surg [Am]. 2005; 30:335-342.

44. Tejwani SG, Markolf KL, Benhaim P: Reconstruction of the interosseous membrane of the forearm with a graft substitute: a cadaveric study. J Hand Surg [Am]. 2005; 30:326-334.

45. Osterman AL, Culp RW, Warhold LG: Reconstruction of the interosseous membrane using a bone-ligament-bone graft. Presented before the American Academy of Orthopaedic Surgeons, 2000.

46. Ruch DS, Change DS, Koman LA: Reconstruction of longitudinal stability of the forearm after disruption of interosseous ligament and radial head excision (Essex-Lopresti lesion). J South Orthop Assoc. 1999; 8:47-52.

47. Forster RI, Sharkey NA, Szabo RM: Forearm interosseous ligament isometry. J Hand Surg [Am]. 1999; 24:538-545.

48. Chandler JW, Stabile KJ, Pfaeffle HJ, et al: Anatomic parameters for planning of interosseous ligament reconstruction using computer-assisted techniques. J Hand Surg [Am]. 2003; 28:111-116.

49. Skahen JR 3rd, Palmer AK, Werner FW, Fortino MD: The interosseous membrane of the forearm: anatomy and function. J Hand Surg [Am]. 1997; 22:981-985.

50. Fujita M: An anatomical study on the interosseous membrane of the forearm. Nippon Sei Gakkai Zasshi 1995; 69:938-950.

51. Pfaeffle HJ, Tomaino MM, Grewal R, et al: Tensile properties of the interosseous membrane of the human forearm. J Orthop Res. 1996; 14:842-845.

52. Stabile KJ, Pfaeffle J, Saris I, et al: Structural properties of reconstruction constructs for the interosseous ligament of the forearm. J Hand Surg [Am]. 2005; 30:312-318.

53. Matsumoto A, Yoshiya S, Muratsu H, et al: A comparison of bone-patellar tendon-bone and bone-hamstring tendon-bone autografts for anterior cruciate ligament reconstruction. Am J Sports Med. 2006; 34:213-219.

54. Kartus J, Movin T, Karlsson J: Donor-site morbidity and anterior knee problems after anterior cruciate ligament reconstruction using autografts. Arthroscopy. 2001; 17:971-980.

55. Miller MD, Nichols T, Butler CA: Patella fracture and proximal patellar tendon rupture following arthroscopic anterior cruciate ligament reconstruction. Arthroscopy. 1999; 15:640-643.

56. Kohn D, Sander-Beuermann A: Donor-site morbidity after harvest of a bone-tendon-bone patellar tendon autograft. Knee Surg Sports Traumatol Arthrosc. 1994; 2:219-223.

57. Sachs RA, Daniel DM, Stone ML, Garfein RF: Patellofemoral problems after anterior cruciate ligament reconstruction. Am J Sports Med. 1989; 17:760-765.

58. Soubeyrand M, Oberlin C, Dumontier C, et al: Ligamentoplasty of the forearm interosseous membrane using the semitendinosus tendon: anatomical study and surgical procedure. Surg Radiol Anat. 2006; 28:300-307.

59. Marcotte A, Osterman AL: Longitudinal radioulnar dissociation: identification and treatment of acute and chronic injuries. Hand Clin. 2007; 23:195-208.

60. Brockman E: Two cases of disability at the wrist joint following excision of the radial head. Proc R Soc Med. 1930; 21(5): 904-905.

61. Graham TJ, Fischer TJ, Hotchkiss RN, Kleinman WB: Disorders of the forearm axis. Hand Clin. 1998; 14:305-316.

The Ulnar-Shortening Osteotomy

32

Anthony J. Lauder, MD and Thomas E. Trumble, MD

Vague complaints of pain stemming from seemingly innocuous events often make the diagnosis and treatment of ulnar-sided wrist ailments an exercise in frustration for both physicians and patients. Fortunately, widespread interest in the pathological conditions of the ulnar wrist has helped elucidate some of the more common conditions affecting this area. One such condition, often referred to as ulnocarpal abutment or the ulnocarpal impaction syndrome, occurs when excessive loads exist between the distal ulna and ulnar carpus. This overloading stems from the distal ulnar articular surface projecting more distal than the ulnar articular surface of the distal radius. This situation has been termed "ulnar-positive variance" with "ulnar variance" being defined as the difference in length between the distal ulnar corner of the radius and distalmost aspect of the dome of the ulnar head (**Fig. 32-1**). Ultimately, ulnar-positive variance combined with a lunotriquetral tear and a triangular fibrocartilage complex (TFCC) tear make up the triad of ulnar impaction syndrome. Many procedures have been developed to alleviate this degenerative, often debilitating, condition, but the gold standard for correcting ulnar-positive variance is the ulnar-shortening osteotomy. The goals of the shortening procedure are to relieve pain and prevent arthritis by reestablishing a neutral or slightly negative ulnar variance.

Biomechanics of Ulnar Impaction Syndrome

Ulnar impaction syndrome is characterized by pain and swelling that typically develop in patients with excessive loading across the distal ulna. Generally, the radius receives 82% of the load borne through the wrist while the ulna receives 18% of the force. However, Palmer and Werner showed that loads through the distal ulna can change and are directly related to ulnar variance.[1] Increasing ulnar length by 2.5 mm raises ulnar loads to 42%, whereas a decrease in length of 2.5 mm lowers the force seen at the distal ulna to 4.3%. Furthermore, these investigators reported that 73% of wrists with tears of the TFCC had either an ulnar-positive or ulnar-neutral variance, indicating that overloading of the ulnar wrist can ultimately lead to injury and degeneration of the TFCC.

The "TFCC," a term coined by Palmer and Werner in 1981,[2] is a ligamentous and cartilaginous structure found between the distal ulna and ulnar carpus that, along with the bony architecture in this region, helps maintain the relationship of the distal ulna to the distal radius (**Figs. 32-2 and 32-3**). Strong volar and dorsal ligaments, termed the "dorsal and palmar radioulnar ligaments," serve as a capsule surrounding the DRUJ. These ligaments continue onto the horizontal surface of the distal ulna, where they become thickened and serve as limbi for the TFCC. Ultimately,

these ligaments go on to attach to the base of the ulnar styloid. Biomechanical studies have revealed a complex interplay between these ligaments and the motion that occurs at the DRUJ. DiTano and coworkers showed that the palmar radioulnar ligament becomes taut in supination, whereas the dorsal radioulnar ligament tightens with pronation (**Fig. 32-4**).[3] This holds importance for different instability patterns that can occur at the DRUJ.

Historical Results of the Procedure

The first ulnar-shortening osteotomy was described by Milch in 1941.[4] He elected to utilize the procedure on a 17-year-old patient who developed a painful ulnar-positive wrist from a distal radius malunion. Milch's technique entailed resection of a portion of the ulnar shaft with wire fixation at the osteotomy site. Since this initial description, numerous authors have described various osteotomy types, including transverse,[5,6] oblique (of varying degrees),[6-10] sliding (long oblique),[11] and step cut.[12] Several commercially available systems have been developed to facilitate bony contact, compression, and rigid fixation at the osteotomy site.[6,10,11]

Attempting to elucidate which osteotomy provides both stability and rapid healing potential, while remaining easy to perform, can be an arduous task. Many authors have reported good results with any of the osteotomy methods just mentioned. In 1995, Wehbé and colleagues reported on their results for ulnar shortening utilizing a transverse osteotomy and the AO small distractor.[5] In their 24 patients with ulnar impaction syndrome, they had no nonunions and an average time to healing of 9.7 weeks. They did have three delayed unions, but these reportedly healed without incident by 28, 34, and 36 weeks. It should be noted that their criteria for bony healing were quite stringent and if they had used criteria utilized by previous authors their delayed unions would have coalesced by 12, 16, and 20 weeks.

In 2005, Darlis and associates reported their results on 29 patients who underwent a step-cut osteotomy of the ulna for various pathological conditions.[12] Average time to union was 8.3 weeks, and they had no delayed unions or nonunions. Although these authors deem this a simple technique, it does require more cuts than transverse or oblique osteotomies.

Many surgeons today prefer an oblique osteotomy based in large part on a 1993 study by Rayhack and associates.[6] In that study, 23 transverse osteotomies in which a specialized external compression device was utilized were compared with 17 oblique osteotomies in which a cutting guide designed by the lead author was implemented. Average healing times for the transverse osteotomies was 21 weeks compared with 11 weeks for the group with the oblique osteotomies. Furthermore, one nonunion was noted for the transverse group. Importantly, Rayhack and associates also reported on the biomechanical differences between the two con-

333

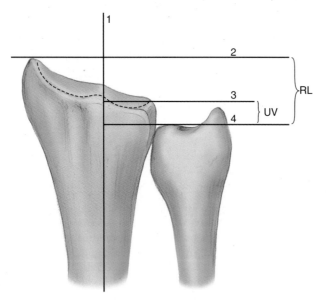

FIGURE 32-1 Ulnar variance is the difference in length between the ulnar corner of the radius (RL) and the articular dome of the distal ulna (UV). *(Adapted from Palmer AK, Werner FW: The triangular fibrocartilage complex of the wrist: anatomy and function. J Hand Surg [Am]. 1981; 6: 154.)*

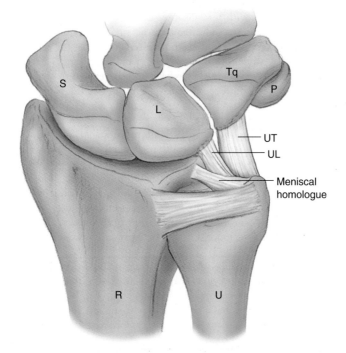

FIGURE 32-2 View from dorsal to palmar of the triangular fibrocartilage complex (TFCC). S, scaphoid; L, lunate; Tq, triquetrum, R, radius; U, ulna; UT, ulnotriquetral ligament; UL, ulnolunate ligament. *(Adapted from Palmer AK. Triangular fibrocartilage complex lesions: a classification. J Hand Surg [Am]. 1989; 14: 595.)*

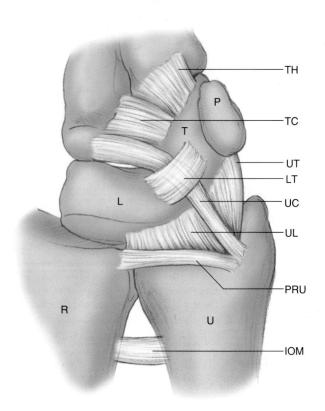

FIGURE 32-3 View looking palmar to dorsal of the volar structures forming part of the TFCC. TC, triquetral capitate ligament; TH, triquetral hamate ligament; LT, lunotriquetral ligament; T, triquetrum; P, pisiform; L, lunate; UL, ulnolunate ligament; UT, ulnotriquetral ligament; UC, ulnocapitate ligament; U, ulna; R, radius; PRU, palmar radioulnar ligament; IOM, interosseous membrane. *(Adapted from Trumble TE: Distal radioulnar joint and triangular fibrocartilage complex. In Trumble TE: Principles of Hand Surgery and Therapy. Philadelphia: WB Saunders, 1999; 129.)*

structs. Cadaveric data revealed no significant difference between the oblique or transverse cuts in regard to anteroposterior or lateral bending strength. The oblique osteotomy was found, however, to be significantly stiffer in torsion.

Several authors utilizing different systems for performing oblique osteotomies have corroborated the excellent results dem-onstrated by Rayhack and associates. Reporting on 27 patients (30 osteotomies), Chun and Palmer described their results for the oblique osteotomy utilizing a freehand technique.[7] The wrists were graded both preoperatively and postoperatively with a modified Gartland and Werley system.[13] Preoperatively, 28 wrists were graded poor and 2 as fair. Postoperatively, 24 wrists were graded excellent with 4 good results, 1 fair result, and 1 poor result. There were no nonunions. Chen and Wolfe also reported good results for the oblique osteotomy utilizing a freehand technique and an AO compression device.[8] Preoperatively, 14 wrists were graded fair and 4 poor whereas, postoperatively, 13 were graded excellent, 3 good, and 2 fair. They also had no nonunions. Most recently, Mizuseki and colleagues reported their results for 24 oblique osteotomies created by their own device.[10] Healing time averaged 8.1 weeks, and they had no nonunions.

Trumble and colleagues combined arthroscopic repairs of the TFCC with ulnar-shortening osteotomies.[14] Their patients regained 83% of their total range of motion and 81% of their grip strength when compared with the contralateral side. In 19 of 21 patients, pain symptoms improved from complaints of pain even with routine activities to having complete relief of pain with all activities postoperatively. The other two patients had decreased levels of pain after surgery but continued to have occasional discomfort with some heavy activities.

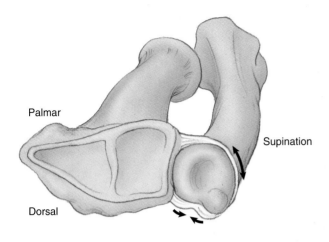

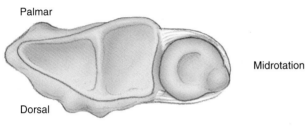

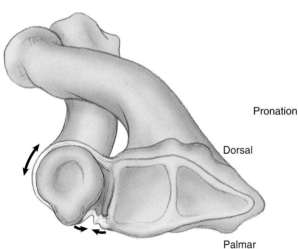

FIGURE 32-4 Axial diagrams of the distal radioulnar joint show that tension in the dorsal and palmar radioulnar ligaments is dependent on forearm rotation. In supination the palmar radioulnar ligament is tight, whereas in pronation the dorsal radioulnar ligament becomes taut. (Adapted from Bedner MS, Arnoczky SP, Weiland AJ. The microvasculature of the triangular fibrocartilage complex: its clinical significance. J Hand Surg [Am]. 1991; 16: 1103.)

Indications

There are many situations in which the ulnar-shortening osteotomy may be indicated. The most common indication is to eliminate the overloading that occurs in an ulnar impaction syndrome. Other indications include tears of the TFCC that cannot be repaired, previous radial head excision, and associated Essex-Lopresti lesions that result in a ulnar-positive variance (provided the intraosseous membrane instability has been corrected either with a radial head implant or bone-ligament-bone graft), attritional lunotriquetral ligament tears, ulnar nonunions, radial malunions resulting in an ulnar-positive variance, and early

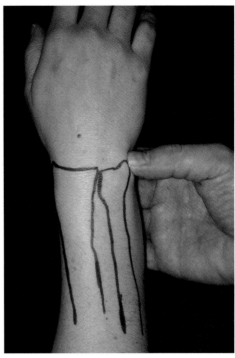

FIGURE 32-5 Patients with overloading of the distal ulna or a pathological process of the TFCC will often have tenderness and/or swelling in an area just distal to the ulnar styloid.

post-traumatic distal radioulnar joint (DRUJ) arthritis. Importantly, a shortening osteotomy can also prove beneficial in patients with signs and symptoms of ulnocarpal impaction but radiographs that demonstrate ulnar-neutral or slightly ulnar-negative variance.

Contraindications

The absolute contraindications for the ulnar-shortening osteotomy are minimal. Certainly, an osteotomy should never be performed in an infectious situation in which the hardware could become a nidus and/or the osteotomy site could go onto an infected nonunion. Along this same line, any patient with open wounds that would leave exposed hardware should be evaluated for soft tissue coverage before an osteotomy. The osteotomy should not be performed in isolation for radial malunions that include deformity other than just shortening. Simply shortening the ulna will not restore a congruent sigmoid notch if the deformity present in the distal radius is not also addressed. Finally, the shortening should not be performed alone in Essex-Lopresti situations where the radial head has been previously excised. In this instance, continued shortening of the radius would be expected unless the osteotomy was performed in conjunction with a radial head replacement.

Surgical Technique
Web Video

32-5

The typical patient who benefits from an ulnar-shortening osteotomy relates a history of ulnar-sided wrist pain that is exacerbated by pronation/supination activities and forceful grip. On examination many patients will have swelling and tenderness localized to the TFCC and distal ulna (**Fig. 32-5**). The ulnar impaction maneuver, performed by moving the distal ulna in a volar and dorsal direction with the wrist in ulnar deviation, can help elicit pain that stems from the TFCC and ulnar impaction

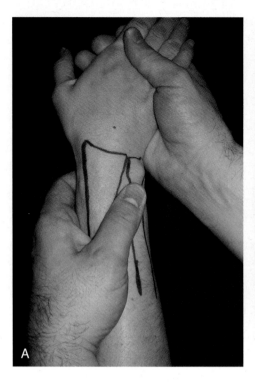
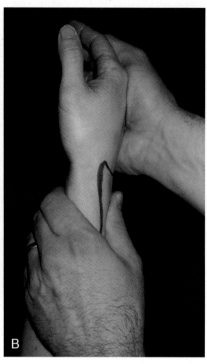

FIGURE 32-6 The ulnar impaction maneuver is performed by ulnarly deviating the wrist (**A**) and translating the carpus in volar and dorsal directions (**B**). This maneuver is positive when pain is elicited.

(**Fig. 32-6**). Another valuable examination maneuver is the ulnar stress test as described by Nakamura and colleagues.[15] This test is considered positive when pain is elicited by axially loading, flexing, and extending a patient's pronated and ulnarly deviated wrist. The "fovea test" is performed by asking the patient to flex the wrist. This allows palpation of the FCU, which facilitates locating the fovea of the TFCC—between the flexor carpi ulnaris and ulnar styloid process. Exclusion of other sources of discomfort, such as pisotriquetral arthritis, DRUJ instability or arthritis, or extensor carpi ulnaris tendinitis or hypermobility heightens the suspicion for a pathological process of the TFCC. Plain radiographs, including posteroanterior and lateral views, should be obtained on every patient. Not only do these help determine the amount of shortening that will be required, but they also help determine if there are any other conditions (i.e., lunotriquetral instability/degeneration) that may need to be addressed. Importantly, one must obtain a true posteroanterior view of the wrist with the shoulder abducted to 90 degrees, elbow flexed to 90 degrees, and wrist in neutral rotation. The significance of a true posteroanterior view stems from the fact that rotation at the wrist can increase (pronation) or decrease (supination) ulnar variance. With this in mind, a posteroanterior view of a pronated wrist can be helpful in patients who develop pain during activities that require pronation (i.e., hammering, typing). These patients may not be experiencing symptoms until their ulnar variance becomes positive with pronation.[16] Plain radiographs of the contralateral wrist may be helpful for determining the amount one wants to shorten the ulna. Contralateral views are not as useful, however, when that wrist is also ulnar positive. Magnetic resonance imaging or arthrography may be a reasonable adjunct to the radiographic evaluation when the surgeon suspects an acute tear of the TFCC that possibly can be repaired.

The required and optional equipment needed for the ulnar-shortening osteotomy is minimal. The procedure, as it will be described here, does require an ulnar-shortening system from Trimed (Valencia, CA). Other equipment required for this procedure includes a radiolucent lateral armboard, a fluoroscopy machine, a wire driver and drill, a lobster claw reduction forceps, a set of baby Hohmann retractors, and a sagittal saw and saw blade (0.4 mm thick; 25 mm long). Occasionally in the revision cases it is helpful to have the 3.5-mm AO Small Fragment Set (Synthes, Paoli, PA).

The patient is placed in the supine position with a pneumatic tourniquet as high as possible on the arm. The arm in its entirety should rest comfortably on a radiolucent hand table.

After exsanguination of the arm and inflation of the tourniquet, a skin incision is made along the subcutaneous border of the ulna. This incision should begin 1 to 2 cm proximal to the ulnar styloid and continue proximally for 15 cm. Incisions at or distal to the ulnar styloid must be made carefully to avoid injury to the dorsal sensory branch of the ulnar nerve. The incision is continued between the interval separating the extensor carpi ulnaris and the flexor carpi ulnaris. The periosteum of the ulna is then incised and both muscles are reflected using an elevator and baby Hohmann retractors. Care must be taken to avoid injury to the ulnar artery and nerve, which lie just radial to the flexor carpi ulnaris. A substantial portion of each muscle must be reflected to adequately visualize the osteotomy.

Whenever possible the plate should be applied to the volar surface of the ulna (**Fig. 32-7**). Not only is there more soft tissue padding, but this side also tends to be the flattest surface of the ulna, allowing for the best plate-to-bone contact. If the volar surface is not practical, then the surgeon should choose the flattest side that is still amenable to adequate soft tissue coverage. Occasionally, it is necessary to utilize plate benders to contour the plate to account for variations in ulnar shape. Plates can also be bent to overcompensate for the normal curvature of the ulna. This will help prevent gapping at the osteotomy site at the time compression is applied.

The position of the lag screw depends on both the arm being operated on and the location of the plate. For a right arm osteotomy and a volarly placed plate the lag screw hole will be distal to the osteotomy site. With dorsally set plates in the right arm the

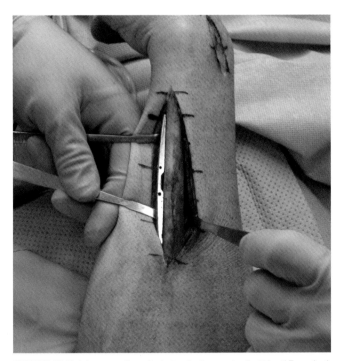

FIGURE 32-7 Intraoperative photograph demonstrating the 15-cm incision and volar plate placement. Most often the volar surface is the broadest and flattest for plate application. Baby Hohmann retractors protect the underlying soft tissues.

lag screw will be proximal to the osteotomy. The opposite is true for left-sided plates in which for volar plates the lag screw will be proximal and for dorsal plates the screw starts distally. Regardless of the orientation of the plate or which ulna is being osteotomized, it is critical that the two small holes on the side of the plate be easily accessible for mounting the cutting guides.

The plate is provisionally secured to the ulna with the help of the ulnar plate clamp. Using the 2.3-mm drill bit, 3.2-mm diameter self-tapping screws are used to fix the plate to the ulna on the same side as the lag screw. When dealing with brittle bone, the 2.3-mm drill holes can be tapped to precut screw threads. A fourth screw is placed in the slotted screw hole to affix the plate both proximal and distal to the planned osteotomy site. This screw should be placed at the end of the slot farthest from the lag screw. This allows for compression after the osteotomy is completed. At this point the combination pin/drill guide is applied. Two 0.062-inch Kirschner wires (K-wires) are placed in the slots of the guide that are away from the lag screw hole (**Fig. 32-8**). The shorter (50 mm) K-wire is placed first, followed by the longer (100 mm) wire. The differing K-wire lengths and the guide ensure the pins will remain parallel during insertion. The pin/drill guide is now removed.

Correlating to measurements made from preoperative radiographs for ulnar variance, a cutting guide is selected for the intended amount of resection (2 to 5 mm). Marked "A" and "B," these cutting guides are designed with pegs that can only be inserted so that the osteotomy cuts are made perpendicular to the path of the planned lag screw. Guide A is placed first. This guide defines the width of the osteotomy and is marked as either A-2, 3, 4, or 5 mm (**Fig. 32-9**). Five millimeters is usually the maximum correction required, but it can be more in certain trauma situations. After placing baby Hohmann retractors around the ulna to protect the adjacent soft tissues, the osteotomy is completed. Use of saline irrigation is recommend to cool the saw blade and prevent thermal injury. Guide A is then replaced with the finish cutting

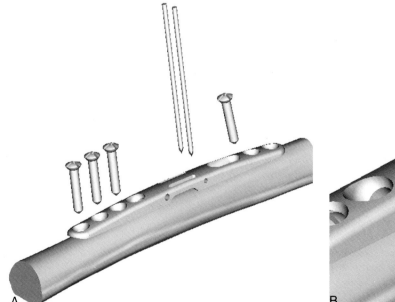
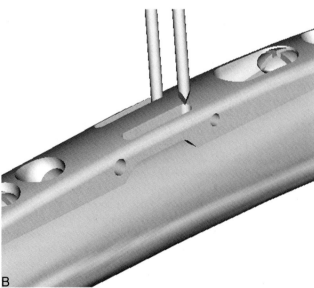

A   B

FIGURE 32-8 **A,** The plate is initially secured with three screws on the same side as the lag screw. On the other side, a screw is inserted into the slot at the point farthest from the lag screw. Similar to the slot screw, two 0.062-inch K-wires are inserted in separate slots at a point farthest from the lag screw. **B,** Close-up view of the K-wires being inserted at a point farthest from the lag screw. Inserting the K-wires and slot screw away from the lag screw will allow for in-line compression after the osteotomy is completed.

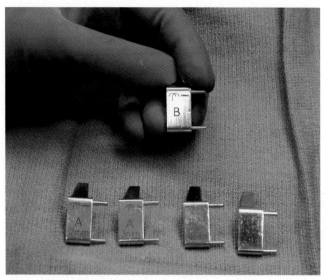

FIGURE 32-9 "A" and "B" guides for completing the osteotomies. Note that the A guides are available for 2-, 3-, 4-, or 5-mm resections.

guide B. Once the sequential osteotomies have been completed the bone wafer is detached from its soft tissue attachments and excised (**Fig. 32-10**). Of paramount importance for the procedure is to keep the plate firmly fixed to the ulna to ensure parallel osteotomy cuts. Therefore, screws should be checked during the osteotomy and retightened as necessary to prevent plate slippage.

The peg of the bone compression clamp is inserted into the side of the plate. The cannulated portion of the clamp is then used as a drill guide to place a third 0.062-inch K-wire low on the bone between the slotted hole and the two parallel K-wires previously inserted. The position of this third wire creates compression forces perpendicular to the osteotomy. The screw in the slotted hole is then loosened to allow compression at the osteotomy using the bone compression clamp (**Fig. 32-11**). Once compression has been achieved, the slot screw should be retightened. At this time radiographs should be obtained to determine if the ulnar variance has been corrected to neutral or slightly negative. It is important to check that plate contact has not changed due to a changing radius of curvature of the ulna from shortening. If this does occur, the plate may need to be bent a second time to afford better conformity and plate contact.

To insert the lag screw the pin/drill guide can be reapplied or the surgeon can choose to drill the hole freehand. A 3.2-mm drill bit is used first for the near cortex (**Fig. 32-12**). This is followed by the 2.3-mm drill bit, which is sent through the far cortex. The lag screw should be tapped to guarantee good purchase of the screw threads. A lag screw of appropriate length (normally 18 to 20 mm) is inserted. The final two screws adjacent to the slotted hole are inserted, followed by removal of the drill guide, compression clamp, and three K-wires. Final radiographs should be obtained to ensure proper screw lengths (**Fig. 32-13**).

The wound is then irrigated and the tourniquet released to check for active bleeding. Wound margins can be injected with bupivicaine and epinephrine for both hemostasis and postoperative analgesia. A drain is placed, and the fascial interval between the flexor carpi ulnaris and extensor carpi ulnaris is closed to avoid muscle herniations. The subcutaneous and skin layers are closed separately with interrupted sutures. A long arm, well-padded splint is then applied.

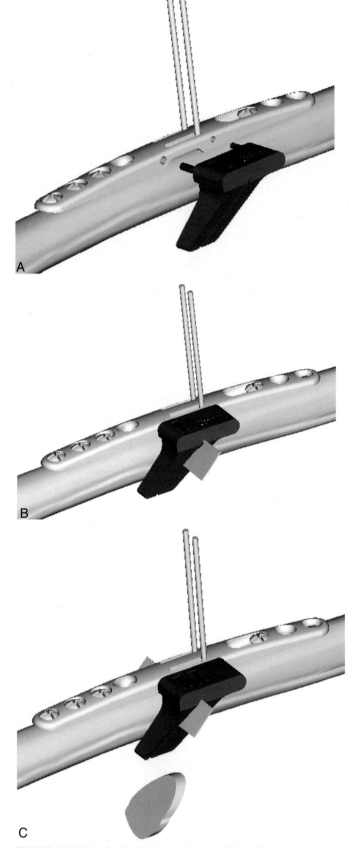

FIGURE 32-10 **A**, Application of guide A, which will determine the amount of ulnar shortening. Note the guide slides directly into the side of the plate. **B**, Completion of the first osteotomy through guide A. **C**, Completion of the second osteotomy through guide B and wafer removal.

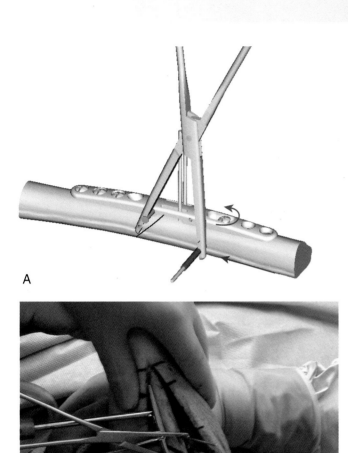

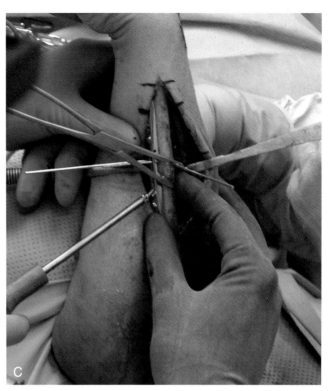

FIGURE 32-11 **A,** Graphic depiction of the bone compression clamp in position and compressing the osteotomy as the plate slides on the slot screw and K-wires. **B,** Intraoperative photograph showing the compression clamp in place before compressing the osteotomy. **C,** Intraoperative photograph demonstrating compression at the osteotomy site while a lag screw is being inserted.

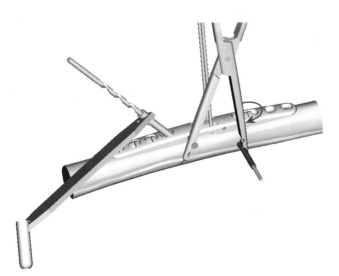

FIGURE 32-12 Graphic depiction of the hole preparation for the lag screw. Note the compression across the osteotomy site with the bone compression clamp. The slotted screw has been loosened, allowing the plate to slide proximally.

Patients are seen at 2 weeks for their first postoperative visit when sutures are removed. Compliant patients are fitted with a removable long arm splint fabricated by one of our hand therapists. This allows for removal during showers and commencement of elbow flexion and extension exercises. Noncompliant patients are placed into a long arm cast. At 6 weeks, radiographs are obtained and gentle wrist range of motion exercises are started if there are early signs of bony consolidation. If there are more signs of bony union at 9 weeks, then the patients are instructed to begin gentle strengthening exercises.

Complications

In a properly performed osteotomy the complications are minimal. The most commonly reported adverse outcome is hardware prominence and tenderness.[8,10,12] In our series of 17 osteotomies we found that four patients ultimately required plate removal owing to ongoing problems with hardware prominence. Other possible complications include infection, delayed union, nonunion, and nerve palsies. In our patients we did not experience any of these situations. The risk of delayed or nonunions can be

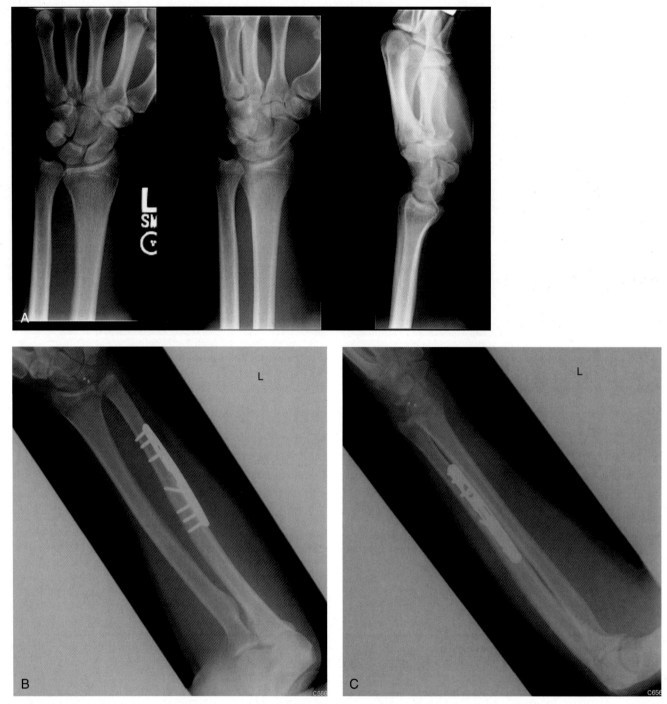

FIGURE 32-13 A, Preoperative radiographs show ulnar-positive variance in a patient with a long-standing history of ulnar-sided wrist pain. Postoperative anteroposterior (**B**) and lateral (**C**) views illustrating a healed osteotomy and ulnar-negative variance.

TABLE 32-1 Qualitative Outcomes with the Trimed System (Valencia, CA)

Feature	Preoperative	Postoperative	% Contralateral
Wrist flexion/extension (degrees)	110.00	116.47	98.26
Wrist radial/ulnar deviation (degrees)	36.47	43.82	95.92
Wrist pronation/supination (degrees)	133.24	136.76	96.70
Grip strength (kg)	26.41	34.06	93.69
Pain (visual analog scale 1-10)	5.88	0.71	NA
Disabilities of the Arm, Shoulder, and Hand (DASH) scores	65.4	10.4	NA

NA, Not applicable.

minimized by avoiding thermal injury during the osteotomy and ensuring good apposition and compression when securing the plate. Nerve palsies can be avoided by the careful placement of retractors during the osteotomy and plate placement. Furthermore, when incisions are made distal to the ulnar styloid, extreme care should be taken to identify and protect the dorsal sensory branch of the ulnar nerve as it courses from volar to dorsal.

Results

Seventeen patients were followed for a minimum of 12 months after undergoing shortening osteotomies with the Trimed system. Overall, the results were quite good, comparing favorably with other studies utilizing similar systems. Preoperative and postoperative range of motion, grip strength, pain, and Disabilities of the Arm, Shoulder, and Hand (DASH) scores are tallied in **Table 32-1**. Bony union, defined as bridging of the trabecular bone and cortical margin blurring, was achieved at an average of 7.41 weeks. The average shortening was 4.12 mm.

Summary

The ulnar-shortening osteotomy has become the gold standard for alleviating symptoms that stem from the overloading of the ulnar wrist that occurs with ulnar-positive variance. Although the technique can be technically demanding, especially when freehand cuts are made, the complications are few. Certainly, any number of systems and techniques can be utilized to create the osteotomy. Probably more important than the advantages or disadvantages of any technique is the surgeon's comfort level with his or her particular approach. Regardless of the technique utilized, the goal with any shortening is to obtain an ulnar-neutral or slightly ulnar-negative variance with good apposition and compression at the osteotomy site.

REFERENCES

1. Palmer AK, Werner FW: Biomechanics of the distal radio-ulnar joint. Clin Orthop Relat Res. 1984; 187:26-35.
2. Palmer AK, Werner FW: The triangular fibrocartilage complex of the wrist—anatomy and function. J Hand Surg [Am]. 1981; 6:153-162.
3. DiTano O, Trumble TE, Tencer AF: Biomechanical function of the distal radioulnar and ulnocarpal wrist ligaments. J Hand Surg [Am]. 2003; 28:622-627.
4. Milch H: Cuff resection of the ulna for malunited Colles' fracture. J Bone Joint Surg [Am]. 1941; 23:311-313.
5. Wehbé MA, Mawr B, Cautilli DA: Ulnar shortening using the AO small distractor. J Hand Surg [Am]. 1995; 20:959-963.
6. Rayhack JM, Gasser SI, Latta LL, et al: Precision oblique osteotomy for shortening of the ulna. J Hand Surg [Am]. 1993; 18:908-918.
7. Chun S, Palmer AK: The ulnar impaction syndrome: follow-up of the ulnar shortening osteotomy. J Hand Surg [Am]. 1993; 18:46-53.
8. Chen NC, Wolfe SW: Ulna shortening osteotomy using a compression device. J Hand Surg [Am]. 2003; 28:88-93.
9. Labosky DA, Waggy CA: Oblique ulnar shortening osteotomy by a single saw cut. J Hand Surg [Am]. 1996; 21:48-59.
10. Mizuseki T, Tsuge K, Ikuta Y: Precise ulna-shortening osteotomy with a new device. J Hand Surg [Am]. 2001; 26:931-939.
11. Horn PC: Long ulnar sliding osteotomy. J Hand Surg [Am]. 2004; 29:871-876.
12. Darlis NA, Ferraz IC, Kaufmann RW, et al: Step-cut ulnar-shortening osteotomy. J Hand Surg [Am]. 2005; 30:943-948.
13. Gartland JJ Jr, Werley CW: Evaluation of healed Colles' fractures. J Bone Joint Surg Am. 1981; 63:895-907.
14. Trumble TE, Gilbert M, Vedder N: Ulnar shortening combined with arthroscopic repairs in the delayed management of triangular fibrocartilage complex tears. J Hand Surg [Am]. 1997; 22:807-813.
15. Nakamura R, Horii E, Imaeda T, et al: The ulnocarpal stress test in the diagnosis of ulnar-sided wrist pain. J Hand Surg [Br]. 1997; 22:719-723.
16. Minami K, Kato H: Ulnar shortening for triangular fibrocartilage complex tears associated with ulnar positive variance. J Hand Surg [Am]. 1998; 23:904-908.

Arthroscopic Wafer Resection

Adrian Butler, MD and Randall Culp, MD

33

Ulnar impaction syndrome or ulnocarpal abutment refers to impaction of the ulnar head against the ulnar carpus, which results in persistent ulnar-sided wrist pain. Additional symptoms may include decreased range of motion, weakness of grip, and clicking of the wrist.[1] A positive or neutral ulnar variance is present in 70% of cases as seen on standardized radiographs.[2] However, ulnar-negative wrists may present with dynamic ulnar impaction with forceful grip, axial load, forearm pronation, and wrist ulnar deviation.[1,3] A positive ulnar variance may be a normal anatomical variant or result after a traumatic injury or abnormal development. Frequent causes include distal radius malunion with loss of radial height, premature distal radial physeal closure, and proximal radial migration after radial head excision. Developmental causes include Madelung's deformity and multiple enchondromatoses, among others, that affect the distal radius.[4,5]

Injury to the triangular fibrocartilage complex (TFCC) occurs early in the disease process and has been staged by Palmer as a class II TFCC abnormality (**Box 33-1**).[6,7] Chronic ulnar impaction results in a degenerative TFCC wear, chondromalacia of the lunate or ulnar head, attenuation or tearing of the lunotriquetral interosseous ligament, and, lastly, osteoarthritis of the ulnar carpus. This spectrum of findings has been termed "ulnar impaction syndrome." TFCC traumatic injuries or class I injuries respond well to repair or débridement.[6] However, TFCC tears in degenerative ulnar impaction syndrome have a failure rate as high as 25% with TFCC débridement alone.[8-11]

Treatment for ulnar impaction syndrome has focused on mechanically unloading the ulnar side of the wrist. Palmer and Werner demonstrated that load distribution across the distal radius and ulna is dependent on ulnar variance.[12] In an ulnar-neutral wrist, 82% of force transmission crosses the radiocarpal joint and 18% crosses the ulnocarpal joint. With 2.5 mm of ulnar lengthening, the force across the ulnocarpal joint increases to 41.9%. When the ulna is shortened 2.5 mm from neutral, force transmission across the ulnocarpal drops to 4.3% and the radiocarpal force transmission increases to 95.7%. The force across the ulnocarpal joint is constant in the native wrist regardless of ulnar variance.[5,13] This is because the thickness of the TFCC is variable. It is thicker in an ulnar-negative wrist and thinner in an ulnar-positive wrist. Disruption of the ulnar variance from its native state will alter the ulnocarpal mechanics. Procedures designed to mechanically unload the ulnocarpal joint include an ulnar-shortening osteotomy, open wafer resection, and arthroscopic wafer resection. More invasive procedures include distal ulnar resection (Darrach), the Sauvé-Kapandji procedure, and the hemi-resection interpositional arthroplasty. These techniques should be reserved as salvage procedures. Of these, only the Darrach resection completely unloads the ulnocarpal joint.[7,14]

Ulnar shortening has given excellent results in the treatment of ulnar impaction syndrome. Milch first described an ulnar shortening in 1941 for a malunited Colles fracture.[15] Subsequent modification of the subperiosteal cuff resection by substituting the AO-ASIF principles of rigid plate fixation produced excellent to good results in 93% of patients treated with an ulnar shortening osteotomy for ulnar impaction syndrome.[5,16-18] On average, 3 months of postoperative immobilization is required. Complications from an ulnar-shortening osteotomy include extensor carpi ulnaris tendinitis from hardware irritation and delayed union and nonunion of the osteotomy. Tendinitis necessitating removal of the plate has been reported to be as high as 52%.[19] Delayed union (>3 months) of the osteotomy has been reported in 18% to 22% of cases.[20]

An open wafer distal ulnar resection was first published by Feldon and associates in 1992.[2] This procedure does not require internal fixation, and it does not require union of an osteotomy. However, it is contraindicated in patients with degenerative arthritis or instability of the distal radioulnar joint (DRUJ) or an ulnar variance greater then 4 mm positive. It is performed through a dorsal approach between the fifth and sixth extensor compartments, as described by Bowers. A radially based, U-shaped flap of the DRUJ capsule is created to expose the DRUJ, TFCC, and proximal articular surfaces of the lunate and triquetrum. After inspection, an osteotome is used to remove 2 to 4 mm of the ulnar head, including articular cartilage and subchondral bone. Care is taken to preserve the styloid process and all TFCC attachments. In addition, the majority of the cartilage articulating with the sigmoid notch of the radius is retained to preserve DRUJ function (forearm rotation). Débridement or repair of the TFCC is also performed. Intraoperative fluoroscopy is used to ensure that 2 mm of ulnar-negative variance is created. Good to excellent results have been obtained in 85% to 100% of patients with near full recovery of motion and grip strength.[2,16,21-23] However, tendinitis of the extensor carpi ulnaris sheath occurred in up to 31% of patients.[21] When compared with an ulnar-shortening osteotomy for initial treatment of ulnar impaction syndrome, no clinical difference in outcome has been found.[19]

Arthroscopic wafer distal ulna resection was first reported in the early 1990s for patients presenting with extensive degenerative TFCC tears, chondromalacia of the ulnar head, or arthritis of the DRUJ.[8] In one biomechanical study it was shown that excision of the centrum of the TFCC and resection of the radial two-thirds width of the ulnar head to a depth of subchondral bone revealed statistically significant unloading of the ulnar aspect of the wrist.[7] It was also shown that ulnocarpal force transmission decreased with continued ulnar recession with maximal unloading at 3 mm of subchondral resection where force was reduced

Box 33-1 Classification of TFCC Tears

Class I: Acute (Traumatic Tears)
A. Central perforation
B. Ulnar detachment—with or without ulnar styloid fracture
C. Distal detachment—ulnotriquetral or ulnolunate ligaments detached
D. Radial detachment—from sigmoid notch

Class II: Degenerative (Ulnar Impaction Syndrome)
A. TFCC wear
B. TFCC wear with ulnar and/or lunate chondromalacia
C. TFCC full-thickness tear with ulnar and/or lunate chondromalacia
D. TFCC tear with lunotriquetral ligament tear in addition to ulnar and/or lunate chondromalacia
E. TFCC tear, ulnocarpal arthritis, lunotriquetral ligament tear, and ulnar and/or lunate chondromalacia

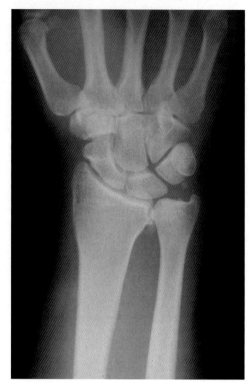

FIGURE 33-1 Posteroanterior radiograph of an ulnar-positive wrist taken with the forearm and wrist in neutral rotation. Ulnar length is measured from the medial radial articular surface to the distal ulnar articular surface.

to 10.8%. No correlation with ulnar variance and resection level was observed. However, a trend was observed between optimal unloading and stage. Stage IIB wrists were unloaded with central TFCC excision. Stage IIC wrists tended to be unloaded after TFCC excision and one-third ulnar articular cartilage resection. Lastly, stage IID wrists were unloaded after resection into subchondral bone.[7] In 12 wrists with ulnar-positive variance, Tomaino found 67% of patients to be completely pain free and 33% to have minimal symptoms at 14 months after arthroscopic wafer resection.[11] All patients were satisfied, and all had a negative ulnocarpal stress test. Preoperative ulnar variance averaged 2 mm positive and was neutral postoperatively. It has also been shown in patients presenting with ulnocarpal abutment syndrome that patients treated initially with an arthroscopic wafer resection had no statistically significant difference in outcome than those treated with arthroscopic TFCC débridement and an ulnar-shortening osteotomy.[20]

Physical Findings

Ulnar impaction syndrome is present equally in both genders and may present at any age. Complaints are classically ulnar-sided wrist pain aggravated by grip, especially with pronation. Ulnar deviation of the wrist may exacerbate the discomfort.

On physical examination, the wrist is frequently benign in appearance. However, there may be associated swelling over the ulnocarpal joint. Wrist and forearm range of motion are usually full and equal to that of the contralateral side unless the symptoms are secondary to a previous injury or congenital malformation. Pain with palpation is usually localized over the ulnocarpal joint and proximal triquetrum. Pain may be elicited with compression of the TFCC by ulnar deviation of the wrist with simultaneous pronation/supination of the ulnocarpal joint (TFCC compression test).[16] If a click is felt or heard, a TFCC tear may also be present.[24,25] Pain may also be produced if a tear of the lunotiquetral ligament is present with ballottement of the lunotriquetral joint.

The remainder of the wrist examination should be negative for other causes of ulnar-sided wrist pain. The extensor carpi ulnaris tendon should be nontender with no evidence of subluxation with supination. Forearm rotation should also be nonpainful and full without evidence of DRUJ instability. There should be no tenderness over the pisotriquetral joint and the hook of the hamate. Ulnar nerve function should be within normal limits, particularly the dorsal sensory branch.

Diagnostic Studies

Imaging studies frequently used to evaluate ulnar-sided wrist pain include radiographs, magnetic resonance imaging (MRI), and computed tomography (CT). Radiographs are frequently used to determine ulnar variance, wrist alignment, and joint integrity. Ulnar variance is assessed on a posteroanterior radiograph with the forearm and wrist in neutral rotation (**Fig. 33-1**). This is easily obtained with the shoulder abducted, elbow flexed 90 degrees, and the wrist lying flat on the radiograph plate.[3] Most patients with ulnocarpal impaction will have an ulnar-positive variance. Cystic changes may be present on both the proximal ulnar lunate and ulnar head. To assess for dynamic ulnar carpal impaction, the posteroanterior radiograph should be obtained with the forearm pronated and with forceful grip.[13] A lateral radiograph should also be obtained to assess for possible volar intercalated segmental instability. Contrast-enhanced MRI may be helpful to assess the integrity of the TFCC, lunotriquetral ligament, and lunate. Increased signal enhancement may be present in the proximal ulnar portion of the lunate and should not be confused with Kienböck's disease, which would involve the entire lunate (**Fig. 33-2**). If malunion or osseous malalignment is suspected, CT with three-dimensional reconstructions may be helpful.

Wrist arthroscopy remains the gold standard for assessing internal derangement of the wrist. It provides both diagnostic as well as therapeutic benefit. Arthroscopy should be considered in

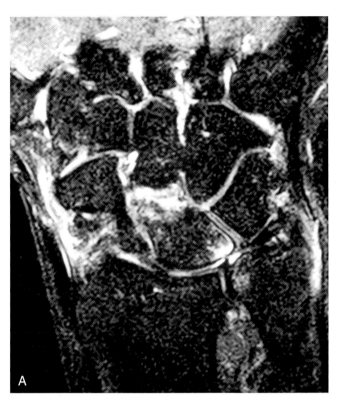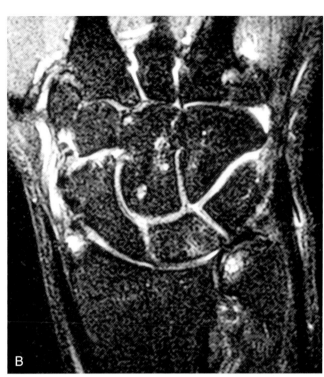

FIGURE 33-2 T2-weighted MR image of a wrist with ulnocarpal impaction syndrome. Note the increased signal in the proximal ulnar portion of the lunate (**A**) and the reciprocal increased signal of the ulnar head (**B**). In addition, the wrist is significantly ulnar positive.

patients with suspected ulnar impaction syndrome who have failed at least 3 to 4 months of conservative management. It allows assessment of the TFCC, extrinsic and intrinsic ligaments, as well as the integrity of the joint surfaces.

Indications

Partial wafer resection of the distal ulna is a procedure designed to treat symptomatic TFC tears associated with a positive or neutral ulnar variance and ulnar impaction syndrome, with a dynamic ulnar-positive variance, or ulnocarpal chondromalacia.[2,4,11,16,17,21-23] In skeletally mature patients with ulnar impaction syndrome who are found to have a TFCC perforation without arthritic change (type II C and D TFCC tears) an arthroscopic wafer resection can be used to shorten the ulna by up to 4 mm.[2,11,16,21] It is still controversial for patients with ulnar impaction syndrome and an intact TFCC (type II A and B lesions) to undergo resection of the TFCC to perform an arthroscopic wafer procedure.

Contraindications

Arthroscopic wafer resection is contraindicated in patients with symptomatic ulnar impaction syndrome who require greater than 4 mm of shortening.[2] It is also not indicated in patients who have instability or degenerative arthritis of the DRUJ.[21] Patients with advanced ulnocarpal arthritis or with significant instability of the wrist will also unlikely benefit from an arthroscopic wafer procedure.[16]

Surgical Technique

With the patient under general anesthesia or sedation with an upper extremity nerve block, a standard wrist arthroscopy is performed. The patient is positioned supine on the operating table with the shoulder abducted 90 degrees and centered on a hand table. An examination under anesthesia is then performed to assess for any instability of the DRUJ in both pronation and supination. A well-padded arm tourniquet is then applied and the upper extremity prepared and draped in the usual sterile fashion. After finger traps are applied, the arm is securely fastened in a well padded traction tower with 10 to 15 lb of traction across the wrist. The forearm is placed in neutral rotation, and the wrist is flexed 10 to 15 degrees (**Fig. 33-3**).

 Web Video 33-1 and 33-2

Standard wrist arthroscopy portals are used. After an Esmarch tourniquet is used to exsanguinate the wrist, the tourniquet is inflated to 250 mm Hg. The 3-4 portal is created first after its location is confirmed with a needle, and the wrist joint is inflated with normal sterile saline. A No. 11 scalpel is used to incise the skin only. This is followed by blunt dissection with a hemostat. A 2.9-mm short, blunt obturator and cannula are then inserted, followed by the 2.7-mm camera. Inflation of the wrist is provided by normal sterile saline pressurized by a pump set to the small joint arthroscopy setting. After the radiocarpal and ulnocarpal joints are inspected, the 4-5 portal is created under direct visualization to avoid iatrogenic injury to the TFCC. A probe is then inserted to aid wrist examination.

Inspection of the chondral surfaces of the scaphoid, lunate, and distal radius is performed. With ulnar impaction syndrome, chondromalacia is frequently present on the ulnar half of the proximal lunate. A reciprocal "kissing lesion" may be present on the ulnar head and may be easily seen if a full-thickness central TFCC tear is present (**Fig. 33-4**). This is also usually accompanied by synovitis, which should be débrided to allow adequate visualization. This is best accomplished with a heat probe and small shaver. Care must be used to avoid débridement of the extensor tendons dorsally.

The radiocarpal, ulnocarpal, scapholunate, and lunotriquetral ligaments are then assessed and probed. Full evaluation of the lunotriquetral ligament requires the camera to be switched to the 4-5 portal or the alternate 6R portal. Suspected scapholunate and lunotriquetral tears can be confirmed by "air arthrogram." This is

accomplished with the camera in the 3-4 portal. Air is then infiltrated into the midcarpal joint with a syringe and the scapholunate and lunotriquetral ligaments simultaneously visualized for any extravasation of air bubbles through either the scapholunate or lunotriquetral ligaments, respectively. Any scapholunate or lunotriquetral ligament tears should be inspected further through radial or ulnar midcarpal portals.

After confirmation of ulnar impaction syndrome, arthroscopic wafer resection can proceed. Using the 3-4, 4-5, and 6R portals, the TFCC tear is débrided with either a suction punch or small arthroscopic shaver (**Fig. 33-5**). The ulnar head is then inspected for evidence of chondromalacia. A small arthroscopic bur is then placed through the 4-5 portal, and the ulnar head is débrided (**Fig. 33-6**). Care is taken to both pronate and supinate the forearm as debridement progresses to ensure removal of both the volar and dorsal portions of the ulnar head (**Fig. 33-7**). After the initial bone resection, a DRUJ portal is created just proximal to the radial attachment of the TFCC. This is created with the aid of a needle to ensure proper placement. The bur is then placed through this portal, and ulnar recession is continued (**Fig. 33-8**). Caution must be used when progressing ulnarly to ensure that the ulnar styloid is preserved. Throughout the recession, alteration of the working portals as well as the viewing and working portals is required to create an even and sufficient ulnar wafer resection. Fluoroscopy is used intermittently throughout and at the conclusion of the case to ensure complete ulnar recession in both pronation and supination. On a forearm-neutral posteroanterior radiograph, the ulna should be at least neutral if it was positive preoperatively (**Fig. 33-9**). On average, 2 to 3 mm of distal ulna should be removed. Once the resection is deemed adequate, the wrist is again examined for full forearm rotation and DRUJ stability. The portal sites are closed, and a soft dressing is applied. Mobilization is started after the first postoperative visit.

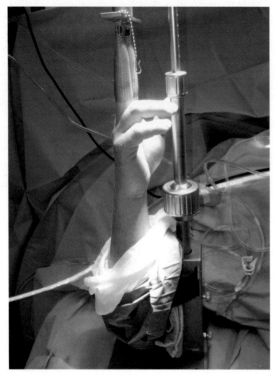

FIGURE 33-3 Example of a standard wrist arthroscopic setup. Note that the forearm rotation is neutral.

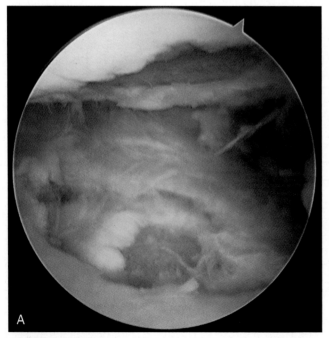

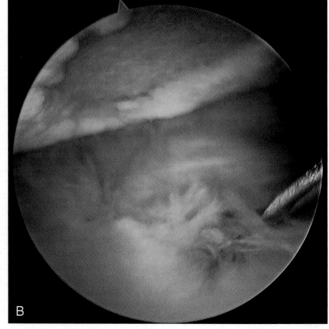

FIGURE 33-4 Intraoperative photograph of the lunate and ulnar head taken through the arthroscope positioned in the 3-4 portal. Note the complete loss of articular cartilage from the proximal ulnar portion of the lunate and the corresponding "kissing lesion" of the ulnar head (**A**) viewed through a large central "degenerative" TFCC tear (**B**).

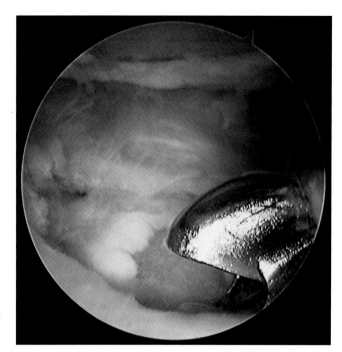

FIGURE 33-5 Intraoperative photograph taken with the arthroscope positioned in the 3-4 portal. A suction punch is used to débride the central TFCC tear back to a stable margin.

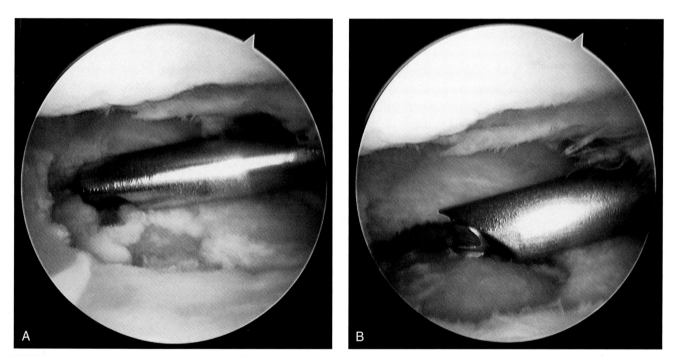

FIGURE 33-6 Intraoperative photographs taken with the arthroscope positioned in the 3-4 portal. An oscillating shaver is used to remove any remaining articular cartilage (**A**). This is followed by a power bur to remove up to 4 mm of ulnar head (**B**). It is imperative to both pronate and supinate the forearm to ensure complete recession of the ulnar head.

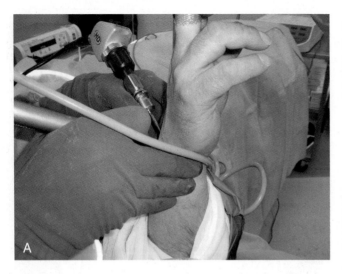

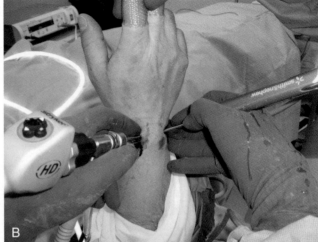

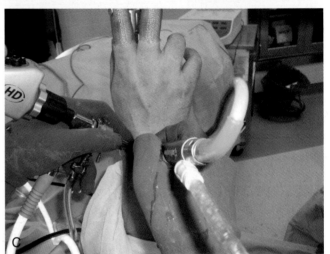

FIGURE 33-7 To ensure complete ulnar head recession, it is frequently necessary to both pronate (**A**) and supinate (**B**) the forearm from the neutral (**C**) position throughout the procedure.

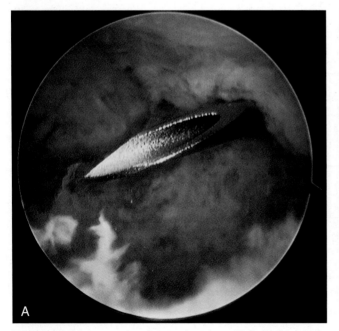

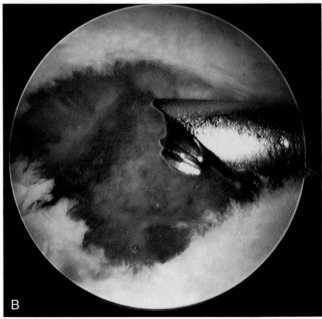

FIGURE 33-8 Intraoperative photographs taken with the arthroscope positioned in the 3-4 portal. A needle is used to ensure proper placement of the DRUJ portal beneath the remaining TFCC (**A**). The arthroscopic bur can then be placed through this portal to complete the ulnar head recession (**B**). Alteration of the working portals is often required to complete the recession.

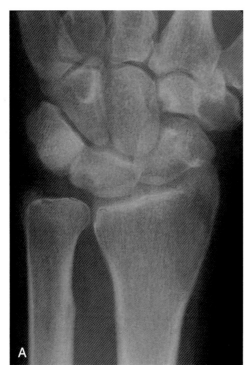 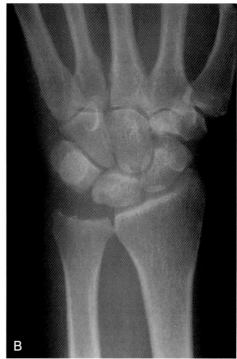

FIGURE 33-9 Posteroanterior radiograph of a wrist in neutral rotation before (**A**) and after (**B**) completion of an arthroscopic wafer procedure.

Results

The senior author has a personal series of 13 consecutive patients treated with an arthroscopic wafer resection with an average follow-up of 4.2 years (range: 3 to 9 years). All patients had a positive TFCC stress test and an average ulnar-positive variance of 2.4 mm (range: 2 to 4 mm) preoperatively. All patients failed conservative management. Intraoperatively, all patients had a central TFCC tear and chondromalacia of the ulnar head and/or ulnar portion of the proximal lunate. The TFCC tears were débrided to a stable margin, and the ulnar heads were resected by 2 to 3 mm. At final follow-up, strength was improved by 18% from preoperative values. All patients reported satisfaction with the procedure, and no revisions were required. The majority of patients (78%) were pain free, and 22% reported only occasional discomfort with strenuous activities. No statistical difference was found between preoperative and postoperative range of motion.

REFERENCES

1. Freidman SL, Palmer AK: The ulnar impaction syndrome. Hand Clin. 1999; 7:295-310.

2. Feldon P, Terrono AL, Belsky MR: The "wafer" procedure. Clin Orthop Relat Res. 1992; 275:124-129.

3. Epner RA, Bowers WH, Guilford WB: Ulnar variance: the effect of wrist positioning and roentgen filming technique. J Hand Surg. 1982; 7:298-305.

4. Le TB, Vaughan C, Bowen A: Ulnar shortening osteotomy. In Gelberman RH, Thompson RC, eds: The Wrist: Master Techniques in Orthopaedic Surgery. Philadelphia: Lippincott Williams & Wilkins, 2002; 307-321.

5. Chun S, Palmer AK: The ulnar impaction syndrome: follow-up of ulnar shortening osteotomy. J Hand Surg [Am]. 1993; 18:46-53.

6. Palmer AK: Triangular fibrocartilage lesions: classification and treatment. J Hand Surg [Am]. 1989; 14:594-606.

7. Wnorowski DC, Palmer AK, Werner FW, Fortino MD: Anatomic and biochemical analysis of the arthroscopic wafer procedure. Arthroscopy. 1992; 8:204-212.

8. Osterman AL: Arthroscopic débridement of triangular fibrocartialge complex tears. Arthroscopy. 1990; 6:120-124.

9. Westkaemper JG, Mitsionis G, Giannakopoulos PN, Sotereanos DG: Wrist arthroscopy for the treatment of ligament and triangular fibrocartilage complex injuries. Arthroscopy. 1998; 14:479-483.

10. Minami A, Ishikawa J, Suenaga N, Kasashima T: Clinical result of treatment of triangular fibrocartilage complex tears by arthroscopic debridement. J Hand Surg [Am]. 1996; 21:406-411.

11. Tomaino MW, Weiser RW: Combined arthroscopic TFCC debridement and wafer resection of the distal ulna in wrists with complex tears and positive ulnar variance. J Hand Surg [Am]. 2001; 26:1047-1052.

12. Palmer AK, Werner FW: Biomechanics of the distal radioulnar joint. Clin Orthop Relat Res. 1984; 187:26-35.

13. Palmer AK, Glisson RR, Werner FW: Relationship between ulnar variance and triangular fibrocartilage complex thickness. J Hand Surg [Am]. 1984; 9:681-683.

14. Werner FW, Glisson RR, Murphy DJ, Palmer AK: Force transmission through the distal radio-ulnar carpal joints:

effect of ulnar lengthening and shortening. Handchir. 1986; 18:304-308.

15. Milch H: Cuff resection of the ulna for malunited Colles' fracture. J Bone Joint Surg 1941; 39:311-313.

16. Loftus JB: Arthroscopic wafer for ulnar impaction syndrome. Tech Hand Upper Extrem Surg. 2000; 4:182-188.

17. Darrow JC, Linscheid RL, Dobyns JH, et al: Distal ulnar recession for disorders of the distal radio-ulnar joint. J Hand Surg [Am]. 1985; 10:482-491.

18. Boulas HJ, Milek MA: Ulnar shortening for tears of the triangular fibrocartilaginous complex. J Hand Surg [Am]. 1990; 15:415-420.

19. Constantine KJ, Tomaino MM, Herndon JH, Sotereanos DG: Comparison of ulnar shortening osteotomy and wafer resection procedure for ulnar impaction syndrome. J Hand Surg [Am]. 2000; 25:55-60.

20. Bernstein MA, Nagle DJ, et al: A comparison of combined arthroscopic triangular fibrocartilage complex débridement and arthroscopic wafer distal ulna resection versus arthroscopic triangular fibrocartilage complex débridement and ulnar shortening osteotomy for ulnocarpal abutment syndrome. Arthroscopy. 2004; 20:392-401.

21. Feldon P, Terrono AL, Belsky MR: Wafer distal ulna resection for triangular fibrocartilage tears and/or ulna impaction syndrome. J Hand Surg [Am]. 1992; 17:731-737.

22. Bilos ZJ, Chamberland D: Distal ulnar head shortening for treatment of triangular fibrocartilage complex tears with ulna positive variance. J Hand Surg [Am]. 1991; 16:1115-1119.

23. Schuurman AH, Bos KE: The ulno-carpal abutment syndrome: follow-up of the wafer procedure. J Hand Surg [Br]. 1995; 20:171-177.

24. Roth JH, Poehiling GG: Arthroscopic "ectomy" surgery of the wrist. Arthroscopy. 1990; 6:141-147.

25. Hornbach EE, Osterman AL: Partial excision of the triangular fibrocartilage complex. In Gelberman RH, Thompson RC, eds: The Wrist: Master Techniques in Orthopaedic Surgery. Philadelphia: Lippincott Williams & Wilkins, 2002; 279-290.

Sauvé-Kapandji Procedure after Distal Radius Fractures

34

Heidi C. Shors, MD and Mark E. Baratz, MD

Injuries to the distal radioulnar joint (DRUJ) with a distal radius fracture can cause ulnar-sided wrist pain, decreased forearm rotation, instability of the ulna, and loss of function. Controversy exists as to the treatment of this disorder. Some of the options include distal ulna resection (Darrach procedure),[1] hemi-resection and interposition arthroplasty,[2] matched distal ulna resection,[3] and the Sauvé-Kapandji procedure.[4] Satisfactory outcomes have been achieved using all of these procedures.[2,3,5-14] Limitations of these procedures can include diminished grip strength, instability of the wrist, rupture of extensor tendons, and ulnar carpal abutment. Consistently good results can be difficult to achieve in young, active patients.[15] In this chapter we discuss the use of the Sauvé-Kapandji procedure for treatment of DRUJ derangement after distal radius fractures.

History

The first description of a pseudarthrosis of the ulna performed for distal radioulnar pathology was recorded by Lauenstein in 1887. In 1921, Baldwin described a similar procedure with fixation of the DRUJ. The first detailed description of a fusion of the DRUJ with resection of bone just proximal to the fusion site was published by Louis Sauvé and Mehmed Kapandji in 1936.[4] Since this publication, there have been several modifications proposed by different authors but the name "Sauvé-Kapandji procedure" has remained.

Indications

Mikkelsen and colleagues[8] used "chronic ulnar wrist pain after Colles' fracture" as the indication for the Sauvé-Kapandji procedure. George and associates[6] stated that "severe and persistent pain in the DRUJ" was the primary indication for the Sauvé-Kapandji procedure. Ulnar-sided wrist pain after distal radius fracture can be the result of a variety of conditions, including DRUJ arthritis, DRUJ instability, and ulnocarpal abutment, all of which are conditions that may be caused or compounded by a malunion of the distal radius. It is our practice to define the pathology and try to restore normal anatomy before proceeding to the Sauvé-Kapandji procedure. For example, ulnar-sided pain in a patient with a malunion of the distal radius, with no arthritis of DRUJ, is offered a corrective osteotomy of the radius. A patient with mild instability of the DRUJ and a radius in at least a neutral palmer tilt is offered an ulnar-shortening osteotomy. If the DRUJ is unstable and there is no arthritis, we will first offer a ligament reconstruction for the DRUJ. Our indications for the Sauvé-Kapandji procedure after distal radius fracture are very specific: (1) active, high-demand patient with DRUJ arthritis and (2) failed ulnar shortening or ligament reconstruction for DRUJ instability.

The Sauvé-Kapandji procedure can be performed after all fractures are healed and nonoperative treatment has failed.

As a general rule, it takes about 6 months before we abandon therapy or injections and proceed to the Sauvé-Kapandji procedure.

Contraindications

The only true contraindication is inadequate bone stock at the DRUJ. Relative contraindications include heavy smoking or medical conditions that might adversely affect bone healing. Patients should understand the limits of the procedure. The Sauvé-Kapandji procedure will not improve extension and flexion of the wrist but is excellent at restoring near-normal forearm rotation. Grip strength is improved but does not return to normal levels, and return to work rates have varied. Pain is generally significantly improved but is still mildly to moderately present with the extremes of activity.[6-9,12,13]

Surgical Technique

Web Video

34-1

An incision is made between the fifth and sixth compartments to expose the distal portion of the ulna and the DRUJ (**Fig. 34-1**). Care should be taken to protect the dorsal sensory branch of the ulnar nerve. The joint capsule is elevated off of the DRUJ (**Fig. 34-2**). Reciprocal surfaces of the DRUJ are resected using a microsagittal saw (**Fig. 34-3**). The resulting space between the head of the ulna and the distal radius is measured (**Fig. 34-4**). A segment of bone of equivalent length is resected from the distal ulna to use as an intercalary graft (**Fig. 34-5**). The head of the ulna can be translated proximally to achieve ulnar-neutral variance (**Fig. 34-6**). When the head is in the desired position, additional ulna is resected to create a space of 10 mm (**Fig. 34-7**).

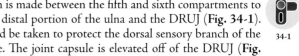

FIGURE 34-1

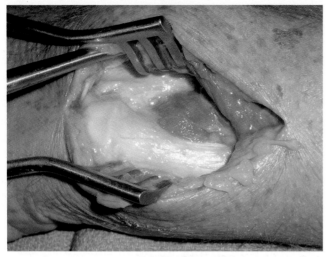

FIGURE 34-2

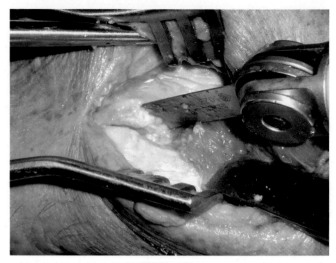

FIGURE 34-3

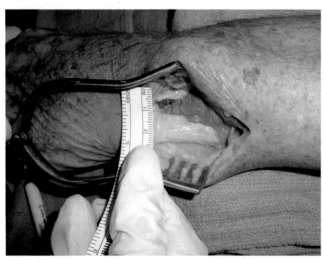

FIGURE 34-4

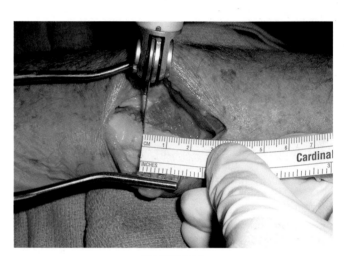

FIGURE 34-5

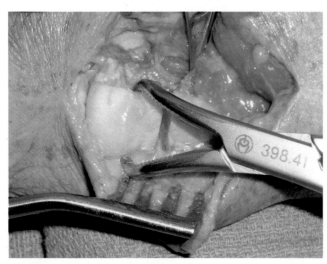

FIGURE 34-6

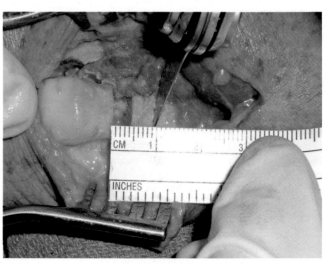

FIGURE 34-7

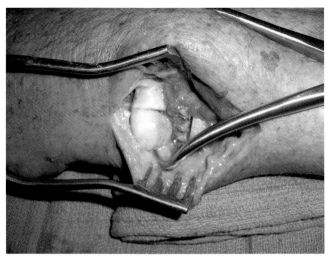

FIGURE 34-8

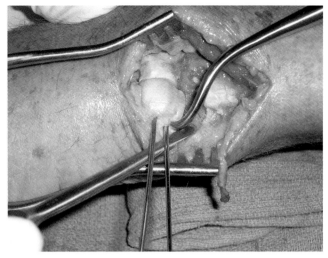

FIGURE 34-9

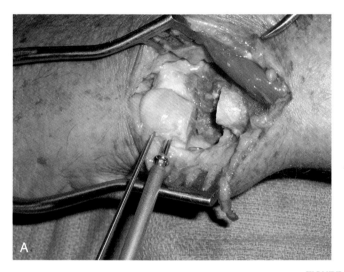

FIGURE 34-10

The initial segment of resected ulna is placed between the head of the ulna and the radius and compressed with a tenaculum (**Fig. 34-8**). The head, graft, and radius are pinned with two cannulated wires spaced sufficiently apart to avoid impingement of the screw heads (**Fig. 34-9**). Wires are measured for the appropriate screw length. Partially threaded 4.0-mm screws are inserted to stabilize the DRUJ (**Figs. 34-10 and Fig. 34-11**).

Variations on the procedure have been described, including placing a portion of the pronator quadratus into the gap to encourage formation of a pseudarthrosis. Some authors have chosen to stabilize the proximal stump of the distal ulna with a distally based slip of the flexor carpi ulnaris or extensor carpi ulnaris.[6,8,13,16]

Postoperatively the limb is immobilized in a long arm cast for 4 weeks with the forearm supinated about 45 degrees. A short arm splint is applied until the fusion site has healed.

Results

No prospective, randomized trials have been performed to study the Sauvé-Kapandji procedure versus other methods

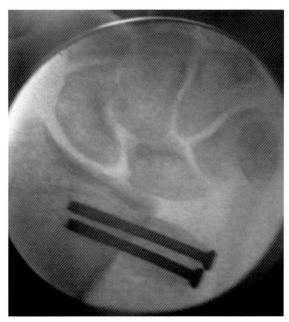

FIGURE 34-11 Posteroanterior postoperative radiograph.

of treatment for DRUJ derangement after distal radius fractures. We identified six articles in which the Sauvé-Kapandji procedure was used to treat DRUJ pathology after a distal radius fracture.[6-10,17]

Indications ranged from persistent ulnar-sided wrist pain after distal radius fracture to salvage of a previously failed procedure. Most series have achieved excellent, reported near-normal forearm rotation (155 degrees arc), mild to moderate pain, unchanged wrist flexion-extension (arc of 80 to 120 degrees), an increased ability to return to work (few can return to 100% capacity of heavy labor work), and 85% satisfaction rating.[4-18] The average Modified Wrist Score was 77, which correlated with a good result.[6,7,9,10]

Complications

The most commonly discussed complication of the Sauvé-Kapandji procedure is instability of the proximal stump. Different methods of stabilization have been proposed using either the pronator quadratus, a slip of the extensor carpi ulnaris tendon (distally based or proximally based), a slip of the flexor carpi ulnaris tendon, or imbrication of the adjacent tissues.[6,8,13,16,19] More recently some surgeons have tried to control stump instability by using an ulnar head prosthesis seated in a cavity created in the remnant of the ulnar head.

REFERENCES

1. Darrach W: Anterior dislocation of the head of the ulna. Ann Surg. 1912; 56:802-803.
2. Bowers WH: Distal radioulnar joint arthroplasty: the hemiresection–interposition technique. J Hand Surg [Am]. 1985; 10:169-178.
3. Watson HK, Ryu J, Burgess R: Matched distal ulnar resection. J Hand Surg [Am]. 1986; 11:812-817.
4. Sauvé L, Kapandji M: Nouvelle technique de traitement chirurgical des luxations récidivantes isolées de l'extrémité inférieure du cubitus. J Chir (Paris). 1936; 47:589-594.
5. Tulipan DJ, Eaton RG, Eberhart RE: The Darrach procedure defended, technique redefined and long-term follow-up. J Hand Surg [Am]. 1991; 16: 438-444.
6. George MS, Kiefhaber TR, Stern PJ: The Sauvé-Kapandji procedure and the Darrach procedure for the distal radio-ulnar joint dysfunction after Colles' fracture. J Hand Surg [Br]. 2004; 29:608-613.
7. Carter PB, Stuart PR: The Sauvé-Kapandji procedure for post-traumatic disorders of the distal radio-ulnar joint. J Bone Joint Surg [Br]. 2000; 82:1013-1018.
8. Mikkelsen SS, Lindblad BE, Larsen ER, Sommer J: Sauvé-Kapandji operation for disorders of the distal radioulnar joint after Colles' fracture. Acta Orthop Scand. 1997; 68:64-66.
9. Jacobsen TW, Leicht P: The Sauvé-Kapandji procedure for posttraumatic disorders of the distal radioulnar joint. Acta Orthop Belg. 2004; 70:226-230.
10. Lamey DM, Fernandez DL: Results of the modified Sauvé-Kapandji procedure in the treatment of chronic posttraumatic derangement of the distal radioulnar joint. J Bone Joint Surg Am. 1998; 80:1758-1769.
11. Zimmerman R, Gschwentner M, Arora R, et al: Treatment of distal radioulnar joint disorders with a modified Sauvé-Kapandji procedure: long-term outcome with special attention to the DASH questionnaire. Arch Orthop Trauma Surg. 2003; 123:293-298.
12. Low CK, Chew WYC: Results of Sauvé-Kapandji procedure. Singapore Med J. 2002; 43:135-137.
13. Minami A, Iwasaki N, Ishikawa J, et al: Stabilization of the proximal ulnar stump in the Sauvé-Kapandji procedure by using the extensor carpi ulnaris tendon: long-term follow-up studies. J Hand Surg [Am]. 2006; 31:440-444.
14. Gordon L, Levinsohn DG, Moore SV, et al: The Sauvé-Kapandji procedure for the treatment of post-traumatic distal radioulnar joint problems. Hand Clin. 1991; 7:397-403.
15. Bain GI, Pugh DMW, MacDermid JC, et al: Matched hemiresection interposition arthroplasty of the distal radioulnar joint. J Hand Surg [Am]. 1995; 20:944-950.
16. Field J, Majkowski RJ, Leslie IJ: Poor results of Darrach's procedure after wrist injuries. J Bone Joint Surg Br. 1993; 75:53-57.
17. Inagaki H, Nakamura R, Horii E, et al: Symptoms and radiographic findings in the proximal and distal ulnar stumps after the Sauvé-Kapandji procedure for treatment of chronic derangement of the distal radioulnar joint. J Hand Surg [Am]. 2006; 31:780-784.
18. Sanders RA, Frederick HA, Hontas RB: The Sauvé-Kapandji procedure: a salvage operation for the distal radioulnar joint. J Hand Surg [Am]. 1991; 16:1125-1129.
19. Rothwell AG, O'Neill L, Cragg K: Sauvé-Kapandji procedure for disorders of the distal radioulnar joint: a simplified technique. J Hand Surg [Am] 1996; 21:771-777.

Hemi-resection Interposition Arthroplasty

35

David S. Zelouf, MD

In the setting of advanced articular involvement of the distal radioulnar joint (DRUJ), a salvage or ablative procedure is recommended. Ablative procedures of the distal ulna include the hemi-resection interposition technique (HIT) arthroplasty,[1] the Sauvé-Kapandji procedure,[2] the matched resection,[3] and the Darrach procedure.[4] The author has no personal experience with the matched resection procedure, but it is conceptually similar to the HIT procedure. Implant arthroplasty of the DRUJ is yet another alternative, and favorable early results have been reported using the implant developed by van Schoohoven and colleagues in the setting of a failed salvage procedure.[5]

The HIT procedure was developed by William H. Bowers in 1981 as an integral part of managing the rheumatoid ulnar wrist. The principle of the procedure is to maintain a strong soft tissue connection of the ulna to the carpus and radius while removing the damaged joint surface. Although originally designed primarily for the rheumatoid wrist, the HIT procedure has also been used successfully in the nonrheumatoid wrist and, in particular, as a reconstructive option in the setting of distal radial malunion.[6-8] It has also been successfully employed in patients affected by symptomatic, primary osteoarthritis of the DRUJ.

Ablative procedures are championed by others, especially in the setting of a relatively young patient with a distal radial malunion in conjunction with a nonsalvageable DRUJ. The Sauvé-Kapandji procedure was first reported by Louis Sauvé and Mehmed Kapandji in 1936 and combines a DRUJ arthrodesis along with a surgical pseudarthrosis between the proximal ulna and ulnar head. The principle of the procedure is to maintain a radioulnar joint surface, thus providing a more physiological pattern of force transmission from the hand to the forearm. Instability of the proximal stump remains problematic at times, similar to the Darrach procedure.

Indications

Choosing between ablative procedures is often a matter of personal preference, but certain principles should be employed to aid in the decision-making process. If the sigmoid notch is incongruous or arthritic, an ablative procedure is usually required. The same is true for the ulnar head. If the articular surface of the ulnar head is deficient, once again an ablative procedure is most often appropriate. None of the distal radioulnar joint salvage procedures is entirely predictable with regard to restoration of painless and stable pronation/supination. Some loss of grip strength is also common after any of the DRUJ salvage procedures.

Caveats

The success of the HIT procedure depends on an intact or reconstructable triangular fibrocartilaginous complex (TFCC). The procedure cannot succeed if the TFCC is not a functional structure. This is often the case in advanced rheumatoid arthritis, and the HIT procedure is not recommended in this setting. In such a patient, a Darrach resection or a Sauvé-Kapandji procedure is recommended. In the absence of inflammatory disease, the TFCC is typically intact or reconstructable. In the setting of a markedly malunited distal radius, a peripheral tear is often present but the overall integrity of the ligament typically remains intact.

Conceptually, the HIT procedure preserves the ulnocarpal ligament complex, thus maintaining some stability while simultaneously addressing the problematic DRUJ by removing the involved distal ulnar articular surface. Thus, the resection involves resection of the ulnar articular head while the shaft/styloid relationship is left intact. The ideal nonrheumatoid candidate presents with a painful distal radioulnar joint with or without a distal radius malunion. The procedure is rarely indicated in the acute setting. The TFCC can be partially deficient, but it must be able to be repaired. It is best if the TFCC is intact; and if it is neither intact nor can be repaired, the procedure offers no advantages over a Darrach procedure. The HIT procedure may also be successfully utilized in the setting of a partially treated distal radius fracture associated with a fracture of the ulnar styloid with associated dislocation of the distal ulna (**Fig. 35-1**).

Contraindications

The most significant contraindication for the HIT procedure is the lack of a functional TFCC. The other relative contraindication for the HIT procedure is significant ulnar-positive variance. In this setting, failure to consider postoperative stylocarpal impingement is likely to result in a clinical failure.

Preoperative Considerations

Before considering an HIT procedure, proper radiographs are obtained, including a posteroanterior film in neutral rotation, as well as a grip-loaded posteroanterior view in full pronation to assess variance and estimate the likelihood of postoperative stylocarpal impingement. After excision of the articular surface, the maximum migration of the radius and ulna toward each other is 0.75 cm. If this amount of migration allows the styloid to come within 2 mm of the ulnar-deviated carpus, stylocarpal impingement can be anticipated with a possible clinical failure. Solutions include partial ulnar styloidectomy, osteotomy of the ulnar styloid with shortening and osteosynthesis of the styloid, ulnar shaft shortening with plate fixation, or an interposition anchovy such as the palmaris longus to the radioulnar void.

The HIT Arthroplasty

The procedure is typically performed utilizing general or regional anesthesia under arm tourniquet control. Prophylactic antibiotics are recommended. If a distal radius osteotomy is required, it is

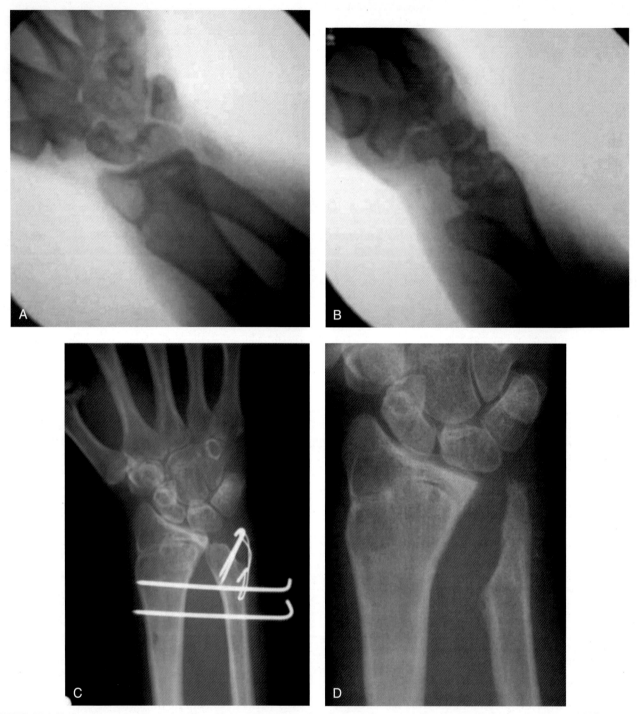

FIGURE 35-1 Preoperative posteroanterior (**A**) and lateral (**B**) radiographs of a partially treated distal radius fracture with ulnar styloid fracture and distal ulna dislocation. **C,** After ORIF of the distal ulna using a tension band technique and DRUJ temporary stabilization with two K-wires. **D,** Despite restoration of reasonable forearm rotation, pain and crepitus persisted, requiring an HIT procedure.

recommended that this be performed first. A separate incision is most often required in this setting.

With the forearm pronated, an angled or straight incision is made over the distal ulna (**Fig. 35-2**). The incision lies dorsal to the dorsal sensory branches of the ulnar nerve. Care is taken to preserve these small branches, which often include both transverse and oblique branches around the DRUJ. The ulnar head presents beneath the retinaculum, between the extensor carpi ulnaris and the extensor digiti minimi (**Fig. 35-3**). The extensor

digiti minimi is used as a guide for fashioning the retinacular flap. In a nonrheumatoid wrist it is recommended that both the retinacular and capsular flaps be ulnar based (**Fig. 35-4**). The retinaculum is incised over the extensor digiti minimi, retracting the tendon radialward. Once the tendon is retracted, the dorsal margin of the sigmoid notch, the DRUJ capsule, and the TFCC are easily identified. The capsule is then detached from the radius reflecting it ulnarward, leaving a 1-mm cuff for possible later repair (**Fig. 35-5**). The capsule is dissected along the head of the

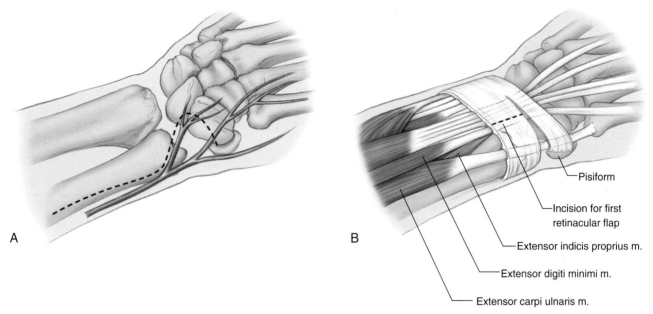

FIGURE 35-2 The incision (**A**) and design of retinacular flaps (**B**).

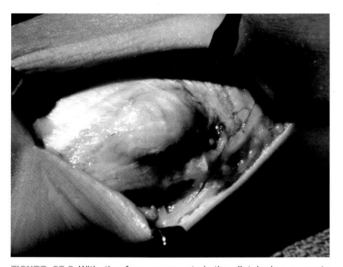

FIGURE 35-3 With the forearm pronated, the distal ulna presents between the extensor digiti minimi radialward and the extensor carpi ulnaris ulnarward.

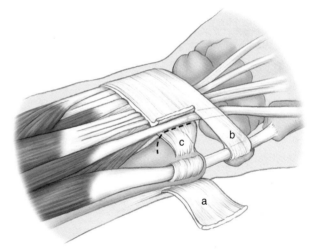

FIGURE 35-4 After reflecting the retinacular flap, the capsule is then incised and reflected ulnarward. a, proximal retinaculum; b, distal retinaculum; c, DRUJ capsule.

ulna subperioseally beneath the extensor carpi ulnaris sheath. For more distal exposure, the distal aspect of the dorsal retinaculum can also be reflected as an ulnarly based flap, with care taken to avoid disrupting the dorsal fibers of the TFCC (**Fig. 35-6**). In the nonrheumatoid wrist, it is not necessary to violate the extensor carpi ulnaris subsheath.

At this point, if the articular surface is sufficiently involved, the ulna articular surface is removed with small, flat osteotomes and a rongeur (**Figs. 35-6 and 35-7**). I recommend starting with a flat osteotome from distal to proximal, removing the dorsal half of the ulna head. Care is taken to ensure that the foveal attachment of the TFCC is not disrupted. A second oblique cut is then made once again from distal to proximal after rotating the forearm. It is typically necessary to make a third cut from proximal to distal once again using a small, flat osteotome. This "third cut" removes

the palmar portion of the head, which is easy to miss if one is not careful. A rasp or small rongeur is used to smooth out the remaining bone. The remaining shaft/styloid axis should be round in cross section and resemble a tapering 1-cm diameter dowel. A small laminar spreader is used to facilitate exposure to be sure an adequate resection has been performed, particularly volarward. All osteophytes around the sigmoid notch and all the bone of the ulnar head beneath the articular surface must be excised. Inadequate bone removal can result in a clinical failure.

After completing the bony resection, all remaining synovium is excised and the integrity of the TFCC is inspected. If necessary, the articular disc can be débrided at this point. An assessment of stylocarpal impingement is then performed, typically with the aid of a portable fluoroscopy unit (**Fig. 35-8**). While under fluoroscopy, the radius and ulna are compressed and rotated with the

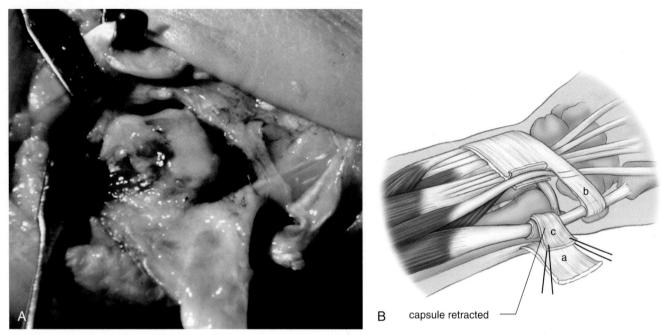

FIGURE 35-5 A and **B,** In this nonrheumatoid wrist, the two retinacular flaps have been reflected ulnarward, allowing visualization of the DRUJ, dorsal limb of the TFC, and, with further dissection, the lunotriquetral joint. a, proximal retinaculum; b, distal retinaculum; c, DRUJ capsule.

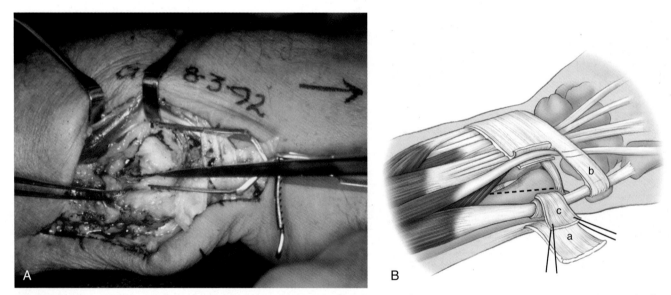

FIGURE 35-6 A and **B,** A small, flat osteotome is used to osteotomize the distal ulna for excision. It is recommended that the first cut be from distal to proximal.

wrist in ulnar deviation. If one remains concerned that the styloid will impinge on the carpus, options include interposing a tendon "anchovy," such as the palmaris longus (**Fig. 35-9**), or performing an ulnar shortening for more obvious degrees of impingement. Available expendable tendons would include the palmaris longus (most common), one half of the flexor carpi radialis, the extensor indicis proprius, or a long toe extensor. The tendon graft is rolled into a ball around a straight clamp and sutured with absorbable 3-0 Vicryl sutures to keep it intact. It is then placed into the cavity after the partial ulnar head resection and sutured to the volar capsule and pronator quadratus to prevent displacement. The dorsal capsule is then anatomically repaired back to the septum between the extensor digiti minimi and the DRUJ.

If one decides that an anchovy is inadequate to prevent impingement and that an ulnar shortening is required, it can be performed at one of three locations. The first and most straightforward location is at the tip of the styloid. This is useful in those cases in which there is a long, hooked styloid. In this instance, the distal aspect of the styloid is exposed and excised. Preservation of the deep fibers of the TFCC attached to the fovea preserves DRUJ stability. The second option is a shortening through the metaphyseal base of the ulnar head at the proximal margin of the head excision, with excision of a wedge of bone and fixation using a compression interosseous wire loop (**Fig. 35-10**). This is technically more demanding. The final alternative is a formal shortening through the proximal ulnar shaft and plate fixation. This is typi-

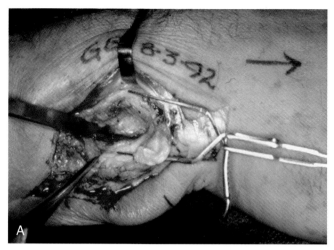
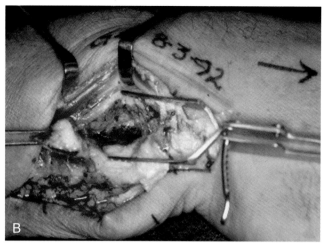

FIGURE 35-7 **A,** The third cut is from proximal to distal, once again using the same flat osteotome. **B,** Resected specimen.

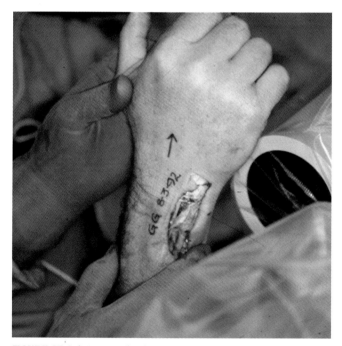

FIGURE 35-8 Intraoperative inspection with the aid of a portable fluoroscopy unit is recommended to assess adequacy of resection and stylocarpal impingement syndrome.

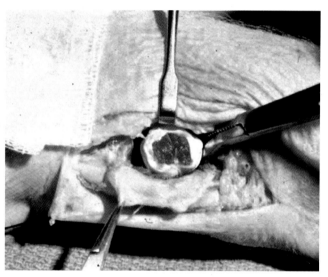

FIGURE 35-9 An "anchovy" prepared from the palmaris longus is inserted into the newly created cavity as a means of preventing stylocarpal impingement.

cally recommended when the preoperative ulnar-positive variance is greater than 3 to 4 mm. When considering stylocarpal impingement, the preoperative variance radiographs are critical. The variance is best determined by an anteroposterior pronated grip radiograph.[9] In borderline cases (preoperative variance between neutral and 2 mm positive), an anchovy may be utilized, but in most cases the capsule and retinaculum are the only materials interposed and are sutured to the volar capsule (**Fig. 35-11**).

Postoperative Care

Typically, the postoperative care depends on what other procedures have been performed. If a corrective distal radius osteotomy has been performed along with a hemi-resection, immobilization may vary depending on the stability of the construct.

In the absence of a distal radius osteotomy, a long-arm plaster splint is utilized for 10 days. The sutures are then removed, and a removable Muenster splint is utilized for 2 to 3 additional weeks. Radiographs are typically obtained at this time. During this period, active elbow and digital motion are encouraged. After approximately 4 weeks, active and gentle passive forearm rotation is begun. If an ulnar shortening is required, a short arm cast is utilized for 4 to 6 weeks while the osteotomy heals. An osteotomy at the site of the ulnar head resection typically heals within 6 weeks, whereas a shortening performed at the shaft level requires a longer period of protection. Supervised hand therapy is most often done, depending on the patient's progress. A return to full activities typically takes 3 to 4 months.

Complications

The most common complication involves stylocarpal impingement. It does not typically occur if it is anticipated and dealt with at the primary procedure. Another potential complication is

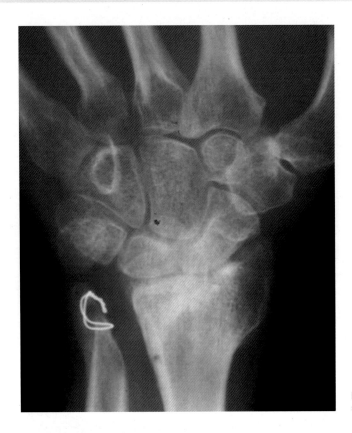

FIGURE 35-10 Postoperative radiograph after HIT procedure with ulnar styloid osteotomy, shortening, and osteosynthesis using a wire loop.

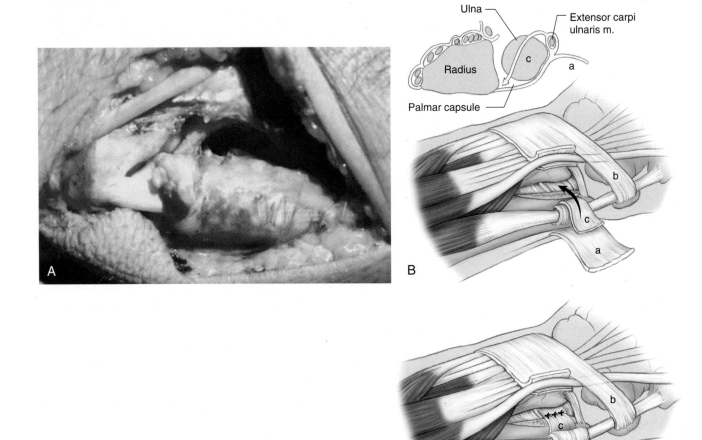

FIGURE 35-11 A to **C**, In this patient, no interposition other than the infolded capsule and retinaculum was required. These are sutured to the palmar capsule. a, proximal retinaculum; b, distal retinaculum; c, DRUJ capsule.

painful and/or restricted forearm rotation. In the absence of sty-locarpal impingement, this is usually the result of inadequate bony resection. Computed tomography obtained in full prona-tion/supination can be helpful in this regard. Another potential complication involves painful instability of the remaining distal ulna. Because of the lack of the "ulnar seat," some degree of insta-bility is inevitable. Most often, however, this does not result in significant symptoms.

Results

In carefully selected cases, the anticipated results are generally good to excellent. Some patients continue to experience mild pain, particularly with heavy use, but most can expect clinical improve-ment within 3 to 6 months. As with most DRUJ salvage proce-dures, a return to heavy labor is not anticipated. In patients with significant ongoing symptoms after an appropriate HIT proce-dure, a DRUJ prosthesis can be utilized with success.

ACKNOWLEDGMENT
The author wishes to thank William H. Bowers, M.D., for providing some of the photos used in this manuscript.

REFERENCES

1. Bowers WH: Distal radioulnar joint arthroplasty: the hemiresection-interposition technique. J Hand Surg [Am]. 1985; 10:169-178.

2. Sauvé L, Kapandji M: Nouvelle technique de traitment chirur-gical des luxations récidivantes isolées de l'extrémité inférieure du cubitus. J Chir (Paris). 1936; 47:589-594.

3. Watson HK, Gabuzda GM: Matched distal ulnar resection for posttraumatic disorders of the distal radioulnar joint. J Hand Surg [Am]. 1992; 17:724-730.

4. Darrach W: Anterior dislocation of the head of the ulna. Ann Surg. 1912; 56:802-803.

5. Van Schooven J, Fernandez DL, Bowers WH, Herbert TJ: Salvage of failed resection arthroplasties of the distal radioul-nar joint using a new ulnar head prosthesis. J Hand Surg [Am]. 2000; 25:438-446.

6. Van Schoohoven J, Kall S, Schober F, et al: The hemiresection-interposition arthroplasty as a salvage procedure for the arthrotically destroyed distal radioulnar joint. Handchir Microchir Plast Chir. 2003; 35:175-180.

7. Bowers WH: Distal radioulnar joint arthroplasty: current concepts. Clin Orthop Relat Res. 1992; 275:104-109.

8. Fernandez DL: Radial osteotomy and Bowers arthroplasty for malunited fractures of the distal end of the radius. J Bone Joint Surg Am. 1988; 70:1538-1551.

9. Tomaino MM: The importance of the pronated grip x-ray. J Hand Surg [Am]. 2000; 25:352-357.

Ulnar Head Implants: Unconstrained

36

Jörg Van Schoonhoven, MD, PhD

The ulnar head is the keystone for mobility and stability of the ulnar-sided wrist as well as the forearm. It not only is one of the joint partners creating the distal radioulnar joint (DRUJ) but also represents an integral part of the wrist joint. Biomechanically, it represents the only fixed, nonmoving anatomical structure at the wrist level. It, therefore, supplies the bony support around which the radius with the wrist and hand rotates in the DRUJ. Arthrotic destruction of the DRUJ will lead to painful limitation of forearm rotation and reduction of grip strength and therefore compromise hand function. Arthrotic derangement may be the result of intra-articular fractures of the DRUJ either with direct damage of the cartilage of the ulnar head or the sigmoid notch in comminuted fractures or secondary destruction due to intra-articular malunion of the joint line. However, the most common origin consists of the malunited extra-articular distal radius fracture. The dorsal or palmar angulation of the distal radial fragment with loss of the physiological ulnar inclination and shortening of the radius will lead to incongruity of the DRUJ and over time result in arthrotic derangement of this joint. I, therefore, consider the malunited extra-articular distal radius fracture a prearthrotic deformity of the DRUJ.[1]

Several salvage procedures have been described to reduce the pain and restore forearm rotation in patients with symptomatic DRUJ destruction, including ulnar head resection[2-4] and the hemi-resection interposition technique.[5] Partial loss of the ulnar head sacrifices the attachment of the palmar ulnocarpal ligaments and the force transfer from the radius onto the ulnar head. Loss of the ligament attachment will result in a palmar drop of the ulnar-sided wrist with a supination deformity of the hand and a dorsally prominent distal end of the ulna. In a way this is comparable to the well-described caput ulnae deformity in rheumatoid patients. The deformity does not truly represent an "instability of the distal end of the ulna" but an instability of the ulnar-sided wrist. Loss of the bony support of the radius in the DRUJ leads to radioulnar narrowing or impingement during forearm rotation and wrist loading and can radiologically be demonstrated on the transverse loading stress views described by Lees and Scheker (**Fig. 36-1**).[6]

A completely different concept to treat the painfully destroyed DRUJ consisting of fusion of the DRUJ and segment resection proximal to the ulnar head to restore forearm rotation was described by Sauvé and Kapandji in 1936.[7] With this procedure the supination deformity and the instability at the DRUJ level is prevented as the attachments of the ulnopalmar ligaments and the triangular fibrocartilage complex (TFCC) remain. However, in pronation underloading of the hand the dynamic dorsal stabilizers of the radius and the wrist may not be sufficient to prevent palmar drop of the wrist and hand in relation to the distal end of the ulna,

therefore leading again to a dorsally prominent distal ulnar stump. Furthermore, on transverse loading of the hand there is no anatomical structure to prevent the radius to fall onto the distal end of the ulna, resulting in radioulnar impingement (**Fig. 36-2**).[8,9]

The concept to prevent development of this instability using an ulnar head spacer in rheumatoid patients was first described by Swanson.[10] This is no longer recommended because of the high failure rate of the Silastic spacer material and secondary Silastic-induced synovitis.[11-15]

To overcome the secondary "painful instability of the distal ulna," several stabilizing soft tissue procedures using part of the flexor and/or the extensor carpi ulnaris tendon have been described. None of these procedures was found to reliably restore the stability or reduce symptoms in biomechanical[16] or clinical[17,18] studies. Wide resection of the ulna[19] as well as lengthening procedures after excessive shortening of the ulna[20] have been advocated but did not resolve the symptoms in my own or other surgeons' experience.[17] Considering the biomechanical and clinical shortcomings of the above-described resection procedures, Herbert developed the concept of restoring stability to the DRUJ as well as the wrist joint and the continuity of the ulna by means of an ulnar head prosthesis.

Based on the results of anatomical, radiological, and biomechanical studies of the distal ulna, the ulnar head, and the DRUJ between 1992 and 1994, Timothy Herbert developed together with me a two-component modular system for ulnar head replacement in cooperation with Martin-Medizin-Technik (Tuttlingen, Germany). It consists of three sizes of replacement heads and three stem sizes. To restore an adequate length of the ulna after a previous resection arthroplasty, each stem size of the prosthesis is provided with three collar lengths. To avoid the problems associated with cement, particularly in small bones, we decided to use a noncemented stem, allowing osseous integration. Porous-coated titanium was chosen because of its biocompatibility and a modulus of elasticity very similar to that of bone. The head of the prosthesis is composed of ceramic (zirconium oxide) because it was believed to be the most suitable material for articulation with joint cartilage due to its biocompatibility.

Following the development of the prosthesis a three-phase clinical study design was developed. Initially, three patients with painful instability of the wrist and forearm after resection arthroplasty were treated in 1995 with promising early results.[21] The second phase consisted of a prospective multicenter study limited to another 20 patients. Because of the excellent mid-term results of these patients,[22] the prosthesis was released to other surgeons. The third phase consisted of the evaluation of the long-term results, and all patients with a follow-up of more than 5 years are currently under review.

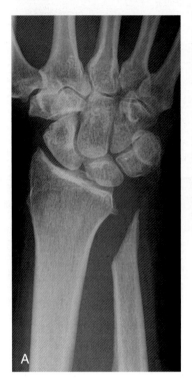

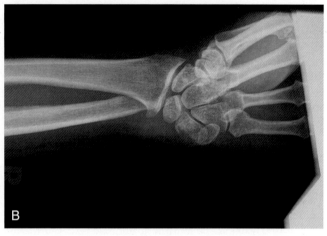

FIGURE 36-1 **A,** Posteroanterior radiograph after hemi-resection inter-position arthroplasty of the DRUJ. **B,** Transverse loading view demonstrating radioulnar impingement.

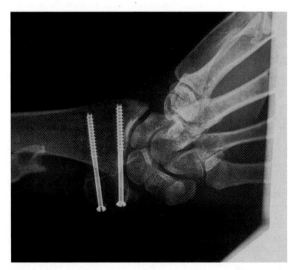

FIGURE 36-2 Radioulnar impingement after a Sauvé-Kapandji procedure.

Indications

Before further outlining the indications for the ulnar head prosthesis, it is important to emphasize that no implant will ever function as well as the original ulnar head. Therefore, ulnar head excision is only justified if the joint surface of the DRUJ is irreversibly destroyed. In any other pathological process of the DRUJ every attempt must be made to restore the DRUJ and therefore prevent the possible development of arthrotic joint destruction.

Originally the procedure was developed to solve the unsolvable and to overcome the problems associated with painful instability of the wrist and forearm after previous resection arthroplasties of

the DRUJ. Increasing experience with this procedure and the lasting excellent results over the past 12 years have led us to extend the indication to other pathological processes. As clinical experience demonstrated that stability of the forearm can be restored with this prosthesis, the indications were extended to primarily use the ulnar head replacement in patients with painful osteoarthritis of the DRUJ.

Post-traumatic Osteoarthrosis of the DRUJ

Distal forearm fractures are the most common cause of problems at the DRUJ. Arthroplasty should be considered only if forearm rotation remains painful after the corrective osteotomy or if there is evidence of irreversible joint damage of the DRUJ at the time of the osteotomy. Anatomical alignment of the radius and the ulna is a prerequisite for ulnar head replacement. Any significant radial deformity represents a contraindication for this procedure. In particular, any malunion of the radial or ulnar shaft must be corrected either before or at the time of ulnar head replacement. Mild deformities of the radial metaphysis (10 degrees of dorsal angulation) may be accepted but any more significant or a palmar malangulation of the radial metaphysis requires correction to allow reconstruction of the DRUJ with the ulnar head prosthesis. In patients with significant painful arthrosis of both the radiocarpal and distal radioulnar joints, partial (i.e., radioscapholunate) or complete fusion of the radiocarpal joint and ulnar head replacement may be performed at the same time.

Other Indications

In *acute trauma*, primary ulnar head replacement may be considered in cases with irreducible, comminuted fractures of the ulnar head requiring ulnar head excision.

Primary osteoarthrosis of the DRUJ is a rare condition but represents an ideal indication for ulnar head replacement because

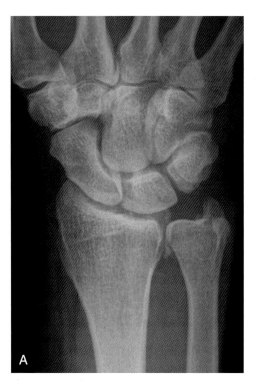 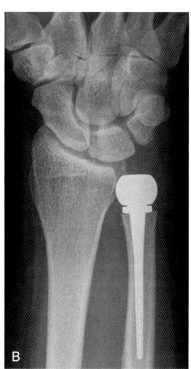

FIGURE 36-3 A, Radiograph of a 55-year-old patient with painful arthrosis of the DRUJ. **B,** Radiograph 46 months after primary ulnar head replacement.

there is no additional DRUJ pathological process that must be addressed at the time of surgery. It frequently affects middle-aged active patients who expect normal performance of the wrist and hand in their professional and private life (**Fig. 36-3**). The same applies for patients with a *giant cell tumor of the ulnar head* requiring ulnar head resection.

The DRUJ is frequently affected in patients with *rheumatoid arthritis*. I consider ulnar head replacement only in the younger and active rheumatoid patient with the arthrotic or ankylotic type of rheumatoid arthritis, minimal other joint involvement, a stable DRUJ, and a sufficient antirheumatoid medication. Hemiresection arthroplasty of the DRUJ still represents the best treatment option for the majority of rheumatoid patients because either the insufficient stabilizing soft tissues or the osteoporosis will not allow prosthetic ulnar head replacement, and the patients' reduced activity level will most probably not lead to symptoms arising from any instability after this procedure.

Another major indication for ulnar head replacement is as a *revision procedure* in patients with painful instability of the wrist and forearm after previous resection arthroplasties (hemiresection or complete resection of the ulnar head) or a Sauvé-Kapandji procedure. The long-term experience with this difficult group of patients has proved that reconstruction of the DRUJ using the ulnar head prosthesis is an effective method to cure the problem. However, revision surgery is often difficult and less predictable than when the operation is carried out as a primary procedure. In patients with painful instability after a Sauvé-Kapandji procedure two options for reconstruction are available. Resection of the fusion mass and insertion of the prosthesis is recommended if either the fusion has not healed completely or the original fusion has been performed in an ulnar-positive variance situation leading to additional symptoms of ulna impaction syndrome. In all other cases a spherical head, designed by Fernandez and colleagues,[23] may be used to articulate within the previously fused ulnar head after reaming of a socket into the proximal fusion mass.

Age of the patient as such does not affect my decision for the procedure. In particular, young and active patients with a high demand on the performance of their hand and wrist will most likely develop a symptomatic instability after one of the salvage procedures and therefore benefit from primary reconstruction of the DRUJ using the ulnar head prosthesis. Older patients in their retirement frequently have the same expectations for their private and sport activities. Salvage procedures should therefore be reserved for patients with low functional demands, in whom instability is unlikely to become symptomatic.

Contraindications

Ulnar head replacement is contraindicated in marked osteoporosis or cystic bone disease and whenever the bone quality is inadequate to allow osseous integration of the stem of the prosthesis.

Insufficient soft tissues may result in instability of the DRUJ after reconstruction. Therefore, ulnar head replacement is contraindicated in the majority of rheumatoid patients. It may be contraindicated in patients with severe ligamentous laxity or if several operations have been performed previously. In these patients it has to remain an intraoperative decision of the surgeon, and the patient has to be informed before the surgery that the procedure may not be possible.

Persisting instability or dislocation of the DRUJ after an Essex-Lopresti injury or previous radial head excision is a contraindication for ulnar head replacement because in my experience the distal local soft tissue flap is not suitable to resist the forces in these longitudinal instabilities of the forearm and will lead to recurrence of instability or dislocation at the DRUJ.

DRUJ reconstruction should not be carried out unless any deformity of the radius or ulna has been corrected. This may be performed either before or simultaneously with the ulnar head replacement.

Surgical Technique

Preoperative preparation includes radiographs of the wrist in two planes. In revision surgery, radiographs of the opposite wrist are required to determine the individual ulnar variance. In patients with a history of radial or ulnar shaft fractures or elbow involvement, radiographs of both forearms are required to assess the longitudinal alignment of both forearm bones and to decide whether additional corrective osteotomies are necessary.

Radiographic templates are used to plan the appropriate resection level and implant.

The operation is carried out with the patient in a supine position on the operating table and under tourniquet control. The arm is resting in full pronation on a side table. An image intensifier is required to control the resection level of the ulna, the positioning of the prosthesis, and the ulnar variance at the wrist level during the procedure. Small joint power equipment is required for the procedure.

Primary Ulnar Head Replacement

A slightly curved longitudinal incision is placed directly over the DRUJ and the fifth extensor compartment. The skin flaps are raised off the extensor retinaculum. The sensory dorsal branches of the ulnar nerve are identified and protected throughout the procedure. The fifth and sixth extensor compartments are identified, and the fifth extensor compartment is longitudinally opened along the length of the incision. The extensor digiti minimi (EDM) tendon is mobilized and retracted radially, exposing the dorsal capsule of the DRUJ.

An ulnar-based capsuloretinacular flap is outlined and raised as previously described.[21,22,24] It includes the extensor retinaculum, the dorsal capsule of the DRUJ, and the sixth extensor compartment, including the extensor carpi ulnaris tendon. The incision is placed along the floor of the fifth extensor compartment and extends from the dorsal shaft of the ulna proximally to the dorsal ulnocarpal joint distally. The dorsal rim of the TFCC is identified, and the flap is carefully raised in one layer along the dorsal radioulnar ligament toward the ulnar styloid process, completely exposing the ulnar head proximally and the ulnocarpal joint distally. The floor of the sixth extensor compartment should be kept intact or repaired to protect the tendon from direct contact with the prosthesis.

At this stage the bone quality and the soft tissue flap are checked. Additionally, the joint surfaces of the DRUJ are inspected to confirm the diagnosis of osteoarthritis and to make the final decision on ulnar head replacement (**Fig. 36-4**).

The hook of the resection guide is now engaged over the distal end of the radius and the resection level, as preoperatively determined using the radiographic template, is marked on the neck of the ulna (**Fig. 36-5**). With a small power saw the osteotomy is performed perpendicular to the long axis of the ulna.

The ulnar head is now grasped with the bone holder and in a combination of blunt and sharp dissection freed from all the connecting tissues. By rotating the ulnar head the underside of the TFCC is exposed and subperiosteally detached from its insertion on the ulnar head. If there is a united fracture of the ulnar styloid, this should be removed.

After removal of the ulnar head the distal ulna is lifted dorsally using the special soft tissue retractor provided. The medullary canal of the ulnar shaft is opened using the broach and then reamed to the appropriate diameter with the hand reamer according to the preoperatively determined size (**Fig. 36-6**). The reamer

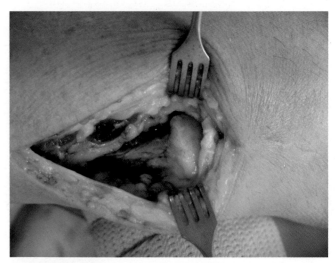

FIGURE 36-4 Arthritically destroyed cartilage of the ulnar head.

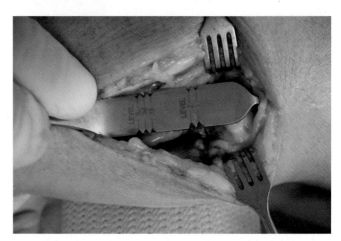

FIGURE 36-5 Determination of the level of the ulnar osteotomy.

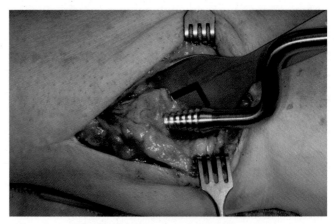

FIGURE 36-6 Reaming of the ulnar shaft.

should completely fit into the medullary canal to allow later insertion of the shaft of the prosthesis.

After inspection, the sigmoid notch is cleared of any scar tissue or osteophytes. In rare cases it may be appropriate to deepen the sigmoid notch using a small power bur. Care should be taken not to open the medullary cavity of the radius.

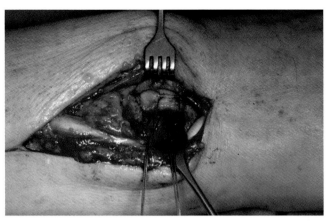

FIGURE 36-7 Transosseous sutures through the dorsal rim of the sigmoid notch for reattachment of the soft tissue flap.

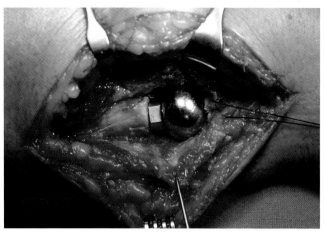

FIGURE 36-8 Insertion of the trial prosthesis and suture for reattachment of the dorsal radioulnar ligament under the soft tissue flap.

Two drill holes are now placed through the dorsal rim of the sigmoid notch, and strong nonabsorbable sutures are passed to allow later reattachment of the flap (Fig. 36-7).

The inner side of the soft tissue "cap" is now inspected. The roof of this cap consists of the TFCC. Any tear should be closed using fine, nonabsorbable sutures. Should there be a major deficiency or tear of the TFCC, this is repaired by means of either a local flap raised from the palmar capsule or from the extensor retinaculum. The floor of the extensor carpi ulnaris tendon sheath is once again inspected. Any tears that occurred during the bone preparation are sutured. Two fine, nonabsorbable sutures are placed through the dorsal rim of the TFCC, allowing later reattachment to the underside of the flap.

The appropriate trial prosthesis is now inserted and reduced into the sigmoid notch (Fig. 36-8). Seating of the head of the prosthesis within the sigmoid notch as well as the tension of the TFCC over the head in full pronation is now examined. The elbow is now flexed into a 90-degree position, and the position of the prosthesis as well as the ulnar variance is checked using the image intensifier. Radiologically, ulnar variance should measure −1 to −2 mm at the wrist level in neutral forearm rotation. If necessary, the trial prosthesis should be removed and a more proximal resection of the ulna is performed. In case of a too-proximal resection of the ulna with excessive ulnar-negative variance, this can be corrected by reverting to a stem with a built-up collar.

The soft tissue flap is now manually advanced over the head of the prosthesis and held down to the dorsal rim of the sigmoid notch. Forearm rotation and stability of the DRUJ are assessed. If the flap is too tight to be attached to the dorsal rim of the sigmoid notch or limits forearm rotation, one should either change to a smaller head size or release the flap. In the case of undue laxity of the flap not allowing stabilization of the DRUJ, a larger head size should be chosen. In these cases ulnar variance has to be reconfirmed radiologically because the larger head will increase the length of the ulna and may require further shortening of the ulna.

After the final determination of the appropriate size of the shaft and head, the arm is rested on the side table again. The definitive prosthesis is implanted using the impactor. The collar of the shaft should completely sit on the distal ulna. Undue forces to implant the shaft should be avoided. If there is any difficulty during implantation, removal of the shaft and further reaming is advised.

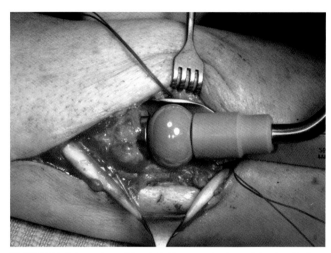

FIGURE 36-9 Insertion of the definitive prosthesis and the head of the prosthesis on the cone of the shaft.

The cone end of the shaft is now cleaned to ensure a good interference fit between the two components; then the head is impacted onto the stem (Fig. 36-9).

The elbow is again flexed into a 90-degree position with the forearm elevated and in 30 degrees of supination. The dorsal rim of the TFCC is reattached to the underside of the flap using the previously placed sutures. The flap is advanced and reattached under the appropriate tension to the radius using the transosseous sutures (Fig. 36-10). The repair is completed by suturing the remainder of the flap to the ulnar rim of the extensor retinaculum of the fourth extensor compartment, leaving the EDM tendon subcutaneous.

Before insertion of a suction drain and wound closure the stability of the DRUJ and the forearm rotation are assessed. Final radiographs and any necessary adjustments are performed.

Revision Surgery after Resection Arthroplasties

In this situation the operative technique is similar to that of a primary procedure with some exceptions.

In revision surgery, radiographs of both wrists have to be available. Analysis of the radiographs includes a determination of the

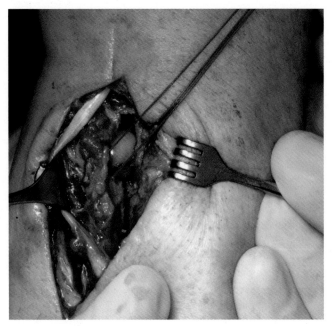

FIGURE 36-10 Reattachment of the soft tissue flap.

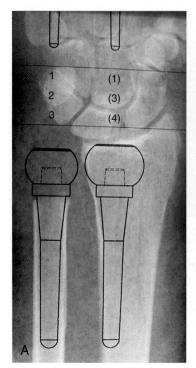
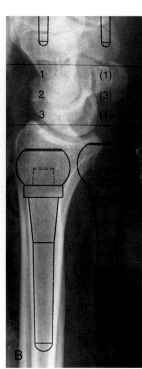

FIGURE 36-11 Radiographic templates for preoperative determination of the adequate type and size of the prosthesis.

individual ulnar variance at the wrist level and the amount of length of the distal ulna that has to be covered to create a new DRUJ. With the use of the radiographic templates, a decision needs to be made whether there remains sufficient ulnar length for a standard stem or whether a revision stem will be required (**Fig. 36-11**). In cases of excessive previous shortening of the ulna a custom-made prosthesis with additional length of the collar of the shaft of the prosthesis may be required.

Whenever possible, the skin incision is placed using the scar from previous surgery. The scar tissue from previous surgery makes definition and preparation of the stabilizing soft tissue flap more difficult than in primary surgery, and some of the scar tissue in the resection cavity has to be used to create a solid flap.

In cases in which a revision or custom-made prosthesis is required, the level of resection of the ulna is best determined by laying the trial prosthesis in the correct position alongside the ulna and then marking off the appropriate level for the osteotomy.

The sigmoid notch has to be completely cleared of any remaining scar tissue to allow a stable reduction.

The anatomical structures defining the flap have to be outlined. The TFCC frequently requires reconstruction.

Revision Surgery after Sauvé-Kapandji Procedures

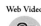
To resolve a painful instability after a Sauvé-Kapandji procedure two options are possible that must be decided on before surgery. Either the arthrodesis of the ulnar head is taken down and a prosthesis is used in a similar manner to that of revision surgery for failed resection arthroplasties or a bony ball-and-socket joint is created underneath the fused ulnar head using the prosthesis with a special spherical head as described by Fernandez and associates.[23]

Removal of the ulnar head is indicated in cases in which fusion of the DRUJ has been performed in an ulnar-positive variance situation, leading to additional symptoms of ulna impaction syn-

drome or if the fusion has not healed completely. In all of these cases a prosthesis with a revision shaft will be required because the previous resection level is far proximal to the neck of the ulnar head (**Fig. 36-12**). In some cases a custom-made shaft may be required to restore the length of the ulna, which must be determined before the surgery using the radiographic templates. The procedure is performed in a similar manner as that for revising a resection arthroplasty with the following exceptions.

Previous surgery is frequently performed using a lateral approach to the ulnar head. In these cases I do not use the scar from the previous surgery but tend to perform the revision using my standard dorsal approach. Creating the soft tissue flap is difficult, and strict subperiosteal dissection of all the soft tissues from the dorsal aspect of the fused ulnar head is advised before resection of the fused ulnar head is performed using small chisels. In cases in which complete fusion of the DRUJ had been achieved, a new sigmoid notch has to be created using small power burs. In cases with incomplete fusion, the sigmoid notch has to be cleared of all remaining osteophytes to create a smooth cavity for the head of the prosthesis. In most patients the TFCC has not been violated from the previous surgery but may be deficient from an ulnar impaction syndrome and require reconstruction.

If the ulnar head has been fused in an anatomical position, stability may be restored by creating a ball-and-socket joint under the fusion mass (**Fig. 36-13**). A longitudinal incision is placed dorsally over the ulnar head extending proximally to the dorsal aspect of the distal end of the ulnar shaft. The distal end of the ulna as well as the proximal end of the fusion mass is exposed. With the use of a special power reamer a spherical cavity is created underneath the proximal end of the fused ulnar head to later contain the spherical head of the prosthesis. Preparation of the ulnar shaft and determination of the appropriate-sized shaft of the prosthesis is performed in a similar fashion to that of a

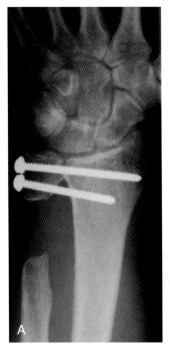
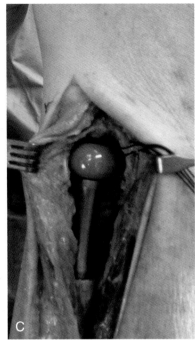
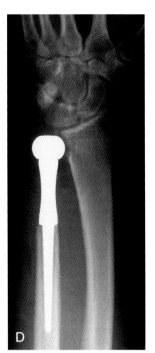
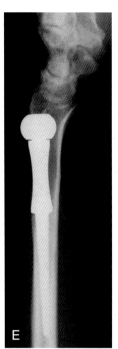
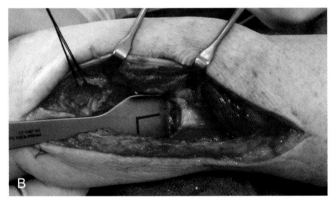

FIGURE 36-12 **A**, Posteroanterior radiograph of a 39-year-old patient with painful radioulnar impingement and symptoms of ulnar impaction syndrome after a Sauvé-Kapandji procedure. **B**, Intraoperative photograph after resection of the fused ulnar head, reaming of a new sigmoid fossa, and preparation of the ulnar shaft. **C**, After insertion of the revision stem of the ulnar head prosthesis. Posteroanterior (**D**) and lateral (**E**) radiographs of the same patient 3.6 years after reconstruction of the DRUJ with the ulnar head prosthesis.

primary procedure. Because in this procedure bony stabilization rather than soft tissue stabilization is the aim, the spherical cavity will have to cover at least one third of the spherical head of the prosthesis. After implantation of the shaft and impaction of the spherical head on the cone of the prosthesis, reduction of the head into the bony cavity may not be possible. Osteotomy of the radius with additional plate osteosynthesis may be needed after reduction of the prosthesis.

Rehabilitation

The wound and soft tissue repair should be protected from undue strain. Therefore, at the end of the operation an above-elbow plaster splint with the elbow in 70 degrees of flexion, the wrist in 20 degrees of extension, and the forearm in 40 degrees of supination is applied. Active mobilizing exercises for the fingers and the thumb are begun the first postoperative day. The suction drain is removed on the second day after surgery. After 2 weeks the suture material is removed and a forearm "gutter" splint is applied, allowing 40 degrees of pronation and supination. After 6 weeks, radiographs are obtained, the splint is removed, and active as well as passive mobilizing exercises are begun to achieve full forearm

rotation. Full unprotected work and activity is allowed after 12 weeks.

Depending on the stability that has been achieved at the end of the operation as well as the quality of the soft tissue repair, this rehabilitation program may be individually modified.

Complications

The following potential complications have been noticed and require particular attention. Most of these complications can be avoided and are due to either wrong patient selection, incorrect planning of the operation, faulty operative technique, or inadequate postoperative immobilization.

Recurrent Instability

The most common cause for this problem is an uncorrected radial deformity, in particular of the radial shaft. The soft tissue flap is not strong enough to overcome a dislocation of the DRUJ caused by a bony deformity.

Failure of the soft tissue flap is most commonly due to improper patient selection. Insufficient soft tissues due to rheumatoid patients or as a result of several previous procedures at the DRUJ

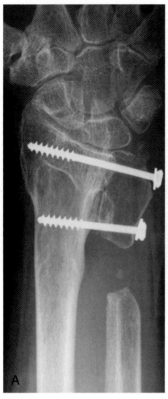
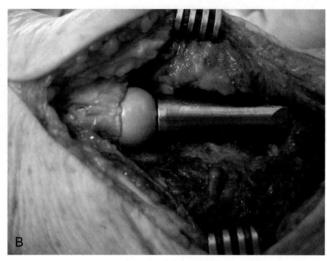
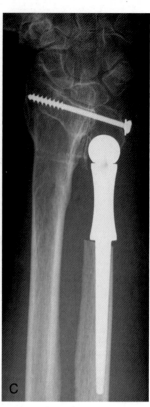

FIGURE 36-13 A, Posteroanterior radiograph of a 67-year-old patient with painful radioulnar impingement after a Sauvé-Kapandji procedure. **B,** Intraoperative demonstration after insertion of a revision stem of the prosthesis into the ulnar shaft and reposition of the spherical head of the prosthesis under the fusion mass by means of a ball-and-socket joint. **C,** Postoperative radiograph of the same patient 27 months after the stabilization using the ulnar head prosthesis.

represent a contraindication for the procedure. This may need to be determined intraoperatively and may necessitate abandoning the procedure. Choice of the correct-sized head of the prosthesis as well as thorough preparation and repair of the flap are crucial for the success of the operation.

Stem Loosening

This problem might occur in patients with severe osteoporosis, which prevents osseous integration of the shaft of the prosthesis.

Other causes include over-reaming of the stem during the operation or selection of an undersized stem that does not allow primary, press-fit stability of the stem in the ulnar shaft.

Secondary loosening of the stem of the prosthesis has been noticed in cases with persistent dislocation of the DRUJ owing to uncorrected radial deformities. This may be explained by the nonphysiological forces and stress applied on the prosthesis.

Ulnar Impaction Syndrome

This problem can always be avoided and is purely due to faulty operative technique. The aim of the procedure is to achieve a DRUJ with an ulnar-negative variance situation of 1 to 2 mm at the wrist level.

Prolonged Pain after the Procedure

Persistent pain for several months after the procedure has been noticed in patients where reaming of the sigmoid notch down to the subchondral bone had to be performed, in particular after a Sauvé-Kapandji procedure. It frequently correlates with radio-

logical signs of remodeling of the sigmoid notch. These symptoms may persist for several months but have always stopped once the bone remodeling process was finalized.

Results

After the development of this prosthesis I started to perform the previously described procedures in 1995. Initially, and until 1999, I only used the prosthesis as a revision procedure in patients with symptomatic instability after previous resection arthroplasties of the DRUJ. All these patients were followed up radiologically and clinically. The lasting and excellent results in this difficult group of patients, and therefore growing confidence in the performance of this prosthesis, led me to start using it as a primary procedure in the treatment of the destroyed DRUJ. My personal series consists of 76 patients whom I have treated with this method.

Clinical Results

At the last follow-up examination, 16 of my 76 patients had a follow-up period of more than 5 years with a mean of 95 (61 to 124) months. All of these patients had suffered from painful instability after a resection arthroplasty of the DRUJ (**Fig. 36-14A,B**). Overall function of their hands had significantly improved after reconstruction of the DRUJ, and all patients would have had the operation again. Twelve patients returned to their original profession, and 4 patients retired due to their age. With the use of a visual analog scale (from 0 to 10), pain was found to be remarkably reduced from a mean of 8.7 preoperatively to 2.0 at the latest follow-up. Preoperative grip strength averaged 42% compared with the contralateral side and increased to a mean

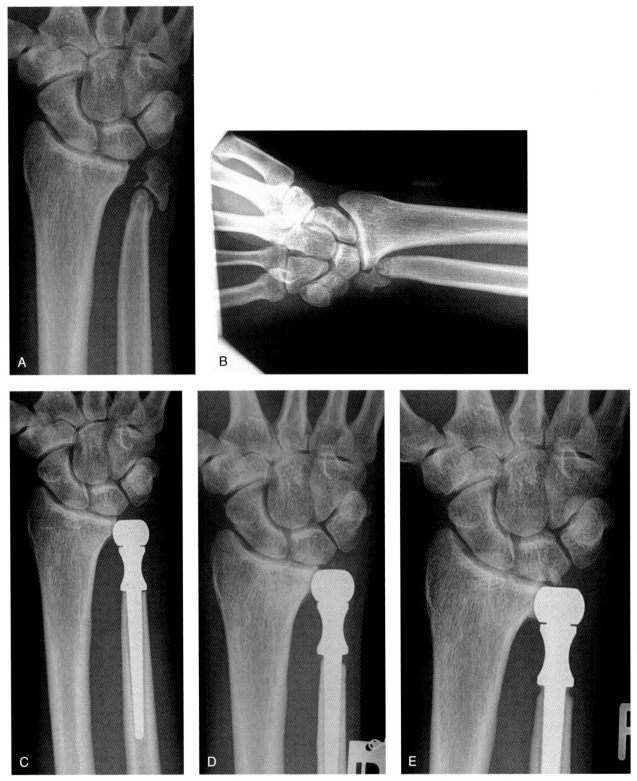

FIGURE 36-14 A, Posteroanterior radiograph of a 36-year-old patient 11 years after a hemi-resection interposition arthroplasty and secondary shortening of the distal ulna. **B,** Transverse loading view of the same patient demonstrating the painful radioulnar impingement. **C,** Posteroanterior view 6 weeks after DRUJ reconstruction. **D,** Posteroanterior radiograph 7 months after ulnar head replacement showing bone resorption of the distal ulna under the neck of the prosthesis as well as initial remodeling of the sigmoid notch toward the head of the prosthesis. **E,** Posteroanterior radiograph 6.3 years after the procedure demonstrating the final remodeling of the sigmoid notch as well as the new bone formation filling the gap under the neck of the prosthesis.

of 74%. Not only was forearm rotation found to be significantly improved after the procedure from a mean of 126 to 144 degrees, but overall wrist range of motion was found to have improved to a similar amount as well. Overall satisfaction with the outcome of the procedure was found to be very high, with a mean of 8.4 on a visual analog scale from 0 to 10.

Radiological Results

It is quite normal to find some early bone resorption at the distal end of the ulna under the collar of the prosthesis (see **Fig. 36-14C, D**). It averaged 2 mm and occurred in 6 of these 16 patients. In 4 patients the resorption area secondarily filled up with new bone over time (see **Fig. 36-14E**). Additionally, it is common to find some reactive bone remodeling at the sigmoid fossa, and I did notice this in 5 of the 16 patients. These bone reactions were harmless and were found to be completed in all patients after 12 to 18 months. Most importantly, there has been no sign of late loosening of the stem of the prosthesis but obvious osseous integration.

REFERENCES

1. Van Schoonhoven J, Prommersberger KJ, Lanz U: The importance of the distal radioulnar joint for reconstructive procedures in the malunited distal radius fracture. Orthopäde. 1999; 28:864-871.

2. Buck-Gramcko D: On the priorities of publications of some operative procedures on the distal end of the ulna. J Hand Surg [Br]. 1990; 15:416-420.

3. Schiltenwolf M, Martini AK, Bernd L, Lukoschek M: Ergebnisse nach Ellenköpfchenresektion. Z Orthop. 1992; 130:181-187.

4. Minami A, Ogino T, Minami M: Treatment of distal radio-ulnar disorders. J Hand Surg [Am]. 1987; 12:189-196.

5. Bowers WH: Distal radioulnar joint arthroplasty: the hemiresection-interposition technique. J Hand Surg [Am]. 1985;10:169-178.

6. Lees VC, Scheker LR: The radiological demonstration of dynamic ulnar impingement. J Hand Surg [Br]. 1997; 22:448-450.

7. Sauvé L, Kapandji M: Nouvelle technique de traitement chirurgical des luxations récidivantes isolées de l'extrémité inférieure du cubitus. J Chir. 1936; 47:589-594.

8. Minami A, Suzuki K, Suenaga N, Ishikawa J: The Sauvé-Kapandji procedure for osteoarthritis of the distal radioulnar joint. J Hand Surg [Am]. 1995; 20:602-608.

9. Carter PB, Stuart PR: The Sauvé-Kapandji procedure for post-traumatic disorders of the distal radio-ulnar joint. J Bone Joint Surg Br. 2000; 82:1013-1018.

10. Swanson AB: Implant arthroplasty for disabilities of the distal radioulnar joint: use of a silicone rubber capping implant following resection of the ulnar head. Orthop Clin North Am. 1973; 4:373-382.

11. Fatti JF, Palmer AK, Mosher JF: The long-term results of Swanson silicone rubber interpositional wrist arthroplasty. J Hand Surg [Am]. 1986; 11:166-175.

12. White RE: Resection of the distal ulna with and without implant arthroplasty in rheumatoid arthritis. J Hand Surg [Am]. 1986; 11:514-518.

13. McMurtry RY, Paley D, Marks P, Axelrod T: A critical analysis of Swanson ulnar head arthroplasty: rheumatoid versus nonrheumatoid. J Hand Surg [Am]. 1990; 15:224-231.

14. Stanley D, Herbert TJ: The Swanson ulnar head prosthesis for post-traumatic disorders of the distal radioulnar joint. J Hand Surg [Br]. 1992; 17:682-688.

15. Sagerman SD, Seiler JG, Fleming LL, Lockerman E: Silicone rubber distal ulnar replacement arthroplasty. J Hand Surg [Br]. 1992; 17:689-693.

16. Petersen MS, Adams BD: Biomechanical evaluation of distal radioulnar reconstructions. J Hand Surg [Am]. 1993; 18:328-334.

17. Bieber EJ, Linscheid RL, Dobyns JH, Beckenbaugh RD: Failed distal ulna resections. J Hand Surg [Am]. 1988; 13: 193-200.

18. Bowers WH: Instability of the distal radioulnar articulation. Hand Clin. 1991; 7:311-327.

19. Wolfe SW, Mih AD, Hotchkiss RN, et al: Wide excision of the distal ulna. J Hand Surg [Am]. 1998; 23:222-228.

20. Watson HK, Gabuzda GM: Matched distal ulna resection for posttraumatic disorders of the distal radioulnar joint. J Hand Surg [Am]. 1992; 17:724-730.

21. Van Schoonhoven J, Herbert TJ, Krimmer H: New concepts for distal radioulnar joint reconstruction using an ulnar head prosthesis. Handchir Mikrochir Plast Chir. 1998; 30:387-392.

22. Van Schoonhoven J, Fernandez DL, Bowers WH, Herbert TJ: Salvage of failed resection arthroplasties of the distal radioulnar joint using a new ulnar head prosthesis. J Hand Surg [Am]. 2000; 25:438-446.

23. Fernandez DL, Joneschild ES, Abella DM: Treatment of failed Sauvé-Kapandji procedures with a spherical ulnar head prosthesis. Clin Orthop Relat Res. 2006; 445:100-107.

24. Van Schoonhoven J, Herbert T: The dorsal approach to the distal radioulnar joint. Tech Hand Up Extrem Surg. 2004; 8:11-15.

Distal Radioulnar Joint Prosthesis

37

L. R. Scheker, MD and B. A. Babb

The forearm has two main forces acting on it: axial load and the force of gravity. Axial load can be represented by a multitude of tasks, including pushing and gripping. Most of the forearm's function can be separated into two components: gripping and load transfer. To grip, the extrinsic muscles of the hand contract, creating axial load passing from the carpus to the radius and to the humerus. Loads are transferred from the hand to the radius and, while supported by the ulna, on to the humerus. These two functions are completely different, and yet they combine to form the normal function of the forearm. The ulna, acting as the axis of the forearm, supports the radius through both flexion and extension of the elbow. The support provided by the ulna allows the radius to rotate in space as it transfers axial load to the humerus.[1,2]

The two bones of the forearm are connected through the radioulnar joint. This bicondylar joint is divided into two parts: the proximal radioulnar joint and the distal radioulnar joint. The focus of this chapter is injury sustained over the distal radioulnar joint (DRUJ). Other than trauma, dysfunction of the DRUJ can be the result of congenital abnormality, degenerative arthritis, inflammatory arthritis, and neoplasm. It must also be noted that excision of the radial head, which allows proximal migration of the radius, will affect the function of the DRUJ, eventually leading to its destruction. All these conditions can create mechanical derangement of the distal radioulnar articulation with serious effects on its biomechanical properties. The DRUJ is involved in approximately 30% of all the distal radius fractures and in all of the Essex-Lopresti and Galeazzi fractures. Distal radius fractures are common, accounting for 60% of all fractures treated in the emergency department.[3]

When anatomical structures of the DRUJ can be repaired to allow a stable, congruent joint, all efforts should be made to do so. In fractures, the malunion may be corrected[4,5] and, if necessary, the ulna may be shortened to change contact between the sigmoid notch and the seat of the ulna, which may help to correct some element of ulna impaction.[6] Post-traumatic and degenerative DRUJ arthritis, as well as some instances of instability with grinding,[7] may be corrected by shortening the ulna by 2.5 mm. The shortened ulna changes the point of contact between the radius and ulna head while also tensioning the triangular fibrocartilage (TFC), which improves stability. In cases of instability without grinding, reconstruction of the ligaments of the TFC may restore function of the DRUJ.[8]

Mechanical derangement of the distal radioulnar articulation has serious effects on its biomechanical properties. The etiological spectrum for this derangement can range from early arthritic erosion to the mutilation that accompanies resection of part or all of the distal ulna.[9] The latter situation, as encountered after Darrach, Watson, Bower, and Sauvé-Kapandji procedures, can lead to a condition known as "ulnar impingement." This condition

occurs because the now unsupported distal end of the radius falls against the adjacent ulnar shaft. It is important to note at this stage that the term "ulnar impingement" conjures up the picture of an ulna that moves and impinges against the radius, but, in reality, the contrary is true.[10]

The ulna is the support of the distal radius and, consequently, loss of this support results in the radius "dropping" and impinging on the distal end of the resected ulna. This is particularly enhanced during lifting of weight in the neutral position. The distal end of the radius rides on top of the head of the ulna while lifting objects with the forearm in the neutral position.[11-13]

Absence of an intact DRUJ, as occurs after any of the previously mentioned resection procedures, causes the radius to make contact with the distal end of the ulna and "hitch a ride" at this point. This impingement may not be evident on regular postero-anterior radiographs, because the forearm is not loaded in this position. A laterally shot posteroanterior view obtained when the person is holding a weight against gravity with the forearm in the neutral position characteristically brings out the impingement (**Fig. 37-1**). With this understanding of the anatomy of the ulna, it is not surprising that ulnar head replacements or hemi-arthroplasties are unable to provide an adequate transfer of force when the forearm is in the loaded position.

Rather than a partial replacement, a prosthesis that replaces the DRUJ must be able to fulfill the joint's functions of transmitting forces during lifting as well as permitting pronation/supination. The APTIS Distal Radioulnar Joint Total Replacement Prosthesis (APTIS Medical, Louisville, KY) has been designed with the specific intention of addressing the issues of transmission of lifting forces as well as permitting stable pronation/supination. This is accomplished by replacing the function of the sigmoid notch, the ulnar head, and the stabilizing characteristics of the TFC.

Indications

Physicians may consider the APTIS prosthesis for patients who experience pain and weakness at the DRUJ that is not improved by nonoperative treatment. Findings may include instability of the ulnar head and radiographic evidence of dislocation with erosive changes of the distal radioulnar joint. Nonreducible fracture of the ulnar head with loss of cartilage or neck fracture with loss of substance may be followed by primary replacement of the joint with the prosthesis. In past cases, the prosthesis has been used after failed ulnar head resection (e.g., the Darrach procedure) or after failed ulnar head arthroplasty.

Patient Selection

Ideal candidates are those individuals in whom the DRUJ cannot be reconstructed. Other requirements are good bone stock with

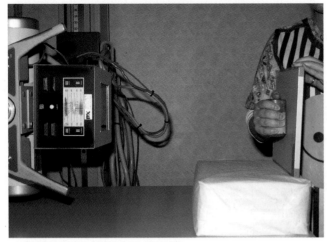

FIGURE 37-1 Method for weight-bearing radiography. The cassette is supported between the body and arm, and the patient does not have to squeeze the cassette. The beam is shot in a horizontal plane, while the patient bears weight.

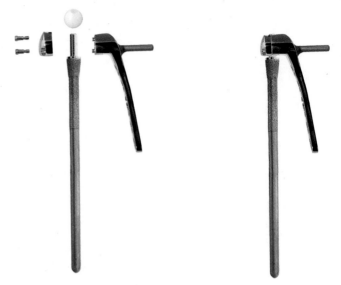

FIGURE 37-2 The components of the prosthesis: the radial plate, the radial plate cover, two screws, the ulnar stem, and the ultra-high-molecular-weight polyethylene (UHMWP) ball.

no history of infection in the area, no systemic disease, and no allergy to nickel. Patients may receive the prosthesis at any time after the skeleton is mature; the timing depends on the individual. In some cases, an individual may sustain a fracture that destroys the DRUJ and it is possible to do an immediate reconstruction. However, because it is not yet available in every institution, a delay may be required to obtain the prosthesis.

Contraindications

Severe osteoporosis, unresolved osteomyelitis, and systemic disease contraindicate the use of the prosthesis. The use of the implant also is contraindicated when bone, musculature, tendons, or adjacent soft tissue is compromised by disease or infection and would not provide adequate support or fixation for the prosthesis. The implant should not be used in patients who have not reached skeletal maturity.

Web Video ## Surgical Technique
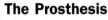
The Prosthesis
37-1

The DRUJ prosthesis is a semi-constrained ball-and-socket joint comprising a radial component and an ulnar component (**Fig. 37-2**).

The radial component (**Fig. 37-3**) provides the socket for the joint and consists of two parts that are assembled intraoperatively. The main part is shaped in the form of a plate with a hemi-socket on the distal end. The body of the plate, with its five screw holes, is contoured to fit against the distal 6 to 7 cm of the interosseous crest, in the area of the sigmoid notch. The plate is fixed to the radius by two means. The first is a peg that is driven into the distal radius in an ulnoradial direction, whereas the second method of fixing the plate involves the use of five specially designed 3.5-mm cortical screws. The hemi-socket, which is part of the plate, is directed ulnarward and is designed to receive the ultra-high-molecular-weight polyethylene ball (UHMWP) of the ulnar component. The other half of the socket, a cover, is separate from the radial component and is fixed to its counterpart on the plate by means of two screws. This assembly encloses the UHMWP ball. The radial component is available in two sizes, small (size

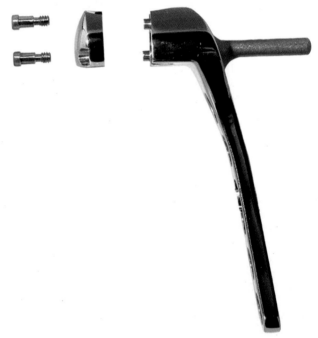

FIGURE 37-3 The radial component is assembled intraoperatively to provide a socket. It comprises a contoured plate, a cover, and two screws.

20) and large (size 30), which fit with the corresponding sizes of the ulnar component.

A fluted stem and the UHMWP ball (**Fig. 37-4**) make up the ulnar component. The ball is placed on the distal end of the stem; this combination replaces the articular surface of the ulnar head. The ulnar stems measure 11 cm in interosseous length, and the distal one third is plasma coated to allow bony ingrowth. A gentle flare at its distal end is present to provide better fixation. The stem is also fluted and slightly tapered to provide rotatory stability and ease of insertion, respectively. The most distal end of the stem bears a highly polished peg or pivot that fits into the hole of the

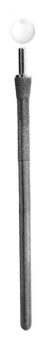

FIGURE 37-4 The ulnar component comprises a fluted stem and an ultra-high-molecular-weight polyethylene (UHMWP) ball.

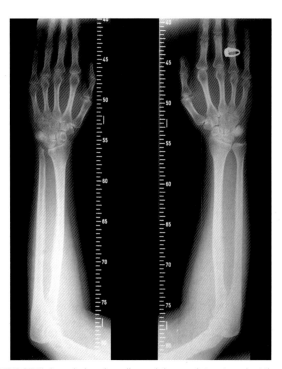

FIGURE 37-5 A graded-scale radiograph is mandatory to select the size of the implant, notably the thickness and length of the ulnar stem. Digital radiographs with a means of measure can also be used.

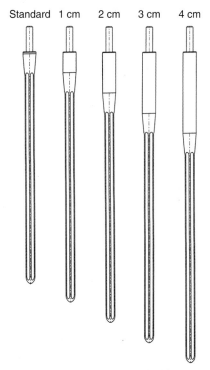

FIGURE 37-6 An ulnar stem template used with graded-scale radiographs determines stem diameter and length. Lengths vary from standard to 4 cm extended.

UHMWP ball. The stems are provided in two diameters, 4.5 mm and 5.0 mm, and have correspondingly sized UHMWP balls. Each size couples with the small and large radial components, respectively.

Preoperative graded radiographs are used to determine whether the large or small prosthesis is most likely needed (**Fig. 37-5**). Digital radiographs can be used if they have accurate measuring capability. The ulna stem size is determined by measuring the narrowest intramedullary diameter of the ulna in its distal 11 cm. A size is chosen that fits this intramedullary diameter best, leaving behind a minimum of 2 mm of cortical bone surrounding the flare of the distal stem. The length of the stem's extraosseous neck, if one is needed, can also be determined preoperatively with the help of a radiographic measuring template (**Fig. 37-6**).

Patient Positioning and Preparation

The procedure can generally be accomplished under axillary block using the standard methods of prepping and draping for the upper extremity. Steri-Drape Wound Edge Protector (3M, St. Paul, MN) is recommended to reduce contact between the skin and the implant. A tourniquet is always used with a pressure setting of about 250 mm Hg (approximately 100 mm Hg above the patient's systolic pressure).

Incision Placement and Dissection

The forearm is placed in full pronation and a 9- to 10-cm hockey stick incision is made above the dorsal lateral aspect of the distal ulna, turning radially just distal to the head of the ulna (**Fig. 37-7**). Dissection can then either follow the interval between the extensor digiti quinti minimi and extensor carpi ulnaris or the interval between the flexor and extensor carpi ulnaris for added protection of the dorsal sensory branch of the ulnar nerve. If the patient has had surgery in the area, the old incision may be incorporated into the exposure. Taking care to protect the dorsal sensory branch of the ulnar nerve, the incision is then carefully

deepened. A fascial/retinacular flap can be created to later provide a barrier between the prosthesis and tendons (**Fig. 37-8**). The extensor carpi ulnaris tendon sheath is then released from the ulnar head to the insertion of the extensor carpi ulnaris. When approaching the ulna between the extensor carpi ulnaris and the

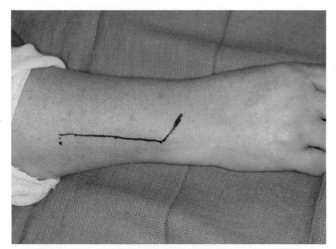

FIGURE 37-7 A hockey-stick incision is placed on the dorsum of the hand between the extensor carpi ulnaris and the extensor digiti quinti minimi.

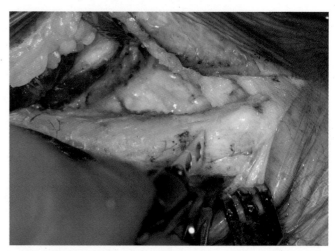

FIGURE 37-9 The head of the ulna is removed just proximal to the distal radioulnar joint, which allows the ulna to be displaced volarly.

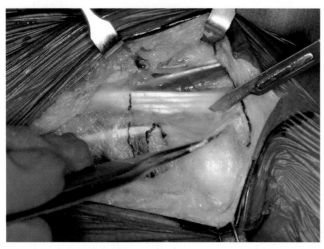

FIGURE 37-8 A dorsal fascial flap is elevated to interpose between the prosthesis and the extensor tendons.

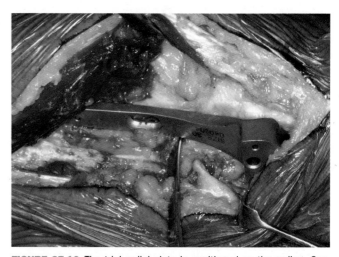

FIGURE 37-10 The trial radial plate is positioned on the radius. Contouring of the radius, if necessary, can be performed with a bur.

extensor digiti quinti, the extensor digiti quinti is elevated from the ulna and interosseous membrane. The extensor mass is also elevated to expose the interosseous crest of the radius.

If present, the head of the ulna is then excised at a level just proximal to the head (**Fig. 37-9**). The radial attachment of the TFC, if found intact, is left undisturbed. If left in situ, this structure can provide a buffering barrier between the prosthesis and the carpus. Excising the ulnar head eases exposure of the radius by allowing the ulnar shaft to be retracted volarward.

Any osteophytes found in the DRUJ are now excised. The dissection then follows dorsally over the ulna, exposing the dorsal surface of the interosseous membrane. The interosseous membrane is elevated 8 to 9 cm from the distal radius along its interosseous crest.

The trial radial plate is then placed over the interosseous surface of the radius. The distal end of the trial plate should be in the area of the sigmoid notch, with the volar edge of the body of the plate aligned with the volar edge of the radius (**Fig. 37-10**). In cases with radial deformity or a prominent volar lip, a bur can be used to contour the radius for better trial positioning. A minimum of 3 mm is required to separate the distal end of the trial plate and the radiocarpal joint. This space is needed to

prevent carpal impingement during ulnar deviation. Proximal positioning is limited by radial width because the radial plate peg is designed to remain within the radius. The volar-facing edge of the trial plate should be on the same plane as the volar surface of the radius. Positioning of the trial plate should also ensure that the plate is not tilted dorsalward or volarward.

Temporary fixation of the trial plate can be accomplished by using 0.045-inch Kirschner wires (K-wires). Both posteroanterior and lateral positioning is confirmed with an image intensifier (**Fig. 37-11**). After position confirmation, a 2.5-mm drill bit with the provided guide is used to drill a transverse hole through the sliding guide hole of the trial plate (**Fig. 37-12**). A depth gauge is used to measure the length of the screws and a 3.5-mm tap is used. None of the screws should more than pierce the outer cortex to prevent possible radial nerve irritation. The oval hole allows for final positioning adjustments, if necessary.

Positioning of the trial plate is again checked and adjustments made if needed. Once the final position is confirmed, the distal K-wire is removed and, using power, the radial peg drill bit is passed through the center distal guide hole of the trial plate. This creates a hole that will accommodate the radial peg portion of the prosthesis (**Fig. 37-13**).

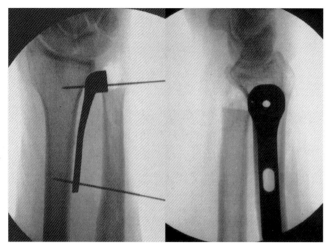

FIGURE 37-11 With an image intensifier, the position of the trial radial plate is evaluated in posteroanterior and lateral views, with carpal clearance and lateral alignment confirmed, respectively.

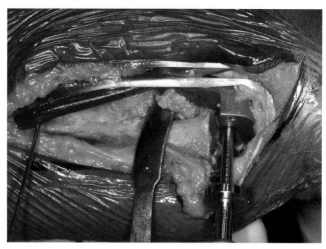

FIGURE 37-13 A dedicated drill bit is used to drill for the radial peg. A stopping plate prevents penetration through the radius.

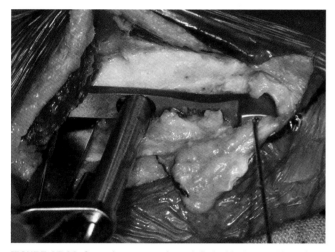

FIGURE 37-12 Once the surgeon is satisfied with the position of the trial radial plate, a 3.5-mm screw is placed in the oval hole. The oval or sliding hole allows final positioning adjustments.

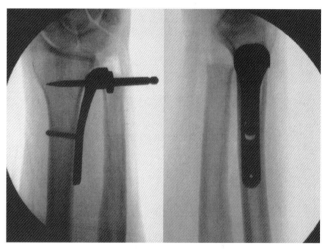

FIGURE 37-14 Image intensifier posteroanterior and lateral views are required before accepting final position of the plate.

Adequacy of the final position of the trial component is then confirmed (**Fig. 37-14**). Once satisfied, the trial component is removed and replaced with the radial plate component. Care should be taken to avoid interposition of soft tissue between the plate and the bone. A plastic impactor is provided to protect the face of the plate while using a mallet, if needed, for the radial peg's insertion (**Fig. 37-15**). Next, the 3.5-mm screw that was used in the trial plate's oval hole will be applied to the radial plate's oval hole. Up to four additional 3.5-mm screws can be used to complete fixation.

It is prudent to keep the most distal screw short to prevent it from potentially impinging against the transverse peg. For this purpose, an 18-mm screw is recommended for use in all cases. Once all screws have been inserted, their length is verified before approaching the ulna (**Fig. 37-16**).

Resection of the Distal Ulna

With the forearm fully pronated, a specially designed measuring device is inserted along the ulna and into the hemi-socket of the radial component. The device employs correspondingly sized,

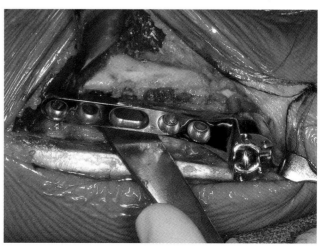

FIGURE 37-15 The permanent plate replaces the trial plate.

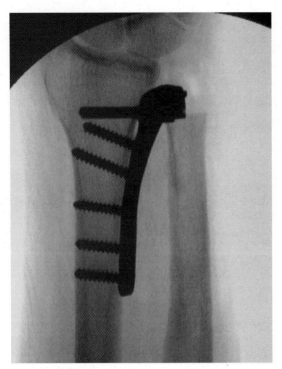

FIGURE 37-16 Radial plate fixation is confirmed noting screw length; avoiding excessive length will prevent radial nerve irritation.

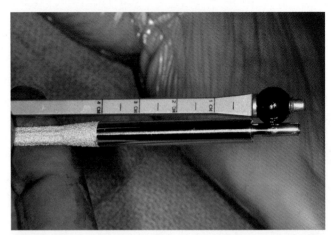

FIGURE 37-18 As an example, the measuring device is placed next to a 4-cm extended ulnar stem. Note the polished extraosseous portion of the stem.

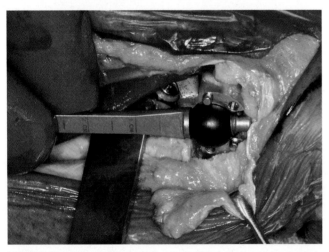

FIGURE 37-17 A measuring device marked in increments is placed in the radial plate socket to determine the proper length of the ulna before the final resection is made.

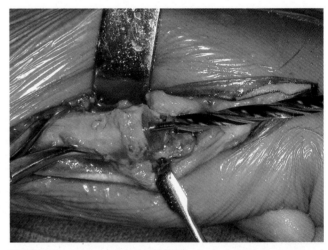

FIGURE 37-19 A cannulated drill bit following a guidewire is introduced 11 cm inside the ulna.

removable balls (black for small and blue for large) and enables the surgeon to assess the exact amount of ulnar shaft to be resected. Ulnar resection should be performed through good bone stock. With the measuring device in place, the proximal edge of the metal lip below the ball indicates the appropriate resection level for a standard-length ulnar stem (**Fig. 37-17**). Once assembled, 1 mm of tolerance should be evident between the ball and the base of the ulnar stem. An extended stem with a suitably lengthened extraosseous neck can then be used when too much bone has been lost due to injury or previous surgery (**Fig. 37-18**).

For cases with additional ulnar loss (e.g., after trauma or after Darrach or Sauvé-Kapandji procedures), the measuring device is marked in 1-cm increments. This allows the selection of an appropriate length of extended stem (see Fig. 37-18). If the ulnar length falls between marks, it will be resected to the next closest proximal mark. This length should be determined preoperatively using the template.

After the appropriate length of the distal ulna has been resected, a 0.062-inch guidewire is inserted into its medullary canal to act as a centralizing guide. Travel of the guidewire should be confirmed with an image intensifier. A cannulated drill bit (either small or large) is then inserted over the guidewire and the medullary canal drilled to a marked length of 11 cm (**Fig. 37-19**).

Next, the medullary reamer of corresponding size (20 or 30) is inserted into the canal and drilled down until its shoulder comes into contact with the distal end of the ulnar shaft (**Fig. 37-20**). This completes preparation of the ulnar shaft.

The medullary canal and surrounding soft tissue is profusely and thoroughly irrigated using gravity irrigation. Next, the ulnar stem component is introduced. A plastic impactor is used to protect the polished distal peg of the ulnar stem (**Fig. 37-21**). If all procedures have been followed, the standard-length stem

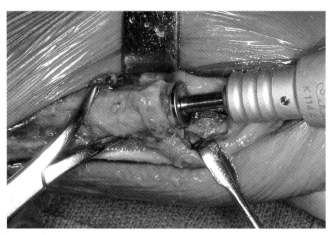

FIGURE 37-20 A reamer is introduced into the ulna until its shoulder reaches the distal end.

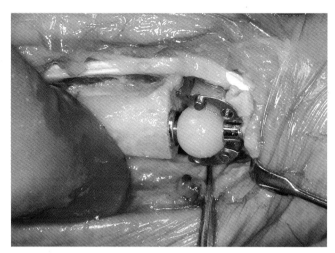

FIGURE 37-22 The UHMWP ball is placed on the ulnar stem and into the radial socket.

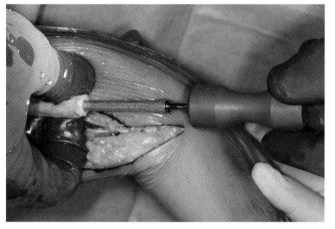

FIGURE 37-21 The ulnar stem is introduced into the ulna, and a plastic impactor is used to protect the stem when using a mallet.

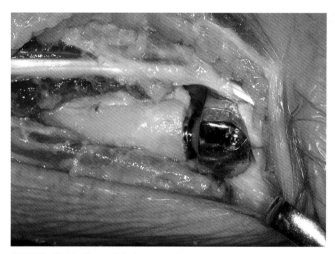

FIGURE 37-23 The radial plate cover is secured in place, and assembly is completed.

should be impacted flush with the distal end of the ulna shaft. When an extended stem is indicated, it is impacted until the plasma coating is within the ulna. In cases in which more ulna is resected than intended, care should be taken not to overinsert the selected stem. Leaving a portion of the plasma coating proud of the distal ulna is an option. When in its final position, the distal end of the stem should be no more proximal than the distal end of the radial plate.

The ulnar component is completed by placing the UHMWP ball over the distal peg of the ulnar stem. This combination replaces the function of the ulna head. The ball and stem are then positioned within the hemi-socket of the radial component, effectively replacing the two articular surfaces of the DRUJ (**Fig. 37-22**).

Finally, the cover is positioned over the radial socket and secured with the two screws provided (**Fig. 37-23**). This encapsulates the UHMWP ball, which recreates the stabilizing effects of an intact TFC and completes the prosthesis.

An image intensifier is once again used to confirm adequacy of the overall position of the completed prosthesis (**Fig. 37-24**). The forearm is moved through a full range of pronation/supination, ensuring free movement. If full motion is not evident, check for any contact of the ulna with the radial plate. If necessary, the ulna can be trimmed to allow full motion. It may also be necessary

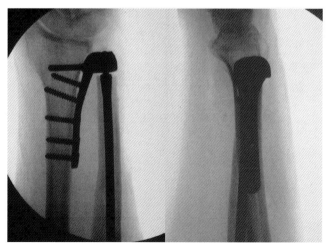

FIGURE 37-24 Final posteroanterior and lateral views before closure.

to release more of the interosseous membrane if it is causing restriction of motion.

The fascial/retinacular flap is now used to cover the prosthesis and create a barrier for the tendons (**Fig. 37-25**). The tourniquet is released, complete hemostasis is secured, and the wound is closed in a layered fashion. The skin is closed with interrupted sutures. It is recommended that a prophylactic antibiotic be used for approximately 5 days.

A bulky soft tissue dressing is applied with the forearm in neutral position. Immediate limited motion can begin according to patient tolerance. The dressing remains in position for 2 weeks, at which time the sutures are removed and full range of motion exercises are encouraged. Therapy is initiated, if necessary, with active range of motion. Without the possibility of dislocation, patients can both move through a full range of motion and bear weight (**Fig. 37-26**).

Practical Tips

+ Always ensure proper placement of the radial plate. A bur can be used to help seat the plate by reducing the prominence of the volar lip of the sigmoid notch.
+ Never overinsert the ulnar stem. The distal end of the stem should be no more proximal than the distal end of the radial plate.
+ Always plan a barrier flap to be positioned between the radial plate and the extensor carpi ulnaris.

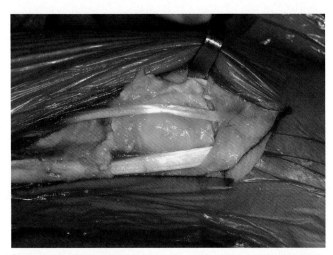

FIGURE 37-25 The fascial flap is positioned between the extensor tendons and the implant.

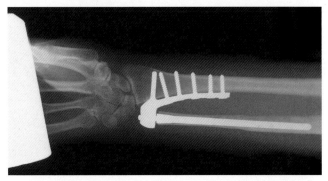

FIGURE 37-26 Radiograph of a patient demonstrating lifting against gravity after placement of the prosthesis.

+ Release the extensor carpi ulnaris sheath to its distal insertion.
+ Irrigate the entire wound profusely before closure to lessen the possibility of heterotopic bone formation.
+ Use bulky soft tissue dressing and allow the patient to move as much as tolerated early. Once the dressing is fully removed, full range of motion should be initiated with weight bearing as tolerated.

Potential Pitfalls

The use of unscaled radiographs for templating can cause an improper size selection. This would be evident in either the medullary canal being too small or too large for the selected ulnar stem. If too small, the ulna could be severely damaged. If too large, the ulnar stem would not seat well and the additional play may cause loosening. Selection of the appropriate radial plate is also important. If the plate is too large its peg may pass through the radius, causing radial nerve irritation, and/or its width could place it more dorsally than desired, causing potential tendon wear.

If the stem is overinserted, its press-fit design will prevent it from being retracted from the ulna. Leaving the stem proximal will leave the ball partially unsupported, resulting in excessive wear. If left too proximal, the stem may dislocate from the ball/plate interface. If necessary, the radial plate can be moved proximally to meet the stem.

Allowing direct tendon contact with the plate by not creating a barrier flap or releasing the extensor carpi ulnaris sheath could lead to excessive tendon wear.

Fixation screw protrusion through the radius may cause radial nerve irritation.

Controversies

The use of the tourniquet may lead to hematoma if the tourniquet is not released before the wound is closed. It is necessary to obtain careful hemostasis.

Complications

In two known cases, infection resulted in the removal of the prosthesis. In one case, antibiotic beads were placed at the site and a new prosthesis was applied 6 months later. Motor vehicle accidents caused the ulnar stems to break in two cases. In both cases, the stems were replaced and the patients regained function and continue unremarkably. In two cases, heterotopic bone led to a restriction in motion. Both cases were treated with excision through irrigation and immediate range of motion. No recurrence has been evident. Osteophyte formation and tendinitis have been seen when a fascial flap has not been placed between the extensor carpi ulnaris and the prosthesis.

Results

The need for a device to completely replace function of the DRUJ became evident as patient after patient entered the clinic after multiple DRUJ reconstruction and salvage procedures. These patients were at a loss after experiencing an average of 5.5 surgical procedures in an attempt to relieve their pain and instability. Some of the patients with unreconstructable DRUJs had undergone nearly all the described soft tissue, resection, stabilization, and implant arthroplasties combined, none of which provided long-term stability and pain relief. The device described in this

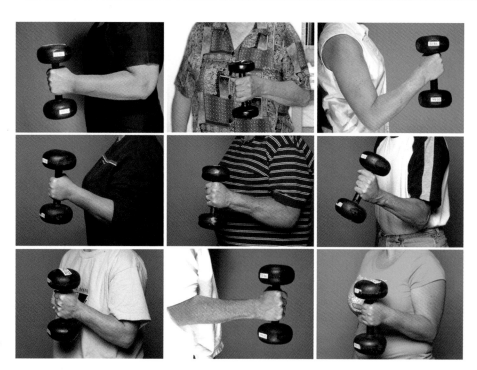

FIGURE 37-27 Various patients demonstrate the ability to bear weight.

chapter was developed as an answer for these patients. It is the only device that replaces the function of three parts of the DRUJ. By replacing the function of the ulnar head, the sigmoid notch, and the TFC, all factors in the joint that could cause instability and pain are eliminated. Preoperatively and postoperatively, the patients were asked to demonstrate not only range of motion but also function, including grip strength and weight-bearing ability. To our knowledge, no current published studies using any other technique test for a patient's functional ability to bear weight or even measure grip strength (**Fig. 37-27**). All patients receiving the total DRUJ demonstrated acceptable range of motion (**Fig. 37-28**) and, more importantly, increased pain-free functional abilities. This improvement included increased grip strength and weight bearing. The goal is not only to relieve pain but also to allow persons with a previously destroyed DRUJ to become once again a functional asset to themselves and society.

If all else, including soft tissue techniques and ulnar shortening, fails, rather than a partial replacement (i.e., replacement of the ulnar head), a total DRUJ replacement like the one presented here is necessary because it will reproduce the function of the sigmoid notch, the ulnar head, and the TFC. We have had experience with over 200 patients who had deranged distal radioulnar joints as a consequence of trauma, congenital abnormality, degenerative arthritis, inflammatory arthritis, and, most frequently, after ulnar head resection had been performed and failed. It has been shown that excision of the head of the ulna leads to impingement and pain with supination and lifting.[10] The majority of these patients have had between 2 and 14 procedures on the DRUJ, from partial excision of the DRUJ to wide excision of the ulna, passing through all the techniques of soft tissue stabilization available. Once the total replacement has taken place, the patient has been able to stop taking prescription pain medications and return to a productive life. More than 10 centers have had experience with this device with similar results to ours.

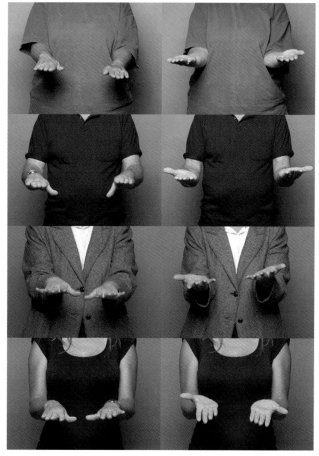

FIGURE 37-28 Various patients demonstrate range of motion, pronation, and supination.

REFERENCES

1. Hagert CG: The distal radioulnar joint. Hand Clin. 1987; 3:41-50.

2. Hagert CG: The distal radioulnar joint in relation to the whole forearm. Clin Orthop Relat Res. 1992; 275:56-64.

3. Ark J, Jupiter JB: The rationale for precise management of distal radius fractures. Orthop Clin North Am. 1993; 24:205-210.

4. Wagner H: Proceedings: Corrective surgery after lesions of the distal end of the radius (author's transl). Langenbecks Arch Chir. 1973; 334:211-219. German.

5. Viegas SF: A new modification of corrective osteotomy for treatment of distal radius malunion. Tech Hand Upper Extremity Surg 2006; 10:224-230.

6. Rayhack JM: Ulnar shortening. Tech Hand Upper Extremity Surg 2003; 7:52-60.

7. Scheker LR, Severo A: Ulnar shortening for the treatment of early post-traumatic osteoarthritis at the distal radioulnar joint. J Hand Surg [Br]. 2001; 26:41-44.

8. Scheker LR, Belliappa PP, Acosta R, German DS: Reconstruction of the dorsal ligament of the triangular fibrocartilage complex. J Hand Surg [Br]. 1994; 19:310-318.

9. Bieber EJ, Linscheid RL, Dobyns JH, Beckenbaugh RD: Failed distal ulna resections. J Hand Surg [Am]. 1988; 13: 193-200.

10. Lees VC, Scheker LR: The radiological demonstration of dynamic ulnar impingement. J Hand Surg [Br]. 1997; 22: 448-450.

11. Shaaban H, Giakas G, Bolton M, et al: The distal radioulnar joint as a load-bearing mechanism—a biomechanical study. J Hand Surg [Am]. 2004; 29:85-95.

12. Shaaban H, Giakas G, Bolton M, et al: The load-bearing characteristics of the forearm: pattern of axial and bending force transmitted through ulna and radius. J Hand Surg [Br]. 2006; 31:274-279.

13. Shaaban H, Giakas G, Bolton M, et al: Contact area inside the distal radioulnar joint: Effect of axial loading and position of the forearm. Clin Biomech 2007; 22:313-318.

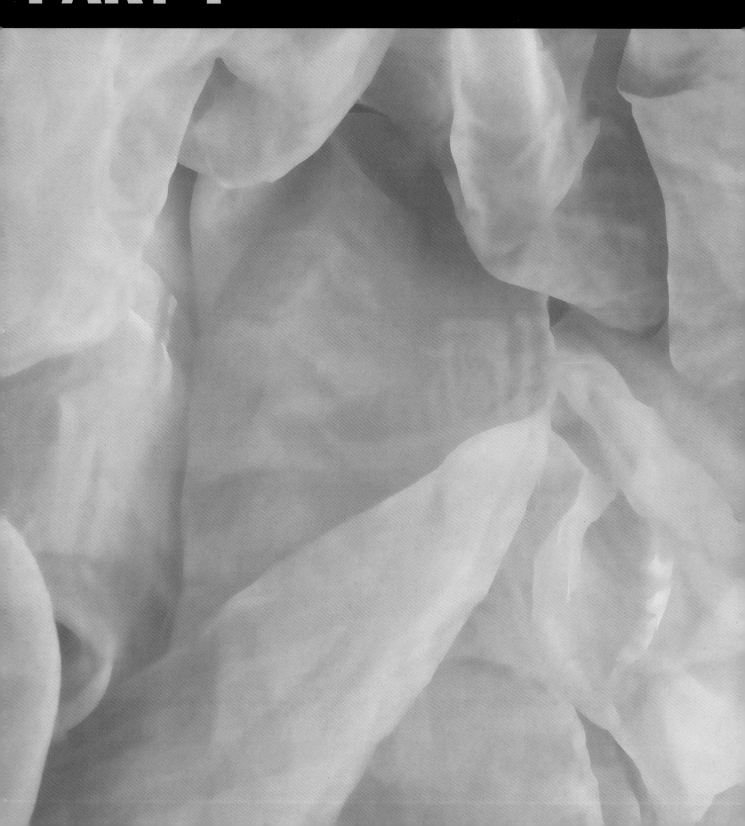

PART 7 CARPAL LIGAMENT INJURY

Carpal Anatomy

Jennifer Moriatis Wolf, MD and Alexander Y. Shin, MD

38

Historical Background

The bones that make up the carpal wrist have names with ancient origins. The name of the scaphoid is derived from the Greek word *scaphe*, which means "boat" or "trough."[1] The lunate was previously named the semilunar due to its resemblance to the moon, and the translation of lunate is "crescent shaped." The capitate is also known as the os magnum because it is the largest bone in the carpus. Finally, the pisiform translates to "pea," which matches the size and shape of this bone.

Much of the modern original work in the anatomy of the wrist was performed by Landsmeer, whose painstaking dissection was the basis for the names of many wrist ligaments. Landsmeer published his atlas of hand anatomy[2] and coauthored a landmark paper with Berger describing the extrinsic ligament anatomy of the carpus.[3]

Osseous Anatomy

The wrist is the link between the forearm and the hand. The carpus is made up of 15 bones excluding the sesamoids and supernumerary bones (**Fig. 38-1**). These include the distal radius and ulna, the two rows of the carpus, and the bases of the five metacarpals. The carpal rows are divided into the proximal and distal carpal rows. In the proximal carpal row are found the scaphoid, lunate, triquetrum, and pisiform. The pisiform articulates only with the triquetrum, because it lies volar to it and is enveloped by the flexor carpi ulnaris tendon except on its deep surface (**Fig. 38-2**). The pisiform is considered by many to be a sesamoid bone but provides an important lever arm for the flexor carpi ulnaris tendon. The trapezium, trapezoid, capitate, and hamate make up the distal carpal row from radial to ulnar in the wrist. The hook of the hamate extends volarly 1 to 2 cm radial and distal to the pisiform and serves as the attachment site for several ligaments.[1] The five metacarpal bases articulate with this row of carpal bones.

The carpus includes three specific joint types: the radiocarpal joint, the midcarpal joint, and the carpometacarpal joints. The radiocarpal joint is composed of the distal articular surface of the radius in addition to the triangular fibrocartilage complex. The distal radius has two articular facets, named after the carpal bone they contact—the scaphoid and lunate facets, respectively.[4] The facets on the radius are divided by the interfossal ridge, which is often a raised portion of the radius but can also have a fibrous ridge to it. The distal radius and triangular fibrocartilage complex articulate as a whole with the proximal carpal row, which forms a convex articular facet.

The midcarpal joint contains three articulations. On the radial side is the scaphotrapezial-trapezoid joint; centrally the scaphoid and lunate articulate with the capitate; and ulnarly the hamate and triquetrum form a helicoid joint.

The carpometacarpal joints vary widely in their degree of stability. The base of the first metacarpal and trapezium comprise a unique "saddle" joint that has a remarkable degree of motion due to the anatomy of these bones. In comparison, the index and middle carpometacarpal joints are tightly interlocked with little motion due to their tight capsular and ligamentous structure. The ring and small carpometacarpal articulation is less restrained, with a greater degree of motion.

Finally, the distal radioulnar joint forms a separate and distinct joint through the sigmoid notch of the radius into which fits the distal ulna. The radius rotates around the stable ulna with supination and pronation.

Ligamentous Anatomy

All of the ligaments of the wrist are intracapsular with the exception of three ligaments: the transverse carpal ligament, or flexor retinaculum, the pisohamate ligament, and the pisometacarpal ligament. Nearly all the wrist ligaments are contained within capsular sheaths of loose connective tissue and fat. This often makes it difficult to visualize individual ligaments when approaching the carpal joints surgically. From within the joints, the ligaments can be viewed as distinct structures, best seen during wrist arthroscopy or visualizing the volar ligaments via a dorsal approach between the carpal bones.[5,6]

Web Video

38-1

There are two general categories of ligaments: intrinsic and extrinsic. Intrinsic ligaments have their origin and insertions within the carpus, with a large area of insertion onto cartilage rather than bone and much less elastic fibers compared with extrinsic ligaments. These ligaments tend to avulse from insertion or origin rather than rupture in mid substance. The extrinsic ligaments of the wrist form connections between the forearm and the carpus. These ligaments are stiffer with lower ultimate yield compared with intrinsic ligaments.

Extrinsic Carpal Ligaments

The extrinsic ligaments of the carpus provide support and form the linkage between the long bones of the forearm and the eight carpal bones. The volar extrinsic ligaments form an inverted "V"-shaped configuration and are best visualized during wrist arthroscopy. In fact, visualization of the ligaments from outside the wrist joint is nearly impossible as the capsule of the wrist blends the extrinsic ligaments together. These ligaments include the radioscaphocapitate, long radiolunate, radioscapholunate, and short radiolunate ligaments on the radial carpus. The ulnolunate, ulnolunocapitate, and ulnotriquetrocapitate ligaments form the volar ulnar ligamentous complex (**Fig. 38-3**).

On the radial side of the wrist, the radioscaphocapitate ligament originates in a broad sheet from the tip of the radial styloid to the midscaphoid fossa and inserts on the distal scaphoid pole, acting as a support to the waist of the scaphoid. The next ulnar

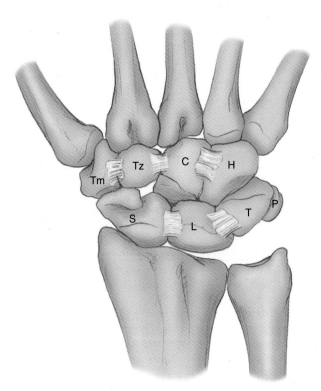

FIGURE 38-1 Osseous anatomy of the carpus. The carpus is made up of 15 bones excluding the sesamoids and supernumerary bones. Tm, trapezium; Tz, trapezoid; C, capitate; H, hamate; S, scaphoid; L, lunate; T, triquetrum; and P, pisiform. *(Courtesy of Mayo Foundation.)*

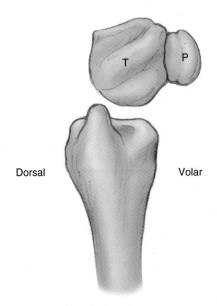

FIGURE 38-2 The pisiform (P) articulates only with the triquetrum (T), because it lies volar to it and is enveloped by the flexor carpi ulnaris tendon except on its deep surface. *(Courtesy of Mayo Foundation.)*

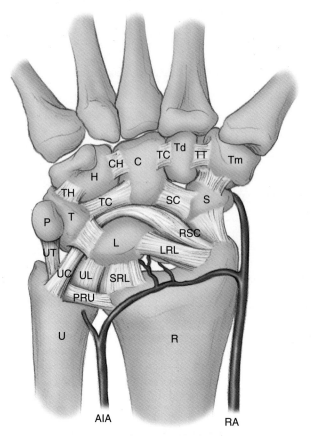

FIGURE 38-3 The extrinsic carpal ligaments include the radioscaphocapitate (RSC), long radiolunate (LRL), radioscapholunate, and short radiolunate (SRL) ligaments on the radial carpus. The ulnolunate (UL), ulnolunocapitate (UC), and ulnotriquetrocapitate (UT) ligaments form the volar ulnar ligamentous complex. *(Courtesy of Mayo Foundation.)*

ligament is the long radiolunate ligament, which originates from the remaining portion of the scaphoid fossa of the radius and attaches to the radial volar aspect of the lunate.[3] Abutting the long radiolunate ligament is the radioscapholunate ligament (or ligament of Testut), which is not actually a true ligament but is rather a capsular tissue through which course blood vessels, including terminal branches of the anterior interosseous artery.[7] This structure goes through the volar capsule and attaches dorsally into the scapholunate interosseous ligament. Finally, the short radiolunate ligament has its origin from the lunate fossa and inserts onto the radial side of the lunate (**Fig. 38-4**).[8]

The ulnocarpal complex includes the most superficially located ulnocapitate ligament, which originates from the ulnar fovea, passing volarly to support the lunotriqetral interosseous ligament, and inserts partially onto the capitate and mostly blends into the radioscaphocapitate ligament. The ulnolunate and ulnotriquetral ligaments are interdigitated proximally as they originate from the palmar radioulnar ligament and then split to attach distally to the lunate and triquetrum, respectively.[8]

Based on the definition of extrinsic ligaments connecting to bones outside the carpus, there is a single dorsal extrinsic ligament, the dorsal radiocarpal or radiotriquetral ligament. The dorsal intercarpal ligament, which lies at the same level but connects the scaphoid, trapezium, and trapezoid to the triquetrum, is often classified as an extrinsic ligament. This ligament complex, which forms a lateral "V" shape, has been shown to indirectly stabilize the scaphoid dorsally during wrist range of motion (**Fig. 38-5**).[9]

The distal radioulnar joint ligaments provide important stability to this construct. The triangular fibrocartilage complex includes the dorsal and palmar radioulnar ligaments (**Fig. 38-6**). The dorsal

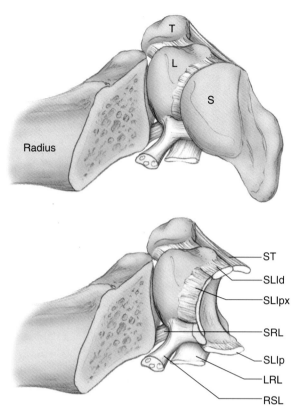

FIGURE 38-4 View of the volar radiocarpal ligaments from within the wrist. S, scaphoid; L, lunate; T, triquetrum; ST, scaphotriquetral ligament; SLId, dorsal portion of scapholunate ligament; SLIpx, palmar and intermediate portion of scapholunate ligament; SLIp, palmar segment of scapholunate ligament; RSL, radioscapholunate ligament (ligament of Testut); LRL, long radiolunate ligament; SRL, short radiolunate ligament. *(Courtesy of Mayo Foundation.)*

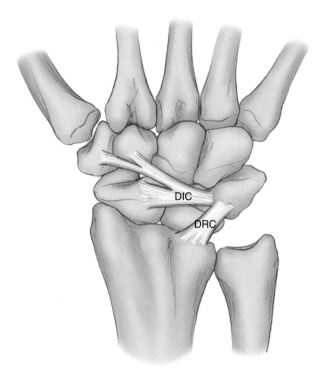

FIGURE 38-5 The dorsal radiocarpal (DRC) and dorsal intercarpal (DIC) ligament complex. This ligament complex, which forms a lateral V shape, has been shown to indirectly stabilize the scaphoid dorsally during wrist range of motion. These ligaments form the interval through which a ligament-sparing capsulotomy is performed. *(Courtesy of Mayo Foundation.)*

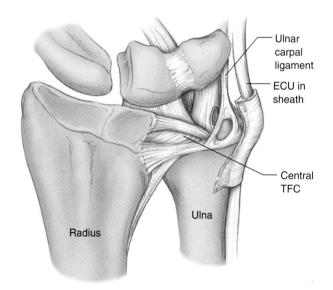

FIGURE 38-6 The triangular fibrocartilage complex includes the TFC disc, the extensor carpi ulnaris (ECU) subsheath, the ulnocarpal ligaments, and the volar and dorsal radioulnar ligaments. *(Courtesy of Mayo Foundation.)*

radioulnar ligament originates at the dorsal rim of the radius at the sigmoid notch and inserts into the ulnar fovea and ulnar styloid. This ligament also contributes fibers to the subsheath of the extensor carpi ulnaris through a separate extension of its most superficial portion. The palmar radioulnar ligament has a volar origin, also at the level of the sigmoid notch of the radius. This ligament also inserts onto the ulnar styloid and fovea, and its fibers blend with those of the dorsal radioulnar ligament at that level. The superficial portion of the palmar radioulnar ligament then forms the ulnolunate and ulnotriquetral ligaments, with the fibers angulating distally. At the level of the ulnar styloid is found the ligamentum subcruentum, defined by Henle as the loose vascular tissue surrounding the volar prestyloid recess.[10] On the dorsal side of the wrist, proximal to the dorsal radioulnar ligament, is found a metaphyseally based ligament that courses distally to interdigitate with the dorsal radioulnar ligament. This is the dorsal radial metaphyseal arcuate ligament,[11] which also contributes to the extensor carpi ulnaris subsheath (see Fig. 38-6).

Intrinsic Carpal Ligaments

In the proximal carpal row, the intrinsic ligaments include the scapholunate interosseous ligament (SLIL) and lunotriquetral interosseous ligament (LTIL) (**Fig. 38-7**). Each of these ligaments is divided histologically into different segments: the dorsal, volar, and proximal portions. In the SLIL, studies have shown that the dorsal region is the thickest and strongest, with the

palmar segment being thin and obliquely oriented. The proximal segment is made up of fibrocartilage, with no collagen fibers. The LTIL, in contrast, is thickest volarly and interdigitates with fibers of the ulnocapitate ligament as it passes volarly over the LTIL. The dorsal region is thin and the proximal portion is, like the SLIL, made up of fibrocartilage.[11]

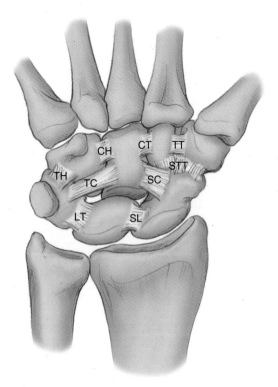

FIGURE 38-7 The intrinsic carpal ligaments. TH, triquetrohamate ligament; CH, capitohamate ligament; CT, capitotrapezoid ligament; TT, trapeziotrapezoid ligament; STT, scaphotrapeziotrapezoid ligament; SC, scaphocapitate ligament; SL, scapholunate ligament; LT, lunotriquetral ligament; and TC, triquetrocapitate ligament. (Courtesy of Mayo Foundation.)

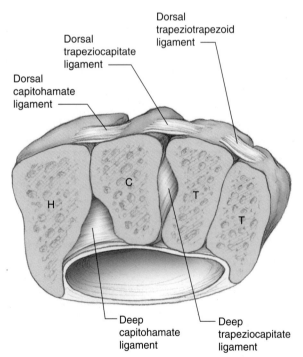

FIGURE 38-8 The intercarpal ligaments of the distal carpal row include the dorsal, palmar, and deep portions of the trapeziotrapezoid, trapeziocapitate, and capitohamate ligaments. (Courtesy of Mayo Foundation.)

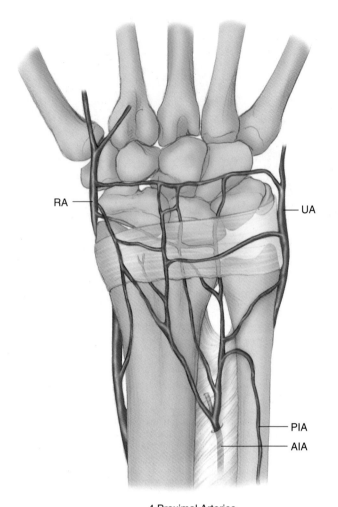

4 Proximal Arteries

FIGURE 38-9 Four extraosseous vessels contribute nutrient vessels to the distal radius and ulna. RA, radial artery; AIA, anterior interosseous artery; PIA, posterior interosseous artery; UA, ulnar artery. (Courtesy of Mayo Foundation.)

In the distal carpal row, the trapeziotrapezoid, trapeziocapitate, and capitohamate ligaments comprise the intrinsic ligaments. Again, each ligament is made up of a dorsal and volar region. The trapeziotrapezoid ligament covers the entire length of the respective carpal bones. In contrast, the trapeziocapitate and capitohamate ligaments insert on the body of the capitate because of the need for proximal extension of the capitate head and neck. A thick deep trapeziocapitate ligament courses at an angle through a notch between the trapezoid and capitate. Similarly, the capitohamate ligament has a deep component that is quite thick and strong, lying within a depression at the volar distal edge of the capitate and hamate articulation. It also extends to the third and fourth metacarpal bases (**Fig. 38-8**).[8]

Between the two rows course the palmar midcarpal ligaments, running from the scaphoid and triquetrum to the bones of the distal carpal row (see **Fig. 38-7**). The arcuate ligament forms the central third of the palmar midcarpal capsule and is composed of the blended fibers of the radioscaphocapitate and ulnocapitate ligaments. These form an important support to the head of the capitate. On the radial side of the midcarpal joint, the scaphotrapeziotrapezoid ligament attaches to the radial and ulnar sides of

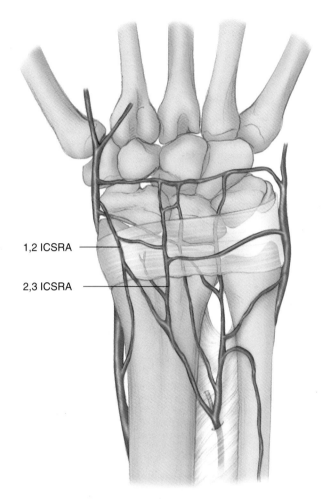

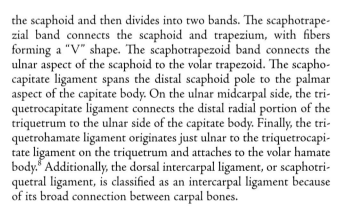

2 Superficial Arteries

FIGURE 38-10 There are two consistent intercompartmental vessels that lie superficial to the retinaculum and are described as supraretinacular. These two vessels, the 1,2 and 2,3 intercompartmental supraretinacular arteries (1,2 and 2,3 ICSRA), are located on the retinaculum between their named compartments. *(Courtesy of Mayo Foundation.)*

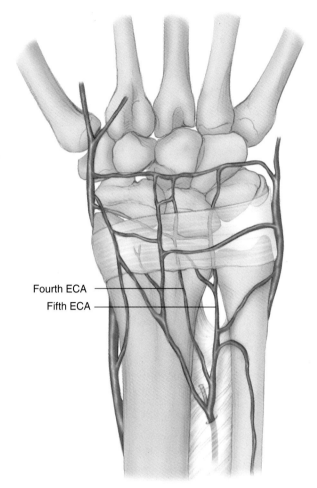

2 Deep Arteries

FIGURE 38-11 Two consistent vessels are found in the fourth and fifth compartments. They lie on the surface of the radius in the floor of the fourth and fifth extensor compartments and are named the fourth and fifth extensor compartment arteries (Fourth and Fifth ECA). *(Courtesy of Mayo Foundation.)*

the scaphoid and then divides into two bands. The scaphotrapezial band connects the scaphoid and trapezium, with fibers forming a "V" shape. The scaphotrapezoid band connects the ulnar aspect of the scaphoid to the volar trapezoid. The scaphocapitate ligament spans the distal scaphoid pole to the palmar aspect of the capitate body. On the ulnar midcarpal side, the triquetrocapitate ligament connects the distal radial portion of the triquetrum to the ulnar side of the capitate body. Finally, the triquetrohamate ligament originates just ulnar to the triquetrocapitate ligament on the triquetrum and attaches to the volar hamate body.[8] Additionally, the dorsal intercarpal ligament, or scaphotriquetral ligament, is classified as an intercarpal ligament because of its broad connection between carpal bones.

Vascular Anatomy

There are four orthograde sources of blood flow to the wrist. These four extraosseous vessels contribute nutrient vessels to the distal radius and ulna and include the radial, ulnar, anterior and posterior interosseous arteries. The anterior interosseous artery divides into anterior and posterior divisions proximal to the distal radioulnar joint. The posterior division and the radial artery form

the primary sources of orthograde blood flow to the distal radius (**Fig. 38-9**).[12]

The vessels supplying the dorsal radius and ulna are best described by their relationship to the extensor compartments of the wrist and extensor retinaculum. They are considered intercompartmental when located between compartments and compartmental when lying within an extensor compartment. There are two consistent intercompartmental vessels that lie superficial to the retinaculum and are described as supraretinacular. These two vessels, the 1,2 and 2,3 intercompartmental supraretinacular arteries, are located on the retinaculum between their named compartments (**Fig. 38-10**).[12,13]

Two consistent vessels are found in the fourth and fifth compartments. They lie on the surface of the radius in the floor of the fourth and fifth extensor compartments and are named the fourth and fifth extensor compartment arteries (**Fig. 38-11**).[12,13]

On the volar aspect of the arm, the palmar carpal arch arises approximately 1.5 cm proximal to the radial styloid and courses volar to the pronator quadratus. It anastomoses with the anterior interosseous artery and continues as the ulnar carpal artery to then anastomose with the ulnar artery. In its path it gives off many

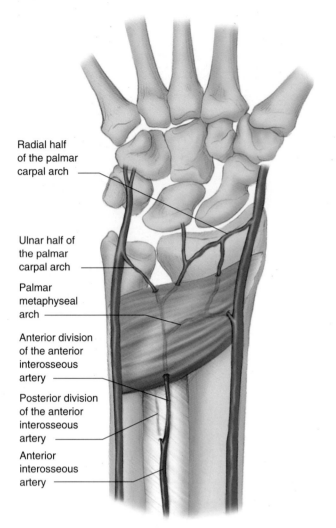

Radial half
of the palmar
carpal arch

Ulnar half of
the palmar
carpal arch

Palmar
metaphyseal
arch

Anterior division
of the anterior
interosseous
artery

Posterior division
of the anterior
interosseous
artery

Anterior
interosseous
artery

FIGURE 38-12 The volar blood supply to the wrist is derived from both the radial and ulnar arteries, which form the radial and ulnar carpal arches. *(Courtesy of Mayo Foundation.)*

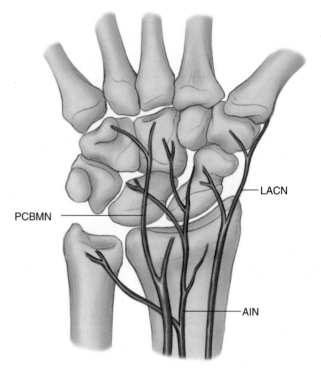

LACN

PCBMN

AIN

FIGURE 38-13 The volar innervation to the wrist. PCBNN, palmar cutaneous branch of the median nerve; LACN, lateral antebrachial cutaneous nerve; AIN, anterior interosseous nerve. *(Adapted from Van de Pol GJ, Koudstaal MJ, Schuurman AH, Bleys RL: Innervation of the wrist joint and surgical perspectives of denervation. J Hand Surg [Am]. 2006; 31:28-34.)*

branch of the radial nerve supplies articular branches to the periosteum and capsule. The superficial radial nerve also contributes articular branches to the dorsal capsule and to the periosteum, as does the dorsal sensory branch of the ulnar nerve (**Fig. 38-14**).[17]

cortical perforating branches and supplies the proximal radiocarpal joint at that level (**Fig. 38-12**).[14]

Nerve Anatomy

The carpus is innervated by articular branches of the anterior and posterior interosseous nerves, the superficial radial nerve, the palmar cutaneous branch of the median nerve, and the dorsal and motor branches of the ulnar nerve. In addition, the dorsal, lateral, and medial cutaneous nerves of the forearm have been variably shown to contribute articular twigs to the wrist.[15]

On the volar side of the wrist, the anterior interosseous nerve has several small branches that travel deep to the pronator quadratus muscle and enter the volar wrist capsule but do not penetrate to the periosteum.[16,17] On the radial volar wrist, the lateral antebrachial cutaneous nerve gives off branches to the wrist capsule and periosteum. The palmar cutaneous branch of the median nerve has an articular branch that terminates in the intercarpal ligaments. Finally, the ulnar nerve has been described as having one or two articular branches on the volar ulnar side of the carpus (**Fig. 38-13**).[17]

At the dorsal carpus, the posterior interosseous nerve is the dominant source of wrist innervation. This terminal

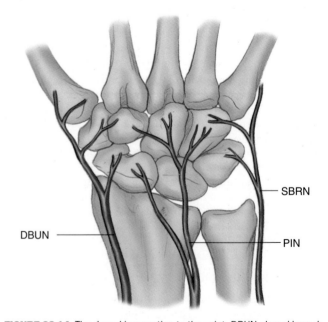

SBRN

DBUN

PIN

FIGURE 38-14 The dorsal innervation to the wrist. DBUN, dorsal branch of the ulnar nerve; SBRN, superficial branch of the radial nerve; PIN, posterior interosseous nerve. *(Adapted from Van de Pol GJ, Koudstaal MJ, Schuurman AH, Bleys RL: Innervation of the wrist joint and surgical perspectives of denervation. J Hand Surg. 2006; 31A:28-34.)*

REFERENCES

1. Eathorne SW: The wrist: clinical anatomy and physical examination—an update. Prim Care. 2005; 32:17-33.

2. Landsmeer JMF: Atlas of Anatomy of the Hand. Edinburgh: Churchill Livingstone, 1976.

3. Berger RA, Landsmeer JM: The palmar radiocarpal ligaments: a study of adult and fetal human wrist joints. J Hand Surg [Am]. 1990; 15:847-854.

4. Stuchin SA: Wrist anatomy. Hand Clin. 1992; 8:603-609.

5. Bettinger PC, Cooney WP 3rd, Berger RA: Arthroscopic anatomy of the wrist. Orthop Clin North Am. 1995; 26: 707-719.

6. Berger RA: Arthroscopic anatomy of the wrist and distal radioulnar joint. Hand Clin. 1999; 15:393-413.

7. Berger RA, Blair WF: The radioscapholunate ligament: a gross and histologic description. Anat Rec. 1984; 210:393-405.

8. Berger RA: The anatomy of the ligaments of the wrist and distal radioulnar joints. Clin Orthop Relat Res. 2001:32-40.

9. Viegas SF, Yamaguchi S, Boyd NL, Patterson RM: The dorsal ligaments of the wrist: anatomy, mechanical properties, and function. J Hand Surg [Am]. 1999; 24:456-468.

10. Kauer JM: The articular disc of the hand. Acta Anat (Basel). 1975; 93:590-605.

11. Berger RA: The ligaments of the wrist: a current overview of anatomy with considerations of their potential functions. Hand Clin. 1997; 13:63-82.

12. Sheetz KK, Bishop AT, Berger RA: The arterial blood supply of the distal radius and ulna and its potential use in vascularized pedicled bone grafts. J Hand Surg. 1995; 20:902-914.

13. Shin AY, Bishop AT: Vascular anatomy of the distal radius: implications for vascularized bone grafts. Clin Orthop Relat Res. 2001;383:60-73.

14. Haerle M, Schaller HE, Mathoulin C: Vascular anatomy of the palmar surfaces of the distal radius and ulna: its relevance to pedicled bone grafts at the distal palmar forearm. J Hand Surg [Br]. 2003; 28:131-136.

15. Buck-Gramcko D: Denervation of the wrist joint. J Hand Surg [Am]. 1977; 2:54-61.

16. Svizenska I, Cizmar I, Visna P: An anatomical study of the anterior interosseous nerve and its innervation of the pronator quadratus muscle. J Hand Surg [Br]. 2005; 30:635-637.

17. Van de Pol GJ, Koudstaal MJ, Schuurman AH, Bleys RL: Innervation of the wrist joint and surgical perspectives of denervation. J Hand Surg [Am]. 2006; 31:28-34.

Chronic Volar-Flexed Intercalated Segment Instability

39

John Stanley, MD

The definition of instability of the wrist has been described by the International Wrist Investigators' Workshop as "the inability of the carpus to maintain its normal anatomical relationships under physiological loading." Dobyns and colleagues,[1] and more recently the International Wrist Investigators' Workshop, have suggested a number of terms that describe the patterns of instability:

Carpal instability nondissociative (CIND; pure midcarpal instability—the VISI pattern)

Carpal instability dissociative (CID; scapholunate and ulnar midcarpal instability—the DISI pattern)

Carpal instability complex (CIC; translocation injury)

Carpal instability adaptive (CIA; secondary to distal radial malunion)

It is now accepted that the stability of the carpus is wholly dependent on the integrity of the interosseous and capsular ligaments of the wrist joint and not on any inherent stability conferred by bone shape or position.[2]

One might look at the effects of failure of these ligaments by using an analogy of the coiled spring. This concept, proposed by Garcia-Elias, identifies that the scaphoid, the lunate, and the triquetrum are intimately connected and, as Kapandji has described,[3]

there is a variable geometry of the proximal row of the carpus as the loaded wrist is moved. Thus, the scaphoid flexes, extends, pronates, supinates, and translates. The lunate flexes, extends, and translates but does not pronate or supinate. Finally, the triquetrum flexes and extends much less than the lunate but does not pronate or supinate and although it does translate, it does not articulate with the distal radius and barely articulates with the triangular fibrocartilage complex (TFCC). The scaphoid has a long lever arm by comparison to the lunate and triquetrum and therefore has a profound effect on the biomechanics of the wrist. Using the coiled spring analogy, axial loading of the intact wrist requires the rotational moment of the scaphoid to be balanced by the opposite rotational moment of the triquetrum, with the lunate acting as the torque converter in its position as the intercalated segment of the proximal row. Failure of the scapholunate ligament gives rise to the potential for the scaphoid to flex under the axial loading but, of course, the triquetral/lunate complex rotational moment is unopposed and the lunate and triquetrum extend, giving rise to the radiographic appearance of dorsiflexed intercalated segment instability (DISI). If, however, the lunate is separated from the triquetrum, the rotational moment of the scaphoid takes the lunate into flexion, thus creating the radiographic appearances of volar-flexed intercalated segment instability (VISI) (**Fig. 39-1**).[4-7]

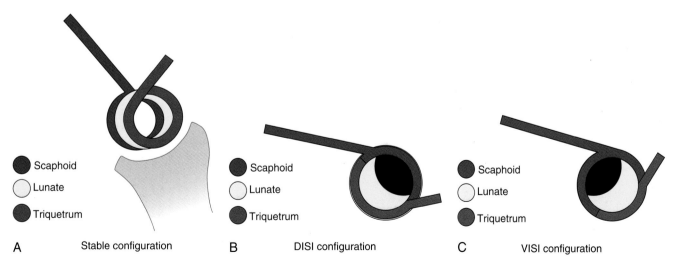

FIGURE 39-1 **A,** The spring theory. The proximal row of the carpus can be represented as a spring indicating the relationship between the three bones. **B,** The spring theory in DISI. When the scaphoid and lunate are disconnected, the scaphoid falls into flexion because of its long lever arm. The lunate and triquetrum fall into extension, giving rise to the appearance of DISI on the lateral radiograph. **C,** The spring theory in VISI. When the proximal and distal rows are disconnected, the longer lever arm of the scaphoid prevails. If there is lunotriquetral dissociation, the lunate goes with the scaphoid into flexion, giving rise to the VISI appearance on the lateral radiograph.

The work of Mayfield and Johnson[8] has shown us that there are patterns of ligamentous injury, through a radial-sided applied force, in which, with the wrist loaded in extension and ulnar deviation, axial loading resulted in sequential ligament disruption. In effect, these injuries occurred as a result of applying what might be described as a proximal row supination force to the cadaver specimens. This is translated into the in vivo injury when, as a result of falling on the outstretched hand, the *thenar* eminence (**Fig. 39-2**) contacts the ground first and thereafter the protective pronation reflex of the forearm forces the hand, and therefore the carpus, into supination, resulting in either a pronator quadratus fracture in the child, a Colles' type fracture in the elderly, a scaph-oid fracture in the young male, and a scapholunate, perilunate lesser arc, type of soft tissue injury in most adults. The sequence of ligament failure in this pattern of injury is well recognized and described elsewhere.

The so-called reverse Mayfield sequence, or the proximal row pronation injury, occurs as a result of the forces acting on the hand as the *hypothenar* eminence strikes the ground first (**Fig. 39-3**). The patterns of injury are complex in that there are many more ligament attachments to the triquetrum than to the scaph-oid. The act of falling on the outstretched hand when the heel of the hand strikes the ground concentrates the forces that now act on the ulnar side of the carpus and therefore through

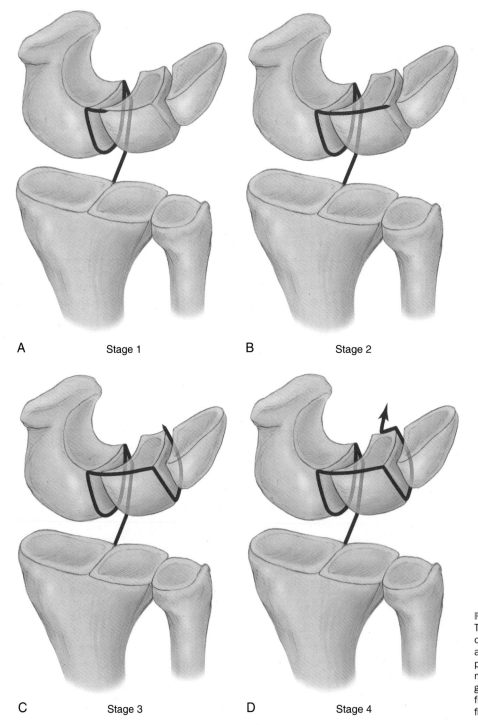

A   Stage 1

B   Stage 2

C   Stage 3

D   Stage 4

FIGURE 39-2 The Mayfield sequence. **A,** The first stage of the sequence is disruption of the scapholunate joint progressing from anterior to posterior. **B,** The second stage is progressive disruption of the dorsal attachments to the lunate. **C,** The third stage progresses through the triquetrolunate joint from posterior to anterior. **D,** The fourth and final stage is dislocation of the lunate.

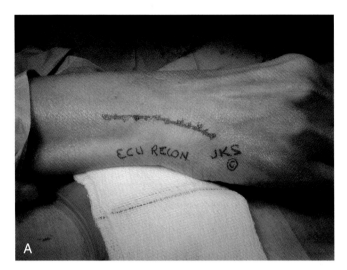

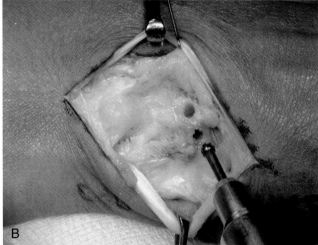

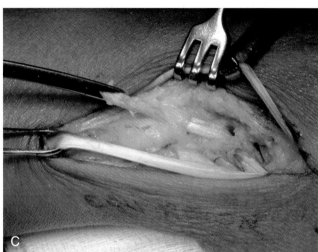

FIGURE 39-3 Operative sequence of ECU reconstruction. **A,** The incision along the fifth compartment. **B,** The triquetrum is exposed, and two bur holes are created. **C,** One third of the ECU is detached proximally and left attached distally. Then this is taken through the triquetrum and the dorsal aspect of the TFCC.

the pisiform to the triquetrum. The position of the pisiform on the volar aspect of the triquetrum results in this pair of bones decelerating rapidly, but the momentum of the individual suffering the injury drives the ulna toward the ground, which results in the forces being transmitted to the structures on the ulnar side of the wrist. There is a tendency to thus force the hand into a pronation attitude with reference to the distal radius and ulna. The ulnar head continues to approach the ground, which leads to a dorsal shearing force that may detach the posterior aspect of the TFCC from the dorsal ulnar carpal ligaments, giving rise to a separation of these two structures. This does not involve a true tear of the TFCC.

Any disruption of connections between the scaphoid and the lunate or the lunate and triquetrum can prevent the wrist from supporting physiological loading without collapsing.[5] The proximal row variable geometry system becomes dyskinetic, that is, it is not in the appropriate configuration in most positions of the loaded wrist. It is accepted from anatomical studies that the most important part of the scapholunate interosseous ligament lies dorsally and the most important part of the triquetrolunate interosseous ligament lies anteriorly.[7] This allows each of the bones to have its own axis or rotation different from the others and also for each bone to move within its limits set down by these two ligaments.

Ulnar midcarpal instability is traumatic, degenerative, or idiopathic.[9-12] The traumatic version is acute or chronic; the degenerative version is chronic and usually defined as part of the ulnar abutment syndrome; and the idiopathic version is related to hyperlaxity and pathological hyperlaxity, as exhibited in Ehlers-Danlos syndrome.

The clinical features of ulnar midcarpal instability are ulnar-sided pain and a sagging carpus. The posterior sag is a very characteristic one and is related to the detachment of the posterior part of the posterior TFCC from the ulnar carpal ligaments, a greater feel of the dorsal tubercle of the triquetrum as this bone flexes, the clunking wrist, tenderness over the lunotriquetral interval, a positive Regan shuck test, and, often, a positive Lichtman pivot shift test.[13]

The arthroscopic features can be defined as a significant step-off between the lunate and the triquetrum when viewed on midcarpal arthroscopy (**Fig. 39-4**).

A possible sequence of events is proposed arbitrarily divided into discrete steps based on the known patterns of injury seen (**Fig. 39-5**):

Stage 1: There is separation attenuation or detachment of the posterior aspect of the TFCC from the ulnar carpal ligaments.

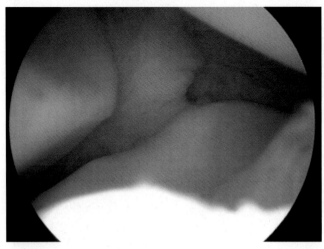

FIGURE 39-4 The lunotriquetral joint. This arthroscopic view of the left wrist demonstrates disruption of the lunotriquetral joint and a large facet on the lunate—the hamate facet.

Stage 2: The injury passes between the triquetrum and the lunate from dorsal to palmar and when it reaches the palmar point the triquetrum becomes truly separate from the lunate in terms of its interosseous ligament connections.

Stage 3a: The injury can then pass through the ulnar hamate ligaments, giving rise to a peritriquetral instability.

Stage 3b: The injury may travel through the midcarpal joint, giving rise to full ulnar midcarpal instability.

Stage 4a: The true reverse Mayfield sequence is rare and is seen when the injury becomes a true perilunate injury.

Stage 4b: The injury can travel through the whole of the midcarpal joint and may give rise to full midcarpal instability.

Treatment Options for Specific Patterns of Instability
Ulnar Midcarpal Instability (Carpal Instability Dissociative)

The treatment options for the management of chronic lunotriquetral instability are limited.[14] An alternative to ligament reconstruction or augmentation is intercarpal fusion, which can give rise to a significant loss of wrist motion.[9] At all levels of the problem the treating physician should respond to the patient's symptoms and, as in any other nonprogressive musculoskeletal problem, the starting point is reassurance and lifestyle modification supported by orthoses and physical therapy in the acute phase or in the acute exacerbation of a chronic injury. Posterior ligament surgery in the form of an extensor carpi ulnaris reconstruction; anterior ligament surgery, which has been described both by Lichtman and by Garcia-Elias; and intercarpal fusions can be performed in cases unresponsive to conservative management. Limited wrist arthrodeses can significantly distort carpal motion, and the results can be disappointing.

Triquetrohamate fusion is ideal for patients with a peritriquetral instability, but this affects a very small number of patients.[15]

Capitolunate fusion will cure the midcarpal instability part of the problem but does not address the persistent detachment of the posterior part of the TFCC and, therefore, only partially solves the problem.

Four-corner fusion serves much the same purpose but is more reliable than capitolunate fusion in terms of achieving fusion.

Total wrist fusion is an extreme management of ulnar midcarpal instability, but the presence of degenerative changes and unremitting pain despite conservative measures would lead to the consideration of a full wrist fusion.

Extensor Carpi Ulnaris Tenodesis for Lunotriquetral Instability

We have described a technique for a ligament augmentation of the dorsal aspects of the ulnar carpal ligament complex, the ECU tenodesis.[16] The operation is shown in **Figure 39-6**.

The skin incision is over the line of the fifth extensor compartment; through the fifth compartment the extensor digiti minimi is exposed and retracted. The extensor retinaculum is reflected from the dorsal aspect of the triquetrum, revealing the ECU and its inner sheath, which is opened. Two holes are drilled through the dorsal cortex of the triquetrum using a rose bur to prevent perforation of the volar cortex (the pisotriquetral joint). The ECU tendon is exposed proximally, and a strip of the first third of the tendon is detached proximally and stripped toward the hand as far as the insertion, leaving it attached distally. The harvested tendon having been passed through the two holes in the triquetrum, distal to proximal, is then tunneled through the posterior aspect of the TFCC and then through the dorsal capsule of the distal radioulnar joint; it is then reattached to itself in the groove of the ulnar head. This ECU loop stabilizes the ulnar carpal complex. Pulling on the ECU, which in the normal course of events because of its position would tend to displace the wrist forward, now tends to reduce the wrist, bringing the triquetrum back toward the TFCC. This is probably not a dynamic tendon transfer because attachment to the dorsal ligaments prevents any active glide and in effect there has been a reconstruction of the dorsal ulnar carpal ligaments.

We have reviewed 46 of these procedures. In the review group there was no gender bias, the average age was 30, the dominant wrist was treated in 33% of patients, and significant trauma was recalled by the patients in 43 cases.[16]

Using the Mayo Wrist Score, in 72% recovery was excellent or good; in 15% it was satisfactory, which meant that although there was sufficient improvement for the patient to believe that the operation was worthwhile, these patients were still left with residual symptoms; and in 13% the patients had no improvement.

The patient dissatisfaction was 13%; that is, 87% of the patients were satisfied but those who failed to improve at all were disappointed with the surgery. The remainder stated that they would happily proceed to have the operation done on their other wrist if necessary or would recommend it to a friend.

Patient selection is crucial, and arthroscopy best identifies the problem and excludes other intra-articular pathological processes. The selection criteria for inclusion were ulnar-sided wrist pain after a fall on the outstretched hand with prominence of the triquetrum to palpation, tenderness over the triquetrolunate joint, a positive Regan shuck test, and evidence of lunotriquetral instability on arthroscopy. Contraindications were full midcarpal instability, previous surgery, and the presence of a full reverse Mayfield injury.

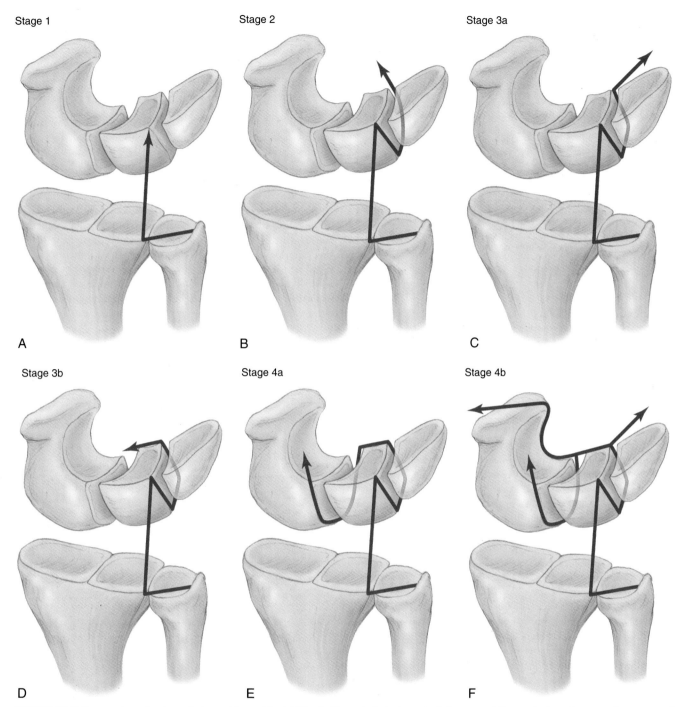

Stage 1

Stage 2

Stage 3a

A

B

C

Stage 3b

Stage 4a

Stage 4b

D

E

F

FIGURE 39-5 Proposed mechanism of ulnar midcarpal instability. **A,** Stage 1: Detachment of ulnar carpal ligaments from the posterior aspect of the TFCC. **B,** Stage 2: Lunotriquetral ligament disruption. **C,** Stage 3a: Peritriquetral instability. **D,** Stage 3b: Disruption of the volar ulnar carpal ligaments. **E,** Stage 4a: Progressive damage to the scapholunate ligaments (the reverse Mayfield). **F,** Stage 4b: The complete disruption of the proximal and midcarpal joint system.

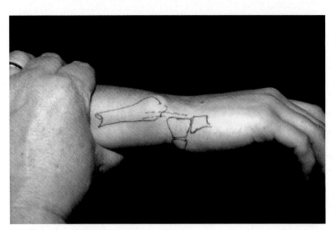

FIGURE 39-6 Ulnar midcarpal instability. Note the volar "sag" of the carpus on the ulnar side secondary to disruption of the dorsal ligament TFCC relationship.

Lunotriquetral instability as a result of proximal row *pronation* injuries can be effectively treated with soft tissue reconstruction. Stage 2, 3a, and 3b pronation injuries are suitable for this procedure. This grading is done at the time of arthroscopy. The procedure is less effective in injuries to the triquetrolunate joint as a result of a *supination* pattern of injury of the carpus. Tensioning of the repair must be performed with the wrist in neutral, not in ulnar, deviation; the surgery is simple, the operating room time is short, and, more importantly, the procedure is reversible. The cosmetic appearance of the scar is very acceptable.

Ligament augmentation has a success rate that will improve with better patient selection. The best results of the series were seen in patients with a stage 2, 3a, or 3b proximal row pronation injury. Modest results were seen in those patients with a Mayfield stage 3 injury with a residual lunotriquetral instability; that is, they had a radial-sided injury. Those with significant full midcarpal instability of stage 4a and 4b also failed the procedure. The failures in the study have also been related to overtensioning of the repair and overambitious expectations of both the surgeon and the patient.

There is an alternative method of repairing the lunotriquetral interval, using a complex reconstruction described from the Mayo Clinic. Garcia-Elias and others have recommended the volar and dorsal approach, repairing both the anterior part of the lunotriquetral internal and the triquetrohamate ligament. This basically is the pisohamate ligament, which runs deep from the pisotriquetral joint to the hook of the hamate at its base. The triquetrocapitate ligament also is reconstructed. Future developments in arthroscopic-assisted surgery may allow earlier diagnosis and intervention, and the techniques of arthroscopic capsular shrinkage may be sufficient to reduce the symptom level to acceptable levels in the milder cases.[17]

True Midcarpal Instability Nondissociative

True midcarpal instability does not involve any injury to the intrinsic scapholunate or triquetrolunate interosseous ligaments; and because there is no such injury there is no dissociation between the individual bones of either the proximal or the distal rows of the carpus. The instability arises between the proximal and distal rows, and therefore the term "carpal instability nondissociative" is applied. This is related to problems where the extrinsic capsular ligament system fails to adequately maintain the

relationship of the proximal row to the distal row and thus allows the distal row to fall into its default position, which forces the proximal row into flexion. This gives rise to the so-called tilting teacup or VISI pattern (**Fig. 39-7**). Ligament reconstruction (or more accurately augmentation or substitution) is unreliable in these circumstances, and one of the limited fusions may be required.

Limited wrist arthrodesis can be in the form of lunotriquetral fusion,[18] triquetrohamate fusion, capitolunate fusion, lunotriquetral-capitohamate fusion (LTCH or so-called four-corner fusion), and radiolunate fusion (the Chamay fusion).

The future for ligament reconstruction in the ulnar midcarpal dissociative type of injury is for better identification of the injury pattern and earlier intervention in a repair and reconstruction mode rather than salvage in the chronic injury. Primary repair of the identifiable injured ligaments, in particular the detachment of the posterior TFCC from the dorsal ulnocarpal ligaments and the repair of the anterior ulnocapitate and radioscaphocapitate ligaments, can give satisfactory results in appropriate cases, but limited wrist arthrodesis may be necessary in the severe or recalcitrant case.

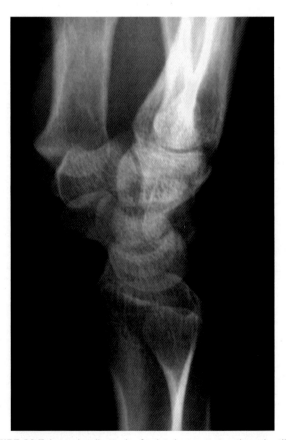

FIGURE 39-7 Lateral radiograph of wrist demonstrates the volar tilt of the lunate that occurs in midcarpal instability.

REFERENCES

1. Linscheid RL, Dobyns JH, Beckenbaugh RD, et al: Instability patterns of the wrist. J Hand Surg [Am]. 1983; 8:682-686.
2. Viegas SF, Patterson RM, Ward K: Extrinsic wrist ligaments in the pathomechanics of ulnar translation instability. J Hand Surg [Am]. 1995; 20:312-318.
3. Kapandji A: [Biomechanics of the carpus and the wrist]. Ann Chir Main. 1987; 6:147-169.
4. Moritomo H, Murase T, Goto A, et al: In vivo three-dimensional kinematics of the midcarpal joint of the wrist. J Bone Joint Surg Am. 2006; 88:611-621.
5. Tang JB, Xie RG, Yu XW, Chen F: Wrist kinetics after lunotriquetral dissociation: the changes in moment arms of the flexor carpi ulnaris tendon. J Orthop Res. 2002; 20:1327-1332.
6. Trumble TE, Bour CJ, Smith RJ, Glisson RR: Kinematics of the ulnar carpus related to the volar intercalated segment instability pattern. J Hand Surg [Am]. 1990; 15:384-392.
7. Wiesner L, Rumelhart C, Pham E, Comtet JJ: Experimentally induced ulnocarpal instability: a study on 13 cadaver wrists. J Hand Surg [Br]. 1996; 21:24-29.
8. Mayfield JK, Johnson RP, Kilcoyne RK: Carpal dislocations: pathomechanics and progressive perilunar instability. J Hand Surg [Am]. 1980; 5:226-241.
9. Ambrose L, Posner MA: Lunate-triquetral and midcarpal joint instability. Hand Clin. 1992; 8:653-668.
10. Shin AY, Battaglia MJ, Bishop AT: Lunotriquetral instability: diagnosis and treatment. J Am Acad Orthop Surg. 2000; 8:170-179.
11. Trail IA, Stanley JK, Hayton MJ: Twenty questions on carpal instability. J Hand Surg [Br]. 2007; 32:240-255.
12. Weiss LE, Taras JS, Sweet S, Osterman AL: Lunotriquetral injuries in the athlete. Hand Clin. 2000; 16:433-438.
13. Alexander CE, Lichtman DM: Ulnar carpal instabilities. Orthop Clin North Am. 1984; 15:307-320.
14. Lichtman DM, Bruckner JD, Culp RW, Alexander CE: Palmar midcarpal instability: results of surgical reconstruction. J Hand Surg [Am]. 1993; 18:307-315.
15. Rao SB, Culver JE: Triquetrohamate arthrodesis for midcarpal instability. J Hand Surg [Am]. 1995; 20:583-589.
16. Shahane SA, Trail IA, Takwale VJ, et al: Tenodesis of the extensor carpi ulnaris for chronic, post-traumatic lunotriquetral instability. J Bone Joint Surg Br. 2005; 87:1512-1515.
17. Moskal MJ, Savoie FH 3rd, Field LD: Arthroscopic capsulodesis of the lunotriquetral joint. Clin Sports Med. 2001; 20:141-153.
18. Goldfarb CA, Stern PJ, Kiefhaber TR: Palmar midcarpal instability: the results of treatment with 4-corner arthrodesis. J Hand Surg [Am]. 2004; 29:258-263.

Kinematics of the Lunotriquetral Joint

40

Marco J.P.F. Ritt, MD, PhD

Lunotriquetral injury is less frequently seen with distal radius fracture than one of the triangular fibrocartilage complex (TFCC) or scapholunate ligament injuries. One of the problems with lunotriquetral disorders is that most patients have normal imaging studies and fall under the broad and often vexing category of patients with ulnar-sided wrist pain. However, these disorders can have devastating effects on carpal mechanics and, unless properly treated, disruptions of the lunotriquetral supporting ligaments may result in substantial instability of the carpus. Knowledge of these effects and potential consequences will aid the treating physician in offering the patient the best possible outcome.

Functional Anatomy

Joint Anatomy

The lunotriquetral joint is part of the proximal carpal row, forming the articulation between the ulnar surface of the lunate and the radial surface of the triquetrum. The articulating surfaces of the lunate and triquetrum are flat and semilunar. In neutral position of the wrist, the orientation of the plane of the joint is nearly orthogonal to the frontal plane of the forearm and approximately 20 degrees oblique to the sagittal plane. In the coronal plane the joint is positioned somewhat distal to the scapholunate joint.

The lunotriquetral joint is also under the influence of the radiocarpal and the midcarpal joints. The convex proximal surfaces of the lunate and triquetrum articulate with the hybrid radiocarpal articulation: the lunate fossa of the distal radius and the triangular disc of the TFCC. Usually, no more than 50% of the lunate articulates with the triangular disc.

The relevant midcarpal articulation is between the distal articular surfaces of the lunate and triquetrum and the proximal surfaces of the capitate and hamate. A sagittal ridge can divide the lunate articular surface into a radial and ulnar fossa, and in these cases the proximal surface of the hamate articulates with the lunate. The incidence of this type II lunate varies considerably and is reported in 27% to 63% of adults.[1,2] Otherwise, the distal surface of the lunate is concave in both coronal and sagittal planes.

The hamate-triquetral articulation has a helicoid or screw-shaped configuration. The plane of the joint is not parallel to the articular surface of the distal hamate with the fourth and fifth metacarpals but is situated at a substantial angle (reported as high as 90 degrees[3]).

Ligament Anatomy

The lunotriquetral joint is stabilized by an intricate arrangement of ligaments (**Fig. 40-1**). The *intrinsic* (both origin and insertion

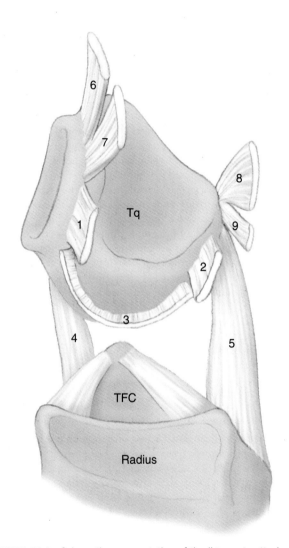

FIGURE 40-1 Schematic representation of the ligaments attached to the triquetrum (Tq) as seen from the radial side, the lunate having been removed. The LTq joint is linked directly by three structures: palmar LTq ligament (1), dorsal LTq ligament (2), and proximal LTq membrane (3). The ulna is connected with the triquetrum by means of the palmar ulnotriquetral ligament (4). The radiotriquetral ligament (5) is wide and fan shaped and is key in the prevention of carpal collapse. The midcarpal joint is constrained palmarly by two fascicles: the triquetrum-hamate ligament (6) and the triquetrum-capitate ligament (7), both of which are important midcarpal stabilizers. The triquetrum is connected dorsally with the trapezium and trapezoid by means of the dorsal intercarpal ligament (8) and with the scaphoid by means of the dorsal scaphotriquetral ligament (9). TFC, triangular fibrocartilage. *(Adapted from Garcia-Elias M, Ritt MJPF. Lunotriquetral dissociation: Pathomechanics. Atlas Hand Clinics, 9(1), 2004: 7-15, with permission.)*

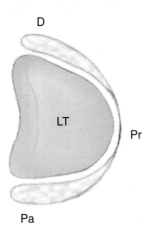

D

LT

Pr

Pa

FIGURE 40-2 Lunotriquetral joint interface. LT, lunotriquetral joint surface; D, dorsal subregion of the lunotriquetral joint; Pr, proximal subregion; Pa, palmar subregion.

are within the carpus) lunotriquetral ligament is "C" shaped and is actually composed of three discrete regions: true ligaments dorsally and palmarly with collinear fascicles of collagen and a proximal region composed of fibrocartilage (**Fig. 40-2**). This proximal region has a wedge-shaped cross-sectional geometry and is reminiscent of a meniscus. In normal subjects there should be no communication between the midcarpal and radiocarpal joints but the proximal region of the lunotriquetral joint can be perforated by age. Because the proximal membrane contributes very little to the overall lunotriquetral stability, a defect at this level is not a sign of instability but can be a normal physiological, albeit age-related, finding, caused by wear. Mikic[4] found up to 55% of lunotriquetral perforations past the third decade.

There are several *extrinsic* (connecting the carpus with the radius or ulna) ligaments constraining the lunotriquetral joint; and from a functional point of view these may be subdivided into two major groups: radioulnocarpal ligaments and midcarpal ligaments.

Radioulnocarpal Ligaments

Most extrinsic ligaments across the radioulnocarpal joint are obliquely oriented relative to the longitudinal axis of the forearm. Based on this, they may be subdivided into two groups: ligaments that prevent excessive passive supination of the proximal row relative to the forearm (anti-supination ligaments) and ligaments that control passive pronation (anti-pronation ligaments).[5,6]

Three ligaments act synergistically to prevent the proximal row to passively supinate beyond normal. The first is the palmar ulnotriquetral ligament that originates at the fovea near the base of the ulnar styloid. In approximately 90% of normal adults, the ulnotriquetral ligament is split distally to form an orifice that connects the radiocarpal and pisotriquetral joints.[7] Second is the ulnolunate ligament that arises from the palmar edge of the triangular fibrocartilage (TFC) and runs obliquely toward its distal insertion into the anterior aspect of the lunate. Palmar to the ulnolunate and ulnotriquetral ligaments is the ulnocapitate ligament, which reinforces both these ligaments before passing anterior to the lunotriquetral joint, where it interdigitates with the fibers of the palmar region of the lunotriquetral interosseous ligament. It arises from the ulna at the fovea where the dorsal and

palmar radioulnar ligaments also attach. Third, the dorsal radiotriquetral ligament is a wide, fan-shaped ligament that connects the dorsal edge of the distal radius to the dorsal rim of the triquetrum.[8-12]

There are two major ligaments preventing the proximal row to passively pronate beyond normal: the radioscaphocapitate ligament, which originates on the palmar margin of the radial styloid process and inserts into the capitate, and the long radiolunate ligament, which emerges from the palmar edge of the radius and inserts into the palmar surface of the lunate. None of these structures is directly inserted into the triquetrum, thus explaining this bone's relative vulnerability against pronation torques.

Midcarpal Ligaments

The ulnar limb of the arcuate ligament, also known as the palmar triquetrum/hamate/capitate ligamentous complex, strongly connects the triquetrum to the distal carpal row.[10,13-16] It consists of a group of fan-shaped fascicles formed by dense collagen fibers that links the distal anterior edge of the triquetrum to the palmar aspects of the hamate and capitate. This ligament can be regarded as an anti-supination ligament. The only dorsal midpalmar crossing ligament is the dorsal intercarpal ligament. It arises from the dorsal ridge of the triquetrum, courses transversely along the distal edge of the lunate, and fans out to insert on the dorsal rim of the scaphoid, the trapezium, and the trapezoid bones.[8,10,17] This ligament can be characterized as an anti-pronation ligament.

There is no dorsal or ulnar ligament between the triquetrum and hamate. Because the midcarpal joint is not a true hinge articulation, there are no vertically oriented ligaments. Their absence is functionally substituted by the extensor carpi ulnaris tendon, which is a thick sheath that may act as a dynamic joint stabilizer.[18]

Mechanics
Material and Constraint Properties

Results of material property testing of the lunotriquetral ligament showed that the palmar region of the ligament is not only thicker but indeed stronger than the dorsal portion of the ligament (average yield strengths: 301 N and 121 N, respectively).[19] The palmar region was found to constrain primarily translation, whereas the dorsal region provides the majority of rotational constraint. The fibrocartilaginous proximal region failed at 64 N and was the least important constraint in all directions. The morphology and material and constraint properties of the lunotriquetral ligament are the exact opposite as found in the scapholunate ligament.[20] In a way, the lunate could be thought of as a "torque-suspended" bone between the scaphoid and the triquetrum, much in the manner of a spring. This "torque suspension" concept, for which there is now sufficient evidence, is of importance for the discussion and understanding of dorsiflexed intercalated segment instability (DISI) and volar-flexed intercalated segment instability (VISI).

Recently, immunohistochemical analysis of wrist ligament innervation showed that sensory important ligaments were primarily related to the triquetrum while mechanically important ligaments were primarily located in the radial, force-bearing column of the wrist. The triquetrum and its ligamentous attachments are regarded as key elements in the generation of the proprioceptive information necessary for adequate neuromuscular wrist stabilization.[21]

Kinematics

The bones of the proximal carpal row form a highly functional adaptable unit, permitting a large range of motion of the hand: flexion/extension, radioulnar deviation, and even some rotation. During hand motions, the proximal carpal row undergoes adaptive geometric changes, dictated by the geometry of the articular surfaces of the carpal bones as well as ligament functions.

The scaphoid is forced to flex palmarly, largely based on its bony geometry, and the lunate is passively forced to follow this motion. There is a strong tendency by the lunate to rotate dorsally owing to its dorsopalmar wedge shape. The shape of the scaphoid, aided by the peripheral location of the interosseous scapholunate ligament, results in a large moment arm, which forces the lunate to follow against its tendency and which therefore demonstrates less flexion than the scaphoid. In its turn, the lunate moves the triquetrum via the interosseous lunotriquetral ligament during scapholunate interaction. These motions and tendencies to move are arrested by the scaphoid/trapezium/trapezoid geometry distally. However, the position of the scaphoid, between trapezium and trapezoid, aided by the specific geometry of the scapholunate ligament proximally, which follows the lunate, prevents exaggerated dorsal displacement of the proximal pole of the scaphoid. By the difference in curvature at the radiocarpal level, the lunate demonstrates less flexion than the scaphoid. Extension is facilitated by the wedge-shaped proximal part of the scaphoid, the tendency of the lunate to move into the same direction according to its wedge shape, and the helicoid articular facet of the triquetrum with the hamate. Geometrically, a helicoid facet represents a surface generated by the rotation of a plane or twisted curve about a fixed line, so that each point of the curve traces out a circular helix with the fixed line as axis. Besides facilitating extension of the wrist, this geometry of the triquetrohamate joint plays a role in ulnar deviation of the wrist as the triquetrum is allowed to extend as it glides distally on the hamate. Aided by the oblique shape of the lunotriquetral interface, the lunate is forced to follow the triquetral motion and extends, taking the scaphoid along into erect position.

In radial deviation of the wrist, the scaphoid is forced to flex over the palmar radioscaphocapitate ligament largely because of its bony geometry. This motion is transmitted by the scapholunate ligament, and the lunate is forced to flex. Transmission of this inclination by the lunotriquetral ligament, aided by the helicoid triquetrohamate surface, causes the triquetrum to flex.

All the above mechanisms make it necessary for the proximal carpal bones to take very specific positions, with small pronation/supination motions and mainly ulnar deviation as conjunct motion to flexion/extension of the wrist. In 60 degrees and 30 degrees of wrist extension, the lunate extended 29.7 degrees and 15.4 degrees and the triquetrum 39.3 degrees and 20.1 degrees, respectively. With 60 degrees and 30 degrees of flexion, the lunate flexed 23.0 degrees and 11.5 degrees and the triquetrum 30.6 degrees and 15.5 degrees, respectively, with simultaneous ulnar deviation of both lunate and triquetrum. In extension/flexion motion of the wrist there is some progressive pronation of the triquetrum. Thus, the total arc of lunotriquetral intercarpal motion in the sagittal plane was 16.8 degrees, with the wrist moving from 60 degrees of extension to 60 degrees of flexion. With radial and ulnar deviation of the wrist, the magnitude of the conjunct motion of both the lunate and triquetrum is greater than the primary motion: that is, flexion/extension motion of these carpals is greater than the prime radioulnar deviation motion.[22]

These results are all in broad agreement with previous in vitro studies[23-25] concerning normal carpal kinematics as well as with more recent in vivo studies.[26,27]

Most recently it has been demonstrated that the kinematics of a type I lunate are different from those of a type II lunate during radioulnar deviation of the wrist: wrists with a type I lunate show statistically greater scaphoid translation with radial deviation, whereas wrists with a type II lunate show statistically greater scaphoid flexion with radial deviation.[28,29]

It is obvious that the intercalated lunate is in need of constraints on both sides to counteract the just-mentioned torques. Although the connections between triquetrum and lunate are strong, they are not so taut as not to allow mutual mobility. In fact, during maximal radioulnar deviation there is an average 2.5-mm proximal shift of the triquetrum relative to the lunate, ranging from 0 to 5.2 mm.[30] Thus, from a kinematic viewpoint, the lunotriquetral joint is not a functional block without intrinsic mobility.

Mechanisms of Injury
Trauma

There is general agreement that injuries to the lunotriquetral ligaments are part of a spectrum of progressive ligament disruption. This is associated with perilunate dislocation either in the classic direction or more often in the reverse direction.

In the latter situation, isolated injuries to the lunotriquetral ligaments appear as the consequence of a fall backward on the outstretched hand, with the arm being externally rotated and the wrist positioned in radial deviation and extension. In such circumstances, the impact concentrates on the pisiform. The triquetrum, already in extended position, is translated dorsally but the lunate does not follow: it is effectively constrained by the radius and the long radiolunate ligament. Furthermore, it is likely that this mechanism, with concomitant midcarpal pronation, is able to tighten the ulnocarpal ligamentous complex to a point where isolated failure of the lunotriquetral fibers may occur, whereas the radiocarpal ligaments are spared. Substantial shear stress appears at the lunotriquetral joint, causing progressive stretching and, ultimately, tear of the different lunotriquetral stabilizing ligaments. Complete rupture of the strong palmar portion of the lunotriquetral ligament rarely occurs unless there is additional violent pronation of the distal row, by which the palmar triquetrum/hamate/capitate ligament adds the extra destabilizing force that is required for this strong part of the ligament to fail. Supporting this theory is the fact that the palmar lunotriquetral and triquetrum/hamate/capitate ligament are seldom both disrupted.

Frequently encountered associated regional injuries are a combination of a partial or complete rupture of the lunotriquetral ligaments, a peripheral tear of the TFCC, and a distal avulsion of the ulnotriquetral ligament. The mechanism of injury may be similar to the just discussed mechanism for the isolated lunotriquetral injury except for the presence of radial deviation and pronation as the predominant torque-inducing vectors. It is reported that this combination of injuries is not unusual, and it is easy to miss any one of its components.[31] Avulsion fracture of the palmar rim of the triquetrum as documented by Smith and Murray[32] should be interpreted as a subtle sign of a more extended lunotriquetral injury and would correlate well with the previously described concept of a "reversed Mayfield perilunate dislocation model" discussed by Viegas and coworkers.[33]

In other circumstances the progression of injury seems to follow a more direct perilunate destabilization process, as described in the well-known paper by Mayfield.[34] This classic pattern of progressive perilunate instability begins with palmar to dorsal disruption of the scapholunate interosseous ligament. In these instances, injury to the lunotriquetral ligaments occurs in stage III, after rupture of the scapholunate ligaments (stage I) and the lunocapitate dislocation (stage II). Lunotriquetral dissociation is an integral part of a progressive perilunate dislocation, but it is difficult to imagine as an isolated finding according to this classic progression pattern. Perhaps isolated lunotriquetral instability represents a residual problem from a previous perilunate injury in which the scapholunate problem heals spontaneously or with intervention.

Acute lunotriquetral ligament injury is less frequently seen with distal radius fracture than one of the TFCC or scapholunate ligament injuries. Still, partial or complete lunotriquetral ligament disruption is reported to be associated with intra-articular fractures in a considerable number of cases, ranging from 7% to 24%.[35-37] Because additional disruption of the palmar arcuate ligament and/or the dorsal radiocarpal ligaments is necessary to produce a VISI stance, this pattern is seldom seen acutely in distal radius fractures.

Degeneration

A lunotriquetral instability pattern may also appear as the consequence of an ulnocarpal abutment resulting in degeneration of (mainly) the proximal portion of the lunotriquetral ligament by a wear mechanism. Patients without history of trauma, inflammatory arthritis, or ulnocarpal abutment also may have degenerative lunotriquetral lesions because this region is prone to age-related degeneration.[4] In both situations the lunotriquetral joint is not dissociated and no progressive derotational changes will develop.

Injury to the Lunotriquetral Supporting Ligaments: Effects on Carpal Kinematics*

In the laboratory, several attempts to ascertain the consequences of lunotriquetral ligament disruptions have been made.[14,15,25,38] The first published investigation of the role of the lunotriquetral ligaments in the carpal kinematics was reported by Reagan and associates,[39] who also were the first to analyze a series of such ligament injuries. They showed that in patients with severe lunotriquetral sprains there was often a static VISI deformity and abnormal motion of the carpus. That clinical study also showed that on lateral radiographs the longitudinal axis of the triquetrum, which in normal subjects exhibits an average 16 degrees of flexion relative to the longitudinal axis of the lunate, shows an extension posture of more than 14 degrees in severe lunotriquetral disruption: this is a more than 30-degree change in the lunotriquetral angle compared with normal. Reagan and associates[39] also described an increased proximal migration of the triquetrum on ulnar-deviated posteroanterior radiographs.

In 1990, Viegas and coworkers[33] showed that even in partial disruptions of the lunotriquetral ligament there is increased motion between the elements of the lunotriquetral joint, a finding later confirmed by Horii and colleagues[25] using biplanar radiog-

raphy. All intercarpal joints have altered kinematics after complete lunotriquetral ligament sectioning. The changes were especially marked at the lunotriquetral joint, with the lunate adopting a palmar-flexed position and the triquetrum rotating into supination. Li and associates[40] concluded that the palmar lunotriquetral ligament is the major stabilizer of the lunotriquetral joint during wrist extension and that the rest of the lunotriquetral ligament provides stability during ulnar deviation.

Horii and colleagues[25] and Viegas and coworkers[33] emphasized the importance of the dorsal radiotriquetral and scaphotriquetral ligaments in the prevention of a global carpal collapse when the lunotriquetral ligaments are disrupted. In most studies, a carpal collapse, typically in the form of a VISI pattern, occurred only when the ligaments were sectioned in association with complete lunotriquetral ligament division. Li and associates[40] did not observe a static or dynamic VISI deformity after sectioning only the lunotriquetral ligaments.

More recently, Ritt and colleagues,[38] from the Mayo Clinic, reported on a series of cadaver specimen using stereoradiographic techniques to study carpal kinematics after different sequences of lunotriquetral ligament sectioning. According to that investigation, neither the isolated section of the proximal lunotriquetral membrane nor the disruption of both proximal and dorsal regions of the lunotriquetral capsule creates any significant change in carpal alignment (stage II in **Table 40-1**) or carpal motion. From a kinematic viewpoint, partial tears of the proximal lunotriquetral membrane need not be treated because they have minimal mechanical consequences. In contrast, when the palmar lunotriquetral ligament is sectioned selectively, significant changes in carpal kinematics occur. Although the intrinsic tendency of the scapholunate complex to rotate into flexion is still balanced (no carpal malalignment yet at this stage), increased lunotriquetral instability becomes evident, especially in ulnar deviation. Only after dividing the dorsal radiotriquetral and scaphotriquetral ligaments does carpal malalignment occur in a consistent fashion: lunate and triquetrum supinate, flex, and radially deviate (stage IV in **Table 40-1**). The strong dorsal radiotriquetral and scaphotriquetral ligaments can act as rotational constraints for the lunotriquetral joint in the absence of the dorsal lunotriquetral ligament.

One factor that should be taken into account is the effect of cyclic loading on the generation of abnormal patterns of motion. Horii and colleagues[25] applied "some degree of manipulation" after sectioning of the ligaments. It may require secondary attenuation from prolonged cyclic loading to produce the clinical findings. Ritt and colleagues[38] simulated gradual attenuation of the remaining ligaments by repetitively loading the joint before analyzing carpal motion. The values of static carpal malalignment changed dramatically: the static malalignment increased in magnitude (stage V in **Table 40-1**).

Most laboratory attempts to explain the pathomechanics of one particular injury have an important drawback: the experiments cannot simulate what happens in living systems in which healing and remodeling have a great effect on the end results. Nevertheless, from most of these cadaver studies, results of which seem to be in accordance with the observations made in clinical practice, one can conclude the following:

- Injury to the proximal and dorsal lunotriquetral ligaments does not cause significant alteration in carpal mechanics.
- After division of all palmar and dorsal lunotriquetral ligaments, substantial kinematic dysfunction, sufficient to induce trau-

*This section is reprinted from Garcia-Elias M, Ritt MJPF: Lunotriquetral dissociation: pathomechanics. Atlas of Hand Clinics 2004; 9(1):7-15.

TABLE 40-1 Carpal Alignment (Degrees) Relative to the Radius (Changes from Intact Stage) at Neutral Wrist Position*

Bone	Stage†	Axis of Rotation		
		X (+) Pronation (−) Supination	Y (+) Flexion (−) Extension	Z (+) Ulnar deviation (−) Radial deviation
Scaphoid	Stage I	0.3	−0.2	−0.6
	Stage II	−1.7	1.0	−0.2
	Stage III	−1.3	−0.2	−0.8
	Stage IV	−1.3	−1.3	−2.2
	Stage V	**−2.6**	**3.8**	−1.4
Lunate	Stage I	1.0	−1.2	0.6
	Stage II	−0.8	1.2	−0.9
	Stage III	**−2.3**	1.2	−1.4
	Stage IV	**−3.5**	0.2	−1.9
	Stage V	**−3.6**	**9.0**	**−2.5**
Triquetrum	Stage I	−0.5	−1.1	0.7
	Stage II	−1.4	0.0	−0.2
	Stage III	1.0	0.5	−1.5
	Stage IV	−0.7	0.4	**−2.0**
	Stage V	**−5.2**	**7.1**	**−3.2**

*Larger, bold numbers indicate statistical significance from intact stage.
†Stage I: intact specimen; stage II: section of the proximal and dorsal LTq ligaments; stage III: complete section of all intrinsic lunotriquetral ligaments; stage IV: section of lunotriquetral and dorsal radiotriquetral ligaments; stage V: as in stage IV after cyclic loading.
Modified with permission from Ritt MJPF, Linscheid RL, Cooney WP, et al: The lunotriquetral joint: kinematic effects of sequential ligament sectioning, ligament repair, and arthrodesis. J Hand Surg [Am]. 1998; 23:432-445.

matic synovitis, may appear but not static deformity (dynamic VISI deformity arises only on cyclic loading).

- When the secondary lunotriquetral joint stabilizers (dorsal radiotriquetral and scaphotriquetral ligaments) are divided, a highly dysfunctional static VISI deformity arises.

REFERENCES

1. Dharap AS, Lutfi I, Abu-Hijleh MF: Population variation in the incidence of the medial (hamate) facet of the carpal bone lunate. Anthropol Anz. 2006; 64:59-65.
2. Galley I, Bain GI, McLean JM: Influence of lunate type on scaphoid kinematics. J Hand Surg. 2007; 32:842-847.
3. Mastella DJ, Zelouf DS: Anatomy of the lunotriquetral joint. Atlas Hand Clin. 2004; 9:1-6.
4. Mikic ZD: Arthrography of the wrist joint. J Bone Joint Surg Am. 1984; 66:371-378.
5. Ritt MJPF, Stuart PR, Berglund LJ, et al: Rotational stability of the carpus relative to the forearm. J Hand Surg [Am]. 1995; 20:305-311.
6. Wiesner L, Rumelhart C, Pham E, Comtet JJ: Experimentally induced ulno-carpal instability: a study on 13 cadaver wrists. J Hand Surg [Br]. 1996; 21:24-29.
7. Berger RA: Arthroscopic anatomy of the wrist and distal radioulnar joint. Hand Clin. 1999; 15:393-413.
8. Viegas SF, Yamaguchi S, Boyd NL, Patterson RM: The dorsal ligaments of the wrist: anatomy, mechanical properties, and function. J Hand Surg [Am]. 1999; 24:456-468.
9. Ambrose L, Posner MA: Lunate-triquetral and midcarpal joint instability. Hand Clin. 1992; 8:653-668.
10. Feipel V, Rooze M: The capsular ligaments of the wrist. Eur J Morphol. 1997; 35:87-94.
11. Garcia-Elias M: Soft-tissue anatomy and relationships about the distal ulna. Hand Clin. 1998; 14:165-176.
12. Hogikyan JV, Louis DS: Embryologic development and variations in the anatomy of the ulnocarpal ligamentous complex. J Hand Surg [Am]. 1992; 17:719-723.
13. Lichtman DM, Noble WH III, Alexander CE: Dynamic triquetrolunate instability: Case report. J Hand Surg [Am]. 1984; 9:185-188.
14. Lichtman DM, Schneider JR, Swafford AR, Mack GR: Ulnar midcarpal instability—clinical and laboratory analysis. J Hand Surg. 1981; 6:515-523.
15. Trumble TE, Bour CJ, Smith RJ, Glisson RR: Kinematics of the ulnar carpus related to the volar intercalated segment instability pattern. J Hand Surg [Am]. 1990; 15:384-392.
16. Weaver L, Tencer AF, Trumble TE: Tensions in the palmar ligaments of the wrist: I. The normal wrist. J Hand Surg [Am]. 1994; 19:464-474.
17. Mizuseki T, Ikuta Y: The dorsal carpal ligaments: their anatomy and function. J Hand Surg [Br]. 1989; 14:91-98.
18. Zancolli ER: Localized medial triquetral-hamate instability: anatomy and operative reconstruction-augmentation. Hand Clin. 2001; 17:83-96.
19. Ritt MJPF, Bishop AT, Berger RA, et al: Lunotriquetral ligament properties: a comparison of three anatomic subregions. J Hand Surg [Am]. 1998; 23:425-431.
20. Berger RA, Imaeda T, Berglund L, An KN: Constraint and material properties of the subregions of the scapholunate interosseous ligament. J Hand Surg [Am]. 1999; 24:953-962.
21. Hagert E, Garcia-Elias M, Forsgren S, Ljung BO: Immunohistochemical analysis of the wrist ligament innervation in relation to their structural composition. J Hand Surg [Am]. 2007; 32:30-36.

22. Kobayashi M, Berger RA, Nagy L, et al: Normal kinematics of carpal bones: a three-dimensional analysis of carpal bone motion relative to the radius. J Biomech. 1997; 30:787-793.

23. Berger RA, Crowninshield RD, Flatt AE: The three-dimensional rotational behaviors of the carpal bones. Clin Orthop Relat Res. 1982; 167:303-310.

24. De Lange A: A kinematic study of the human wrist joint. Thesis, University of Nijmegen, the Netherlands, 1987.

25. Horii E, Garcia-Elias M, An KN, et al: A kinematic study of lunotriquetral dissociations. J Hand Surg. 1991; 16:355-362.

26. Moojen TM, Snel JG, Ritt MJ, et al: In vivo analysis of carpal kinematics and comparative review of the literature. J Hand Surg. 2003; 28:81-87.

27. Moojen TM, Snel JG, Ritt MJ, et al: Three-dimensional carpal kinematics in vivo. Clin Biomech. 2002; 7:506-514.

28. Nakamura K, Beppu M, Patterson RM, et al: Motion analysis in two dimensions of radial-ulnar deviation of type I versus type II lunates. J Hand Surg. 2000; 25:877-888.

29. Galley I, Bain GI, McLean M: Influence of lunate type on scaphoid kinematics. J Hand Surg. 2007; 32:842-847.

30. Garcia-Elias M, Pitágoras T, Gilabert-Senar A: Relationship between joint laxity and radio-ulno-carpal joint morphology. J Hand Surg [Br]. 2003; 28:158-162.

31. Melone CP, Nathan R: Traumatic disruption of the triangular fibrocartilage complex: pathoanatomy. Clin Orthop Relat Res. 1992; 275:65-73.

32. Smith DK, Murray PM: Avulsion fractures of the volar aspect of triquetral bone of the wrist: a subtle sign of carpal ligament injury. AJR Am J Roentgenol 1996; 166:609-614.

33. Viegas SF, Patterson RM, Peterson PD, et al: Ulnar-sided perilunate instability: an anatomic and biomechanic study. J Hand Surg [Am]. 1990; 15:268-278.

34. Mayfield JK: Patterns of injury to carpal ligaments: a spectrum. Clin Orthop Relat Res. 1984; 187:36-42.

35. Leibovic SJ, Geissler WB: Treatment of complex intra-articular distal radius fractures. Orthop Clin North Am. 1994; 25:685-706.

36. Kolkin L: Wrist arthroscopy. Paper presented at the AAOS annual meeting, Washington, DC, 1992.

37. Geissler WB, Fernandez DL: Percutaneous and limited open reduction of the articular surface of the distal radius. J Orthop Trauma. 1991; 5:255-264.

38. Ritt MJPF, Linscheid RL, Cooney WP, et al: The lunotriquetral joint: kinematic effects of sequential ligament sectioning, ligament repair, and arthrodesis. J Hand Surg [Am]. 1998; 23:432-445.

39. Reagan DS, Linscheid RL, Dobyns JH: Lunotriquetral sprains. J Hand Surg [Am]. 1984; 9:502-514.

40. Li G, Rowen B, Tokunaga D, et al: Carpal kinematics of lunotriquetral dissociations. Biomed Sci Instrum. 1991; 27:273-281.

The Dorsal Ligaments of the Wrist

41

Naoya Yazaki, MD, Rita M. Patterson, PhD, and Steven F. Viegas, MD

Relatively little attention or significance had been given to the dorsal ligaments of the wrist until more recent studies described the anatomical and mechanical properties of the dorsal radiocarpal ligament and the dorsal intercarpal ligament of the wrist[1] and subregions of the scapholunate[2-4] and lunotriquetral[5] interosseous ligaments. An explanation of the functional design of the dorsal wrist ligament configuration was also offered recently.[6] Dorsal approaches to the wrist have also generally ignored the ligament anatomy. Even commonly referenced and used illustrations and diagrams of the dorsal ligaments of the wrist are anatomically inaccurate.[7,8]

The specific anatomy of the dorsal radiocarpal (DRC) and dorsal intercarpal (DIC) ligaments of the wrist has been reported, but relatively little attention or importance has been ascribed to these ligaments in the past. The DRC has also been referred to in the literature as the dorsal radiotriquetral and the dorsal radio-lunotriquetral ligament[9-11] (**Fig. 41-1**). The distal attachments of the DRC ligament have been described by a number of authors.[9-14] Some describe the ligament attaching onto the lunate,[9,11,12,14] others describe it attaching onto the lunate and the scaphoid,[10] whereas others report it attaching onto the lunate and capitate.[13] Berger and Garcia-Elias[9] described the DRC ligament attaching to the lunate and intermingling with fibers of the lunotriquetral ligament. The attachment of the DRC ligament

proximally was described by all of those authors as being proximally at the dorsal aspect of the radius and its distal attachment, at least in part, including the dorsal tubercle of the triquetrum.[9-14] A number of authors[9-14] have reported that the DRC ligament was found to consistently have an osseous attachment proximally, at the dorsal aspect of the radius, and, distally, at the dorsal tubercle of the triquetrum. It was also found to consistently have an osseous attachment onto the distal ulnar aspect of the dorsal lunate and dorsal portion of the lunotriquetral interosseous ligament, as described by Berger and Garcia-Elias[9] and Viegas and colleagues (**Fig. 41-2**). There were no attachments onto the scaphoid for the DRC ligament, but there was a dorsal branch or branches of the DRC ligament from the radius to the triquetrum that passed over, but did not attach to, the dorsal aspect of the proximal scaphoid, which may offer some dorsal support to the scaphoid in type II and III DRC ligaments as classified by Viegas

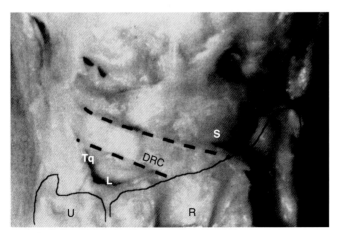

FIGURE 41-1 View of the dorsal radiocarpal ligament. DRC, dorsal radiocarpal ligament; R, radius; U, ulna; S, scaphoid; L, lunate; Tq, triquetrum. *(From Viegas SF, Yamaguchi S, Boyd NL, Patterson RM: The dorsal ligaments of the wrist: anatomy, mechanical properties and function. J Hand Surg [Am]. 1999; 24: 456-468, with permission.)*

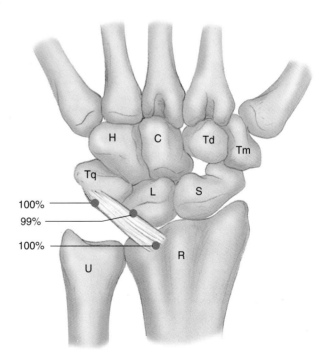

FIGURE 41-2 Anatomy and the osseous/ligamentous attachments of the DRC. *(From Viegas SF, Yamaguchi S, Boyd NL, Patterson RM: The dorsal ligaments of the wrist: anatomy, mechanical properties and function. J Hand Surg [Am]. 1999; 24: 456-468, with permission.)*

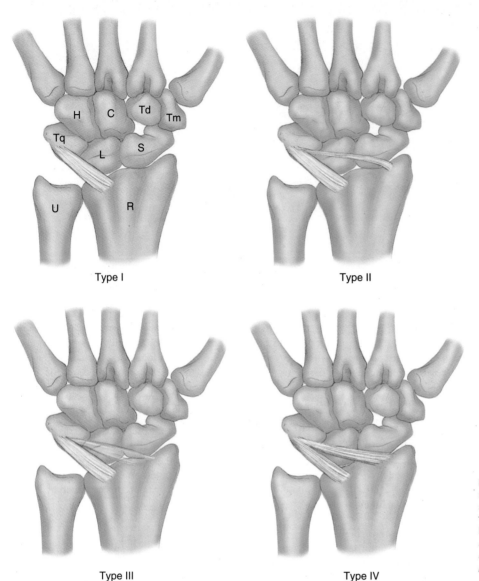

Type I   Type II

Type III   Type IV

FIGURE 41-3 The four types of the dorsal radiocarpal ligament. R, radius; U, ulna; S, scaphoid; L, lunate; Tq, triquetrum; Tm, trapezium; Td, trapezoid; C, capitate; H, hamate. *(From Viegas SF, Yamaguchi S, Boyd NL, Patterson RM: The dorsal ligaments of the wrist: anatomy, mechanical properties and function. J Hand Surg [Am]. 1999; 24: 456-468, with permission.)*

and colleagues.[6] This anatomical classification system (**Fig. 41-3**) was a modification of Mizuseki's classification[10] (**Fig. 41-4**) of the DRC ligament. Types I and IV are classified the same as his classification types 1 and 4. Mizuseki[10] described that type 2, in addition to type 1, fibers have thin deltoid fibers covering the scaphoid, converging onto the triquetrum. Viegas and colleagues[1] stated that these thin deltoid fibers were not detected in the dorsal structures.

Function of the DRC ligament has been proposed by a number of authors.[10,12,13,15] The DRC ligament has been attributed to maintaining the lunate in apposition to the distal radius.[16] The direction of the fibers of the DRC ligament implies that the triquetrum is prevented from ulnar translation by the DRC ligament and the volar radiolunotriquetral ligament.[10] The DRC ligament also functions as a stabilizer and pronator of the wrist. When the forearm pronates, the DRC ligament draws the attached carpus and hand passively into pronation.[12,13] Some biomechanic and kinematic studies have been performed on the DRC ligament. In a 1990 anatomical and biomechanical study by Viegas and colleagues[17] that was designed to better understand the patho-anatomy and pathomechanics involved in volar intercalated

segment instability (VISI) deformity of the wrist, it was found that the DRC must be attenuated or disrupted for a static VISI to develop. In fact, that study demonstrated that disruption of the DRC alone would result in a nondissociative static VISI deformity. Horii and associates,[18] in 1991, also confirmed the importance of the DRC in stabilizing the carpus and preventing a static VISI deformity.

A limited number of anatomical and biomechanical papers on the dorsal intercarpal ligament (**Fig. 41-5**) have been published. The osseous attachments of the DIC ligament have been described by a number of authors.[9,10,13,19,20] Mizuseki and Ikuta described the DIC as having attachments on the dorsal tubercle of the triquetrum and trapezoid, on the capitate, and at the dorsal rough groove of the scaphoid.[10] Berger and Garcia-Elias[9] reported that the DIC attached to the triquetrum and the scaphoid and, to a lesser degree, on the dorsal surface of the trapezoid. Savelberg and coworkers[19] found that the DIC attached to the triquetrum, the scaphoid, and the trapezium. Viegas and colleagues[6] also classified the various anatomical types of DIC ligaments and found that the DIC ligament was composed of two sections. One section consisted of a more distal section of generally thinner fibers

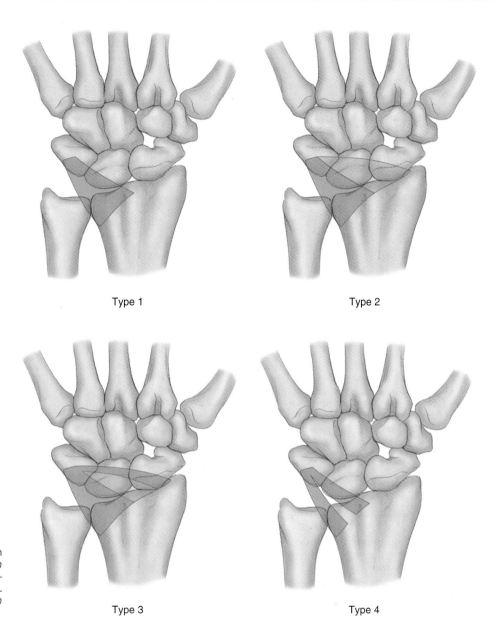

FIGURE 41-4 Mizuseki's classification of the dorsal radiocarpal ligament. *(From Mizuseki T, Ikuta Y: The dorsal carpal ligament: their anatomy and function. J Hand Surg [Br]. 1989; 14:91-98, with permission.)*

Type 1 Type 2 Type 3 Type 4

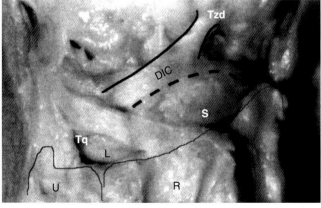

FIGURE 41-5 View of the dorsal intercarpal ligament. DIC, dorsal intercarpal ligament; R, radius; U, ulna; S, scaphoid; L, lunate; Tq, triquetrum; Td, trapezoid. *(From Viegas SF, Yamaguchi S, Boyd NL, Patterson RM: The dorsal ligaments of the wrist: anatomy, mechanical properties and function. J Hand Surg [Am]. 1999; 24: 456-468, with permission.)*

extending from the dorsal tubercle of the triquetrum to the dorsal aspect of the trapezoid or capitate. Another, more proximal thicker section extended from the dorsal tubercle of the triquetrum to the dorsal distal aspect of the lunate to the dorsal groove of the scaphoid and then to the proximal rim of the trapezium. They found that the attachment to the lunate of the DIC ligament was a consistent finding (**Fig. 41-6**). In 1997, Berger and Bishop described a surgical approach to the dorsal aspect of the wrist that they called a fiber-splitting or ligament-sparing approach.[21] The dorsal arm of this approach follows what Berger previously described as the dorsal scaphotriquetral ligament.[3] However, this would not spare the attachments of the DIC ligament, which Viegas and coworkers[6] have demonstrated attach to the scaphoid, lunate, and triquetrum.

Smith[20] classified the DIC ligament using three-dimensional Fourier transform magnetic resonance imaging techniques. His classification is similar to that of Viegas and colleagues[6] (**Fig. 41-7**), but the reported incidence of each type was different. Smith[20] reported the incidence of three types of DIC ligaments—

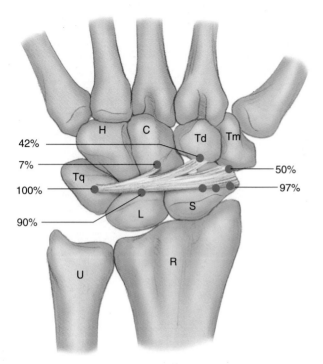

FIGURE 41-6 Anatomy and the osseous/ligamentous attachments of the DIC. *(From Viegas SF, Yamaguchi S, Boyd NL, Patterson RM: The dorsal ligaments of the wrist: anatomy, mechanical properties and function. J Hand Surg [Am]. 1999; 24: 456-468, with permission.)*

stated that the scaphotriquetral ligament (proximal DIC fibers) did have an important role in the transverse stabilization of the proximal carpal row.

It can be difficult to accurately delineate the anatomy and measure the dimensions of the ligaments of the wrist. Viegas and colleagues[6] used a combination of meticulous dissections of both fresh and embalmed specimens to complete the task of detailing the ligament anatomy. That, in combination with observations from previous anatomical and biomechanical studies, has afforded the opportunity to gain some insight into the anatomy and function of the ligaments of the wrist. Despite this, the task of accurately detailing where one structure ends and another begins, particularly in the presence of the normal variability of human anatomy, remains challenging and may offer a reason for some of the variability in the literature.

Recently, Nagao and associates[22] quantified and visually depicted the three-dimensional attachment sites of the carpal ligaments using a combination of detailed dissection, computed tomographic (CT) imaging, and a three-dimensional digitization technique. They visually demonstrated that the DIC ligament attaches to the dorsal aspect of scaphoid, lunate, and triquetrum and how the DIC ligament partially overlaps with portions of the dorsal scapholunate interosseous (SLIO) and lunotriquetral interosseous (LTIO) ligaments (**Fig. 41-8**).

The mechanical properties of the dorsal ligaments of the wrist have been reported.[16,19] The strongest ligaments are the palmar radiotriquetral ligament (210 N) and the DRC ligament (240 N).[16] Only the DRC ligament and palmar radiocapitate ligament appear to have a relatively high Young's modulus, about 93 megapascal (Mpa) and 83 Mpa, respectively.[19] The DIC ligament, on average, has a Young's modulus of 47.5 Mpa.[19] Viegas and colleagues[6] suggest that the DRC and DIC ligaments collectively deliver indirect dorsal radioscaphoid stability. They also explain that the combined mechanical properties of the DIC and the dorsal SLIO ligaments have mechanical strength (162.4 ± 64.7 N) comparable with the DRC (143.3 ± 41.5 N).

Dorsal ligamentous structures are important in maintaining carpal stability and alignment and in affording normal carpal kinematics, in addition to playing an important role in preventing

type 1, 14%; type 2, 44%; and type 3, 38%—which is comparable to Viegas and colleagues'[1] type C, 25.6%; type A, 30.0%; and type B, 44.4%, respectively. Smith[20] believed that the main portion of the DIC ligament consisted of deep fibers, whereas the superficial fibers were very thin and were not considered to be an important stabilizer of the carpus. Mizuseki and Ikuta[10] believed that the DIC ligament was always thin and seemed to be of little anatomical importance. Fahrer[13] believed the DIC ligament was much less developed than the palmar structures. Berger and Garcia-Elias[9]

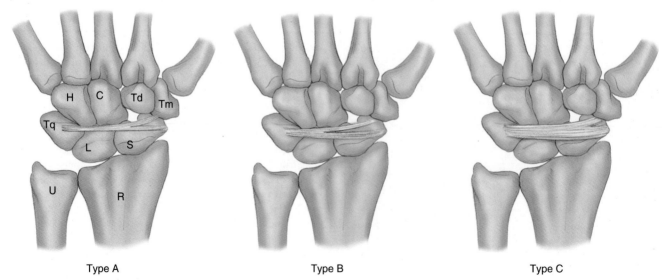

|Type A|Type B|Type C|

FIGURE 41-7 The three types of the dorsal intercarpal ligament. R, radius; U, ulna; S, scaphoid; L, lunate; Tq, triquetrum; Tm, trapezium; Td, trapezoid; C, capitate; H, hamate. *(From Viegas SF, Yamaguchi S, Boyd NL, Patterson RM: The dorsal ligaments of the wrist: anatomy, mechanical properties and function. J Hand Surg [Am]. 1999; 24: 456-468, with permission.)*

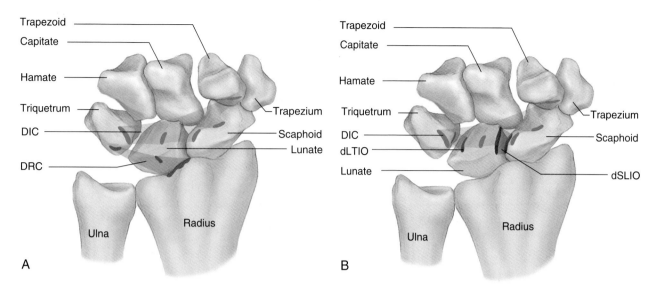

FIGURE 41-8 A and **B,** A dorsal view of the three-dimensional models of a left wrist joint. *Colored areas* indicate ligament attachment and *transparent colored areas* show the path of the ligament(s). DRC, dorsal radiocarpal ligament; DIC, dorsal intercarpal ligament; dSLIO, dorsal portion of the scapholunate interosseous ligament; dLTIO, dorsal portion of the lunatotriquetral interosseous ligament.

the loss of integrity of the dorsal complex and the development of VISI deformities and in dorsal intercalated segment instability (DISI), according to some reports.[1,6]

The DRC and DIC ligaments (along with the dorsal intercarpal interosseous ligaments of the proximal carpal row) form a construct that is elegant in its biomechanical design and is complex, yet simple, in its way of delivering indirect dorsal stabilization to the scaphoid at its proximal pole. The DRC and the DIC (along with the dorsal intercarpal interosseous ligaments of the proximal carpal row) together act effectively as a dorsal radioscaphoid ligament that has the ability to vary its length by changing the angle between the two arms of the lateral "V" construct formed by the DRC and DIC ligaments, while maintaining its stabilizing effect (**Fig. 41-9**). This lateral "V" configuration of the DRC and DIC construct allows dorsal stability of the proximal pole of the scaphoid while still allowing a threefold increase in the distance between the DRC radial attachment and the DIC

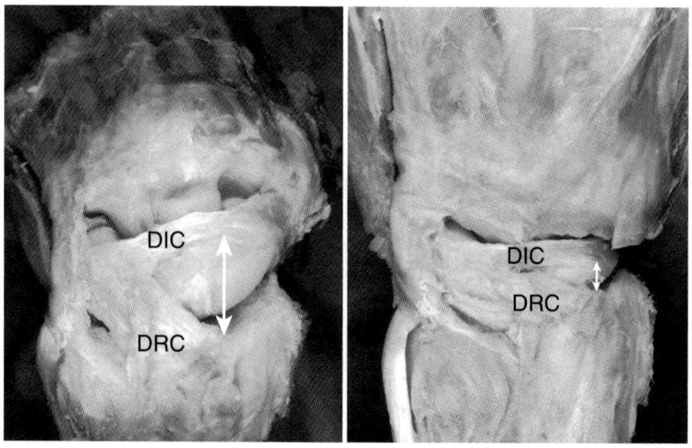

scaphoid attachment (**Fig. 41-10**). This unique design allows dorsal stability of the scaphoid throughout the range of motion of the wrist, which would require changes in the length of a dorsal radioscaphoid ligament, if one existed or could be surgically constructed, far greater than any single fixed ligament could accommodate. To maintain the dorsal stability of the scaphoid, the DRC and the individual intercarpal components or linkages of the proximal carpal row and the DIC ligament have to maintain their integrity.

Viegas and colleagues[6] report that, in the clinical setting, they have observed scapholunate dissociations in which the DIC ligament is partially (**Fig. 41-11**) or completely avulsed off the scaphoid. It has also been observed clinically that the dorsal SLIO and the DIC ligaments are most often avulsed off the scaphoid, rather than off the lunate. Pigeau and associates,[23] using arthroscopy and CT, also found the dorsal SLIO ligament was most commonly avulsed off the scaphoid in cases of scapholunate dissociations. This coincides with the findings of the biomechanical portion of the study by Viegas and colleagues[1] in which the location of failure of the DIC and the dorsal SLIO ligaments, when tested in combination, was also at the scaphoid. In some cases, the DIC has also been avulsed from its lunate attachment (**Fig. 41-12**), in which case the surgical repair/reconstruction should also include reattachment or reconstruction of the DIC to both the scaphoid and the lunate (**Fig. 41-13**). It is very important to recognize the combined role and strength of the dorsal component of the SLIO ligament complex and the DIC ligament in the function and strength of the scaphoid and lunate. In addition, the repair or reconstruction must reestablish the DIC attachments at the scaphoid and the lunate, in addition to its other attachments. Different authors[6,8,17] have reported using the DIC ligament as part of the surgical repair/reconstruction in the treatment of a scapholunate dissociation. Garcia-Elias and associates have described a method of reconstructing the distal arm of the lateral "V" construct with a portion of the flexor carpi radialis tendon.[24]

Previous studies of the SLIO and the LTIO ligaments have better detailed the histological and mechanical properties of the

FIGURE 41-9 Lateral "V" configuration of the DRC and DIC ligament. The distance between the osseous attachments of the DRC and DIC ligaments (*arrow*) in wrist flexion is approximately three times larger than that in extension.

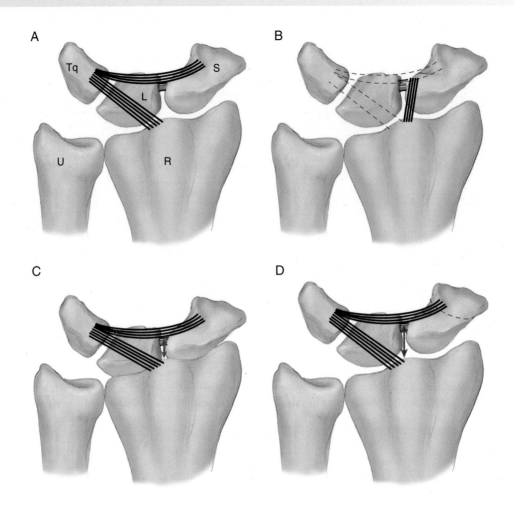

FIGURE 41-10 A, Lateral "V" configuration of the dorsal radiocarpal (*parallel lines*) and the dorsal intercarpal ligaments (*curved lines*) that function as (**B**) a dorsal radioscaphoid ligament (*parallel black lines*) while allowing (**C**) the linear dimensions (*arrow*) from the distal radius to the scaphoid to change as much as three times its length from wrist extension where the lateral V of the DRC/DIC forms a small angle to (**D**) wrist flexion where the lateral V of the DRC/DIC forms a large angle. *(From Viegas SF, Yamaguchi S, Boyd NL, Patterson RM: The dorsal ligaments of the wrist: anatomy, mechanical properties and function. J Hand Surg [Am]. 1999; 24: 456-468, with permission.)*

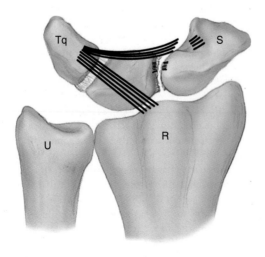

FIGURE 41-11 Disruption of the membranous and dorsal components of the scapholunate interosseous ligament and the portion of the dorsal intercarpal ligament that attaches to the dorsal groove of the scaphoid. This injury pattern can often be found in patients with DISI injuries. *Parallel gray lines,* DRC ligament; *black curved lines,* DIC ligament. *(From Viegas SF, Yamaguchi S, Boyd NL, Patterson RM: The dorsal ligaments of the wrist: anatomy, mechanical properties and function. J Hand Surg [Am]. 1999; 24: 456-468, with permission.)*

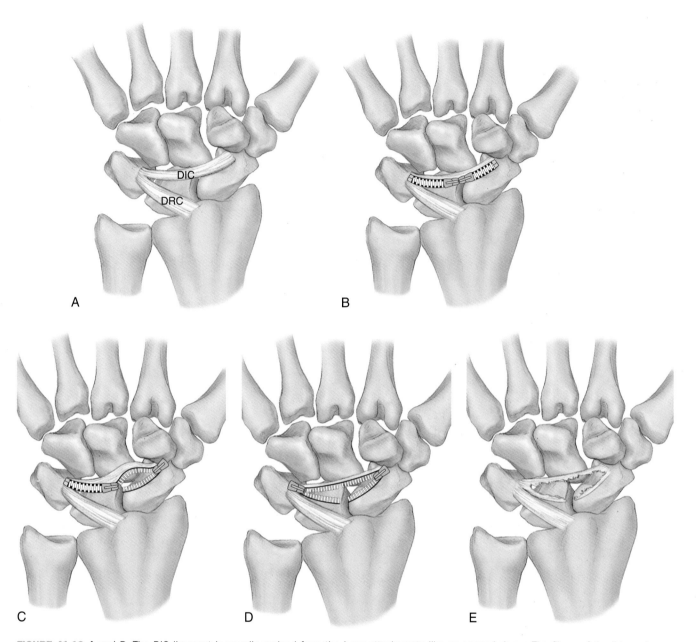

FIGURE 41-12 A and **B,** The DIC ligament is usually avulsed from the bony attachments like an opened zipper. The fibers of the ligaments are sometimes split and rarely disrupted. **C,** When the DIC ligament is detached from the proximal aspect of the scaphoid, but remains attached to the lunate, the scaphoid and lunate may be unstable in the loaded condition, but the scapholunate dissociation may not be apparent in an unloaded condition. **D** and **E,** Then avulsion of the ligament from the lunate will lead to a static scapholunate dissociation. Hence, in the treatment of acute scapholunate dissociation, reattachment of the DIC ligament is required, in addition to that of the SLIO ligament.

subregions of the interosseous ligaments.[2-4] Both the LTIO and the SLIO ligaments have been shown by Berger and associates[2-4] to have three subregions, with the central or proximal portions of both having a membranous portion that is less substantial, both histologically and mechanically, than the dorsal or volar components (**Fig. 41-14**). This may offer additional information to explain the mobility between the bones of the proximal carpal row, which allows for greater intercarpal motion within the proximal carpal row than within the distal carpal row. This may allow the dorsal subregions of the SLIO and the LTIO ligaments to be considered functionally as part of the dorsal ligaments and the volar subregions of the SLIO and the LTIO ligaments to be considered a part of the volar ligaments.

Mitsuyasu and coworkers[25] found that complete disruption of the scaphoid from the lunate when the lunate still has an intact LTIO, and the DIC attachments to the lunate and the triquetrum are also intact, results in dynamic scapholunate instability (SLI). However, a wrist will not develop a static SLI with a DISI deformity until the DIC ligament is attenuated and/or disrupted from the lunate (**Fig. 41-15**). These results suggest that the treatment of SLI should address not only the SLIO ligament but also the DIC ligament at both its scaphoid and lunate attachments. Mitsuyasu and coworkers[25] suggested that the role of the DIC ligament and the effect of its partial or complete disruption at the scaphoid and the lunate may be a key component in the anatomical difference between a dynamic and a static SLI with DISI. A

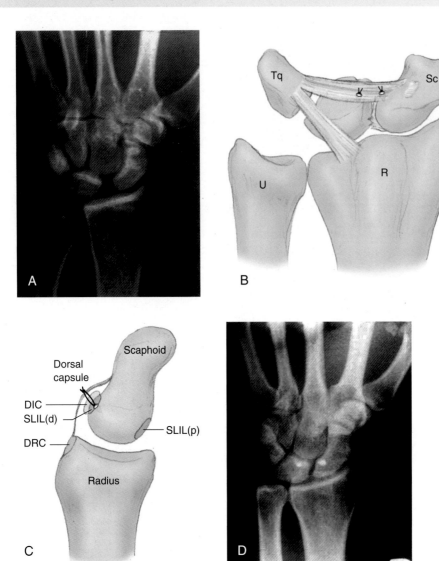

FIGURE 41-13 **A,** Radiograph of a 31-year-old left-handed surgeon's left wrist, injured in a fall he sustained while skating. He developed a painful, symptomatic scapholunate instability. **B,** Reconstruction of the dorsal complex and reestablishment of the indirect dorsal stability of the scaphoid using suture anchors to reattach the DIC to the lunate and to reattach the DIC and the dorsal component of the scapholunate interosseous ligament to the scaphoid from which it is often found to be avulsed in DISI injuries. **C,** Lateral view of a scaphoid with the suture anchor in the scaphoid showing the suture fixing first the dSLIL and DIC and then using the same suture to repair the capsule. **D,** Postoperative image of the patient in **A** who underwent the same type of repair/reconstruction. *(From Viegas SF, Yamaguchi S, Boyd NL, Patterson RM: The dorsal ligaments of the wrist: anatomy, mechanical properties and function. J Hand Surg [Am]. 1999; 24: 456-468, with permission.)*

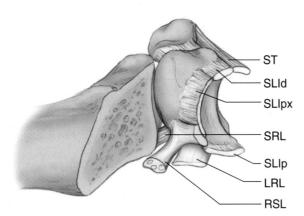

FIGURE 41-14 The three subregions of the scapholunate interosseous ligament. LRL, long radiolunate ligament; SRL, short radiolunate ligament; three subregions of the scapholunate interosseous ligament (SLId, dorsal subregion; SLIpx, proximal subregion; SLIp, palmar subregion); RSL, radioscapholunate ligament; ST, scaphotriquetral ligament. *(From Berger RA, Imeada T, Berglund T, An KN. Constraint and material properties of the subregions of the scapholunate interosseous ligament. J Hand Surg [Am]. 1999; 24: 953–962, with permission.)*

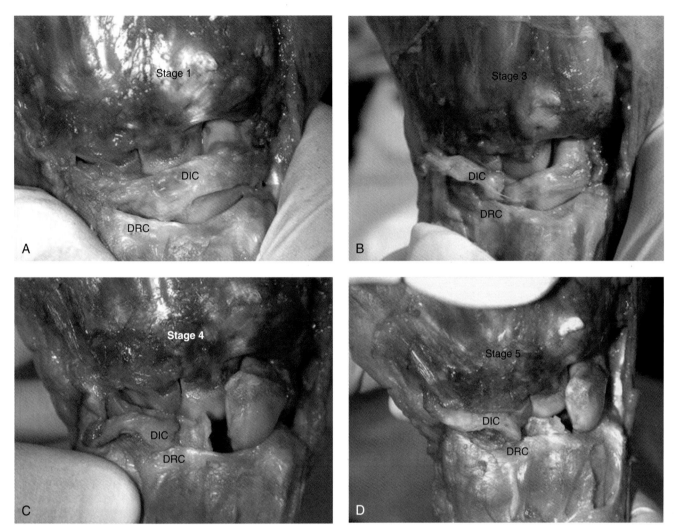

FIGURE 41-15 Mitsuyasu and associates designed their study to clarify the pathomechanics of the scapholunate instability. Six stages of increasing instability were developed by sectioning progressively the following structures through a dorsal capsular incision. **A,** Stage 1: Only capsulectomy was performed. Stage 2: The palmar and membranous portions of the SLIO ligament were sectioned. **B,** Stage 3: The DIC ligament was detached from its attachment on the scaphoid and trapezium. **C,** Stage 4: The dorsal portion of the SLIO ligament was sectioned but the DIC ligament was still attached to the lunate; the resulting carpal instability showed a flexed posture of the scaphoid and a widened scapholunate gap, but only when loaded. **D,** Stage 5: The DIC ligament was detached from its attachment on the lunate. The scaphoid flexion, the lunate extension, and the widening of the scapholunate interval occurred even in unloaded conditions. Stage 6: The LTIO ligament was completely sectioned. There was no apparent effect or further destabilization of the scaphoid or lunate. *(From Mitsuyasu H, Patterson RM, Shah MA, et al: The role of the dorsal intercarpal ligament in dynamic and static scapholunate instability. J Hand Surg [Am]. 2004; 29:279-288, with permission.)*

possible explanation of why SLI can progress from a dynamic to a static instability with disruption or avulsion of the DIC off the lunate, even when all three subregions of the LTIO are intact, is because, as Ritt and colleagues[5] have described, the dorsal subregion of the LTIO is weaker and less restrictive than the volar subregion. This would mean that the loss of the additional dorsal stability between the triquetrum and lunate that the DIC ligament affords would allow the lunate to assume a slightly extended posture, rotating at the more constraining volar LTIO subregion, subsequently allowing the capitate to further load the lunate into even more extension, increase the scapholunate gap, and shift the scaphoid into a flexed, dorsally subluxed posture.

New and more detailed information on the DRC and the DIC ligaments offers an explanation of the unique way that they act together, in their lateral "V" design, to deliver indirect dorsal stability with relative freedom of motion. This is a new perspective on the dorsal ligaments of the wrist that takes a more global view of how their anatomy and function act together. The information

appears to suggest that the dorsal ligaments of the wrist play a greater and more important role in carpal stability and carpal kinematics than was previously recognized. The information on the DIC ligament also better explains the anatomical progression of scapholunate instability from the clinically recognized dynamic to static scapholunate carpal instability. It is hoped this information will provide a better understanding of carpal kinetics and kinematics and afford a better understanding of the pathomechanics in various wrist injuries, including DISI and VISI injuries, and the repair or reconstruction needed to treat them.

ACKNOWLEDGMENTS

The authors gratefully acknowledge Kristi Overgaard for her editorial assistance and Randal Morris for his assistance with Figure 41-12, which was illustrated by Dr. Steven Viegas. This chapter was modified from Viegas SF: The dorsal ligaments of the wrist. Hand Clin. 2001; 17:65-75 with permission.

REFERENCES

1. Viegas SF, Patterson RM, Peterson PD, et al: Ulnar-sided perilunate instability: an anatomic and biomechanic study. J Hand Surg [Am]. 1990; 15:268-278.

2. Berger RA: The gross and histologic anatomy of the scapholunate interosseous ligament. J Hand Surg [Am]. 1996; 21:170-178.

3. Berger RA: The ligaments of the wrist: a current overview of anatomy with considerations of their potential functions. Hand Clin. 1997; 13:63-82.

4. Berger RA, Imeada T, Berglund LJ, An KN: Constraint and material properties of the subregions of the scapholunate interosseous ligament. J Hand Surg [Am]. 1999; 24:953-962.

5. Ritt MJ, Bishop AT, Berger RA, et al: Lunotriquetral ligament properties: a comparison of three anatomic subregions. J Hand Surg [Am]. 1998; 23:425-431.

6. Viegas SF, Yamaguchi S, Boyd NL, Patterson RM: The dorsal ligaments of the wrist: anatomy, mechanical properties and function. J Hand Surg [Am]. 1999; 24:456-468.

7. Regional Review Course in Hand Surgery. Rosemont, IL: American Society of Surgery of the Hand. 1985; 12:12-15.

8. Slater RR, Szabo RM, Bay BK, Laubach J: Dorsal intercarpal ligament capsulodesis for scapholunate dissociation: biomechanical analysis in a cadaver model. J Hand Surg [Am]. 1999; 24:232-239.

9. Berger RA, Garcia-Elias M: General anatomy of the wrist. In An KN, Berger RA, Cooney WP, eds: Biomechanics of the Wrist Joint. New York, Springer-Verlag, 1991; 1-22.

10. Mizuseki T, Ikuta Y: The dorsal carpal ligaments: their anatomy and function. J Hand Surg [Br]. 1989; 14:91-98.

11. Taleisnik J: The ligaments of the wrist. J Hand Surg. 1976; 1:110-118.

12. Bogumill GP: Anatomy of the wrist. In Lichtman DM, ed: The Wrist and Its Disorders. Philadelphia: WB Saunders, 1988; 14-26.

13. Fahrer M: Introduction to the anatomy of the wrist. In Tubiana R, ed: The Hand. Philadelphia: WB Saunders, 1981; 130-135.

14. Kaplan EB, Taleisnik J: The wrist. In Spinner M, ed: Kaplan's Functional and Surgical Anatomy of the Hand. 3rd ed. Philadelphia: JB Lippincott, 1984; 154-178.

15. Mayfield JK: Wrist ligaments: anatomy and pathogenesis of carpal instability. Orthop Clin North Am. 1984; 15:209-216.

16. Mayfield JK, Williams WJ: Biomechanical properties of human carpal ligaments. Orthop Trans. 1979; 3:143-144.

17. Viegas SF: Ligamentous repair following acute scapholunate dissociation. In Gelberman RH, ed: Master Techniques in Orthopaedic Surgery; The Wrist. 2nd ed. New York: Lippincott–Raven, 2000; 163-175.

18. Horii E, Garcia EM, An KN, et al: A kinematic study of luno-triquetral dissociations. J Hand Surg [Am]. 1991; 16: 355-362.

19. Savelberg HH, Kooloos JG, Huiskes R, Kauer JM: Stiffness of the ligaments of the human wrist joint. J Biomech. 1992; 25:369-376.

20. Smith DK: Dorsal carpal ligaments of the wrist: normal appearance on multiplanar reconstructions of three-dimensional Fourier transform MR imaging. AJR Am J Roentgenol. 1993; 161:119-125.

21. Berger RA, Bishop AT: A fiber-splitting capsulotomy technique for dorsal exposure of the wrist. Tech Hand Up Extrem Surg. 1997; 1:2-10.

22. Nagao S, Patterson RM, Buford WL Jr, et al: Three-dimensional description of ligametous attachments around the lunate. J Hand Surg [Am]. 2005; 30:685-692.

23. Pigeau I, Sokolow C, Romano S, Saffar P: Evaluation of scapho-lunate ligament by arthro-CT scan. Presented at the 54th annual meeting of the American Society of Surgery of the Hand in Boston, Massachusetts, September 4, 1999.

24. Garcia-Elias M, Lluch AL, Stanley JK: Three-ligament tenodesis for the treatment of scapholunate dissociation: indications and surgical technique. J Hand Surg [Am]. 2006; 31:125-134.

25. Mitsuyasu H, Patterson RM, Shah MA, et al: The role of the dorsal intercarpal ligament in dynamic and static scapholunate instability. J Hand Surg [Am]. 2004; 29:279-288.

Midcarpal Instability

42

Carlos Heras-Palou, MD

The first description of a "snapping wrist," diagnosed as anterior midcarpal subluxation,[1] was recorded in 1934, although "dorsal luxation of the capitate" had been presented in a congress in Paris in 1919. The article by Lichtman and colleagues[2] in 1981 brought this particular condition to the attention of orthopaedists. Of all the forms of carpal instability, midcarpal instability (MCI) has been the most confusing. The two main reasons for this are that MCI is a mixed bag of conditions, and that their pathophysiology is not well understood. The management of MCI remains controversial. **Table 42-1** provides a summary of MCI.

The term MCI covers a range of conditions characterized by a painful clunk, usually felt in ulnar deviation of the wrist. It has been suggested that the term "instability of the proximal carpal row" would be a more accurate description[3] because the mechanical problem is a carpal instability nondissociative, affecting the radiocarpal or the midcarpal joints or both. The scaphoid, lunate, and triquetrum move like one unit, but not in a predictable, smooth manner.

Most patients with MCI respond to nonoperative treatment. Combinations of immobilization, splints, anti-inflammatories, activity modification, and exercise have been prescribed with diverse success. Surgical treatment suggested for MCI includes soft tissue stabilizations, limited carpal arthrodesis, corrective osteotomies, and arthroscopic thermal capsulorrhaphy. The role of proprioception in carpal instability is starting to be recognized, but is not yet fully understood.

What Causes the Clunk?

Clunking of the wrist can be caused by congenital laxity of the wrist ligaments, bone or joint dysplasia, lunotriquetral injury, distal radius malunion, or insufficiency of the extrinsic ligament affecting the radiocarpal or the midcarpal joint or both. In a normal wrist, during radial deviation, the proximal carpal row goes into flexion, and during ulnar deviation it extends, in a smooth transition (**Fig. 42-1A**). In a wrist with palmar MCI, there is palmar subluxation of the capitate head with the wrist in radial deviation in the midcarpal joint, and the proximal carpal row remains flexed until terminal ulnar deviation, at which time it is suddenly forced into extension. This sudden extension causes the so-called catch-up clunk felt by the patient and often clearly seen and heard by observers (**Fig. 42-1B**).

Classification of Midcarpal Instability

Lichtman and Wroten[4] proposed a classification of MCI that includes intrinsic MCI, which is caused by ligamentous insufficiency, and extrinsic MCI, secondary to distal radius fractures. Intrinsic MCI is subdivided further into palmar, dorsal, and combined, depending on the direction of displacement. This classification is helpful in understanding the spectrum of conditions that constitute MCI, and in defining the boundaries between them.

Caputo and coworkers[5] believe that only conditions with a static or dynamic volar intercalated segment instability (VISI) of the proximal carpal row constitute MCI. Their definition of MCI is more restrictive than generally accepted. These authors have classified MCI depending on whether the cause of the instability lies on the ulnar side or on the radial side of the wrist. Ulnar-sided MCI corresponds to palmar MCI without significant symptoms (type I) or with significant symptoms (type II). Radial-sided MCI manifests with a rotary subluxation of the scaphoid, with either an intact scapholunate ligament (type III) or a scapholunate ligament disruption (type IV).

Palmar Midcarpal Instability

Patients with palmar MCI present with a painful clunk of the wrist, often with a history of trivial injury or no trauma at all. Sometimes they can demonstrate the clunk voluntarily "to the amusement of friends, and consternation of doctors."[6] In the author's experience, this is the most common form of MCI.

Pathomechanics of Palmar Midcarpal Instability

Palmar MCI is considered to be caused by insufficiency of some of the extrinsic wrist ligaments. Ligaments do not work in isolation, but in a synergistic manner, where groups of ligaments resist certain forces. The extrinsic ligaments in the wrist form an antisupination sling and an antipronation sling, both running around the carpus in opposite directions (**Fig. 42-2A**).

On the volar aspect of the wrist, the ligaments are organized in the shape of a proximal "V" and a distal "V." The proximal "V" is formed by the ligaments from the radius to the lunate and from the volar band of the triangular fibrocartilage complex to the lunate. The distal "V," also called the arcuate ligament, is formed mainly by the radiocapitate and scaphocapitate ligaments on the radial side, and the ulnotriquetral, ulnocapitate, triquetrohamate, and triquetrocapitate ligaments, which are also known as the triquetrohamate capitate ligament, on the ulnar side. Between the two "Vs" there is the loose "space of Poirier."

On the ulnar side of the wrist, the dorsal radiotriquetral, which is also known as the dorsal radiocarpal ligament, and the volar triquetrohamate capitate ligaments prevent the proximal carpal row from falling into a VISI alignment. The ligaments act as a sling from the dorsum of the radius, around the triquetrum, and onto the volar aspect of the capitate. This has an antisupination action on the wrist (**Fig. 42-2B**). If these ligaments fail, the

417

TABLE 42-1 Summary Table for Midcarpal Instability (MCI)*

	Ligaments Involved	Static Alignment	Fluoroscopy	Conservative Treatment	Operative Treatment
Palmar MCI (ulnar sided)	Dorsal rad-triq Volar triq-cap Volar triq-ham	VISI	"Clunk" seen	Splint Strengthen FCU and hypothenar	ECRL tenodesis
Palmar MCI (radial sided)	Volar rad-cap Dorsal scaph-triq Volar scaph-cap	VISI	"Clunk" seen STT opens	Strengthen FCR	FCR tenodesis Modified Brunelli
Dorsal MCI	Volar radiocarpal ligaments	Normal	Often clunk, dorsal displacement	Activity modification and strengthening	Tighten space of Poirier
Combined MCI	Volar and dorsal extrinsic ligaments	VISI	Clunk and dorsal displacement Radiocarpal opens	Strengthen FCR, FCU, and hypothenar	Radiolunate arthrodesis
Extrinsic MCI	Malunion radius	DISI	Often clunk, dorsal displacement	Splint	Corrective osteotomy of distal radius

*In each of the groups there is a wide spectrum of severity. The treatment of midcarpal instability is controversial. The treatments in this table are the author's recommendation. DISI, dorsal intercalated segment instability; ECRL, extensor carpi radialis longus; FCR, flexor carpi radialis; FCU, flexor carpi ulnaris; STT, scaphotrapeziotrapezoid; VISI, volar intercalated segment instability.

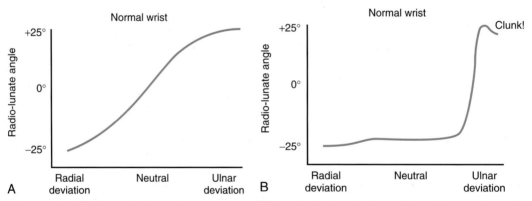

FIGURE 42-1 **A,** In a normal wrist, the proximal carpal row moves smoothly from flexion to extension, as the wrist moves from radial to ulnar deviation. **B,** In palmar midcarpal instability, the proximal row remains flexed until nearly the extreme of ulnar deviation, when it suddenly jumps into extension, causing a catch-up clunk.

carpus has a tendency to fall into a VISI alignment and into intercarpal supination. The proximal row loses its normal transition from flexion to extension during ulnar deviation of the wrist, causing a clunk.

The distal scaphoid has ligaments to the capitate and to the trapezium. If these ligaments fail, there is a tendency for the scaphoid to flex and to take with it the lunate and the triquetrum, causing a VISI alignment. There is a ligamentous sling, which starts with the volar radiocapitate ligament, follows around the triquetrum, connects to the dorsal scaphotriquetral ligament, and goes around the scaphoid ending with the volar scaphocapitate ligament (**Fig. 42-2C**). This sling goes round the wrist causing an antipronation effect. Failure of this mechanism may cause flexion of the proximal row, starting on the radial side, and a tendency toward intercarpal pronation. This would cause radial-sided palmar midcarpal instability.

Several studies have attempted to reproduce carpal instability in cadaver models. Biomechanical studies[2] reported that sectioning the dorsal radiotriquetral and the triquetrohamate portion of the triquetrohamate capitate ligament did not produce frank instability or a clunk. Further division of the triquetrocapitate portion of the triquetrohamate capitate ligament produced a clunk similar, but not identical, to clunks observed in patients. Other studies have shown that sectioning either the ulnar arm of the distal volar "V" ligaments or the dorsal radiotriquetral ligament can produce a VISI and mechanical changes typical of palmar MCI.[7,8]

Assessment of Palmar Midcarpal Instability

The symptoms of a patient presenting with a clunking wrist range from none at all to severe. Looking at the wrist from the ulnar side, a palmar sag can be seen, which reduces with ulnar deviation

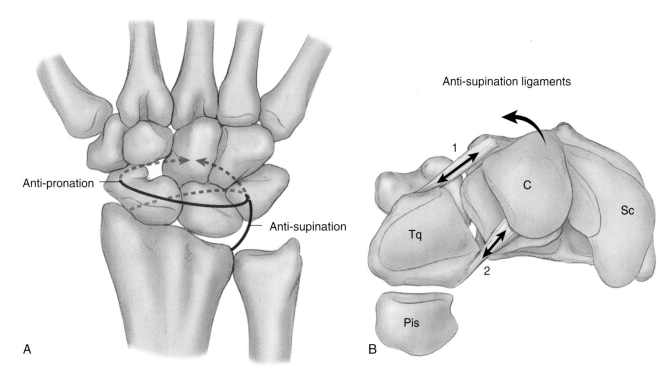

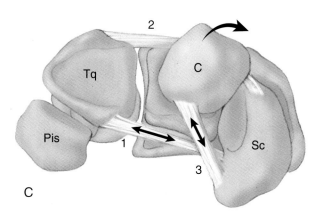

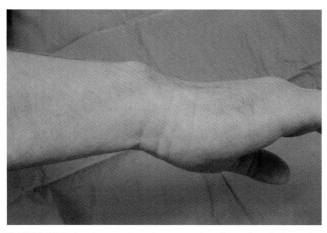

FIGURE 42-2 **A,** The ligaments in the wrist form two slings that go around the carpus in opposite directions, providing stability in all positions of the range of movement. **B,** The antisupination sling is formed by the dorsal radiotriquetral ligament (*1*) and the volar triquetrohamate and triquetrocapitate (*2*). **C,** The antipronation sling is formed by the volar radiocapitate ligament (*1*) and its connections to the triquetrum, dorsal triquetroscaphoid (*2*), and volar scaphoid capitate (*3*). *(Courtesy of Dr. Marc Garcia-Elias.)*

of the wrist (**Fig. 42-3**). The midcarpal shift test, described by Lichtman,[2] reproduces the patient's wrist instability. This test is done by placing the patient's wrist in neutral with the forearm pronated. A palmar force is applied to the hand at the level of the distal capitate. The wrist is simultaneously loaded axially and deviated ulnarly. The test is positive if a painful clunk occurs that reproduces the patient's symptoms.

Plain radiographs generally show a VISI pattern, but no dissociation between the bones of the proximal carpal row (**Fig. 42-4**). If there is a dissociation between lunate and triquetrum, this is a type of carpal instability dissociative and not MCI (**Fig. 42-5**).

Fluoroscopy is diagnostic, and it is useful to record it so that radiation exposure can be minimized. Recording also allows the examiner to watch the video as many times as it takes to understand the mechanical problem, and it provides a permanent record of the most important diagnostic test.

On a mini-C-arm, a lateral view of radioulnar deviation of the wrist shows the typical jump of the proximal row from flexion to

FIGURE 42-3 A palmar sag can be seen, when the carpus is in a volar intercalated segment instability alignment, in patients with midcarpal instability.

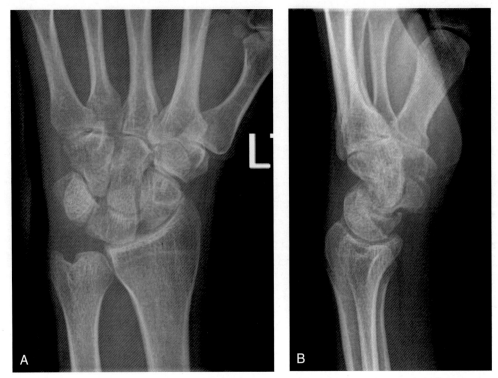

FIGURE 42-4 A and **B**, Plain radiographs show a volar intercalated segment instability alignment of the carpus. There is no dissociation. This is typical of palmar or combined midcarpal instability.

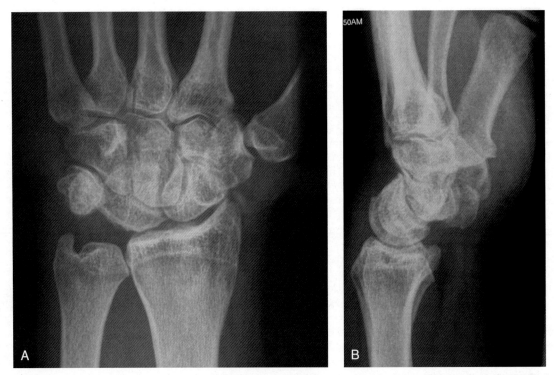

FIGURE 42-5 A and **B**, In this case, there is a volar intercalated segment instability alignment, but also a dissociation between the lunate and triquetrum. This is not midcarpal instability; it is a static lunotriquetral instability.

extension. The examiner should perform a "passive palmar displacement" and a "passive dorsal displacement" of the wrist, and observe if there is displacement and opening at either joint. This maneuver establishes if the laxity is at the midcarpal joint or radiocarpal or both. On the posteroanterior view, radioulnar deviation needs to be observed, to rule out any scapholunate or lunotriquetral dissociation, and to look for any opening of the scaphotrapeziotrapezoid (STT) joint, which would indicate laxity of the ligaments on the radial side of the wrist.

The main role of arthroscopy in the assessment of MCI is to exclude other pathology, in particular lunotriquetral dissociation, and to assess the joint surfaces before reconstructive surgery. It is easy to perform arthroscopy of a wrist with MCI because there is a lot of space owing to the laxity of the joint, and sometimes there is synovitis. The synovitis is most often found on the dorsal aspect of the radiocarpal and the midcarpal joints. No particular ligaments seem to be injured on inspection. In long-standing cases, there may be some degenerative changes of the proximal lunate or the proximal hamate.

Treatment of Palmar Midcarpal Instability

Conservative treatment is often successful, particularly in milder cases of palmar MCI. Training of the flexor carpi ulnaris and the hypothenar muscles with isometric contractures can improve symptoms. These exercises generate a dorsally directed force toward the triquetrum, through the pisiform, which may support the ulnar side of the wrist and decrease instability. Attempts to train proprioception and gain strength using hand-held gyroscopes (Powerball, NSD, South Africa) have helped in some patients.

Arthroscopic thermal capsulorrhaphy has been used for MCI with promising early results. Standard portals for the radiocarpal and midcarpal joints and a 2.3-mm VAPR probe (DePuy Mitek, Leeds, UK) have been used. The objective is to shrink the relevant ligaments, followed by immobilization of the wrist in a cast for 6 weeks. All the volar extrinsic wrist ligaments should be treated in an attempt to tighten the arcuate ligament. There are no published series on this form of treatment as yet. At present, it should still be considered an experimental treatment.

For palmar MCI, published studies support the use of limited carpal arthrodesis over soft tissue stabilizations.[9,10] Triquetrohamate,[11] four-corner arthrodesis,[12] and STT[5] fusions have been proposed. The downside of these procedures is that they block the midcarpal joint, preventing the useful movement in the "dart throwing" arc, from dorsoradial to palmar-ulnar.

If a particular ligament is found to be the cause of the instability, augmentation seems to be the most sensible option. In palmar MCI in which the pathology is ulnar-sided, the author's limited experience with the procedure proposed by Garcia-Elias and Geissler[13] has produced excellent results. This technique uses half the extensor carpi radialis brevis tendon to recreate the ulnar limb of the arcuate ligament and the dorsal radiotriquetral ligament.

If the cause of palmar MCI is on the radial side, conservative treatment including exercises to strengthen the flexor carpi radialis should be tried. Failing that, a modified Brunelli reconstruction using half of the flexor carpi radialis tendon would recreate the ligaments across the STT joint and the dorsal scapholunate ligament, providing a good alternative to an arthrodesis.[13]

Dorsal Midcarpal Instability

Patients with dorsal MCI present with clicking and pain in the wrist, related to dorsal subluxation of the midcarpal joint. The pathomechanics differ from palmar MCI. In dorsal MCI, the capitate is reduced when the wrist is in neutral radioulnar deviation and subluxates dorsally in ulnar deviation. It is not a "catch-up" clunk, but more of a subluxation click. When the wrist moves from extreme ulnar deviation toward neutral, the capitate relocates, and this may be accompanied by a click or a clunk.

There are two subgroups in this type of MCI. The first subgroup manifests typically without a history of trauma, with pain and clicking of the wrist, precipitated by tight grasping, particularly with the forearm in supination; this has been named the capitolunate instability pattern.[14] In a reported series of 11 patients, plain radiographs seemed normal, but doing a dynamic dorsal displacement under fluoroscopy revealed the diagnosis in all patients. To perform the test, the examiner applies dorsally directed force to the scaphoid tuberosity, with longitudinal traction and flexion of the wrist. X-rays show a dorsal subluxation of the proximal row with characteristic dorsal subluxation of the capitate from the lunate. This test reproduces the patient's symptoms. Ten of 11 patients became asymptomatic with conservative treatment. This condition was attributed to laxity of the radiolunate ligaments and extrinsic ligaments of the scaphoid.

The second group of patients with dorsal MCI, called chronic capitolunate instability, present with post-traumatic chronic wrist pain, weakness, and wrist clicking, and a history of an extension wrist injury. In the report of a series of 12 patients, radiographs were normal except in 1 patient with a dorsal intercalated segment instability pattern.[15] Under fluoroscopy, dorsal subluxation of the capitate on the lunate could be shown by pushing the capitate dorsally. This caused apprehension, and the patients recognized the click caused by the sudden movement of the lunate dorsal and ulnar. Of the 12 patients, 11 underwent surgery to suture the volar radiocapitate ligament to the radiotriquetral ligament, in an attempt to close the space of Poirier. Surgery was generally successful at stabilizing the wrist, although some extension was lost. This condition has been attributed to traumatic attenuation of the palmar radiocapitate ligament. Dorsal MCI seems to be related to insufficiency of the ligaments in the antipronation sling.

Treatment of Dorsal Midcarpal Instability

The two subgroups of dorsal MCI probably represent different stages of the same spectrum. Patients presenting with a short duration of symptoms and no history of trauma tend to improve with conservative treatment.

In the rare cases when surgery is required, the author recommends the method described by Johnson and Carrera.[15] Through a volar approach, the space of Poirier is obliterated using a strong nonabsorbable suture, accepting certain loss of extension of the wrist.

Combined or Palmar-Dorsal Midcarpal Instability

Some patients present with a combination of palmar MCI and a positive passive dorsal displacement test, usually in a wrist with marked laxity. In a series of 14 such patients presenting with wrist pain and weakness, half of them had a history of trauma.[16] Radiographs showed a VISI deformity. Doing a dorsal displacement test showed subluxation of the capitolunate joint and in some cases subluxation of the radiolunate also. These patients did not improve with nonoperative treatment, and they underwent surgery to obliterate the space of Poirier. This was done by sutur-

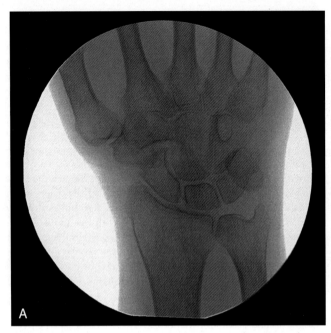
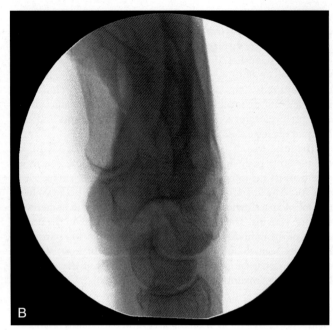

FIGURE 42-6 **A** and **B,** This patient underwent excision of the distal one fourth of the scaphoid as treatment for scaphotrapeziotrapezoid osteoarthritis. This procedure was successful in eliminating the pain. A few weeks after the surgery, the patient developed clicking when gripping and pain localized to the dorsum of the wrist. Doing a dynamic dorsal displacement test shows dorsal subluxation of the distal row, indicative of dorsal midcarpal instability.

ing the radiocapitate ligament to the long radiolunate on the radial side, and the capitotriquetral to the lunotriquetral on the ulnar side. The authors reported excellent outcome in eight cases, good in five, and fair in one.

Treatment of Combined Midcarpal Instability

Patients with combined dorsal and palmar MCI usually have marked laxity of the wrists, and they should be treated nonoperatively as far as possible. The reported result of surgery in multidirectional instabilities is unsatisfactory.[3] This coincides with the author's experience that patients with very lax wrists do not do well with soft tissue surgery.

If all conservative measures fail, and the patient is very symptomatic, the best option is a radiolunate arthrodesis as originally proposed by Halikis and colleagues.[17] This procedure orientates the lunate appropriately and abolishes the "proximal row instability," providing an excellent range of movement in these patients.

Extrinsic Midcarpal Instability

The cause of extrinsic MCI is not primarily in the ligaments, but a bony abnormality with secondary insufficiency of the ligaments. The common reason is the malalignment of a distal radius malunion, but rarely STT osteoarthritis can be a cause.

Carpal malalignment secondary to malunion of distal radial fractures was recognized in the 1970s.[6] In 1984, Taleisnik and Watson[18] reported 13 patients with symptoms of instability and wrist pain, 6 of them with recurrent voluntary midcarpal subluxation. Nine patients were treated by corrective osteotomy of the radius, which resulted in symptom relief and stabilization of the wrists. The one patient whose wrist was stabilized by ligament reconstruction presented with a recurrence of the voluntary midcarpal subluxation.

Caputo and coworkers[5] no longer consider this condition to be MCI. They prefer the term "dorsal radius angulation carpal overload," considering that the cause of the instability is the repet-

itive overload of the midcarpal joint as a result of the reversal of the normal palmar tilt of the distal radius. This cause is supported by the fact that the instability often manifests months after the injury. The ligaments in the wrist are developed to resist volar and ulnar directed forces, but are inadequate to resist dorsal or radial directed forces such as the ones present after a distal radius malunion.

An alternative explanation for this instability is insufficiency of the volar extrinsic wrist ligaments resulting from the reversal of the volar tilt of the radius.[4] The secondary malalignment of the carpus shortens the distance these ligaments span, causing relative laxity and creating a situation similar to dorsal MCI. The instability immediately disappears when the carpal bones realign after a corrective osteotomy. Perhaps another contributing factor is that the mechanism of injury in a distal radius fracture is the same one that can cause an injury of the volar extrinsic wrist ligaments.

There also is a relationship between STT osteoarthritis and dorsal MCI.[19] It seems that shortening of the scaphoid can cause extension of the proximal carpal row into a dorsal intercalated segment instability, which can be made worse with certain treatments, such as excision of the distal pole of the scaphoid (**Fig. 42-6**).

Treatment of Extrinsic Midcarpal Instability

For extrinsic MCI with significant symptoms, surgery should address the cause of the problem. In the case of distal radius malunion, the bone anatomy usually can be restored by a corrective osteotomy of the radius. The results are predictably good.

REFERENCES

1. Mouchet A, Belot J: Poignet a'ressaut: subluxation mediocarpienne en avant. Bulletin et Memories de la Societe Nationale de Chirurgie. 1934; 60:1243-1244.

2. Lichtman DM, Schneider JR, Swafford AR, et al: Ulnar midcarpal instability—clinical and laboratory analysis. J Hand Surg [Am]. 1981; 6:515-523.

3. Wright TW, Dobyns RL, Linscheid RL, et al: Carpal instability non-dissociative. J Hand Surg [Br]. 1994; 19:763-773.

4. Lichtman DM, Wroten ES: Understanding midcarpal instability. J Hand Surg [Am]. 2006; 31:491-498.

5. Caputo AE, Watson HK, Weinzweig J: Midcarpal instability. In Watson HK, Weinzweig J, eds: The Wrist. Philadelphia: Lippincott Williams & Wilkins, 2001.

6. Linscheid RL, Dobyns JH, Beabout JW, et al: Traumatic instability of the wrist: diagnosis, classification, and pathomechanics. J Bone Joint Surg Am. 1972; 54:1612-1632.

7. Trumble T, Bour CJ, Smith RJ, et al: Kinematics of the ulnar carpus related to the volar intercalated segment instability pattern. J Hand Surg [Am]. 1990; 15:384-392.

8. Viegas SF, Patterson RM, Peterson PD, et al: Ulnar-sided perilunate instability: an anatomic and biomechanic study. J Hand Surg [Am]. 1990; 15:268-277.

9. Lichtman DM, Bruckner JD, Culp RW, et al: Palmar midcarpal instability: results of surgical reconstruction. J Hand Surg [Am]. 1993; 18:307-315.

10. Trumble T, Bour CJ, Smith RJ, et al: Intercarpal arthrodesis for static and dynamic volar intercalated segment instability pattern. J Hand Surg [Am]. 1988; 13:384-390.

11. Rao SB, Culver JE: Triquetrohamate arthrodesis for midcarpal instability. J Hand Surg [Am]. 1995; 20:583-589.

12. Goldfarb CA, Stern PJ, Kefhaber TR: Palmar midcarpal instability: the results of treatment with 4-corner arthrodesis. J Hand Surg [Am]. 2004; 29:258-263.

13. Garcia-Elias M, Geissler WB: Carpal instability. In Green DP, Hotchkiss RN, Pederson WC, et al, eds: Green's Operative Hand Surgery. 5th ed. Churchill Livingstone, 2005; 535-604.

14. Louis DS, Hankin FM, Greene TL, et al: Central carpal instability—capitate lunate instability pattern: diagnosis by dynamic displacement. Orthopaedics. 1984; 7:1693-1696.

15. Johnson RP, Carrera GF: Chronic capitolunate instability. J Bone Joint Surg Am. 1986; 68:1164-1176.

16. Aspergis EP: The unstable capitolunate and radiolunate joints as a source of wrist pain in young women. J Hand Surg [Br]. 1996; 21:501-506.

17. Halikis MN, Colello-Abraham K, Taleisnik J: Radiolunate fusion: the forgotten partial arthrodesis. Clin Orthop Relat Res. 1997; 341:30-35.

18. Taleisnik J, Watson HK: Midcarpal instability caused by malunited fractures of the distal radius. J Hand Surg [Am]. 1984; 9:350-357.

19. Tay SC, Moran SL, Shin AY, et al: The clinical implications of scaphotrapezium-trapezoidal arthritis with associated carpal instability. J Hand Surg [Am]. 2007; 32:47-54.

Perilunate Injuries of the Wrist

Hamid R. Redjal, MD and Gregory H. Rafijah, MD

43

Perilunate injuries of the wrist include a spectrum of carpal dislocations and fracture-dislocations. These are rare injuries that often involve high-energy trauma, such as motor vehicle accidents, falls from a height, and industrial accidents. Despite the severity of trauma, initial diagnosis of these injuries tends to be delayed in 16% to 25% of cases.[1] Young men are most frequently affected by these injuries. In one study[1] of 166 perilunate injuries, the average age was 32 years with 97% males affected.[1,2]

A pure perilunate injury involves a dislocation of the carpus from the lunate and constitutes a purely ligamentous injury to the wrist. The lunate is strongly bound to the radius and ulna by stout capsular ligaments, and only in severe end-stage perilunate injuries does the lunate dislocate from the radius. Pure perilunate dislocations are considered lesser arc injuries because the traumatic force results in a circular disruption of ligaments close to the body of the lunate.

Greater arc injuries occur when the force takes a path around the lunate of greater circumference. Greater arc injuries are perilunar fracture-dislocations of the wrist that combine ligament ruptures, bone avulsions, and carpal bone fractures in a variety of clinical forms. Greater arc perilunate fracture-dislocations most commonly involve the scaphoid, but also may include fractures of the radial and ulnar styloids, capitate, and triquetrum in any combination. Of perilunate dislocations, greater arc injuries are more common, with approximately two thirds of perilunate dislocations classified as greater arc injuries.[1,3] The trans-scaphoid perilunate dislocation is the most common variant of this type of injury encountered in all published series. Of greater arc perilunate fracture-dislocations, 95% include a fracture through the middle third of the scaphoid. Usually the proximal fragment of the scaphoid remains attached to the lunate even if it has undergone a palmar dislocation; however, 3.8% of trans-scaphoid perilunate injuries may include a complete scapholunate ligament rupture.[1,3-5] Fracture of the capitate also is occasionally encountered and is present in approximately 8% of all fracture-dislocations of the wrist.

Mechanism and Patterns of Injury

Perilunate injuries are a spectrum of carpal injuries that are the result of high-energy trauma. The mechanism of injury is typically hyperextension, ulnar deviation, and intercarpal supination of the wrist. Indirect forces typically cause perilunate injuries when the point of rotation is distal to the radius and there is more stress on the carpal bones. In very young patients, such a force typically results in a physeal injury to the distal radius, and in older patients with osteopenic bone, a distal radius fracture typically occurs through the soft bone of the distal radius. This probably explains why perilunate injuries are typically seen in young

patients with good bone quality who are involved in high-energy activities.

Mayfield[3,6,7] described a spectrum of progressive perilunar instability that has greatly enhanced understanding of these injuries. Perilunate injuries are divided into four stages based on the concept of a sequential pattern of traumatic intercarpal wrist instability.

All perilunate injuries except the very rare "reverse perilunate" begin with injuries on the radial side of the wrist and progress ulnarward. The first stage in lesser arc injuries is scapholunate dissociation followed by lunocapitate dislocation with lunotriquetral disruption and finally lunate dislocation from the radius. A lesser arc injury is a purely ligamentous injury that typically manifests with dorsal dislocation of the capitate from the lunate and rarely with lunate dislocation toward the carpal tunnel.

Mayfield also noted that carpal fractures may occur in perilunate injuries in lieu of ligament ruptures. In these cases, the force is concentrated on the carpus away from the lunate as it progresses from radial to ulnar, which results in the carpal bone fractures. The injuries that result are called greater arc injuries because the route of injury includes a path more remote from the lunate than lesser arc injuries (**Fig. 43-1**).

Progressive perilunar instability as described by Mayfield has four stages that follow a common sequence after exposure of the wrist to forceful hyperextension with a strong supination torque (**Fig. 43-2**). Stage I injuries result in scapholunate dissociation.[6,7] Hyperextension of the scaphoid places a strong torque on the lunate and its ligaments. The extrinsic palmar and dorsal ligaments tightly stabilize the lunate, and the force is concentrated on the scapholunate ligament, which ultimately begins to tear from palmar to dorsal. If the force is strong enough, the scapholunate ligament completely ruptures, completing stage I.

In stage II injuries, there is sufficient force to dislocate the midcarpal joint with the capitate typically dislocating dorsal to the lunate. Midcarpal dislocation requires additional injury to the extrinsic ligaments, including the scaphocapitate and radioscaphocapitate. The space of Poirier, which is a deficiency in the palmar wrist capsule between radial and ulnar capsular ligaments, is opened by the progressive injury with a palmar capsular rent that exposes the midpalmar joint. In stage III injuries, the force continues in an ulnar direction with rupture of the lunotriquetral ligament and may include additional capsular injuries to the ulnolunate ligaments.

In stage IV injuries, the lunate is forced volarly to dislocate into the carpal tunnel through the opened space of Poirier. Isolated volar dislocations of the lunate are the end stage of the spectrum of progressive perilunar instability. Lunate dislocations are divided into three types. Type 1 lunate dislocations result in

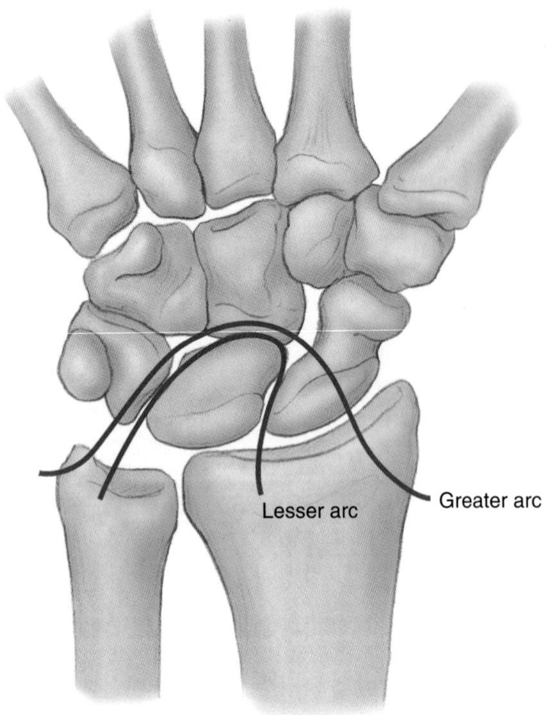

FIGURE 43-1 Greater and lesser arc injuries of the wrist. Lesser arc injuries result in a disruption of ligaments that bind the carpus to the lunate. The path of injury passes close to the body of the lunate and results in a purely ligamentous injury to the wrist. Greater arc injuries occur following a force that disrupts the carpus in a path further away from the lunate. Greater arc injuries may often include carpal bone fractures and avulsion fractures of the radial and ulnar styloids in a variety of combinations.

a lunate that has rotated palmarly up to 90 degrees. Type 2 lunate dislocations produce a lunate with more than 90 degrees of palmar rotation as it is hinged on the short radiolunate ligament. Type 3 injuries result in dislocation of the lunate into the carpal tunnel. Reverse perilunar instabilities result from hyperpronation of the wrist and may be the mechanism for rare perilunate injuries with palmar dislocation of the midcarpal joint.[3]

In greater arc injuries, the variable pattern of fracture might include avulsion of the radial styloid or fracture of the scaphoid, capitate, triquetrum, or ulnar styloid. The most common pattern observed in greater arc injuries is the trans-scaphoid perilunate fracture-dislocation. The trans-scaphoid variant is observed in 60% of perilunate wrist injuries.[1,3,6] The scaphoid fracture is through the waist in 60% to 72% of cases.[1,3] The scaphoid may fracture at any level, however, including the proximal pole.

Fracture of the capitate may occur and be part of the "scapho-capitate" syndrome.[3,6,8-10] This injury consists of a variation of a greater arc perilunate fracture-dislocation, in which the scaphoid and the capitate are fractured. The capitate fracture typically occurs proximally at the proximal neck of the bone. Complete rotation of the capitate fragment is typical with the proximal fragment often rotated 90 to 180 degrees. The mechanism of the fracture seems to involve a direct impact of the capitate against the dorsal lip of the radius with the wrist in a hyperextended and ulnarly deviated position. Rotation of the proximal capitate fragment is a result of the return of the distal fragment to its neutral position after dislocation (**Fig. 43-3**).

Greater and lesser arc injuries usually manifest with ligament ruptures on the ulnar side of the lunate, including complete rupture of the lunotriquetral ligament. Greater arc perilunate injuries may manifest with fractures of the triquetrum. Triquetral fractures may occur in any plane, but the most common pattern is a sagittal split in the body of the triquetrum or an avulsion fracture of the proximal pole.

Fractures of the radial or ulnar styloids also may be observed in greater arc perilunate injuries. These are typically smaller avulsion fractures, but may be of significant size and include the origins of major wrist stabilizers, such as the triangular fibrocartilage complex or radioscaphocapitate ligaments.

Presentation and Diagnosis

Patients who present with a perilunate fracture-dislocation have obvious pain and swelling of the hand and wrist. A full musculoskeletal examination and screening for concomitant axial or appendicular skeleton injuries is important because these represent high-energy injuries, and the patient may have sustained additional trauma.

Patients may present with symptoms of median or ulnar nerve compression. The incidence of acute carpal tunnel syndrome manifesting with perilunate injury ranges from 16% to 46%.[11] Most patients have resolution of nerve compression after closed reduction, but persistent nerve dysfunction after closed reduction may require urgent surgical decompression. Close attention should be paid to the patients' neurovascular status, and the status of the median nerve in particular should be carefully established before and after reduction.

A standard four-view wrist series should be diagnostic of perilunate injuries and exhibit typical features. Most importantly, the dislocation of the midcarpal joint is best appreciated on the lateral view where lunocapitate dissociation can be easily visualized. The position of the lunate is best determined on the lateral view, which may reveal malrotation or dislocation of the lunate (**Fig. 43-4**).

In perilunate injury, one also may appreciate on the anteroposterior view that there are radiographic breaks in the smooth arcs between the carpal rows described by Gilula.[12] These arcs are named after Gilula, the radiologist who described the concept of the greater and lesser arc injuries. Additionally, the carpus appears foreshortened with loss of carpal height. Malrotation of the lunate produces a "triangular-shaped" lunate that overlaps the capitate on the anteroposterior radiograph (**Fig. 43-5**). A cortical ring sign of the scaphoid consistent with rotary subluxation of the scaphoid also may be noted on the anteroposterior radiograph. Additionally, wrist films should be inspected for associated fractures of the radial styloid, scaphoid, capitate, hamate, triquetrum, and ulnar styloid, which may represent a greater arc injury.

Sixteen percent to 25% of perilunate injuries are initially missed in the emergency department and manifest as chronic dislocations. Herzberg and colleagues[1] observed that the diagnosis was missed in 41 cases of 166 greater arc injuries. Suspicion for the injury and careful interpretation of the radiographs should prevent any delay in diagnosis. Perilunate injuries tend to occur as a result of high-energy trauma, however, and patients may have more serious injuries that distract the physician from the injured wrist. Such a scenario also may contribute to a delay in the diagnosis of a perilunate injury.

Initial Treatment

In the acute trauma setting, an urgent reduction of the carpus should be performed. Closed reduction in the emergency depart-

Stage

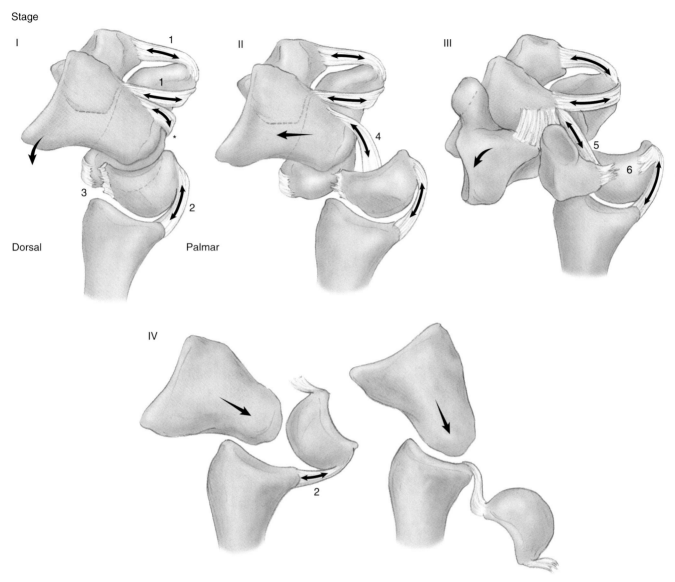

Dorsal

Palmar

FIGURE 43-2 **The four stages of perilunar carpal instability. Stage I:** As the distal carpal row is forced into extension (*arrows*), the scaphotrapezio-capitate ligaments (*1*) pull the scaphoid into extension, opening the space of Poirier (*asterisk*). The lunate is constrained by the short radiolunate ligament (*2*), and the hyperextension force of the scaphoid results in concentration of energy to the scapholunate ligament. A scapholunate liga-ment rupture or scaphoid fracture may occur. The scapholunate ligament usually ruptures from palmar to dorsal with complete dissociation noted when the dorsal portion of the scapholunate ligament fails (*3*). **Stage II:** Midcarpal dislocation may occur with the capitate usually moving dorsal to the lunate. The midcarpal translation is limited by the integrity of the radioscaphocapitate ligament (*4*). **Stage III:** If hyperextension and intercarpal supination progresses, the ulnar carpal ligaments (*5*) and the lunotriquetral interosseous ligament (*6*) may fail. **Stage IV:** In end-stage injury, addi-tional hyperextension forces the capitate to push the lunate palmarly through the torn volar capsule and the space of Poirier. The lunate may dislo-cate into the carpal tunnel hinged on the intact short radiolunate ligament (*2*).

ment is the best way to restore carpal alignment initially and should be attempted. A closed reduction is usually obtainable and allows definitive surgery to be delayed to an optimal time and place.

Closed Reduction

After placing the wrist in traction for approximately 10 minutes to relax muscle spasm, thumb pressure should be maintained volarly on the lunate, and the wrist should be hyperextended. With longitudinal traction, the wrist should be flexed while press-ing on the lunate. This dorsally directed pressure on the palmar surface of the lunate is crucial to avoid pushing the lunate further volarly into the carpal tunnel. A palpable snap may be heard as

the capitate reduces to the lunate. The wrist is then splinted in a neutral position, allowing for active digital motion. Postreduction radiographs should be taken to evaluate the accuracy of reduction and to help visualize injuries that might not have been appreciated on the prereduction or traction x-rays.

Occasionally, closed reduction cannot be obtained because of lunate dislocation or dorsal capsular interposition.[13] In irreducible cases, urgent open reduction with carpal tunnel release should be performed to relieve pressure on the median nerve and to restore carpal alignment. Another emergent indication for surgery is an open perilunate injury. Eight percent of perilunate injuries are open cases[1,3] and are typically more severe. Open injuries are more likely to have a poor outcome because of a greater amount of

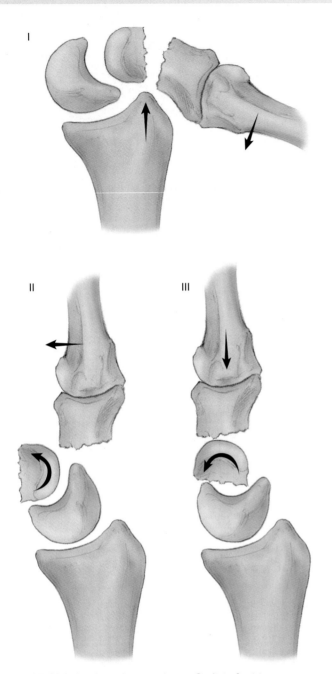

FIGURE 43-3 **Scaphocapitate syndrome.** Capitate fractures may occur with fracture of the scaphoid in greater arc perilunate injuries. The capitate fracture is usually through the neck and may occur after extreme wrist extension (I). The final wrist position after injury may result in the capitate rotated up to 180 degrees with the articular surface facing cancellous bone (II and III).

trauma and energy absorption than closed cases. Open injuries require emergent surgical irrigation and débridement in addition to open reduction.

Acute post-traumatic carpal tunnel syndrome may occur after perilunate injury and be observed in a quarter of patients treated initially.[1,14] The immediate solution is to proceed with closed reduction of the dislocated wrist in the emergency department. If median nerve symptoms persist or worsen after closed reduction of the perilunate dislocation, the surgeon should proceed with urgent decompression of the carpal tunnel to decrease the pres-

sure caused by soft tissue swelling and hematoma formation around the median nerve.

Although gross closed reduction of perilunate injuries is possible, an absolutely anatomical reduction is difficult to obtain and hold with simple immobilization. Closed reduction and immobilization has been recommended as definitive treatment by a few authors. Most studies note that an initially acceptable closed reduction loses its alignment over time.[3,15]

Closed Reduction and Pinning of Perilunate Injuries

Some authors have advocated closed reduction and percutaneous pinning of perilunate injuries as definitive treatment, and satisfactory results have been reported.[1,2] The overall quality of reduction and accuracy of internal fixation are greatly enhanced by an open approach. Closed reduction and pinning should be reserved for patients who refuse open reduction or have a contraindication to open surgery, such as long-term anticoagulation therapy. If after closed reduction there is residual intercarpal widening of more than 3 mm or scapholunate angle more than 80 degrees, a poor prognosis can be expected with closed treatment, and open reduction should be recommended.[3]

Open Reduction and Fixation of Perilunate Injuries

There is a consensus in the literature that open reduction of perilunate injuries provides the patient with the best possible prognosis.[1-3,6,12,15-22] Open reduction allows the surgeon to assess fully the injury to the wrist, remove loose bone and cartilage fragments, perform direct ligament repair, and visually ensure anatomical realignment of the carpus.[3,6] The clinical benefits after open reduction of perilunate injuries include a lower rate of recurrent instability and maintenance of carpal congruity. Generally, patients treated with open reduction regain better motion, strength, and pain relief than patients treated nonoperatively.

There also is agreement in the literature that prompt surgical treatment improves the prognosis over cases treated with delayed open reduction.[1] Open reduction of perilunate injuries is best performed as soon as possible, but delay up to 1 week does not seem to affect the final result as long as a stable closed reduction has been obtained before surgery. Some series report satisfactory results in patients treated 6 weeks postinjury, but a significant delay to surgery can have a negative impact on the expected outcome.[1,15,23]

A debatable issue regarding the open treatment of perilunate injuries is the surgical approach. Recommendations are mixed on the utility of a dorsal approach, a volar approach, or combined volar and dorsal approach.

Advocates of the dorsal approach note the ability to visualize fully all pathology in perilunate dislocations and perilunate fracture-dislocations. The dorsal approach allows direct reduction and fixation of the carpal bones, interosseous ligaments, and the dorsal capsule.[17,19,24] Visualization of the torn volar capsule is limited with an isolated dorsal approach, however, and the volar capsule is usually left to heal without direct repair. Sohn and associates[19] argued that the volar capsule is usually automatically realigned after anatomical reduction and fixation of the carpus through a dorsal approach, and that the volar capsule heals satisfactorily during the subsequent period of immobilization without direct repair. Knoll and coworkers[24] reported good results in 25

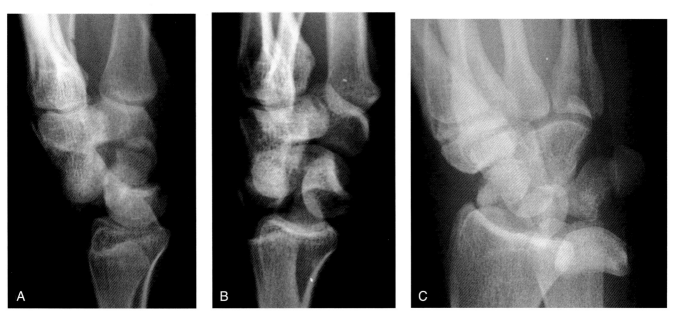

FIGURE 43-4 **A,** The lateral injury film reveals dislocation of the midcarpal joint with dorsal dislocation of the capitate from the lunate. **B,** Midcarpal dislocation accompanied with palmar rotation of the lunate. **C,** Palmar dislocation of the lunate (Mayfield stage 4).

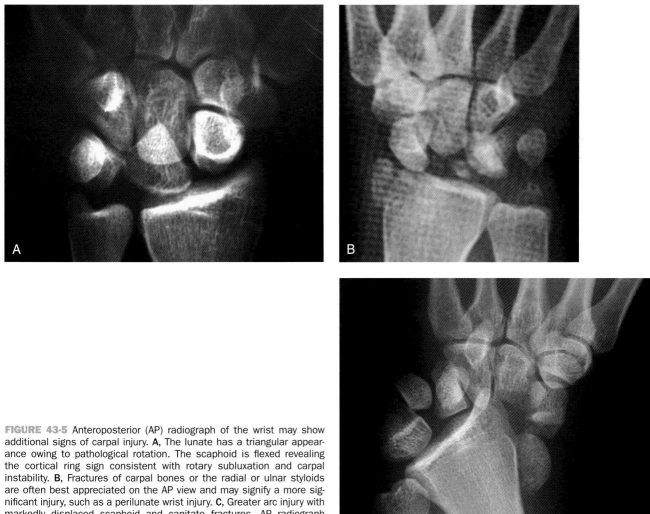

FIGURE 43-5 Anteroposterior (AP) radiograph of the wrist may show additional signs of carpal injury. **A,** The lunate has a triangular appearance owing to pathological rotation. The scaphoid is flexed revealing the cortical ring sign consistent with rotary subluxation and carpal instability. **B,** Fractures of carpal bones or the radial or ulnar styloids are often best appreciated on the AP view and may signify a more significant injury, such as a perilunate wrist injury. **C,** Greater arc injury with markedly displaced scaphoid and capitate fractures. AP radiograph shows the degree of radial displacement in this case. The lunate remains reduced to the radius despite the severity of injury consistent with a perilunate mechanism of injury.

trans-scaphoid perilunate fracture-dislocations of the wrist treated with an isolated dorsal approach. Adkison and Chapman[15] noted that initially in their experience they approached the wrist volarly, but found that the volar approach made it difficult to visualize the full scope of wrist pathology after a perilunate injury. These authors now favor the dorsal approach for perilunate injuries of the wrist.

Hee and colleagues[23] reported on 63% good to excellent results after open reduction of trans-scaphoid perilunate injuries treated with an isolated volar approach, including internal fixation of the scaphoid. Several authors recommend combined dorsal and volar surgical incisions to manage perilunate injuries.[3,6,11,16,25] Trumble and Verheyden[11] reported on 22 isolated perilunate ligamentous injuries to the wrist with good results using dorsal and volar approaches. They noted that the volar approach was helpful with joint reduction and placement of internal fixation, and allowed for carpal tunnel release.

Regardless of approach, the goal of surgical treatment of perilunate injuries is to obtain a stable and accurate anatomical joint reduction. Most commonly, Kirschner wires (K-wires) are used as the principal internal fixation device of choice, but compression screws may be used for large fracture fragments. Typically, scaphoid fractures are treated with compression screws and bone grafting as needed. Intercarpal gaps are usually reduced and held together with K-wires, but the use of temporary screw fixation and cerclage wire[11,14,24] to keep these gaps closed has been reported as alternative choices of internal fixation.

Authors' Preferred Methods

Lesser Arc Injuries

Pure perilunate injuries are probably best treated with combined volar and dorsal approaches, especially in stage IV injuries (lunate dislocation). When a volar approach is made, open reduction of the dislocated lunate is performed, and complete carpal tunnel release is provided as an additional benefit. The volar approach also makes it possible to repair the torn volar capsule, which is a principal site of injury in these cases. The volar capsule is repaired with 3-0 nonabsorbable sutures.

The dorsal approach is made through a longitudinal midline incision at Lister's tubercle, and an approach is made to the wrist through the third dorsal extensor compartment. The dorsal capsule is usually torn, and the arthrotomy is frequently through this rent. The joint is inspected to appreciate the scope of damage, and a complete débridement of any tiny loose osteocartilaginous fragments is performed.

The position of the lunate is reduced to its position on the radius, and if necessary, a temporary K-wire is inserted between radius and lunate to secure its position before reducing the adjacent joints. Next, the scaphoid is reduced to the lunate. A K-wire may be inserted into the scaphoid as a joystick to facilitate derotation and allow reduction of the scapholunate interval. The scaphoid is usually in a flexed orientation, and the K-wire joystick can help to rotate the scaphoid into an extended position alongside the lunate. Next, the scapholunate interval is reduced, and temporary use of bone reduction forceps may be needed to maintain alignment while inserting internal fixation. The correct alignment should result in excellent apposition of the dorsal and distalmost fibers of the scapholunate interosseous ligament. The preliminary radiograph should show no residual intercarpal gap and restoration of the scapholunate angle (30 to 60 degrees). When the position is confirmed to be acceptable, the scapholunate interval

is stabilized with two 0.062-inch K-wires inserted from the scaphoid into the lunate. An additional 0.062-inch K-wire is inserted from the distal scaphoid into the capitate to prevent rotary subluxation of the scaphoid and subsequent loss of reduction (**Fig. 43-6**).

If the scapholunate ligament has good residual substance, a ligament repair is attempted. The repair may be made through drill holes or augmented with suture anchors. If the ligament is shredded or of otherwise poor quality, however, no attempt for direct repair is made, and the ligament is allowed to heal spontaneously.

After scapholunate repair, the lunotriquetral joint is addressed. The triquetrum must be simultaneously reduced to the lunate and to the spiral groove of the hamate. A dental pick is used to facilitate the reduction of the triquetrum as it is coaxed toward the apex between the lunate and hamate bones. When reduced, the triquetrum is stabilized with two 0.062-inch K-wires inserted from the ulnar border of the wrist and passing across the lunotriquetral and triquetral-hamate joints.

Greater Arc Injuries

Open reduction and internal fixation (ORIF) of perilunate fracture-dislocations is typically performed through an exclusively dorsal approach to the wrist. The dorsal approach provides all the necessary exposure to address fully the pathology present, and stable fixation of the scaphoid fracture sufficiently addresses the injury to the radial side of the wrist. A palmar approach is used only to address median nerve compression if present or to reduce the lunate if dislocated into the carpal tunnel.

Typically, in greater arc injuries, the scapholunate ligament is intact with an associated midwaist fracture of the scaphoid and lunotriquetral dissociation. When the position of the lunate and proximal pole of the scaphoid is reduced to the appropriate position on the radius, the scaphoid can be repaired with internal fixation.

The scaphoid typically is repaired with a headless self-compressing screw if possible. The screw is inserted into the scaphoid fracture antegrade through the proximal pole; excellent fixation is typical (**Fig. 43-7**). The scaphoid fracture may be comminuted or very proximal, however, making it difficult to obtain solid fixation. K-wire fixation is acceptable in these situations, and bone grafting from the distal radius should be obtained if necessary.

Occasionally, the proximal pole of the scaphoid is a free fragment with simultaneous rupture of the scapholunate ligament. Herzberg and colleagues[1] reported that simultaneous scaphoid fracture and scapholunate ligament tear occurred in 3.8% of cases. In these situations, it is probably best to use K-wire fixation for the scaphoid fracture because the presence of a screw in the scaphoid makes scapholunate ligament repair more difficult. After wire fixation of the scaphoid, the scapholunate joint is reduced and stabilized as noted in the technique for lesser arc perilunate repair.

When the capitate is fractured, the open reduction typically proceeds with this bone first (**Fig. 43-8**). The head of the capitate is typically a free osteocartilaginous fragment that has rotated 180 degrees. The fragment can be derotated and repaired with a headless compression screw or with K-wire fixation. Bone grafting from the distal radius may be required. Fractures of the radial or ulnar styloids are usually avulsion fractures that are treated with direct open reduction and pin fixation, although screw fixation also may be considered if the fragments are large.

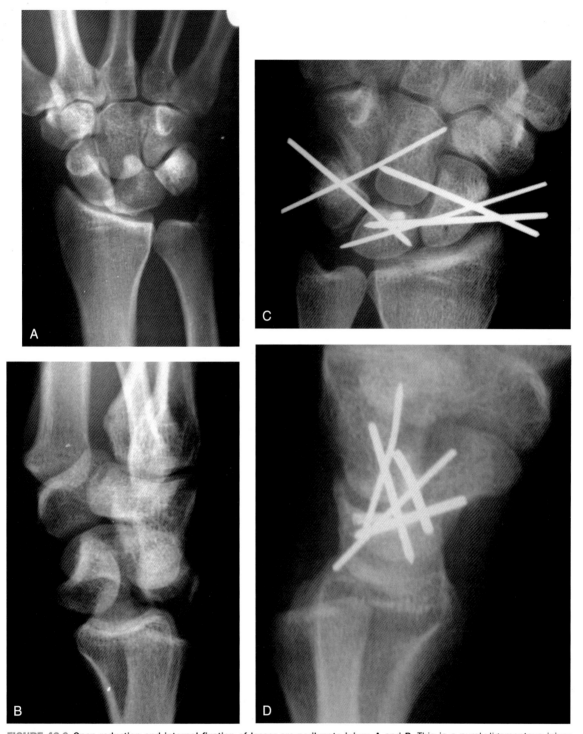

FIGURE 43-6 Open reduction and internal fixation of lesser arc perilunate injury. A and **B,** This is a purely ligamentous injury with midcarpal dislocation noted on the lateral view and triangular shape of the lunate seen on the anteroposterior view. **C** and **D,** Postoperative x-rays after open reduction and internal fixation with Kirschner wires. The scaphocapitate wire is helpful to prevent palmar rotation of the scaphoid. A suture anchor was placed in the lunate to augment scapholunate ligament repair.

Finally, the lunotriquetral joint is reduced and stabilized. In perilunate fracture-dislocation, the lunotriquetral ligament is usually disrupted without fracture, and the lunotriquetral joint is reduced and pinned with 0.062-inch K-wires as noted in the technique of lesser arc perilunate repair. Fracture of the trique-trum may occur in greater arc injury, however. In such cases, the triquetral fracture can be treated with pin or screw fixation depending on the size of the fracture fragments.

Postoperative Care

Pins are cut below the skin, and the wrist is immobilized initially in a short arm splint and bulky hand dressings until suture

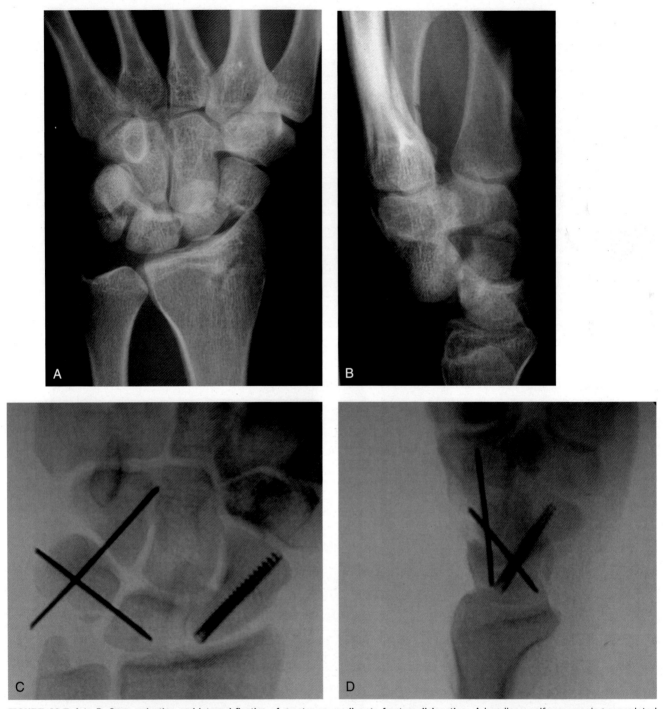

FIGURE 43-7 A to **D**, Open reduction and internal fixation of greater arc perilunate fracture-dislocation. A headless self-compressing cannulated screw is inserted into the scaphoid dorsally and antegrade at the proximal pole. Kirschner wires are used to stabilize the lunotriquetral interval for healing of the lunotriquetral ligament and triquetral fracture.

removal. A short arm cast is used until 10 weeks postoperatively, at which time the pins are removed. Careful surveillance of the scaphoid fracture is required because of the possibility of delayed union or nonunion. The patient is enrolled in an occupational therapy program after cast removal with gradual progression of activities. Twelve to 18 months may be required until the final result is obtained, when pain resolves, and motion and strength have been optimized.[25]

Outcomes

Patients who undergo timely ORIF for perilunate injuries have the most successful outcomes. Most authors agree that the expected recovery of wrist range of motion after ORIF is about a 110-degree arc of flexion and extension with return of approximately 75% of grip strength.[3] Although outcome studies of perilunate injuries have shown suboptimal assessment scores

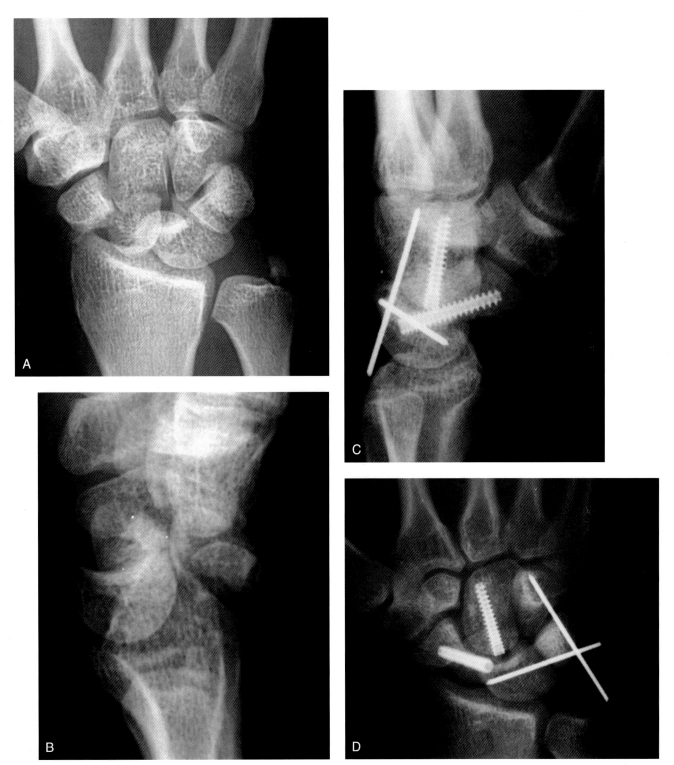

FIGURE 43-8 A to **D, Greater arc perilunate injury with scaphoid and capitate fractures (scaphocapitate syndrome).** Note the fracture of the capitate and the malrotation of the fragment. Open reduction and internal fixation is performed through a dorsal approach with headless cannulated screw fixation of the scaphoid and capitate. The lunotriquetral joint is stabilized with Kirschner wires after open reduction.

consistent with loss of function,[25,26] there also are numerous reports of acceptable patient satisfaction with regards to pain relief and function after ORIF. Hee and colleagues[23] reported 62% excellent and good results in the outcome of 15 patients treated with ORIF. Sotereanos and associates[25] noted that despite loss of motion and grip, 82% of patients were satisfied with the procedure, but only 45% returned to work. Other series report a much more optimistic prognosis for return to work after perilunate ORIF, including a return to employment rate of 80% to 100% with 66% to 92% able to return to their preinjury occupation.[11,19,24,26]

Souer and coworkers[14] compared K-wires with temporary intercarpal screws in 18 patients (9 treated with 3-mm cannulated intercarpal screws and early mobilization at 3 weeks, and 9 treated with intercarpal K-wires and casting for 3 months). The intercarpal screws were removed an average of 5 months and the K-wires an average of 3 months after the initial procedure. Four patients (two in each cohort) had wrist arthrodesis with poor results. Among the 14 remaining patients, the final flexion arc was 97 degrees for patients treated with screw fixation compared with 73 degrees for patients treated with K-wires. The authors concluded that the results of treatment with temporary screws were comparable to the results of treatment with temporary K-wires. The appeal of temporary screw fixation lies in the ability to begin mobilizing the wrist within a few weeks and the absence of pin-related complications. Although superior wrist motion was obtained in the intercarpal screw group, the numbers were too small to provide any definitive conclusions.[14]

Delay to definitive surgical treatment is one of the most significant variables that adversely affect the outcome of perilunate injuries. This is significant because there is frequently a delay in the diagnosis and treatment of perilunate injuries, which may result in a poor outcome. Herzberg and colleagues[1] noted that patients treated with ORIF within 1 week had superior Mayo wrist scores compared with patients treated later, with only fair to poor results reported in patients treated after 45 days. Open injuries also are likely to have a poor outcome. The adverse results after open perilunate injuries is probably a reflection[1] of the more serious initial injury to the wrist, including the greater magnitude of injury to joint surfaces and ligaments.

Poor results in most series have followed cases with residual wrist instability, ulnar translocation of the carpus, and scaphoid nonunion. Despite the serious injury to the wrist in the vicinity of the lunate, reported cases of Kienböck's disease and lunate fragmentation are rare after perilunate wrist injury. The reported incidence of post-traumatic arthrosis at late follow-up is high, however, and is usually identified in the midcarpal joint. The incidence of post-traumatic arthritis after treatment of perilunate injuries is reported to range from 50% to 100% in the literature.[1,14,16,26]

Late Presentation

Too many perilunate injuries are missed at initial presentation, and this creates a very difficult situation for the treating surgeon. Suboptimal results can be expected in these cases, but open reduction should be performed if possible. It is unknown how late in presentation that ORIF can be performed, but there are reports[3] of successful open reduction performed up to 35 weeks postinjury. Some authors have recommended the use of preoperative or intraoperative traction with external fixation to facilitate delayed open reduction.[3]

Siegert and colleagues[27] and others evaluated 16 perilunate dislocations and fracture-dislocations with an average delay to surgery of 17 weeks. Despite the delay in presentation, they were able to perform open reduction in six of these cases with acceptable outcomes. When open reduction was impossible, the authors resorted to lunate excision, proximal row carpectomy, or wrist arthrodesis as primary treatment. Siegert and colleagues[27] noted that patients treated with simple lunate excision had poor results, and this was not recommended as primary treatment of chronic perilunate injuries.

REFERENCES

1. Herzberg G, Comtet JJ, Amadio PC, et al: Perilunate dislocations and fracture dislocations: a multicenter study. J Hand Surg [Am]. 1993; 18:768-779.
2. Herzberg G, Forissier D: Acute dorsal trans-scaphoid perilunate fracture-dislocations: medium term results. J Hand Surg [Br]. 2002; 27:498-502.
3. Garcia-Elias M, Geissler WB: Carpal instability. In Green DP, Hotchkiss RN, Pederson WC, et al, eds: Green's Operative Hand Surgery. 5th ed. Philadelphia: Churchill Livingstone, 2005.
4. Berger RA: The ligaments of the wrist: a current overview of anatomy with considerations of their potential functions. Hand Clin. 1997; 13:63-82.
5. Berger RA: The anatomy of the ligaments of the wrist and distal radioulnar joints. Clin Orthop. 2001; 383:32-40.
6. Grabow RJ, Catalano L: Carpal dislocations. Hand Clin. 2006; 22:485-500.
7. Mayfield JK, Johnson RP, Kilcoyne RF: Carpal dislocations: pathomechanics and progressive perilunar instability. J Hand Surg [Am]. 1980; 5:226-241.
8. Sawant M, Miller J, Heath T: Scaphocapitate syndrome in an adolescent. J Hand Surg [Am]. 2000; 25:1096-1099.
9. Vance RM, Gelberman RH, Evans EF: Scaphocapitate fractures. J Bone Joint Surg Am. 1980; 62:271-276.
10. Weseley MS, Barenfeld PA: Transscaphoid, transcapitate, transtriquetral perilunate fracture dislocation of the wrist: a case report. J Bone Joint Surg Am. 1972; 54:1073-1078.
11. Trumble T, Verheyden J: Treatment of isolated perilunate and lunate dislocations with combined dorsal and volar approach and intraosseous cerclage wire. J Hand Surg [Am]. 2004; 29:412-417.
12. Taleisnik J: The Wrist. New York: Churchill Livingstone, 1985.
13. Jasmine MS, Packer JW, Edwards GS: Irreducible trans-scaphoid perilunate dislocation. J Hand Surg [Am]. 1988; 13:212-216.
14. Souer JS, Rutgers M, Andermahr J, et al: Perilunate fracture-dislocations of the wrist: Comparison of temporary screw versus K-wire fixation. J Hand Surg. 2007; 32:318-325.
15. Adkison JW, Chapman MW: Treatment of acute lunate and perilunate dislocations. J Bone Joint Surg. 1982; 164:199-207.
16. Cooney WP, Bussey R, Dobyns JH, et al: Difficult wrist fractures. Clin Orthop. 1987; 214:136-147.
17. Moneim MS: Management of greater arc carpal fractures. Hand Clin. 1988; 4:457-467.

18. Moneim MS, Hofmann KE, Omer GE: Transscaphoid peri-lunate fracture-dislocation: result of open reduction and pin fixation. Clin Orthop. 1984; 190:227-235.

19. Sohn R, Rafijah G, Jo M, et al: Dorsal only approach for trans-scaphoid perilunate fracture dislocation: a review of results. Poster presented at 60th Annual Meeting of American Society of Surgery of the Hand, San Antonio, Texas, 2006.

20. Soejima O, Iida H, Naito M: Transscaphoid-transtriquetral perilunate fracture dislocation: report of a case and review of the literature. Arch Orthop Trauma Surg. 2003;123(6): 305-307.

21. Green DP, O'Brien ET: Open reduction of carpal disloca-tions: indications and operative techniques. J Hand Surg. 1978; 3:250-265.

22. Green DP, O'Brien ET: Classification and management of carpal dislocations. Clin Orthop. 1980; 149:55-72.

23. Hee HT, Wong HP, Low YP: Transscaphoid perilunate fracture/dislocations—results of surgical treatment. Ann Acad Med (Singapore). 1999; 28:791-794.

24. Knoll VD, Allan C, Trumble TE: Trans-scaphoid fracture dislocations: results of screw fixation of the scaphoid and lunotriquetral repair with a dorsal approach. J Hand Surg [Am]. 2005; 30:1145-1152.

25. Sotereanos DG, Mitsionis GJ, Giannakopoulos PN, et al: Perilunate dislocation and fracture dislocation: a critical analysis of the volar-dorsal approach. J Hand Surg [Am]. 1997; 22:49-56.

26. Hildebrand KA, Ross DC, Patterson SD, et al: Dorsal peri-lunate dislocations and fracture-dislocations: questionnaire, clinical, and radiographic evaluation. J Hand Surg [Am]. 2000; 25:1069-1079.

27. Siegert JJ, Frassica FJ, Amadio PC: Treatment of chronic perilunate dislocations. J Hand Surg [Am]. 1988; 13:206-212.

The Role of Arthroscopy in Scaphoid Fractures

44

Christophe Mathoulin, MD and Vera Sallen, MD

Rationale and Basic Science Pertinent to the Procedure

Classically, it was considered that consolidation of scaphoid fractures could be achieved without surgery. For many years since, however, open reduction and internal fixation has been the recommended and well-accepted treatment for displaced and unstable intra-articular fractures.

The complex morphology and the small size of the scaphoid bone resulted in the development of numerous sophisticated techniques to achieve an anatomical and stable fixation. In 1984, Herbert and Fischer[1] reported their experience using a cannulated screw, which originally was not developed for fixation of scaphoid fractures. In the early 1990s, the first article was published[2] describing inserting cannulated screws with a minimally invasive technique. The main principle was to preserve the surrounding ligaments of the carpal bones to avoid a destabilization of the reduction and to protect the fragile vascularization of the scaphoid bone.[3]

Meanwhile, patients and their referring physicians became more and more demanding. The surgical indication was expanded because of the inconvenience of conservative treatment with its unpredictable economic consequences owing to the long duration of immobilization.

Whipple[4,5] first presented a method with percutaneous screw fixation using a modified Herbert screw combined with image intensifier control and arthroscopic examination of the wrist. This method allowed the surgeon to control the reduction and to assess potential associated lesions.

In the treatment of scaphoid fractures by surgical reduction and internal fixation, some rules have to be respected, as follows: verify the exact fracture reduction, avoid an intra-articular penetration of the screw, maintain the fixation under compression, and allow an early return to activities of daily living. We report our more recent experience of 38 scaphoid fractures treated with an arthroscopically assisted percutaneous screw fixation technique using a cannulated Herbert screw.

Indications

The disabling long cast immobilization in this mostly young and active patient population and the risk of nonunion or malunion favor surgical reduction and internal fixation of scaphoid fractures. The aim is stable fracture fixation allowing early mobilization without compromising consolidation. It is important to neutralize the fracture forces, while compressing the fracture. The minimally invasive technique, and hence limited operative trauma, allows early functional rehabilitation. Arthroscopy helps to reduce the fragments; to control the quality of the reduction; and to assess the position of the screw, especially with regard to the radiocarpal joint.

The ideal candidate for surgery is a patient motivated to return to sports or business activities as soon as possible (e.g., a professional swimmer on the French national team who sustained a scaphoid fracture and was determined to qualify for the Olympic Games at Athens 2004 15 days later). The typical patient is young (mean age in our series 31.5 years), understands the aim of the treatment, and understands its risks and benefits. The delay between fracture and surgery should be as short as possible and not more than 1 month. One should delay immediate surgery if the conditions are not optimal (e.g., cutaneous lesions). In these situations, the wrist should be immobilized until the conditions are perfect.

Contraindications

In uncooperative patients who do not understand the risks and benefits, this method is contraindicated. In comminuted fractures, it is not realistic to achieve an anatomical reduction with this technique. Advanced age, cutaneous lesions, suboptimal operative conditions (e.g., incomplete surgical equipment), and severe associated lesions (e.g., severe scapholunate dissociation) are relative contraindications that can delay the intervention or preclude this type of surgery.

Operative Technique

Web Video

44-1

Under ambulatory conditions, the operation is performed with locoregional anesthesia. The patient is placed in the supine position on a special arm table with a tourniquet on the arm applied as proximal as possible. During the critical parts of the operation, the forearm can be extended using a pad underneath the wrist. Another possibility is to put the wrist under traction with a traction device, which is placed outside the arm table still allowing positioning the image intensifier. A retrograde (from distal to proximal) screw fixation is aimed. First, the fracture is visualized under arthroscopy using standard portals, leaving the forearm free on the table. Next, a 1-mm pin is placed through a small (5-mm) incision to the distal tuberosity of the scaphoid in a retrograde fashion (**Fig. 44-1**). Then the wrist is put under traction allowing arthroscopic control to verify the exact reduction of the scaphoid.

The arthroscope is introduced through a radial midcarpal portal through which the fracture can be assessed easily. If necessary, a débridement of the articulation can be done with the shaver while cleaning the medial surface of the scaphoid. If the fracture is displaced, reduction of the fragments is possible with a little retractor introduced through the STT midcarpal portal. Under arthroscopic control, the fracture fixation pin is slightly pulled

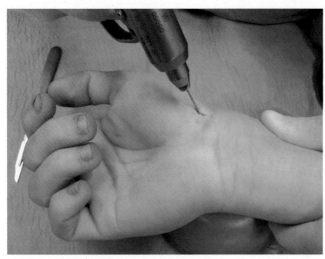

FIGURE 44-1 Percutaneous retrograde pinning of the scaphoid through a small approach centered on the distal tuberosity.

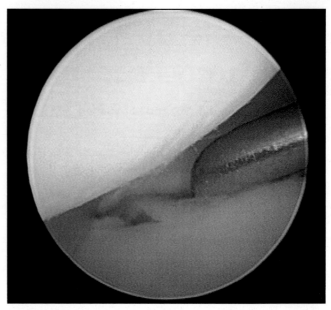

FIGURE 44-3 Mediocarpal arthroscopic view of the same fracture during reduction with a probe after the pin was pulled back distally to the fracture line.

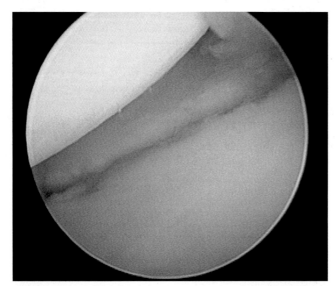

FIGURE 44-2 Mediocarpal arthroscopic view of a displaced scaphoid fracture.

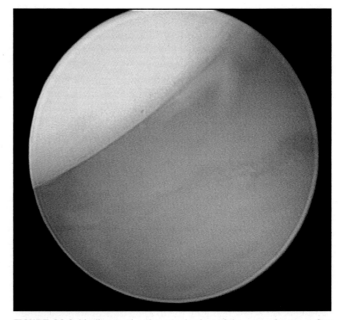

FIGURE 44-4 Mediocarpal arthroscopic view of the same fracture after reduction and stabilization.

back beyond the fracture line, then the fracture is reduced, and the pin is replaced into the proximal fragment (**Figs. 44-2, 44-3, and 44-4**). As soon as a satisfactory reduction is achieved, the hand is removed from the traction device, and the wrist is positioned on a pad on the arm table.

Under fluoroscopic control, the hole for the screw is tapped. If a resorbable screw is chosen, a double-sized trephine, drilling proximal with a 3-mm part and distal with a 3.5-mm part at the same time, is used. The two different screw threads are separately prepared mechanically to avoid the phenomenon of blockage in torsion with a resorbable screw. This avoids the risk of implant fracture (**Fig. 44-5**). The screw is inserted over the guidewire. Again under arthroscopic control, the radiocarpal compartment is visualized through the 3,4 portal; this allows the surgeon to verify the absence of an intra-articular penetration of the screw head at the level of the proximal pole (**Fig. 44-6**).

The entire radiocarpal compartment is inspected to assess potential associated lesions. Midcarpal exploration allows the

inspection of the fracture line to the medial articular surface of the scaphoid and the assessment of the reduction quality. In case of insufficient compression, the screw can be redrilled while visualizing the compressive effect. The scaphotrapeziotrapezoid articulation remains untouched. The resorbable screw has only one size with a long distal part, which allows adaptation to different scaphoid sizes. The surgeon must cut the part that is outside of the bone short at the scaphoid with a mini-oscillating saw (**Fig. 44-7**). The incisions are closed using Steri-strips. Postoperatively, the wrist is left unprotected; a simple anterior splint can be applied after the first dressing to help with postoperative pain.

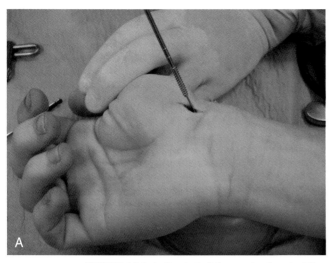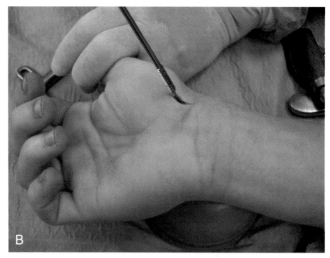

FIGURE 44-5 **A,** Tapping of the proximal part of the scaphoid. **B,** Tapping of the distal part of the scaphoid.

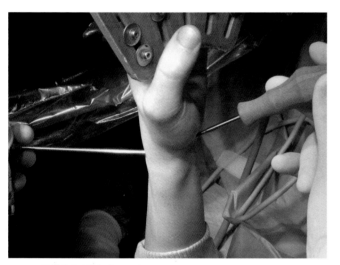

FIGURE 44-6 Screw fixation under arthroscopic control.

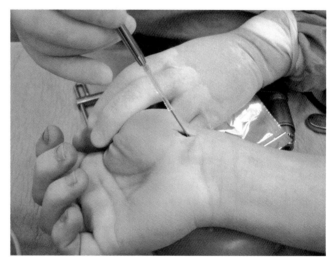

FIGURE 44-7 Placement of the resorbable screw before to cut it easily at the level of the bone.

Important aspects of the operative technique are as follows:

+ Arthroscopic assessment of the midcarpal joint is done to verify the reduction.
+ Partial retrieval of the pin from the distal portion of the scaphoid is done in case of an insufficient reduction. Redirection of the pin is realized under arthroscopic control.
+ Drilling and precise mechanical tapping is separately performed distally and proximally if a resorbable screw is used.
+ Systematic arthroscopic radiocarpal examination at the end of the surgery is done to verify the correct and non–intra-articular position of the screw.

The risks of the procedure are as follows:

+ Breakage of the resorbable screw can occur because of torsion forces if the screw is not tapped correctly.
+ Intra-articular screw positioning with an overlapping screw tip can occur, although the fluoroscopic control seems to be correct. Arthroscopic radiocarpal control at the end of the operation avoids this potential mistake.

+ Scaphoid fixation of a nonreduced or insufficiently reduced fracture can occur.

Complications
Perioperative Complications

Although the intraoperative fluoroscopic result was satisfactory, wrist arthroscopy revealed an overlength of the screw tip because of an intra-articular breakout at the proximal pole of the scaphoid in three cases. The screws had to be changed to shorter ones. This observation confirms the importance of arthroscopic control during this procedure. The guiding pin was broken in the radiocarpal compartment in one patient. Pin removal could be realized under arthroscopic control without any difficulties.

Postoperative Complications

Four patients with nonresorbable screws have had slight anterior pain in the area of the scaphotrapeziotrapezoid joint. Screw removal solved this problem in three patients, whereas slight pain persisted in the fourth patient.

Results

Between 2001 and 2005, 36 patients with 38 isolated scaphoid fractures (two bilateral fractures) underwent arthroscopically assisted percutaneous screw fixation. Thirty patients were men, and six patients were women. The mean age was 34 years (range 17 to 52 years). The dominant side was involved in 75% of the cases. One patient with bilateral fractures was operated the same day; in the other patient, the two operations were performed within 5 days.

All fractures were acute (type B according to the classification of Herbert and Fischer[1]); the mean delay from trauma to surgery was 9 days (range 2 to 30 days). There were mainly waist fractures (type III and IV according to Schernberg's classification[6]); fractures of the proximal pole were not included (**Table 44-1**). The fracture was nondisplaced in 22 cases.

In 16 cases, the reduction could be held with intra-articular arthroscopic maneuvers. Eight resorbable screws and 30 Herbert screws were inserted retrograde from distal to proximal. No remarkable difference in the use of the two screws was noticed. Arthroscopic control was used systematically independent of the perioperative fluoroscopic control. Although there was a satisfying intraoperative fluoroscopic result, wrist arthroscopy revealed an overlength of the screw tip owing to an intra-articular breakout at the proximal pole of the scaphoid in three cases. The screws had to be changed to shorter ones. This observation confirms the interest in the arthroscopic control during this procedure. The guiding pin was broken in the radiocarpal compartment in one patient. Pin removal could be realized under arthroscopic control without any difficulties.

In our series, we have found just a few associated lesions. In one patient, a central perforation of the triangular fibrocartilage complex was débrided with the shaver. In another case, a lesion of the anterior part of the scapholunate ligament without dynamic instability was observed. In this 52-year-old patient, it did not have any therapeutic consequences.

The mean duration of surgery was 32 minutes (range 15 to 70 minutes). The last case had the shortest duration, documenting very well the learning curve of this technique. All patients were reviewed by one examiner independent of the operating surgeon. Postoperative fracture consolidation was assessed radiographically with four x-rays.

The mean follow-up was 29 months (range 6 to 56 months). All fractures healed primarily; nonunion or malunion was not observed. The mean duration of consolidation was 62 days (range 45 to 80 days). The mean duration in originally displaced fractures was 70 days, whereas it was 55 days in originally nondisplaced fractures.

All patients were very satisfied or satisfied with the result. None of the patients regretted choosing this method. The main reason for this high satisfaction rate was the fast functional recovery and the absence of postoperative immobilization. Patients appreciated the small scars, an observation regularly made after most of the endoscopic and arthroscopic procedures.

Return to work was very fast. Twenty patients returned to work immediately. Rapid return to work facilitated patients' decision to choose this technique. Most patients either had an independent occupation or were professional high-level athletes. The mean duration of return to their activities was 21 days (range 0 to 92 days).

The results in terms of pain were excellent. Only five patients had intermittent slight pain. All the other patients were completely pain-free. Four patients with nonresorbable screws have had slight anterior pain in the area of the scaphotrapeziotrapezoid joint. Screw removal solved this problem in three patients, whereas in the fourth patient slight pain persisted.

At final follow-up, 31 of the 34 wrists (two cases with bilateral fractures excluded) reached 90% of the mobility compared with the contralateral side. Comparison of the grip strength measured with a Jamar Dynamometer (Sammons Preston, Inc., Bollingbrook, IL) also confirmed the quality of the recovery (91% of the strength of the healthy contralateral side).

Discussion and Review of Literature

Numerous more recent studies have shown the capability of a percutaneous fixation of scaphoid fractures using cannulated screws.[2,7-9] The various cannulated screw models underline the interest in this method and create competition with the classic conservative method of forearm immobilization for 3 months. Several studies confirm the increased rate of fracture consolidation with this method.[7-10] The time to consolidation in nondisplaced fractures seems to be shorter with percutaneous screw fixation. Shin and coworkers[10] reported in their randomized study (percutaneous screw fixations versus conservative treatment) a consolidation time of 4 to 5 weeks after percutaneous screw fixation. With our results with an average radiological consolidation of less than 2 months in nondisplaced fractures, we can confirm this statement.

In various series, return to professional activities was earlier after screw fixation.[8,10,11,14,21] In our study, the functional recovery also was exceptionally fast. This also might be due to a patient selection bias because many of our patients have chosen this method with regard to their professional and personal duties. It seems to be more logical to propose the percutaneous screw fixation to a motivated and well-informed patient even more when conservative treatment has the risk to fail (e.g., in unstable fractures). The failure rate in terms of consolidation can be 15% after cast immobilization of 3 months.[12,13] In our series, there were no nonunions.

Wrist arthroscopy combined with percutaneous screw fixation allows avoiding certain complications that are relatively frequent in fracture fixation of the scaphoid. Filan and Herbert[13] found 14 intra-articular (Herbert) screw penetrations in their series of 431 patients. In our series, after final arthroscopic control of the radiocarpal joint, we had to change three screws because of breakout of the screw tip out of the scaphoid. Arthroscopic midcarpal examination also allows assessing the quality of fracture reduction after screw fixation.

We agree with Whipple[16] that direct visual examination of the reduction quality is much more efficient than fluoroscopic evaluation. Direct visual control of fracture compression is an additional security for the surgeon. The possibility to diagnose and treat associated lesions with arthroscopic exploration of the wrist

TABLE 44-1 Classification of Scaphoid Fractures According to Schernberg

Displacement	Type II	Type III	Type IV
None	3	14	5
<2 mm		5	4
>2 mm		3	3

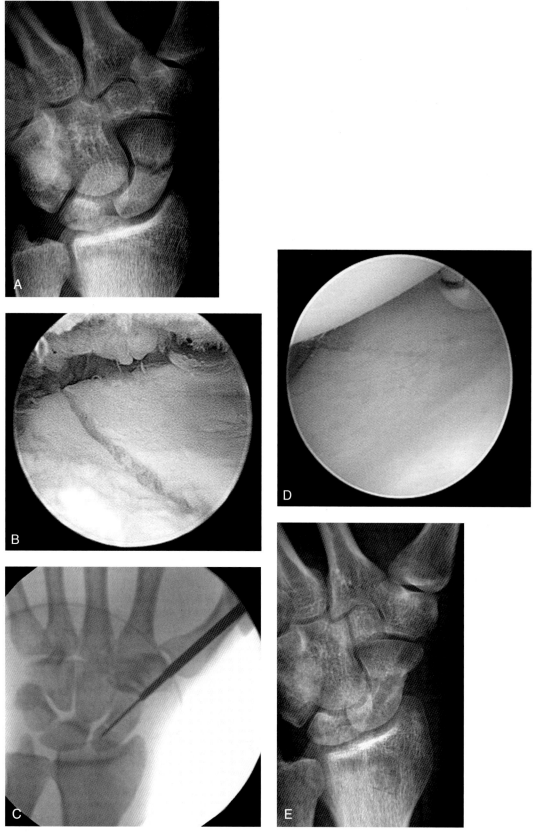

FIGURE 44-8 A, Displaced scaphoid fracture. **B,** Mediocarpal arthroscopic view showing the rotational displacement between the two fragments. **C,** Mediocarpal arthroscopic view showing the reduction after disimpaction of the two fragments with the help of a small curet. **D,** Drilling with fluoroscopic control. **E,** Radiographic control after 60 days showing the consolidated fracture.

was described by many authors.[15,16] Shin and coworkers[10] found 11 intracarpal lesions during arthroscopic exploration in a series of 15 displaced scaphoid fractures that were treated with arthroscopic reduction and percutaneous fixation. Most of them were minor lesions, but the authors also found two complex scapholunate lesions that could be treated with reduction and pinning.

Because of the need for reduction, displaced scaphoid fractures usually required classic open reduction.[17] The possibility to maintain the reduction by external maneuvers justified the use of percutaneous screw fixation.[18] If one could not maintain the reduction, change to an open procedure was indicated.[19] In our series we did not have any problems with the reduction, and all the displaced scaphoid fractures could be reduced and maintained under arthroscopic control (**Fig. 44-8**).

Wrist arthroscopy has found its place for this indication allowing direct and indirect reduction maneuvers. Slade and colleagues[20] described in detail their technique of percutaneous arthroscopically assisted fracture fixation from proximal to distal. The guiding pin is placed with the wrist in hyperflexion and hyperpronation after reduction of the geometric axis of the scaphoid under fluoroscopic control. The screws that were used (Acutrak LLC, Hillsboro, OR) are voluminous, and in our opinion penetration of the screw at the proximal pole may cause a significant cartilage lesion at the scaphoid head. In the case of a fracture type I according to Schernberg, the small-sized proximal fragment has to be fixed with a standard screw. Apart from these specific cases, the technique of screw fixation through a volar approach with the assistance of a small elevator through an STT midcarpal portal to align the fragments always allowed us to verify the reduction without major difficulties. The classic disadvantages of the scaphotrapeziotrapezoid articulation with a volar approach have led to a systematic removal of the screw after 1 year to avoid secondary osteoarthritis.[20] The advent of resorbable screws may have solved this particular problem.[22] We have performed screw removal only in the case of persistent anterior wrist pain. A longer follow-up is necessary to evaluate the potential development of secondary osteoarthritis.

REFERENCES

1. Herbert TJ, Fischer WE: Management of the fractured scaphoid using a new bone screw. J Bone Joint Surg Am. 1984; 66:114-123.

2. Wozasek GE, Moser KD: Percutaneous screw fixation of fractures of the scaphoid. J Bone Joint Surg Am. 1991; 73:138-142.

3. Gelberman RH, Menon J: Vascularity of the scaphoid bone. J Hand Surg [Am]. 1980; 5:508-513.

4. Whipple TL: Stabilization of the fractured scaphoid under arthroscopic control. Orthop Clin North Am. 1995; 26:749-754.

5. Whipple T: Arthroscopic surgery. In: The Wrist. Philadelphia: J.B. Lippincott, 1992.

6. Schernberg F, Elzein F, Gerard Y: Etude anatomo-cliniquedes fractures du scaphoïde carpien. Problème des cals vicieux. Rev Chir Orthop. 1984; 70(II suppl):55-63.

7. Ledoux P, Chahidi N, Moermans JP, et al: Percutaneous Herbert screw osteosynthesis of the scaphoid bone. Acta Orthop Belg. 1995; 61:43-47.

8. Inoue G, Sionoya K: Herbert screw fixation by limited access for acute fracture of the scaphoid. J Bone Joint Surg Br. 1997; 79:418-421.

9. Haddad FS, Goddard NJ: Acute percutaneous scaphoid fixation: a pilot study. J Bone Joint Surg Br. 1998; 80:95-99.

10. Shin A, Bond A, McBride M, et al: Acute screw fixation versus cast immobilisation for stable scaphoid fractures: a prospective randomized study. Presented at the 55th American Society of Surgery for the Hand, Seattle, October 5-7, 2000.

11. Gellman H, Caputo RJ, Carter V, et al: Comparison of short and long arm thumb-spica casts for non displaced fractures of the carpal scaphoid. J Bone Joint Surg Am. 1989; 71:354-357.

12. Kuschner SH, Lane CS, Brien WW, et al: Scaphoid fractures and scaphoid non-union: diagnosis and treatment. Aust N Z J Surg. 1985; 55:387-389.

13. Filan SL, Herbert TJ: Herbert screw fixation of scaphoid fractures. J Bone Joint Surg Am. 1996; 78:519-529.

14. Bond CD, Shin AY, McBride MT, et al: Percutaneous screw fixation or cast immobilization for nondisplaced scaphoid fractures. J Bone Joint Surg Am. 2001; 83:483-488.

15. Shih JT, Lee HM, Hou YT, et al: Result of arthroscopic reduction and percutaneous fixation for acute displaced scaphoid fractures. Arthroscopy. 2005; 21:620-626.

16. Whipple TL: The role of arthroscopy in the treatment of intra-articular wrist fractures. Hand Clin. 1995; 11:13-18.

17. Schernberg F: Les fractures récentes du scaphoïde. Chir Main. 2005; 24:117-131.

18. Cooney WP, Dobyns JH, Linscheid RL: Fractures of the scaphoid : a rational approach to management. Clin Orthop. 1980; 149:90-97.

19. Herbert TJ: Internal fixation of the scaphoid—history. In: Le Scaphoïde. Sauramps, 2004; 125-129.

20. Slade JF 3rd, Grauer JN, Mahoney JD: Arthroscopic reduction and percutaneous fixation of scaphoid fractures with a novel dorsal technique. Orthop Clin North Am. 2001; 32:247-261.

21. Rosati M, Nesti C, Del Grande S, et al: L'osteosintesi con vite cannulata percutanea nelle fratture di scafoide carpale. Riv Chir Mano. 2004; 41:149-157.

22. Martinache X, Mathoulin C: Ostéosynthèse percutanée des fractures du scaphoide carpien avec assistance arthroscopique. Chir Main. 2006; 25:S171-S177.

Arthroscopic Diagnosis of Carpal Ligament Injuries with Distal Radius Fractures

45

Tommy Lindau, MD

Carpal ligament injuries have been found in association with distal radius fractures (**Fig. 45-1**)[1-3] and with scaphoid and other fractures (**Fig. 45-2**).[4,5] In contrast to these injuries, which sometimes are radiographically visible, there are other associated soft tissue injuries involving the median nerve, the radial artery (**Fig. 45-3**), or flexor tendons with ruptures. In addition, numerous articles have highlighted the extent of associated cartilage and ligament injuries with displaced distal radius fractures, especially in nonosteoporotic individuals.[6-10] These injuries occasionally can be found with fluoroscopy or magnetic resonance imaging,[11] but are most often found when the distal radius fracture is managed with wrist arthroscopy as an adjunct.

There has been a tendency to overlook these injuries, in contrast to the awareness of similarly important injuries in the lower extremity (**Fig. 45-4**). To minimize the impact of missed associated injuries, we have to improve our knowledge about them and improve our management of distal radius fractures. We should try to define, classify, and treat the devastating "syndesmosis" injuries of the wrist as soon as possible (**Fig. 45-5**).

Assessment and Decision Making for Associated Injuries

Injuries associated with distal radius fractures should be looked for at least at the following opportunities when the fracture is reviewed and management is discussed:

1. At the time of the fracture when the initial radiographs are reviewed
2. At the fracture clinic during the first week
3. At the fracture clinic at the 10- to 14-day follow-up
4. At the time of surgical treatment
5. At a later follow-up about 3 months after the fracture

At the Time of the Fracture When Initial Radiographs Are Reviewed

There is an obvious difference between patients and their needs, which can be clearly seen already at the initial presentation, where a range of associated, but preexisting conditions can be found (**Fig. 45-6**). Sometimes the associated injuries are obvious, but in most situations the soft tissue injuries are not evident at all (**Fig. 45-7**). We then either have to find them or have to exclude that such associated injuries exist.

At the Initial Presentation, at the Fracture Clinic during the First Week, and at the 10- to 14-Day Follow-up

The radiographs should always be reviewed with the utmost scrutiny regarding degree of displacement, including the ulnar styloid fracture, which may indicate an ulnoradial ligament detachment (peripheral triangular fibrocartilage complex [TFCC] injury) (**Fig. 45-8**). The three carpal arcs of Gilula[12] (**Fig. 45-9**), which are indicative of intercarpal ligament injury, always should be checked.

The most important prognostic factor for a bad outcome after distal fractures is the ulnar-positive variance[13]; there is a 2.5 times increased risk for a bad outcome in nonosteoporotic individuals if the ulnar-positive variance is more than 2 mm. An ulnar-positive variance more than 2 mm also has been shown to give a 3.9 relative risk (95% confidence interval 1.1 to 13.3; $P = .01$) of a grade 3 to 4 scapholunate (SL) ligament injury (Lindau classification system).[7,14]

The second most important prognostic factor is articular involvement; an intra-articular incongruency of more than 1 mm leads to osteoarthritis).[15] An intra-articular fracture also has been shown to be a potentially important factor for a poor outcome in nonosteoporotic patients.[13] Fractures that have a partial intra-articular (AO type B) or combined extra-articular and intra-articular involvement (AO type C) have been shown to increase the risk for a Lindau grade 3 to 4 SL ligament injury[7,14] at the time of injury and to increase the risk for radiographic dynamic or static SL dissociation 1 year after the trauma.[14]

Patient age, metaphyseal comminution of the fracture, and ulnar variance have been shown to be the most consistent predictors of radiographic outcome.[13,16] Dorsal angulation and radial length have not been shown to be associated with a bad outcome,[13,16] which may explain why the AO and Frykman classifications[17] have failed to correlate with the outcome.[18]

An evidence-based algorithm can be very helpful in managing distal radius fractures (**Fig. 45-10**), where the search for associated injuries is added to the general decisions regarding management of the fracture. There is a special emphasis in the algorithm on the differences between nonosteoporotic and osteoporotic patients.[19] The differences are in regard to fracture pattern, associated injuries, treatment alternatives, and outcome, which reflect the future need of patients for their wrists after the injury. Initial assessment also should address the potential risks not obvious on an x-ray, where palmarly displaced fragments especially can cause

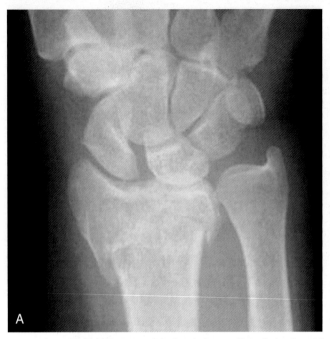

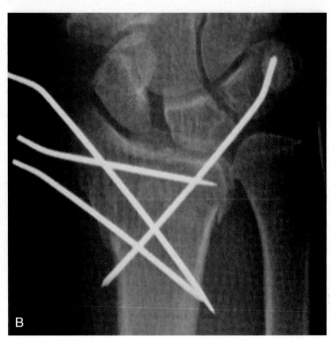

FIGURE 45-1 **A** and **B,** Scapholunate dissociation found before and after treatment of displaced distal radius fracture.

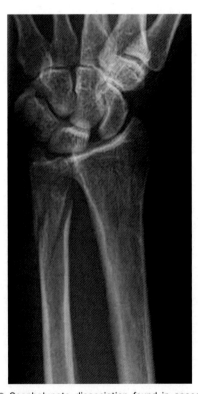

FIGURE 45-2 Scapholunate dissociation found in association with a distal ulnar fracture.

radial artery injuries, flexor tendon ruptures, or median nerve entrapments (carpal tunnel syndrome).

At the Time of Surgical Treatment

If surgical treatment is necessary according to the initial assessments and the pathways of the evidence-based algorithm (see **Fig. 45-10**), we have the golden opportunity to assess, find, and treat all injured parts of the wrist.

Arthroscopy—the Gold Standard of Detecting and Treating Associated Injuries

If surgery is necessary, there is a paramount reason to consider arthroscopy as an adjunct to the final treatment. General arthroscopic technique is applied with the following guidelines[2]:

+ Arthroscopy is done after 2 to 5 days.
+ Traction of about 2 to 5 kg is applied.
+ Swelling distorts the anatomical landmarks for the normal portals.
+ Radiocarpal portals are developed around 3-4 (in between the third and fourth extensor compartments).
+ Access to the joint is with blunt technique.
+ Lavage of the joint and additional shaving to clear out debris are performed.

A standard setup is used with a mobile cart with a monitor at the foot end of the patient. Arthroscopy can be done as either a standard vertical setup or with horizontal arthroscopy,[20] which gives the surgeon several options for additional treatment after the initial arthroscopy has been done.

After the joint has been cleared, the arthroscopy-assisted reduction starts by disimpacting the fragments followed by elevating the fragments, securing the reduction with Kirschner wires (K-wires) or percutaneous fixation, and finally verifying the reduction. The joint surface should be reduced by starting with the ulnar fragments because they cause a "double joint incongruency" (i.e., the radiocarpal joint and the distal radioulnar joint [DRUJ]).[2] Various techniques have been described for special fracture situations.

The final fixation of the fragments can be done with a "closed" reduction of the ulnar fragments with a mini-invasive reduction and percutaneous pinning according to the technique recommended by Geissler and colleagues.[21] Kapandji intrafocal pinning[22] is a useful option in selected cases. Another option is an open

Text continued on p. 449

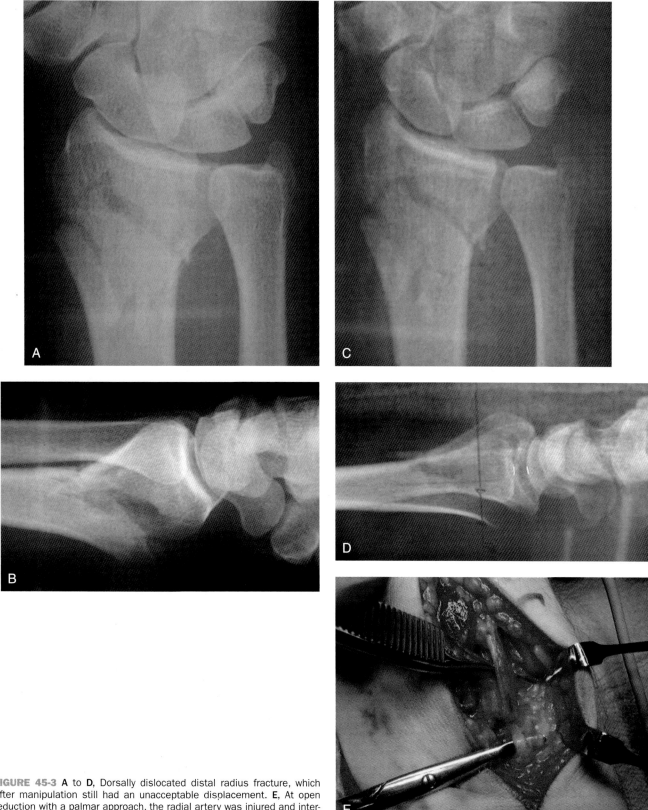

FIGURE 45-3 A to **D,** Dorsally dislocated distal radius fracture, which after manipulation still had an unacceptable displacement. **E,** At open reduction with a palmar approach, the radial artery was injured and interposed in the fracture.

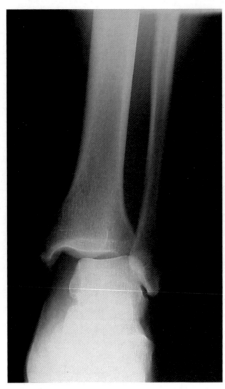

FIGURE 45-4 Syndesmosis injury in an ankle without fracture. This devastating ligament injury is defined and classified and receives full treatment and attention in the orthopaedic community.

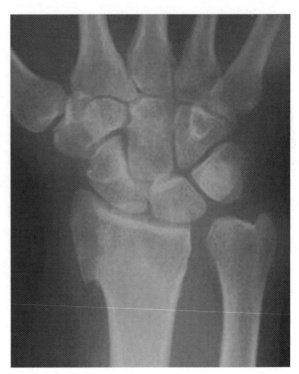

FIGURE 45-5 "Syndesmosis" injury of the wrist with an undetected, untreated ulnoradial ligament (peripheral triangular fibrocartilage complex) tear where the signs of the healed distal radius fracture can be seen.

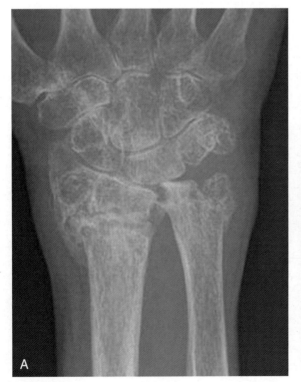

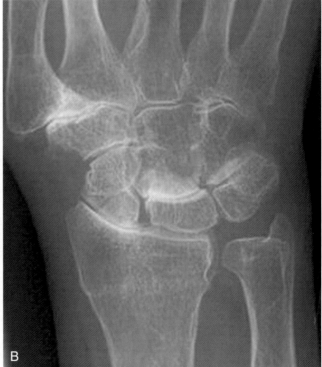

FIGURE 45-6 A and **B,** Preexisting rheumatoid arthritis (**A**) and osteoarthritis (**B**) at the initial presentation of a distal radius fracture. Knowledge of preexisting problems helps the orthopaedist understand how to manage the acute fracture.

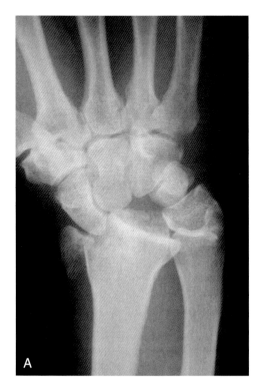

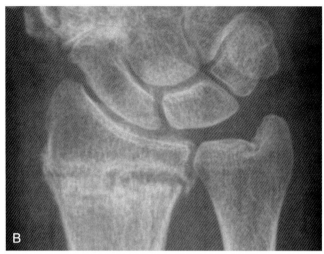

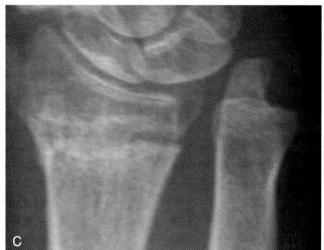

FIGURE 45-7 **A,** Trans-styloid perilunate dislocation with all the signs of the Mayfield chain of intercarpal ligament injuries. **B** and **C,** Distal radial fracture at the initial presentation (**B**) and with stress views reflecting an ulnoradial ligament injury (**C**).

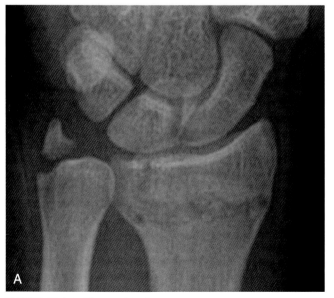

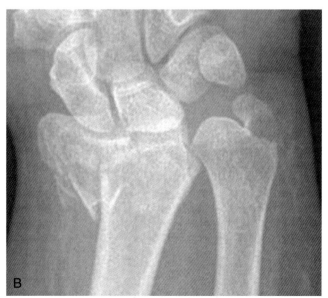

FIGURE 45-8 **A,** Ulnar styloid fracture at the base, which may represent a destabilizing ulnoradial ligament tear causing instability of the distal radioulnar joint. **B,** The ulnar styloid is avulsed in a radial direction as a sign of involvement of the ulnoradial ligament being attached to the avulsed ligaments like two reins.

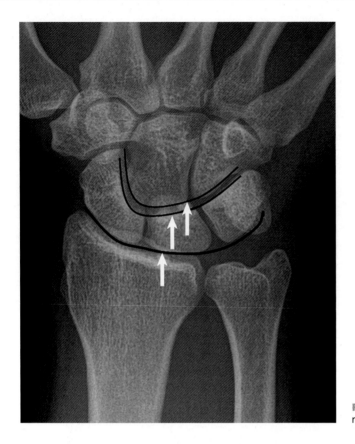

FIGURE 45-9 The three carpal lines of Gilula (*arrows*), which, if disrupted, reveal an intercarpal ligament injury.

DISTAL RADIAL FRACTURES IN DERBY

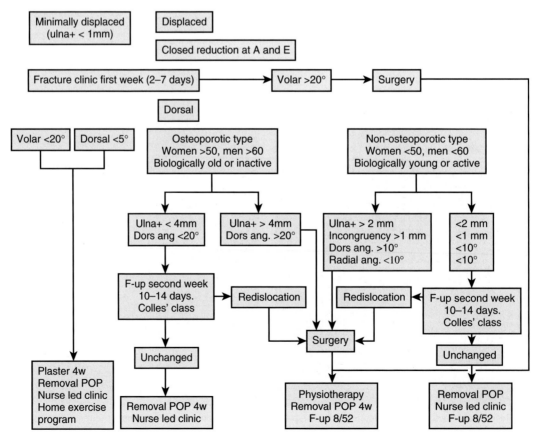

FIGURE 45-10 Evidence-based algorithm with a flow chart for distal radius fractures in adults.

reduction of ulnar-sided fractures, which can be part of managing a combined intra-articular and extra-articular fracture. This can be fixed according to the surgeon's preference with various types of dorsal or palmar plates, including the currently popular locking plates. The final fixation of the extra-articular components of the fracture is facilitated with the horizontal position at the initial arthroscopy, which is converted easily into the final open fixation.[20]

Ulnar Styloid Fractures May Represent a Destabilizing Injury

Fracture of the ulnar styloid has been found with and without a destabilizing injury to the ulnoradial ligament (peripheral tear of the TFCC).[7,9] af Ekenstam and coworkers[23] did not find any statistical difference regarding either redislocation or healing of the styloid or functional outcome of the distal radial fracture. A fracture of the ulnar styloid has not been associated with a development of DRUJ laxity 1 year after the fracture.[24] Consequently, an ulnar styloid fracture is not a good indicator for severity, as stated by Frykman,[17] which probably explains why the Frykman classification[17] has failed to correlate to final outcome.[18]

Ulnar styloid fracture at its base with initial displacement more than 2 mm should be treated with open reduction and internal fixation (see **Fig. 45-7A**).[21,25] Use of open reduction and internal fixation is even more important if the dislocation is in a radial direction (detaching the ulnoradial ligament; see **Fig. 45-8B**) than in an axial, distal direction (detaching the ulnotriquetral collateral ligament; see **Fig. 45-7A**). The fixation can be done with a single K-wire,[26,27] tension band wiring,[21] a wire loop/suture,[26] or screw fixation.[28]

Triangular Fibrocartilage Complex Tears Are the Most Common Destabilizing Injuries

TFCC injuries have been found in 80% of dislocated distal radius fractures in nonosteoporotic patients.[7] They have been associated with shortening (ulna positive) and dorsal angulation of the radius fracture.[9] The most important of these injuries are the tears to the ulnoradial ligaments (peripheral TFCC tears), which have been shown to cause laxity 1 year after the fracture.[24] Peripheral TFCC tears probably should be repaired, which can be done with an arthroscopically assisted technique and reattachment to the fovea (**Fig. 45-11**).[2] A central perforation tear of the TFCC is stable and can be débrided with a suction punch (**Fig. 45-12**).[2]

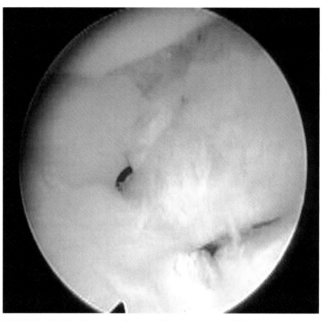

FIGURE 45-11 Triangular fibrocartilage complex (TFCC) reattachment with an arthroscopy-assisted technique showing two sutures that have tightened the avulsed ligament. The radius is seen between 6 and 9 o'clock. The lunate is on top between 11 and 1 o'clock. TFCC is between 5 and 9 o'clock with the ulnar side toward the right.

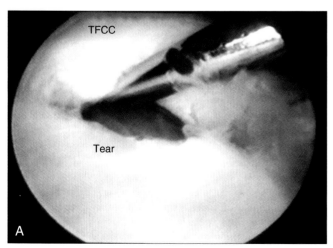

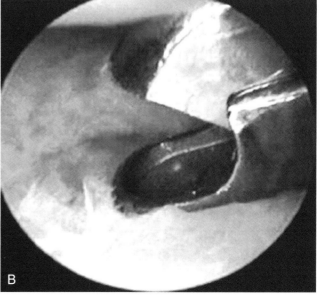

FIGURE 45-12 **A,** Central perforation tear of the triangular fibrocartilage complex (TFCC). Radius in between 4 and 9 o'clock. TFCC above and the probe lifting the torn membranous disc of the TFCC. Dorsal to the right. **B,** Débridement with a suction punch of such a lesion. Dorsal to the right.

TABLE 45-1 Classification System for Interosseous Scapholunate and Lunotriquetral Ligament Injuries and Mobility of the Joints

Grade	Radiocarpal Arthroscopy Ligament Appearance	Midcarpal Arthroscopy	
		Diastasis (mm)	Step-off (mm)
1	Hematoma	0	0
2	As above and/or partial tear	0-1	<2
3	Partial or complete tear	1-2	<2
4	Complete tear	>2	>2

From Lindau T, Arner M, Hagberg L: Intraarticular lesions in distal fractures of the radius in young adults: a descriptive arthroscopic study in 50 patients. J Hand Surg. 1997; 22B:638-643.

Scapholunate Ligament Injury Leads to Scapholunate Dissociation

SL ligament tears have been found in 50% of dislocated distal radius fractures in nonosteoporotic patients.[7] At radiocarpal arthroscopy, the ligament appearance can be assessed, and with comparison of the midcarpal appearance the diastasis and step-off can be measured to classify the grade of SL injury according to Geissler[29] or Lindau[7] (**Table 45-1**). With this assessment, we have shown that a grade 3 to 4 SL ligament injury (Lindau classification[7] [see Table 45-1]) that was found at the time of the distal radial fracture, but not treated, leads to radiographic dissociation 1 year after the injury.[14]

In the absence of prospective randomized studies, it is reasonable to treat grade 3 injuries with reduction of the displaced carpal bones by positioning K-wires in the lunate and the scaphoid. The reduction of the incongruent SL joint is monitored in the midcarpal joint, and the K-wires are secured into the bones. Fluoroscopy can verify the reduction and fixation.[2] The pins should be kept for 6 weeks.

The results with the arthroscopy-assisted technique are encouraging; Whipple[30] showed that 33 of 40 patients maintained reduction and relief of symptoms if the injury was less than 3 months and the gap was less than 3 mm. In contrast, if there was more than 3 months and more than 3 mm of gap, the improvement occurred in only 21 of 40 patients. Time is consequently of the essence in finding these injuries, and if they are found in time, the results are good in 85% after 2 to 7 years.[30] No further long-term studies have been done in this area. Finally, it also seems reasonable to assume that grade 4 injuries, especially injuries with a dissociation already on the trauma films, probably should be treated with an open repair.[2]

Lunotriquetral Ligament Injuries Are Uncommon

Lunotriquetral ligament tears have been found in 10% of dislocated distal radius fractures in nonosteoporotic patients.[7] There are no long-term studies in this area, but complete tears with severe mobility (grade 4 [see Table 45-1][7]) probably have to be pinned for 6 weeks.[2] Pinning of acute lunotriquetral tears has shown to have a good outcome with 16 of 20 patients excellent

or good after 2½ years and 18 of 20 with improved grip strength.[31]

Cartilage Injuries Lead to Osteoarthritis

Subchondral hematoma and cartilage avulsions have been found in one third of patients with dislocated fractures among non-osteoporotic patients.[7] These lesions result in radiographic subchondral bone plate changes and osteoarthritis after 1 year.[32] The implication is that subchondral hematoma after injury is a possible explanation of development of osteoarthritis in other joints. There is currently no treatment other than débridement for these injuries. The most tempting, but unproven, option would be the microfracture treatment used in similar injuries in the knee. If found, these cartilage injuries may lead, however, to changes in treatment in the sense that a comminuted intra-articular fracture might be treated with a partial wrist fusion. It also would give the surgeon an awareness of an expected bad outcome.

Other Options at the Time of Surgical Treatment

In the absence of arthroscopy, a fluoroscopic assessment, including stress views, before reduction and fixation is mandatory to plan the surgical approach appropriately. Fluoroscopy is done with examination with an ulnar and radial deviation to see any gapping between the carpal bones. A traction view also may be tried to see whether the Gilula lines[12] are disrupted. The DRUJ is difficult to assess before the distal radius fracture has been stabilized.

After reduction and fixation of the distal radius fracture, a new assessment of the intercarpal ligaments (see Fig. 45-1) and DRUJ stability (see Fig. 45-7B and C) should be done. The focus should not be on the fracture alone. One should try to avoid overdistracting the soft tissues if external fixation is used (**Fig. 45-13**), and one should try to understand if a fragment may represent the insertion of a crucial radiocarpal stabilizing ligament (**Fig. 45-14**).

At a Later Follow-up about 3 Months after the Fracture

At assessment at approximately 3 months after a moderate to severe distal radius fracture, occasional ache, decreased grip strength at about 50% to 65% of the contralateral hand, and limited range of motion are acceptable. Signs of pain and instability and clicking or clunking of the wrist are unacceptable.

At this stage, one should reassess everything, including all radiographs through the treatment; do a thorough clinical examination; and probably have new x-rays taken. At the clinical examination, one should look for signs of sagging of the hand compared with the distal forearm and look out for a prominent ulnar head (**Fig. 45-15**). This may represent an avulsed dorsal radiotriquetral ligament causing the sagging lateral view and potentially development of a midcarpal instability. The DRUJ should be examined; the stability test has been shown to be useful and reproducible.[33] Additional radiographs, including stress views such as clenched fist views, should be considered and thereafter possibly arthrography, computed tomography, or magnetic resonance imaging depending on access to these imaging modalities. The final option to understand fully the reasons for complicating symptoms and signs 3 months after a distal radius fracture is to do a wrist arthroscopy.

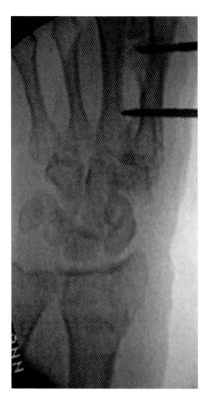

FIGURE 45-13 Distal radius fracture treated with external fixator in which the emphasis has been on reducing the bony fracture only. Ligamentotaxis is overstretching the radiocarpal and intercarpal ligaments.

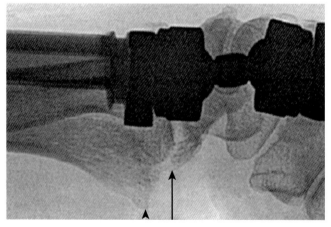

FIGURE 45-14 Distal radial fracture with a palmar fragment that was recognized after the initial reduction and external fixation. It represents the important radiocarpal ligament, which causes radiocarpal instability if it is not detected and addressed with open reduction and internal fixation.

Conclusion

A fall on an outstretched hand may lead to a variety of injuries to the wrist—ranging from a sprain to a full-blown perilunate dislocation (see Fig. 45-7A). There are degrees of injuries and significance in the Mayfield[34] mechanism causing a variety of injuries in the wrist (see Figs. 45-1, 45-7A, and 45-8B). It is our task to assess early and decide what kind of injury we have to treat in every case.

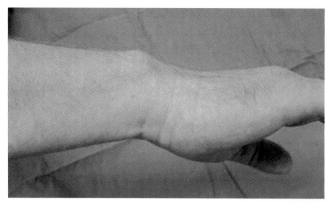

FIGURE 45-15 Sagging of the hand at external examination represents a dorsal radiotriquetral ligament injury, which may lead to midcarpal instability.

We should look for prognostic markers on the initial radiographs, where an ulnar-positive variance more than 2 mm and an intra-articular fracture marks a higher risk of more severe fractures and more associated ligament injuries. This evaluation should be repeated at every follow-up in fracture clinics during the first week and at the 10- to 14-day follow-up. At these early assessments, there is an important role for an evidence-based algorithm (see Fig. 45-10) showing the pathway for each patient according to the appearance of the fracture with an emphasis on whether there are signs of clinical osteoporosis.

If the patient, according to the evidence-based algorithm, is suitable for surgical treatment, the opportunity should not be missed to rule out all important pathology by using arthroscopy. If arthroscopy is unavailable, at least a clinical and fluoroscopic assessment should be done before reduction and after fixation so that every aspect of the wrist injury has been analyzed before the patient leaves the operating room.

We should treat the fracture perfectly, but we must remember that the fracture represents a significant injury to the entire wrist, of which the fracture is the only obvious injury. We must be aware of the risk for associated injuries. Rule them out or find them, then you are doing fine!

REFERENCES

1. Cooney WP 3rd, Dobyns JH, Linscheid RL: Complications of Colles' fractures. J Bone Joint Surg Am. 1980; 62:613-619.
2. Lindau T: The role of wrist arthroscopy in distal radial fractures. Atlas Hand Clin. 2001; 6:285-306.
3. Mudgal CS, Jones WA: Scapho-lunate diastasis: a component of fractures of the distal radius. J Hand Surg [Br]. 1990; 15:503-505.
4. Fisk GR: Carpal instability and the fractured scaphoid. Ann R Coll Surg Engl. 1970; 46:63-76.
5. Vender MI, Watson HK, Black DM, et al: Acute scaphoid fracture with scapholunate gap. J Hand Surg [Am]. 1989; 14:1004-1007.
6. Geissler WB, Freeland AE, Savoie FH, et al: Intracarpal soft-tissue lesions associated with an intra-articular fracture of the distal end of the radius. J Bone Joint Surg Am. 1996; 78:357-365.
7. Lindau T, Arner M, Hagberg L: Intraarticular lesions in distal fractures of the radius in young adults: a descriptive

arthroscopic study in 50 patients. J Hand Surg [Br]. 1997; 22:638-643.

8. Lindau T: Distal radial fractures and effects of associated ligament injuries. Thesis. Lund: University of Lund, 2000.

9. Richards RS, Bennett JD, Roth JH, et al: Arthroscopic diagnosis of intra-articular soft tissue injuries associated with distal radial fractures. J Hand Surg [Am]. 1997; 22:772-776.

10. Shih JT, Lee HM, Hou YT, et al: Arthroscopically-assisted reduction of intra-articular fractures and soft tissue management of distal radius. J Asia-Pacific Fed Soc Surg Hand. 2001; 6:127-135.

11. Spence LD, Savenor A, Nwachuku I, et al: MRI of fractures of the distal radius: comparison with conventional radiographs. Skeletal Radiol. 1998; 27:244-249.

12. Gilula LA: Carpal injuries: analytic approach and case exercises. AJR Am J Roentgenol. 1979; 133:503-517.

13. Beumer A, Adlercreutz C, Lindau T: Early prognostic factors for a bad outcome in non-osteoporotic distal radius fractures. Presented as a poster at IFSSH meeting, Sydney, Australia, 2007.

14. Forward D, Lindau T, Melsom D: Intercarpal ligament injuries associated with fractures of the distal radius: arthroscopic assessment and 12 month follow-up. J Bone Joint Surg Am. 2007; 89:2334-2340.

15. Knirk JL, Jupiter JB: Intra-articular fractures of the distal end of the radius in young adults. J Bone Joint Surg Am. 1986; 68:647-659.

16. Mackenney PJ, McQueen MM, Elton R: Prediction of instability in distal radial fractures. J Bone Joint Surg Am. 2006; 88:1944-1951.

17. Frykman G: Fracture of the distal radius including sequelae, shoulder-hand-finger syndrome, disturbance in the distal radio-ulnar joint and impairment of nerve function. Acta Orthop Scand. 1967; 38(Suppl 108):83-88.

18. Flinkkilä T, Raatikainen T, Hämäläinen M: AO and Frykman's classifications of Colles' fracture: no prognostic value in 652 patients evaluated after 5 years. Acta Orthop Scand. 1998; 69:77-81.

19. Lindau T, Aspenberg P, Arner M, et al: Fractures of the distal forearm in young adults: an epidemiologic description of 341 patients. Acta Orthop Scand. 1999; 70:124-128.

20. Lindau T: Wrist arthroscopy in distal radial fractures with a modified horizontal technique. Arthroscopy 2001; 17(1), E5.

21. Geissler WB, Fernandez DL, Lamey DM: Distal radioulnar joint injuries associated with fractures of the distal radius. Clin Orthop. 1996; 327:135-146.

22. Kapandji A: [Internal fixation by double intrafocal plate: functional treatment of non articular fractures of the lower end of the radius] (author's transl). Ann Chir. 1976; 30(11-12):903-908.

23. af Ekenstam F, Jacobsson OP, Wadin K: Repair of the triangular ligament in Colles' fracture: no effect in a prospective randomized study. Acta Orthop Scand. 1989; 60:393-396.

24. Lindau T, Adlercreutz C, Aspenberg P: Peripheral tears of the triangular fibrocartilage complex cause distal radioulnar joint instability after distal radial fractures. J Hand Surg [Am]. 2000; 25:464-468.

25. May MM, Lawton JN, Blazar PE: Ulnar styloid fractures associated with distal radius fractures: incidence and implications for distal radioulnar joint instability. J Hand Surg [Am]. 2002; 27:965-971.

26. Mikic DJZ: Treatment of acute injuries of the triangular fibrocartilage complex associated with distal radioulnar joint instability. J Hand Surg [Am]. 1995; 20:319-323.

27. Shaw JA, Bruno A, Paul EM: Ulnar styloid fixation in the treatment of posttraumatic instability of the radioulnar joint: a biomechanical study with clinical correlation. J Hand Surg [Br]. 1990; 15:712-720.

28. Hauck RM, Skahen J III, Palmer AK: Classification and treatment of ulnar styloid nonunion. J Hand Surg [Am]. 1996; 21:418-422.

29. Geissler WB: Arthroscopically assisted reduction of intra-articular fractures of the distal radius. Hand Clin. 1995; 11:19-29.

30. Whipple TL: The role of arthroscopy in the treatment of scapholunate instability. Hand Clin. 1995; 11:37-40.

31. Osterman AL, Seidman GD: The role of arthroscopy in the treatment of lunatotriquetral ligament injuries. Hand Clin. 1995; 11:41-50.

32. Lindau T, Adlercreutz C, Aspenberg P: Cartilage injuries in distal radial fractures. Acta Orthop Scand. 2003; 74:327-331.

33. Lindau T, Runnquist K, Aspenberg P: Patients with laxity of the distal radioulnar joint after distal radial fractures have impaired function, but no loss of strength. Acta Orthop Scand. 2002; 73:151-156.

34. Mayfield JK, Johnson RP, Kilcoyne RF: The ligaments of the human wrist and their functional significance. Anat Rec. 1976; 186:417-428.

Open Scapholunate Ligament Repair

46

Mark S. Cohen, MD

Rationale

Dissociation between the carpal scaphoid and lunate is the most common pattern of wrist instability.[1-3] Because scapholunate dissociation leads to progressive degenerative arthritis of the wrist,[2,4,5] reduction and internal fixation is the preferred method of treatment, particularly in the acute setting.[6-10] Owing to the small surface area and the high loads placed on the repaired ligament, a variety of capsular reconstructions (capsulodeses) have been described to augment scapholunate ligament repair. These procedures use the dorsal capsule or the dorsal radiocarpal and dorsal intercarpal ligaments, or both the capsule and ligaments, to help keep the scaphoid out of pathological flexion and the lunate out of excessive extension (**Fig. 46-1**).

Indications

Indications for direct ligament repair and capsulodesis include a documented dissociation with an adequate ligament still available for repair at the time of surgery, a reducible scapholunate relationship, and the absence of degenerative changes within the carpus. Although these procedures are best when performed early, some data suggest that the results do not depend on the interval between injury and surgical repair.[11] Additional reconstructive options to treat scapholunate dissociation are discussed in subsequent chapters, including using the flexor carpi radialis tendon as a tenodesis

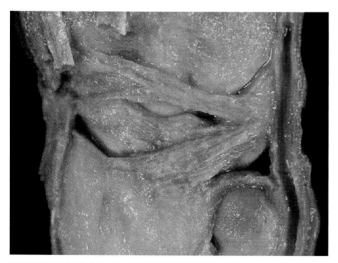

FIGURE 46-1 Cadaver specimen depicting the dorsal wrist ligaments. Note the dorsal radiocarpal ligament spanning from the radius to the triquetrum. The dorsal intercarpal ligament originates on the triquetrum and inserts into the trapezium and distal scaphoid. These ligaments are used in a variety of fashions to augment scapholunate ligament repair (capsulodesis).

and a screw, rather than smooth pins, to maintain the scaphoid and lunate relationship. Partial wrist fusions, such as between the scaphoid, trapezium, and trapezoid (scaphotrapeziotrapezoid fusion) or between the scaphoid and capitate (scaphocapitate fusion), which were previously popular are falling out of favor for scapholunate dissociation.

Contraindications

The main contraindication to direct ligament repair of a scapholunate dissociation is arthritic changes within the carpus. When the scaphoid and lunate become dissociated, a progressive pattern of wrist arthritis ensues. Wear begins at the radial styloid and progresses to involve the entire radioscaphoid articulation and then the midcarpal joint. The degree of arthrosis is not always apparent on plain radiographs of the wrist (**Fig. 46-2**). When degenerative changes are present, most notably in the scaphoid fossa of the radius, alternative salvage options are required, such as a proximal row carpectomy or a midcarpal (four-bone) fusion.

Surgical Technique

Web Video

46-1

The procedure of direct scapholunate ligament repair with dorsal capsulodesis begins with a dorsal longitudinal incision centered over the scapholunate interval. The dorsal retinaculum is divided in line with the third compartment, and the extensor pollicis longus is retracted radially. The posterior interosseous nerve can be found on the radial floor of the fourth dorsal compartment. A neurectomy is performed because this nerve partly innervates the scapholunate ligament.[12] The fourth dorsal compartment is subperiosteally reflected ulnarly to aid in the exposure, but its subsheath is not violated.

The wrist joint is exposed through a straight capsular incision. Care is taken not to elevate the radial capsular flap off of the radius. Alternatively, the radial flap can be elevated in a subperiosteal fashion, but this would need to be secured later to the dorsal aspect of the distal radius to complete the capsulodesis. The dorsal and membranous portions of the scapholunate interosseous ligament are evaluated. The ligament is typically torn off of the scaphoid remaining attached to the lunate. It can avulse off of the lunate, however, and remain attached to the scaphoid. Lastly, one occasionally observes central attenuation within the ligament proper. If there is little or no interosseous ligament remaining for repair, alternative surgical options can be considered.[13-17]

The dorsal aspect of the proximal pole of the scaphoid and corresponding scaphoid facet of the distal radius are inspected for degenerative changes. As noted previously, if significant degeneration exists, one needs to consider a salvage-type operation.[5,18-20] Advanced radioscaphoid arthritis is a contraindication to direct ligament repair. If only slight pointing at the radial styloid exists,

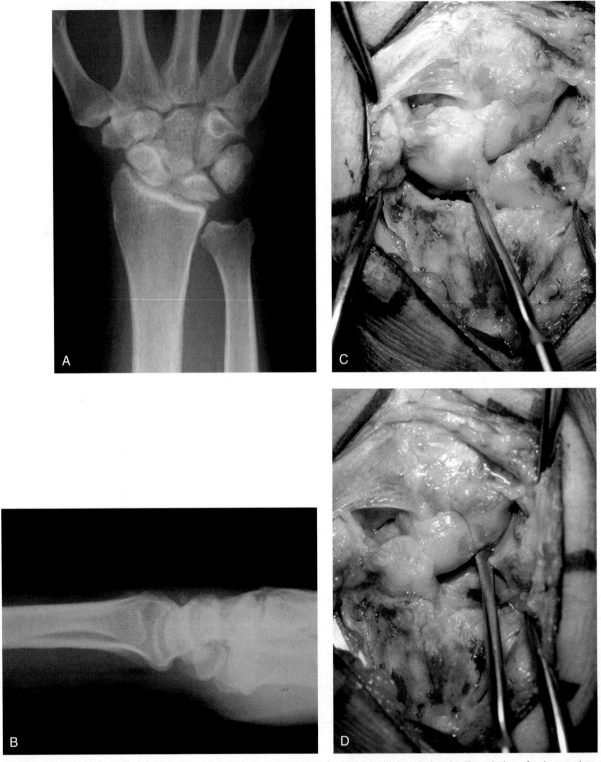

FIGURE 46-2 A and **B,** Posteroanterior (**A**) and lateral (**B**) radiographs of a patient with scapholunate dissociation of unknown duration. Note the extended posture of the lunate on the lateral projection. The frontal film shows pointing at the radial styloid consistent with early wear from the dissociation. The remaining radioscaphoid and midcarpal joints appear unaffected. **C** and **D,** Intraoperative photographs revealing advanced radiocarpal arthritis with complete loss of cartilage in the proximal pole of the scaphoid (**C**) and advanced midcarpal arthritis (**D**). This patient is not a candidate for direct scapholunate ligament repair, and alternative salvage options are required.

however, a limited styloidectomy can be done. Care is taken to protect the radial capsule during subperiosteal dissection for the styloidectomy.

Kirschner wires are inserted in a dorsopalmar direction into the scaphoid and lunate to be used as joysticks. Because signifi-

cant force may be required to reduce the diastasis, 0.062-inch wires are typically used for this purpose. The scaphoid wire is placed in a slightly distal to proximal direction; the lunate pin is angled slightly from proximal to distal to facilitate subsequent rotation of the bones. A narrow trough is created next along the dorsal lunate or scaphoid with a bur or fine rongeur at the site of detachment. Although the repair was originally described using drill holes and Keith needles, newer miniature bone anchors can be used to aid in the repair. With the joint opened, the anchors can be placed (**Fig. 46-3**). It is sometimes easier to place the

anchor sutures into the ligament in their anatomical position before the final fixation. This is especially true for the more proximal sutures, which may be difficult to work with when the bones are reduced, and this area rotates beneath the dorsal rim of the radius.

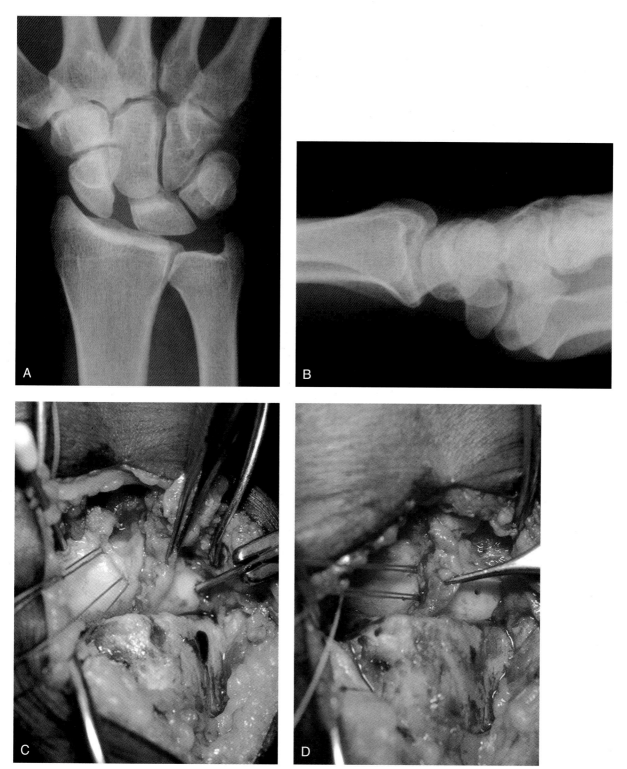

FIGURE 46-3 **A** and **B**, Posteroanterior (**A**) and lateral (**B**) radiographs of a patient with a scapholunate dissociation. **C**, Intraoperative photograph depicting the bone anchors that have been placed into the scaphoid at the site of ligament avulsion. Note the Kirschner wires in the scaphoid and lunate being used as joysticks. **D**, The scapholunate dissociation has been reduced and secured with percutaneous Kirschner wires placed from the scaphoid into the lunate, and from the scaphoid into the capitate. The ligament is seen in the forceps.

Continued

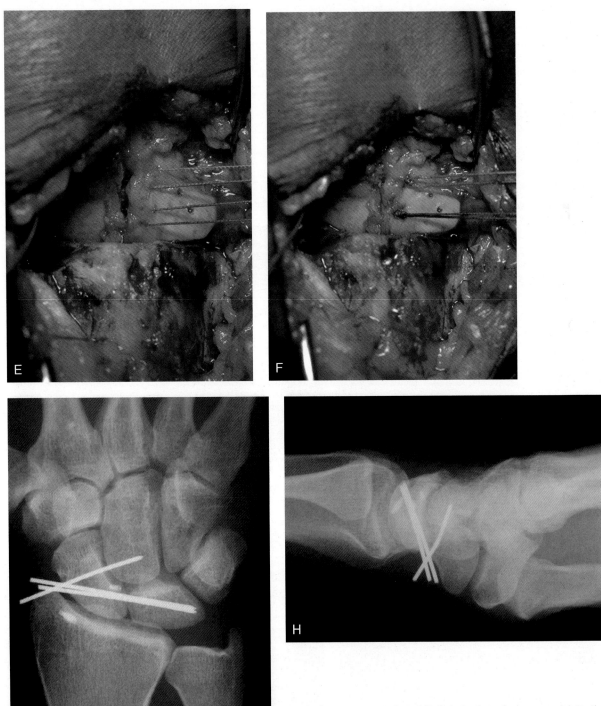

FIGURE 46-3, cont'd **E** and **F,** Sutures have been passed into the ligament (**E**) and tied completing the direct ligament repair (**F**). **G** and **H,** Postoperative posteroanterior (**G**) and lateral (**H**) radiographs. Note the reduction of the scapholunate relationship and the bone anchors in the scaphoid and distal radius for the dorsal capsulodesis performed in a "reverse" fashion in this case.

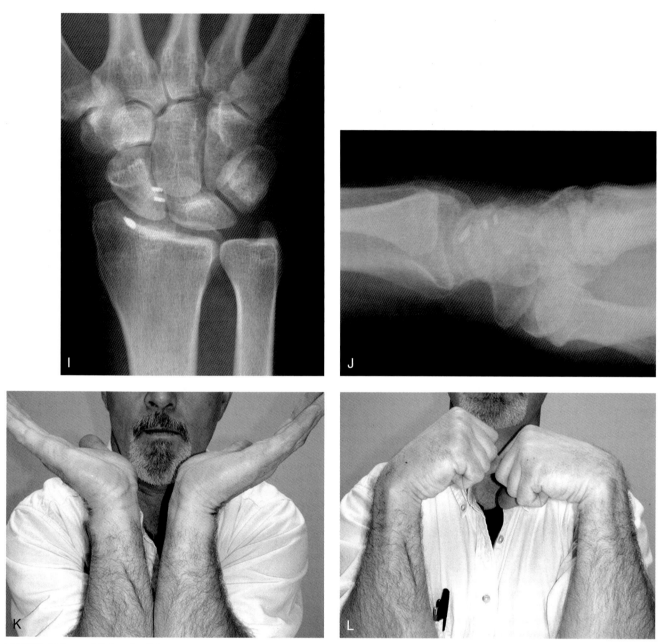

FIGURE 46-3, cont'd **I** and **J**, Follow-up posteroanterior (**I**) and lateral (**J**) radiographs. **K** and **L**, Final wrist extension (**K**) and flexion (**L**) at follow-up. Note the loss of terminal wrist flexion, which is attributed to the capsulodesis.

The joint is next reduced using the Kirschner wires by extending the scaphoid and flexing the lunate. Occasionally, the bones also have to be pulled together, supinating the scaphoid. In addition to flexion, the scaphoid pronates when it dissociates from the lunate.[21,22] After reduction (slight over-reduction may be preferable), the bones are pinned with 0.045-inch Kirschner wires directed from the scaphoid into the lunate and from the scaphoid into the capitate. The reduction is checked and verified under fluoroscopy. With the scapholunate joint reduced, the ligament is repaired to the trough using the bone anchor sutures (see **Fig. 46-3**). If previously placed, these are tied under tension completing the repair. As described by Viegas and DaSilva,[23] the proximal fibers of the dorsal intercarpal ligament can be incorporated into

the repair. This intercarpal ligament passes transversely just distal to the scapholunate ligament and may normally reinforce this bony relationship (**Fig. 46-4**).

When the ligament is directly repaired, a secondary capsulodesis can be added. The original technique of dorsal capsulodesis was described by Blatt in 1987.[7] He used a proximally based strip of the dorsal capsule off the radial aspect of the radius to tether and stabilize the distal scaphoid. Taleisnik modified Blatt's technique to include a direct scapholunate ligament repair and an imbrication of the radial capsule to complete the capsulodesis (**Fig. 46-5**).[11] Securing the radial capsule to the distal scaphoid provides a dorsal tether to resist subsequent scaphoid flexion.[7] Although the capsulodesis was initially described using a palmar

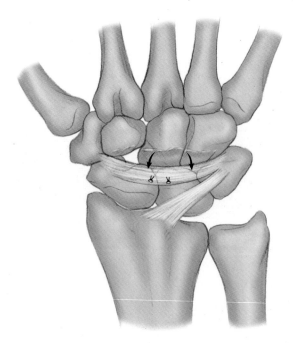

FIGURE 46-4 Diagram depicting the capsulodesis technique of Viegas and DaSilva[23] in which the central aspect of the dorsal intercarpal ligament is pulled proximally and reattached to the scaphoid and lunate in an effort to reinforce the repair and restore anatomy.

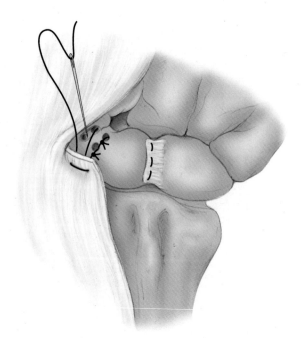

FIGURE 46-5 Schematic diagram of scapholunate ligament repair and capsulodesis as originally described by Taleisnik[11] in which drill holes are placed through the scaphoid to facilitate repair. The newer miniature bone anchors are an alternative to this technique. The radial capsular flap, still attached to the distal radius, is advanced to the distal pole of the scaphoid to complete the capsulodesis. The ulnar capsule is imbricated over the top of this, completing the dorsal capsular reconstruction.

pullout suture, attachment of the radial capsule to the distal scaphoid also can be facilitated using a small bone anchor. Care must be taken to create a trough in the dorsal aspect of the scaphoid distal to the midwaist. This improves the mechanical advantage of the capsulodesis. With the radial capsule pulled distally under tension, the capsule is secured down to the scaphoid trough using the bone anchor sutures or with a pullout suture tied palmarly over a bolster. If a bone anchor is chosen, it is easiest to place it in the center of the trough before reduction and pinning of the scapholunate dissociation. The ulnar capsular flap is used to reinforce the repair by suturing it to the radial capsule. The extensor retinaculum is approximated leaving the extensor pollicis longus outside of the retinaculum, and the skin is repaired in the usual manner.

Alternative capsulodesis reconstructions have been described to augment the direct scapholunate ligament repair. Szabo and coworkers[24,25] have modified the capsulodesis to incorporate the dorsal intercarpal ligament, as is discussed in a subsequent chapter. Kleinman[26] has described using the dorsal intercarpal ligament as a capsulodesis by releasing it ulnarly and repairing it to the distal radius. Walsh and coworkers[27] have described an alternative capsulodesis using the proximal half of the dorsal intercarpal ligament, which is sutured to the lunate. Because this capsulodesis does not cross the radiocarpal joint, it theoretically should not limit wrist flexion to the same degree.

Postoperatively, the wrist is immobilized in a short arm cast for approximately 8 weeks, at which time the Kirschner wires are removed. A gradual range of motion program is started under occupational therapy guidance with interval splinting of the wrist for protection and support. Return of wrist motion is generally slow. Resisted exercises are not allowed until approximately 3 to 4 months postoperatively. Activities requiring wrist extension

against vigorous resistance are not permitted until approximately 6 months after surgery.

Practical Tips

The most difficult aspect of the operation, and possibly most important, is proper reduction of the scaphoid to the proximal and distal rows of the carpus. One method to simplify the pinning is first to pin the capitate to the lunate with a retrograde wire. With a pin provisionally placed in the capitate, the lunate is flexed and pulled radially against the reduced scaphoid. Advancing the pin locks the midcarpal joint in proper position; this simplifies reduction of the scaphoid because there is now only one moving part. The scaphoid is extended and supinated to reduce it to the fixed lunate and capitate. The scaphoid can be pinned with smooth wires.

Using conventional bone anchors, it also is sometimes difficult to reattach the scapholunate ligament directly to the point of bony avulsion. Even if the knot is tightly tied, the ligament may not be completely approximated to the bony trough because it is difficult to "push" tissue down to the bony surface using this technique (**Fig. 46-6**). Newer anchors (originally designed for larger joints such as the shoulder) that are applied by first placing a locking stitch into the ligament edge and then driving this down into the bone may be more effective for scapholunate repair. We have been using these at our institution for several years and have found them to provide a more satisfying repair because they drag the ligament edge directly into the bony trough (see Fig. 46-6).

Finally, another technical difficulty involves proper tensioning of the radial capsule to complete the capsulodesis. Because it is

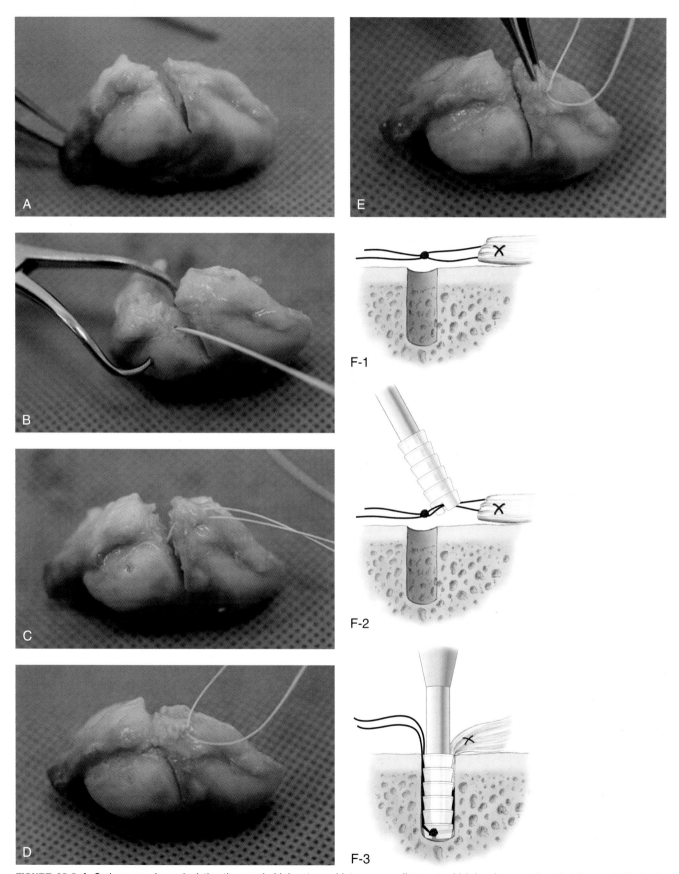

FIGURE 46-6 A, Cadaver specimen depicting the scaphoid, lunate, and interosseous ligament, which has been sectioned at its scaphoid attachment to simulate a ligament rupture. **B,** Conventional bone anchor placed into the insertion point. **C** and **D,** Sutures have been passed into the ligament (**C**) and tied to complete the simulated repair (**D**). **E,** Note how the edge of the ligament is not firmly attached to the bone edge. It can be difficult to "push" tissue to bone using conventional bone anchors for this repair. **F,** Diagram depicting newer V-Tak anchor (Arthrex, Inc, Naples, FL) in which the sutures are first placed into the ligament with a locking stitch. The suture is tied, and the knot is driven into the bone using a fork on the anchor. This delivers the ligament edge to the bone better and completes the repair more securely.

Continued

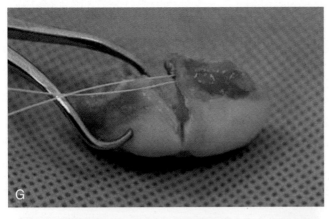

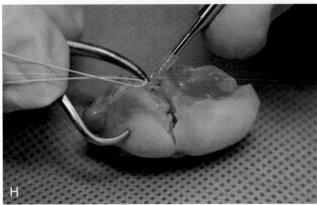
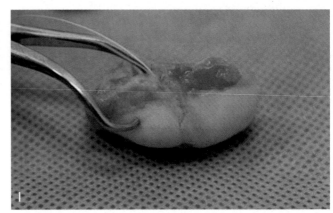

FIGURE 46-6, cont'd **G,** Suture placed in the ligament edge of a specimen with this technique. **H,** Note the bone anchor, which captures the knot and helps drive the ligament edge to the bone. **I,** Final repair using this technique. This latter technique has been shown experimentally to be superior with respect to pullout strength when used for the scapholunate ligament.

occasionally difficult to push the thick dorsal capsular tissue down to the scaphoid trough under tension using a bone anchor (if sutured too tightly, it would not reach, and if too loose, it would not provide an adequate dorsal tether), one can alternatively fix the distal capsule to the scaphoid first. This "reverse capsulodesis" technique also is used if it was decided to perform a radial styloidectomy, or if the radial capsule was subperiosteally dissected off the radius during exposure. In this way, the capsule can be first secured distally under minimal tension. This ensures that the capsule is directly secured to the cancellous trough created in the scaphoid. The radial capsule can be pulled taut proximally and secured to the radius under tension using an additional bone anchor.

Potential Pitfalls

Direct scapholunate repair and capsulodesis is technically demanding, and there are several potential pitfalls. First, it is important to document the absence of arthritis along the scaphoid facet of the distal radius before attempting direct ligament repair. Proper reduction of the scaphoid is essential with adequate pin purchase in the carpus maintaining the reduction. Pin migration during immobilization can occur, and using two pins for the scapholunate joint and one to two pins for the scaphocapitate relationship can be helpful. Lastly, even in the best performed procedure, there are some cases where the scapholunate reduction is lost when the pins are removed, and the wrist is rehabilitated.

There is currently no way to predict which patients are most at risk for this complication.

Results

In 1992, we published our results of direct scapholunate ligament repair using the original capsulodesis as described by Taleisnik.[11] The average time from injury to surgical repair was 17 months. Wrist motion at an average follow-up of 33 months was equal to the unaffected wrist in all planes except flexion ($P < .001$). This limitation is most likely related to the dorsal capsulodesis, which provides a tether limiting terminal scaphoid flexion. Patients must be counseled on the expected loss of terminal wrist flexion even in successful cases. This is rarely a functional problem. Using visual analog scales,[28] peak and general levels of pain were significantly improved at follow-up ($P < .001$). Radiographically, the scapholunate gap was reduced from a mean of 3.2 mm preoperatively to 1.9 mm at follow-up.

Conclusion

Scapholunate dissociation can be treated successfully by direct ligament repair and dorsal capsular augmentation. Requirements include an adequate interosseous ligament identified at surgery and absent degenerative changes at the radioscaphoid articulation. The rationale for soft tissue repair is based on the premise that restoration of the normal intracarpal relationships would halt degenerative changes, while maximizing wrist motion and function. The dorsal capsulodesis provides a checkrein to excessive palmar flexion of the scaphoid. Since its initial description, several variations have been described, all using the dorsal capsule and dorsal wrist ligaments. Although all capsulodesis reconstructions that cross the radiocarpal joint may limit palmar flexion of the wrist, this is not a clinical problem.

REFERENCES

1. Jones WA: Beware of the sprained wrist: the incidence and diagnosis of scapholunate instability. J Bone Joint Surg Br. 1988; 70:293-297.
2. Linscheid RL, Dobyns JH, Beabout JW, et al: Traumatic instability of the wrist. J Bone Joint Surg Am. 1972; 54:1612-1632.
3. Taleisnik J: Carpal instability: current concepts review. J Bone Joint Surg Am. 1988; 70:1262-1267.
4. Sebald S, Dobyns JA, Linscheid RL: The natural history of collapse deformities of the wrist. Clin Orthop. 1974; 104:104-108.
5. Watson HK, Ballet FL: The SLAC wrist: scapholunate advanced collapse pattern of degenerative arthritis. J Hand Surg [Am]. 1984; 9:358-365.
6. Beckenbaugh RD: Accurate evaluation and management of the painful wrist following injury: an approach to carpal instability. Orthop Clin North Am. 1982; 15:289-300.
7. Blatt G: Capsulodesis in reconstructive hand surgery: dorsal capsulodesis for the unstable scaphoid and volar capsulodesis following excision of the distal ulna. Hand Clin. 1987; 3:81-102.
8. Goldner JL: Treatment of carpal instability without joint fusion: current assessment. J Hand Surg [Am]. 1982; 7:325-326.
9. Kleinman WB: Management of chronic rotary subluxation of the scaphoid by scapho-trapezium-trapezoid arthrodesis. Hand Clin. 1987; 3:113-133.
10. Nathan R, Lester B, Melone CP: The acutely injured wrist: an anatomic basis for operative treatment. Orthop Rev. 1987; 6:80-95.
11. Lavernia CJ, Cohen MS, Taleisnik J: Treatment of scapholunate dissociation by ligamentous repair and capsulodesis. J Hand Surg [Am]. 1992; 17:354-359.
12. Berger RA, Blair WF, Crowninshield RD, et al: The scapholunate ligament. J Hand Surg. 1982; 7:87-91.
13. Eckenrode JF, Louis DS, Greene TL: Scaphoid-trapezium-trapezoid fusion in the treatment of chronic scapholunate instability. J Hand Surg [Am]. 1986; 11:497-502.
14. Kleinman WB: Long-term study of chronic scapholunate instability treated by scapho-trapezium-trapezoid arthrodesis. J Hand Surg [Am]. 1989; 14:429-445.
15. Peterson HA, Lipscomb PR: Intercarpal arthrodesis. Arch Surg. 1967; 95:127-134.
16. Watson HK, Black DM: Instabilities of the wrist. Hand Clin. 1987; 3:103-111.
17. Watson HK, Hempton RF: Limited wrist arthrodesis, I: the triscaphoid joint. J Hand Surg. 1980; 5:320-327.
18. Cohen MS, Kozin SH: Degenerative arthritis of the wrist: proximal row carpectomy versus scaphoid excision and four-corner fusion. J Hand Surg [Am]. 2001; 26:94-104.
19. Inglis AE, Jones EC: Proximal row carpectomy for diastasis of the proximal carpal row. J Bone Joint Surg Am. 1977; 59:460-463.
20. Neviaser RJ: On resection of the proximal carpal row. Clin Orthop. 1986; 202:12-15.
21. Kauer JMG: The mechanism of the carpal joint. Clin Orthop. 1986; 202:16-26.
22. Short WH, Werner FW, Fortino MD, et al: A dynamic biomechanical study of scapholunate ligament sectioning. J Hand Surg. 1995; 20:986-999.
23. Viegas SF, DaSilva MF: Surgical repair for scapholunate dissociation. Tech Hand Upper Extrem Surg. 2000; 4:148-153.
24. Slater RR, Szabo RM, Bay BK, et al: Dorsal intercarpal ligament capsulodesis for scapholunate dissociation: biomechanical analysis in a cadaver model. J Hand Surg [Am]. 1999; 24:232-239.
25. Szabo RM, Slater RR, Palumbo CF, et al: Dorsal intercarpal ligament capsulodesis for chronic, static scapholunate dissociation: clinical results. J Hand Surg [Am]. 2002; 27:978-984.
26. Kleinman WB: Dorsal capsulodesis (ligamentodesis) of the wrist. Presented at Advanced Techniques or the Treatment of Carpal Instability, American Society for Surgery of the Hand Annual Meeting, Seattle, October 5, 2000.
27. Walsh JJ, Berger RA, Cooney WP: Current status of scapholunate interosseous ligament injuries. J Am Acad Orthop Surg. 2002; 10:32-42.
28. Huskisson EC: Measurement of pain. Lancet. 1974; 2:1127-1131.

Arthroscopic Treatment of Scapholunate Ligament Tears

47

Steven H. Goldberg, MD, Kongkhet Riansuwan, MD, and Melvin P. Rosenwasser, MD

Scapholunate interosseous ligament (SLIL) injuries are common causes of mechanical wrist pain. Despite an increased knowledge of carpal injuries and improvements in radiological evaluation, the diagnosis of a SLIL tear can be difficult or missed unless the evaluating physician has a high index of suspicion and an appropriate level of understanding of wrist anatomy and injury patterns. Usually a detailed history and physical examination and a series of plain radiographs are sufficient to make a diagnosis of SLIL injury (**Fig. 47-1**). Occasionally, advanced imaging techniques, such as magnetic resonance imaging (MRI) with or without intra-articular contrast enhancement, can be helpful in establishing a diagnosis and evaluating the wrist for associated injuries.[1-3] MRI usually detects large, complete tears better than partial, smaller tears, however, particularly if the tear configuration is oblique to the imaging plane, or the tear is smaller than the distance between contiguous image slices.

After successful introduction in the knee and shoulder, arthroscopy gained popularity as a useful modality to diagnose and treat a wide spectrum of wrist pathology.[4,5] This procedure has become the gold standard for diagnosis of SLIL injuries.[6-8] Arthroscopy is a minimally invasive procedure allowing direct observation of intrinsic and extrinsic carpal ligaments and articular cartilage integrity under static and dynamic conditions. Comprehensive and accurate diagnosis and treatment of all carpal injuries can be done concurrently.

Because a delayed or missed diagnosis of an SLIL tear can lead to progressive carpal instability and predispose the patient to a predictable pattern of carpal arthritis called scapholunate advanced collapse (SLAC),[9-11] we believe that wrist arthroscopy should be considered early during the evaluation and management of a patient with a suspected SLIL injury. It should be used selectively, however, for patients with significant symptoms, for patients with a mechanism of injury consistent with SLIL injury, and for patients in whom conservative treatment has failed or in whom acute operative management is indicated.

Anatomy of the Scapholunate Complex

The wrist is a complex structure comprising multiple small joint articulations with stability resulting from a complex linkage of intrinsic, intercarpal ligaments and extrinsic capsular ligaments. The wrist can be thought of as two separate rows with hand motion being the composite effect of motion between the radius, ulna, proximal carpal row (scaphoid, lunate, and triquetrum) and distal carpal row (scaphoid, trapezium, trapezoid, capitate, and hamate). The scaphoid is uniquely situated in both rows on an oblique axis to stabilize the carpus, while still permitting coordi-

nated relative motion between the two rows and the radius and ulna. The scaphoid is stabilized by many ligaments, including the SLIL, radioscaphocapitate, scaphotrapeziotrapezoid, scaphocapitate, and dorsal intercarpal.[12]

The SLIL is a C-shaped structure connecting the dorsal, proximal, and palmar surface between the scaphoid and the lunate, leaving the distal aspect of the joint bare of soft tissue allowing the evaluation of scapholunate articular congruity, preservation, and instability. This midcarpal visualization is essential in assessing the degree of instability between the two bones and in grading the spectrum of partial to complete injury.[13] The dorsal and palmar portions of the SLIL are true ligamentous structures.[14] The proximal portion is a membranous structure composed mainly of fibrocartilaginous tissue. In the absence of a tear, the transition between the dorsal and the proximal portion is not readily visualized during arthroscopy. Palpation of the SLIL with a probe permits differentiation, however, between the thick, taut dorsal ligament and the softer, thin proximal portion.

A partial SLIL tear may appear as a patulous, convex outpouching, rather than a confluent, barely discernible structure (**Fig. 47-2**). The probe may uncover a complete disruption of the insertion of the SLIL often from the lunate, which could not be perceived with observation alone. Partial tears may require palpation in the radiocarpal joint with a probe to appreciate the laxity and a thorough evaluation of the distal scapholunate joint articular surface congruity in the midcarpal joint to observe subtle incongruity or diastasis. A significant complete intrasubstance SLIL tear is readily visualized in the radiocarpal and the midcarpal joints.

Biomechanical and Kinematic Considerations

The three different portions of the SLIL have different biomechanical properties. The dorsal portion of the SLIL has a highest load at ultimate failure, followed by the palmar portion and then the proximal portion.[15] Serial, sequential ligament sectioning studies in cadavers have shown that the SLIL is the primary ligament scapholunate stabilizer.[16-21] No significant dissociation between the scaphoid and the lunate is shown, however, on static radiographs with an isolated, complete SLIL disruption.[16,22] This is explained by the presence of secondary stabilizers of the scapholunate joint, which must be injured either acutely or chronically to show radiographic instability. Injury to the volar extrinsic (radiolunate and radioscaphocapitate),[16,23] the distal intrinsic (scaphotrapezial),[16,24] or the dorsal intercarpal ligaments and the SLIL is needed to visualize pathological carpal bone rotation radiographically.[25]

463

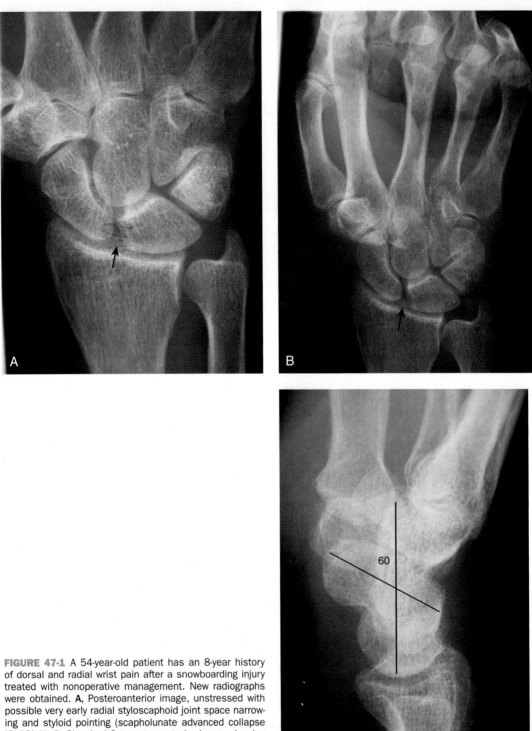

FIGURE 47-1 A 54-year-old patient has an 8-year history of dorsal and radial wrist pain after a snowboarding injury treated with nonoperative management. New radiographs were obtained. **A,** Posteroanterior image, unstressed with possible very early radial styloscaphoid joint space narrowing and styloid pointing (scapholunate advanced collapse [SLAC] 1). **B,** Clenched fist posteroanterior image showing no change in width of scapholunate interval or scapholunate step-off. **C,** Lateral radiograph.

An isolated tear of the SLIL changes carpal loading and kinematics even without demonstrable radiographic abnormalities. Isolated loss of this major stabilizer of the carpus may lead to attenuation of the secondary supporting structures and progressive dissociation and rotation of the scaphoid and the lunate. With axial loading over time and without proximal restraint by the intact scapholunate joint, the capitate can descend proximally, further driving the scaphoid and lunate apart like a wedge. This results in midcarpal instability, loss of carpal height, and increased clinical symptoms as the bones increase their abnormal rotation. Changes in the radiocarpal, intercarpal, and midcarpal joint contact areas and loads in conjunction with the altered kinematics result in predictable SLAC arthritis. This process begins with radial styloid beaking and radial styloscaphoid joint narrowing

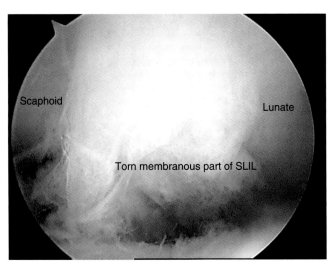

FIGURE 47-2 Intraoperative radiocarpal view of patient in Figure 47-1 showing patulous, lax membranous portion of the scapholunate ligament with a complex, fibrillated palmar tear.

(stage 1), then progresses proximally to alter the radioscaphoid facet proximal pole scaphoid articulation (stage 2), and finally progresses to the midcarpal capitolunate joint (stage 3).[9]

Treatment Options

Several factors need to be considered in clinical decision making about an arthroscopic procedure, not only to diagnose, but also to treat symptomatic scapholunate injuries (**Fig. 47-3**). Acute repairable lesions have heretofore been treated with open suture repair or reattachment with bone anchors. Previous reports have sought to separate acute injuries from chronic by using an arbitrary and unproven 6 weeks as a cutoff, with the implied understanding that only acute injuries could be repaired. Because the patient history is often unreliable regarding the first subtle injury versus the most recent and now symptomatic injury, however, dates alone should not indicate irreparable ligaments. We believe all such presumed SLIL injuries should be evaluated arthroscopically to stage properly and treat all injured structures. Repair, if possible, is preferred. Arthroscopy also has the added advantages that it is real time, can include direct palpation of structures, and can assess the dynamic nature of the instability and its reducibility (neither of which can be known from even the best MRI study).

Stable wrists with symptomatic tears (predynamic radiographic instability) are assumed after obtaining normal static and stress radiographs. Unstable wrists with tears demonstrable on grip films or cineradiography only (dynamic radiographic instability) have abnormal carpal alignment on stress radiographs (e.g., pronated posteroanterior grip), but normal alignment on unloaded routine radiographs. Unstable wrists with static instability on routine plain films (static radiographic instability) are obvious injuries and are not missed. These wrists may have advancing cartilage degeneration, however, which is often underappreciated, especially at the capitolunate joint. The presence of significant polyarticular arthritis changes treatment options and often precludes reconstruction and indicates salvage procedures, which usually fall outside of the purvey of arthroscopy except for a master arthroscopist.

Arthroscopic assessment guides and rationalizes the potential for repair by confirming the degree of injury and the severity of instability.[13] Arthroscopic treatment options include the follow-

ing either in isolation or in combination: ligament débridement, ligament thermal shrinkage, transarticular Kirschner wire (K-wire) fixation, and radial styloidectomy (see Fig. 47-3).

Complete repairable tears in the senior author's (M.P.R.) experience are best managed with open techniques. If the dorsal ligament has been avulsed from its attachment, it can and should be primarily repaired either with transosseous suture or with suture anchor. Depending on the amount of associated soft tissue injuries, this can be augmented with any of the numerous variations on dorsal capsulodesis.[26-28]

SLAC wrist evolution beyond the radial styloid and scaphoid waist articulation often requires more extensive, open surgical procedures. Complete irreparable tears in a young, active patient with a wide scapholunate diastasis and significant carpal malrotation should be considered for any procedure that can realign the carpus and preserve carpal kinematics so that the natural history of end-stage SLAC wrist can be forestalled. One such procedure used by the senior author since 1989 is the reduction and association of the scaphoid and lunate (RASL) creating a SLIL neoligament and protecting the repair with a transosseous scapholunate headless bone screw.

Standard Arthroscopic Technique

Similar patient positioning and technique are used in each of the arthroscopic surgical techniques. The patient is placed supine with the symptomatic arm abducted on a hand table. Regional anesthesia is preferred, and prophylactic intravenous antibiotics are administered. The arm is elevated, and prepared and draped in the usual manner, and a sterile tourniquet is applied to the upper arm. The index and middle fingers are placed in finger traps and suspended from a traction tower with the elbow flexed 90 degrees. The upper arm is strapped to the hand table and traction tower for countertraction. Care is taken to ensure all of the ulnar nerve and all bony prominences are well-padded and protected. Ten pounds of traction is applied.

All arthroscopic portals are outlined with a skin marker before exsanguination so that the superficial veins are noted and avoided during portal creation. The arm is exsanguinated, and the tourniquet is inflated to 250 mm Hg. An 18-gauge needle is used to confirm the location of each arthroscopic portal, ensuring that the entry angle corresponds to the volar tilt and radial inclination of the distal radius. The radiocarpal joint is distended with 3 to 5 mL of normal saline to increase the working space of the joint and reduce the risk of iatrogenic chondral injury.

A no. 11 blade is used to make a push incision through the skin only, which minimizes the chance for an injury to any adjacent cutaneous nerve branches. Then a fine curved hemostat is used to penetrate the capsule bluntly. The hemostat is spread to establish a viewing portal, and a blunt-tipped trocar within a cannula is inserted in a controlled manner with a gentle pressure. If there is any resistance to instrument advancement, the needle should be used to confirm portal location. Iatrogenic damage to the articular cartilage or intercarpal ligaments usually occurs during forced introduction of the trocar at the wrong angle or starting point.

After successful cannula placement, the trocar is removed, and a 30-degree angled, 2.7-mm arthroscope is inserted. Distention of the radiocarpal space is maintained by a pressurized irrigation system through the cannula with outflow through a separately placed 18-gauge needle into the radiocarpal joint in the 1,2 portal or the ulnocarpal joint through the 6R or 6U portals. The 3,4, 4,5, 6U, 6R, midcarpal radial, and midcarpal ulnar portals are

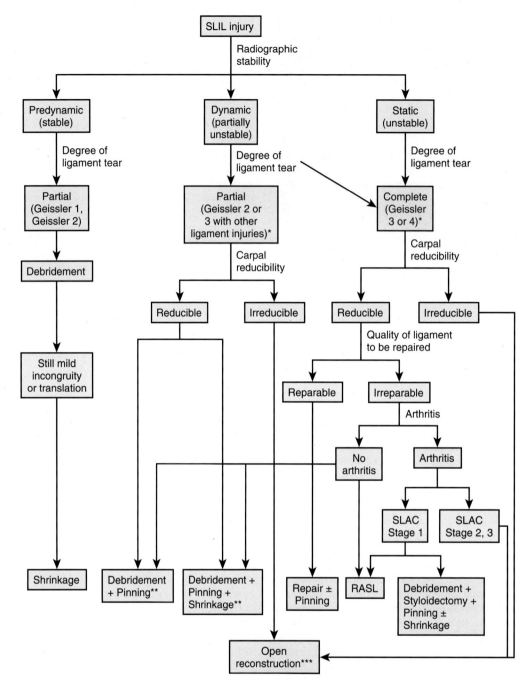

FIGURE 47-3 Algorithm of management of scapholunate ligament tears. *Depending on degree of associated ligament injuries, Geissler grade 2 or 3 can result in dynamic or static instability. **Transarticular Kirschner wire fixation of the scapholunate joint is necessary when carpal malrotation is present so that normal alignment can be maintained after carpal bone reduction. ***Depending on injury pattern, degree of arthritis, and surgeon preference, open reconstruction options include ligament reconstruction by tendon weaves, bone-retinaculum-bone constructs, limited intercarpal fusion, proximal row carpectomy, scaphoidectomy, and four-corner fusion. RASL, reduction and association of scaphoid and lunate procedure; SLAC, scapholunate advanced collapse.

necessary to complete a thorough diagnostic evaluation and allow therapeutic procedures.

Arthroscopic Débridement
Indications

Arthroscopic débridement alone is indicated for acute or chronic partial, but stable tears of the volar or membranous portion of the

ligament in a patient with mechanical symptoms (**Fig. 47-4**). These patients usually have focal reproducible mechanical wrist pain over the dorsal scapholunate joint worsened by activity and normal x-rays. It is common to treat these patients conservatively for several months with splints and activity modification. Persistent symptoms often lead to MRI; imaging rarely provides a definitive diagnosis and does not illuminate the treatment options. Arthroscopy in these patients typically reveals a stable Geissler

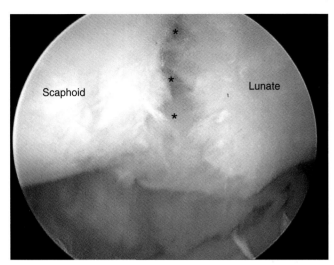

FIGURE 47-4 In the patient from Figures 47-1 and 47-2, the scapholunate joint (*) is visible after débridement of the membranous portion of the scapholunate ligament.

grade 1 or 2 injury pattern with slight midcarpal incongruity and joint widening. Patients' symptoms are due to tears in the substance of the ligament, which, although not destabilizing, create mechanical impingement during wrist motion causing focal dorsal wrist pain and occasionally leading to a synovitis and dorsal capsular thickening. Débridement of these SLIL flap tears in either the dorsal or the membranous portions and partial synovectomy often ameliorate symptoms.

Contraindication to Débridement Alone

An absolute contraindication is a complete reparable tear or a more advanced Geissler instability pattern that was underappreciated in the preoperative evaluation. Static instability patterns with preexistent arthritis are not helped except in a few selected cases of elderly patients with low demand. A staged débridement and synovectomy can be offered with the full understanding that it may fail and necessitate a more comprehensive salvage procedure.

Technique

Evaluation of the instability is central in indicating the appropriate procedure and requires radiocarpal and midcarpal arthroscopy to determine the Geissler grade. If the wrist is stable (Geissler grade 1 or 2 injuries), the tear can be débrided by alternating the arthroscope and working instruments between the 3,4 and 4,5 radiocarpal portals. The torn portion of the SLIL is débrided to stable margins, with care taken to preserve healthy, intact fibers. This is facilitated by using the least aggressive shaver, such as a full radius resector, which would not injure healthy intact tissue. After débridement, it is important to reprobe the midcarpal scapholunate articulation to ensure that stability has not been affected.

Results

Isolated arthroscopic débridement has been reported in several small case series (**Table 47-1**).[5,7,29] Most patients have predynamic or dynamic radiographic instability and Geissler grade 1 or 2 tears. Good pain relief, grip strength improvement, and maintenance of range of motion have been reported. The need for

postoperative immobilization is unclear because some studies treated patients in a soft dressing with immediate motion, and some studies reported wrist immobilization for 6 to 8 weeks.

Radiofrequency Thermal Collagen Shrinkage
Indications

The indications for radiofrequency thermal collagen shrinkage are similar to the indications described in the débridement section. In particular, it may be most useful in partial membranous tears or ligament redundancy. If the surgeon appreciates increased motion between the scaphoid and the lunate, particularly after débridement, without significant rotation, radiofrequency thermal collagen shrinkage can be performed in an attempt to tighten the intact portions of the SLIL and improve carpal kinematics. Additionally, if there is a redundancy or laxity in the SLIL, usually corresponding to Geissler grade 1, radiofrequency thermal collagen shrinkage can be performed with or without débridement based on surgeon judgment.

Contraindications

Radiofrequency thermal collagen shrinkage alone is contraindicated in the presence of significant, unstable flaps of ligamentous tissue because débridement of this tissue is necessary to decrease mechanical symptoms. It also is contraindicated as an isolated procedure in patients with carpal bone rotation, in patients with repairable ligament tears, and in patients with significant arthritis.

Technique

One study describes thermal stabilization using monopolar cautery (Oratec, Mountain View, CA) placed through the 4,5 portal.[30] The probe is applied to the SLIL starting volarly and working dorsally until all the lax and redundant SLIL has been made taut. The authors recommend continuous irrigation with a safety limit on the probe set to 75°C to prevent chondral thermal injury. When midcarpal examination reveals the scapholunate joint congruency without gapping, the thermal shrinkage is complete. The authors believe postoperative immobilization for 4 to 6 weeks is crucial to allow ligament healing and to prevent recurrent laxity.

Another study uses a 2.3-mm bipolar probe (Vapr; Mitek, Westwood, MA), which is placed through the 4,5 portal.[31] The probe was carefully applied to the torn rim of the volar portion of the ligament, the proximal membranous portion, and a small part of the dorsal ligament using multiple strokes similar to a paintbrush until visual color changes occurred. The probe was used intermittently, delivering energy for only a few seconds at a time to allow adequate outflow of warmed fluid. The tissue quality was palpated with a probe to confirm decreased laxity.

The senior author (M.P.R.) often applies the radiofrequency probe (Microblator 30 1.4 mm; Arthrocare, Sunnyvale, CA) to the proximal, membranous portion of the SLIL and the palmar midcarpal ligaments. In the midcarpal joint, the palmar ligamentous tissue at the junction of the scaphoid and lunate corresponds to the distal edge of the palmar SLIL and the radioscaphocapitate ligament (**Fig. 47-5**). Careful, limited, short bursts of thermal energy applied to this palmar midcarpal ligamentous and capsular tissue tightens the scapholunate and scapholunocapitate

TABLE 47-1 Summary of Literature Regarding Arthroscopic Treatment of Scapholunate Interosseous Ligament Injuries

	Westkaemper	Weiss	Ruch	Hirsh	Darlis	Rosenwasser (unpublished)	Whipple	Peicha
No. patients	23 cases	28 cases	7 cases	10 cases	16 cases	8 cases	40 cases	11 cases
Average age	30 yr	32 yr	41 yr	37 yr	34 yr	38 yr	Not mentioned	40 yr
Average length of preoperative symptoms	6 mo	8 mo	>6 mo	2 (<6 mo); 6 (>6 mo); 2 unknown	5 mo	25 mo	Variable	Acute
Clinical instability	6 cases	30 cases	Not mentioned	10 cases	13 cases	4 cases	Not mentioned	7 cases
Radiographic instability							Not mentioned	Not mentioned
Predynamic	23 cases	Not mentioned	7 cases	8 cases	16 cases	5 cases		
Dynamic		8 cases		2 cases		3 cases		
Static		2 cases						
Geissler grade (no.)	1 or 2 (21); 3 (2)	Complete (15)	Not mentioned	2 (10)	1 (2); 2 (14)	1 (1); 2 (7)	Not mentioned	3 or 4 (7)
Procedure (postoperative immobilization)	Débridement (6-8 wk)	Débridement (2 wk)	Débridement (none)	Monopolar thermal shrinkage (4-6 wk)	Débridement + bipolar thermal shrinkage (2 wk)	4 débridement + shrinkage (none); 4 débridement + shrinkage + pinning (6-8 wk)	Temporary pinning (unknown)	Temporary pinning (8 wk)
Average follow-up	15 mo	27 mo	34 mo	28 mo	19 mo	3-8 mo	24-96 mo	36 mo
Outcome	11 excellent; 9 good; 1 fair; 2 poor	67% completed; 85% partial resolved	Good pain relief; minimal loss of motion	9/10 pain resolved; average DASH = 20	8 pain-free; VAS 8-4 mm; grip 80%; flexion/extension 142 degrees	7 good pain relief; minimal loss of motion; 1 finally wrist fusion	85% pain relief if <3 mo and <3 mm of scapholunate diastasis	4 pain relief; 3 mild pain; residual pain may be related to distal radial fractures

DASH, Disabilities of the Arm, Shoulder, and Hand; VAS, visual analog scale.

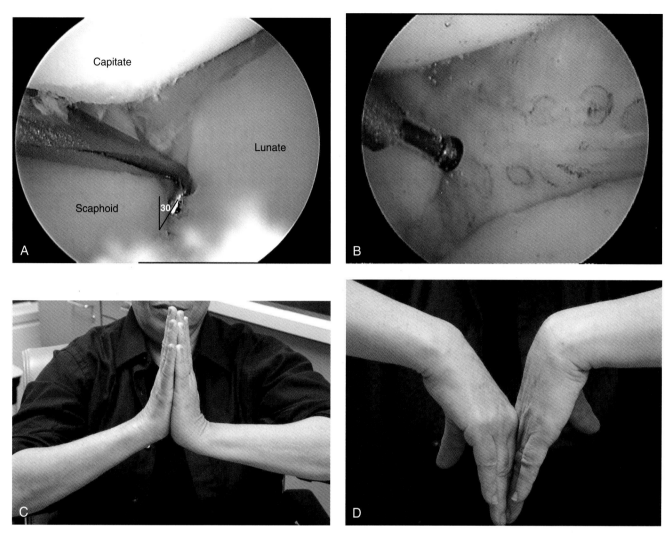

FIGURE 47-5 **A,** Midcarpal joint picture of the patient (from Figs. 47-1, 47-2, and 47-4) with a probe inserted into scapholunate joint and able to rotate greater than 30 degrees, indicating at least a Geissler grade 2 tear. **B,** After thermal capsular shrinkage of the palmar midcarpal ligaments, note the brown color change from **A. C,** Clinical follow-up of patient 4 months after débridement, thermal shrinkage, and temporary Kirschner wire fixation. Wrist extension of 52 degrees (*right*) and 80 degrees (*left*). **D,** Wrist flexion of 40 degrees (*right*) and 55 degrees (*left*).

articulations. This midcarpal application of thermal collagen shrinkage can address proximal row intercarpal and midcarpal instability. Decreased gapping between the scaphoid and the lunate is readily observable. Manual reciprocal palmar-dorsal translation between the scaphoid and lunate before and after thermal shrinkage should be performed without traction to determine if there are any changes in stability after shrinkage. Without reduction of traction, a false increased sense of stability may be appreciated. Additionally, it should be more difficult to insert a probe in the midcarpal scapholunate interval.

Results

There are two published series of 10 and 16 patients treated with monopolar and bipolar electrothermal collagen shrinkage and postoperative immobilization ranging from 2 to 6 weeks (see Table 47-1).[30,31] Complete pain relief ranged from 50% to 90% with preservation of wrist motion and no postoperative radiographic instability.

Arthroscopic-Assisted Temporary Transarticular Wire Placement
Indications

Transarticular pinning has been hypothesized to result in ligament stiffening and the formation of fibrosis along the pin tract, which can lead to joint stability and alleviate symptoms in patients with mild scapholunate instability. This technique may be useful in patients with mild carpal bone malrotation and diastasis from partial SLIL injuries. When carpal bone anatomical position needs to be restored, transarticular pin placement is necessary to hold the bones in the reduced position until soft tissue healing occurs. In patients with partial tears without carpal malrotation in whom the surgeon would like to try to increase stability but does not want to perform radiofrequency thermal collagen shrinkage, or there is minimal remaining ligament to débride, the placement of temporary wires may result in increased scapholunate stability.

Contraindications

There are no absolute contraindications to transarticular wire placement. Wire placement across the intercarpal joints may be unnecessary, however, in the absence of carpal malrotation.

Technique

Using manual pressure applied on the distal scaphoid tubercle, palmar to dorsal, the scaphoid can be rotated out of palmar flexion. Radial to ulnar pressure between the scaphoid and triquetrum can close the scapholunate gap. Fluoroscopy and arthroscopy should be used to confirm anatomical reduction. If the lunate is dorsiflexed on the lateral view, it is impossible to be reduced by closed manipulation. Separate wires can be placed into individual bones and used as joysticks to derotate the scaphoid and lunate. The scaphoid joystick wire is placed obliquely into the scaphoid aiming from distal-dorsal to proximal-palmar so that pressure applied to the wire from distal to proximal causes scaphoid extension. The lunate joystick wire is placed obliquely from proximal-dorsal to distal-palmar so that proximal to distal pressure results in lunate flexion.

After the bones have been derotated, a percutaneous wire is placed across the scapholunate joint from radial to ulnar. Either 0.045-inch or 0.062-inch wires can be used. Pin insertion technique is crucial because the anatomical snuffbox contains the dorsal branch of the radial artery, the cephalic vein, and multiple sensory nerve branches with a narrow safe zone.[32] Wires should be pushed through the skin and down to the scaphoid freehand. Then the wire driver is placed over the wire and turned on. By having the wire tip fixed to the bone before wire rotation by the driver, soft tissue injury is minimized. Several divergent pins can be placed across the scapholunate and scaphocapitate joint in this manner. This is the best way to maintain the reduction of the scapholunate diastasis achieved through derotation.

Results

Two case series have been reported on patients who underwent arthroscopic reduction of the scapholunate joint and temporary transarticular scapholunate joint fixation for isolated SLIL injury or associated with a distal radius fracture (see Table 47-1).[33,34] These types of injuries are very different and do not act the same way clinically over long-term follow-up. Acute injuries recognized and treated after trauma have more predictable outcomes, in contradistinction to chronic injuries with a vague history of significant antecedent trauma; this correlates with the quality of the tissue at the ligamentocapsular injury site and its capacity to heal.

Arthroscopic Débridement, with or without Thermal Shrinkage, with or without Temporary Transarticular Pinning
Indications

SLIL débridement combined with thermal capsular shrinkage is indicated in the context of clinical localizing signs and symptoms, radiographic instability, and arthroscopic grading of injury. Any carpal bone malrotation (dynamic instability) or incongruence requiring reduction should be supported further with temporary transarticular pinning.

Contraindications

This procedure is contraindicated and inadequate for patients with static carpal malalignment. Static carpal malalignment corresponds to chronicity, and that translates to a lack of adequate residual ligament as scaffolding that could foster repair and provide stability and improved carpal kinematics. These patients require supplemental tissue grafting using open or closed techniques, such as various capsulodeses and ligament reconstruction with tendon grafts or bone-ligament-bone constructs or salvage procedures that restrict carpal motion and maintain reduction through limited intercarpal fusions, such as scaphotrapeziotrapezoid. Simple débridement and Kirschner pinning for these static instabilities routinely fail to maintain the correction of carpal alignment achieved at surgery.[26,35,36]

Technique

Ligament débridement, thermal shrinkage, and temporary transarticular pinning are performed together in a similar fashion as described in the previous sections.

Results

To date, there are no published reports detailing the outcomes of patients treated with this protocol. This communication is the opinion of the senior author (M.P.R.), who has performed thermal ligament shrinkage in eight patients with follow-up to an early clinical result. The average age of patients was 38.3 years (range 21 to 54 years) (personal communication) (see **Table 47-1**), and all met the clinical and radiographic inclusion criteria discussed previously. Procedures included ligament débridement (eight), scaphocapitate (four) and scapholunate (four) transarticular pinning (0.045-inch K-wire), dorsal ganglionectomy (one), débridement of the triangular fibrocartilage complex (two), and posterior interosseous neurectomy (one). Predynamic and dynamic radiographic instability was observed in five (predynamic) and three (dynamic) patients. The proximal scapholunate ligament was thermally shrunk in all patients, and the midcarpal palmar ligaments were shrunk in four patients.

Postoperative immobilization was used in the four patients with reducible instability who underwent pinning. Seven of eight patients had pain and symptom resolution. One patient with a workers' compensation claim and a prior wrist arthroscopy complained of persistent pain after thermal capsulorrhaphy done by the senior author (M.P.R.). He was revised to a total wrist arthrodesis, which allowed him to return to work. During intraoperative assessment 12 months after thermal shrinkage, there was no visible evidence of cartilage or ligament injury from the thermal shrinkage.

Arthroscopic Styloidectomy
Indications

Arthroscopic radial styloidectomy eliminates the painful impingement between the distal scaphoid and the radial styloid in stage I SLAC. It is typically done in combination with arthroscopic SLIL débridement. The presence of arthritis indicates longstanding carpal instability with secondary ligament attenuation. Arthroscopic styloidectomy and SLIL débridement alone are usually recommended in older patients with low demand who present with localizing radial wrist pain during activities of daily living. They must be counseled that styloidectomy and débridement may provide only temporary relief of symptoms.

Contraindications

Arthroscopic styloidectomy is contraindicated when arthritis extends beyond the radial styloscaphoid waist articulation, as in stage II or III SLAC wrist. It is not recommended as the definitive intervention in a younger, more active patient with higher demands because it does not treat the underlying chronic instability.

Technique

After diagnostic arthroscopy confirms advanced midcarpal or proximal radioscaphoid arthritis, the working instrumentation portal is the 1,2 portal, which is established between the extensor pollicis brevis and extensor carpi radialis longus tendons. A shielded bur is inserted in the 1,2 portal. Alternatively, the arthroscope may be placed in the 4,5 portal with the bur placed through the 3,4 portal. Radiocarpal synovectomy improves visualization of the radial styloid and volar extrinsic ligaments. Less than 4 mm of styloid should be removed to avoid detachment of the radioscaphocapite ligament. The radioscaphocapite ligament prevents ulnar translation of the carpus. The diameter of the bur helps guide the resection depth, but the degree of resection and decompression also should be assessed with the mini-fluoroscope and in the provocative positions of wrist flexion and radial deviation.

Results

There are no published reports on the outcome of arthroscopic radial styloidectomy in the treatment of SLIL injury and its sequelae. Arthroscopic and open radial styloidectomy were discussed in relation to SLAC wrist in a study by Yao and Osterman,[37] without clinical results.

Reduction and Association of the Scaphoid and Lunate

The RASL procedure was developed as an open reconstructive procedure to reassociate the scapholunate joint and foster a fibrous neoligament by dechondrification of the interface and maintaining the reduction through healing with a headless bone screw, which is placed transarticularly by the senior author (M.P.R.). The procedure can be and is being done arthroscopically, and although the follow-up time is shorter, the results are similar.[38-40]

Indications

The RASL procedure is a technique developed for treatment of a chronic static scapholunate instability in which the ligament is irreparable and the resultant arthritis is focal. It is also indicated in salvage after a failed primary surgical reconstruction such as scapholunate ligament repair, scapholunate pinning, or a dorsal capsulodesis.

The premise of RASL technique is that it is important to maintain the obligatory intercarpal scapholunate rotation, while still controlling the aberrant scaphoid flexion and lunate extension by relinking the joints without fusing them. The crucial elements of a successful RASL procedure are the dechondrification of the opposing surfaces of the scaphoid and lunate; the anatomical reduction of the scaphoid, lunate, and capitate; and the maintenance of this normal carpal alignment during the reparative phase in which the formation of a fibrous neoligament between the scaphoid and the lunate occurs. The planned retention of a headless bone screw (**Fig. 47-6**) augments and protects the fibrous neoligament, while undergoing an expected lucency around the

lunate screw threads as it permits near-physiological motion between the scaphoid and the lunate. This concept has been confirmed by a cadaver biomechanical study in which scapholunate motion after the RASL procedure was found to be preserved within 5 degrees of the preinjury state for all positions of wrist motion.[41]

Contraindications

The RASL procedure is contraindicated in patients with partial tears without instability or with repairable, unstable SLIL tears. Additionally, this procedure would not relieve pain in the presence of advanced radiocarpal or midcarpal arthritis. Limited radial styloscaphoid arthritis is not a contraindication because a radial styloidectomy is an integral part of the procedure to gain access for the placement of the screw in the central axis of rotation of the lunate.

Technique

A longitudinal dorsal skin incision is made just ulnar to Lister's tubercle. The third compartment is opened longitudinally, and the extensor pollicis longus is retracted radially. The fourth compartment is elevated subperiosteally in an ulnar direction. Wrist arthrotomy is performed in a ligament-sparing fashion through a transverse incision parallel and proximal to the dorsal intercarpal ligament. The dorsal radiotriquetral ligament also is preserved.

The radial styloid is approached through a separate, short, longitudinal, radially based incision. Identification and protection of the superficial radial sensory nerve branches and the radial artery are mandatory. Next, the first dorsal compartment retinaculum is incised and reflected, and later is used to imbricate the radial collateral ligament and capsule at closure. The thumb tendons are retracted, and the capsule is opened longitudinally. A limited styloidectomy is performed, preserving the scaphoid fossa and most of the radioscaphocapite ligament origin; this provides access to the radial proximal scaphoid for later screw placement and treats the concomitant radial styloscaphoid arthritis. The dorsal capsulotomy is performed through two transverse windows, which respect the dorsal intercarpal ligament, an important secondary stabilizer of the wrist.

To manipulate the scaphoid and the lunate during reduction, a 0.062-inch K-wire is placed into each bone and used as a joystick. Each K-wire should be placed in an orientation that does not block the guidewire placement in the center axis of rotation of the lunate and the subsequent headless screw fixation. If this is noted in subsequent passes of the guidewire, the joystick K-wire can be repositioned after reduction is obtained. One K-wire is placed distally near the scaphotrapezial joint and directed proximally into the palmar-flexed scaphoid, and another is placed proximally and directed distally in the dorsiflexed lunate. The cartilage of the scaphoid and the lunate at the articulation is burred to induce punctate subchondral bleeding. This bleeding facilitates the ingrowth of vascularity leading to the development of fibrous tissue and a neoligament.

The scapholunate joint is anatomically reduced by derotation reciprocally by performing flexion of the lunate and extension of the scaphoid using the wire joysticks. This also results in reduction of the capitolunate joint, which is anatomical when the cartilage of the capitate proximal pole is no longer visualized. A Kocher clamp is placed on the reduced K-wires to maintain the reduction, which is confirmed fluoroscopically and visually. Then the wire for the cannulated Headless Bone Screw (Hand Innovations, Miami, FL) is inserted through the radial incision just

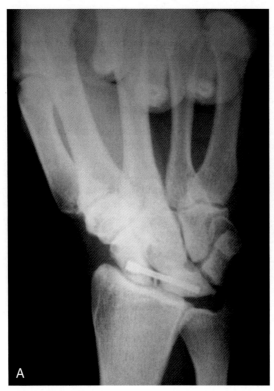 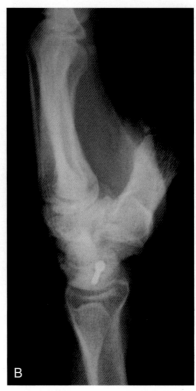

FIGURE 47-6 Two years after RASL procedure, the patient (from previous figures) has 50 degrees of extension and 60 degrees of flexion with no pain or activity restrictions. **A,** Posteroanterior grip view. Note central placement of screw into lunate vertex ulnarly. Expected radiolucent lines are seen around the screw ends within the scaphoid and lunate indicating rotation of the bones around the screw. **B,** Lateral radiograph showing slightly palmar position of screw with maintenance of neutral alignment between the radius, lunate, and capitate. Radiolucent lines also are visualized.

proximal to the scaphoid waist toward the lunate vertex. The wire should pass through the center of the scaphoid and lunate in the coronal and the sagittal planes to establish an isometric rotation point, which nearly restores carpal kinematics. The depth should be measured so that the screw can be countersunk slightly within the scaphoid. The screw is advanced, and fluoroscopy is used to confirm appropriate screw position and length. The K-wires all are removed. Interrupted absorbable sutures are used to close the radial capsule. The first dorsal retinaculum is closed over the relocated tendons. The dorsal wrist capsule is carefully repaired without imbrication, and no capsulodesis is performed to limit motion. The extensor pollicis longus remains transposed from its sheath.

A volar splint is used for comfort for 2 to 3 weeks. Then early, active motion in a supervised occupational therapy program is initiated. Gradual resistance exercises are begun several weeks later with unrestricted activity at 4 o 6 months.

The arthroscopic RASL procedure follows the same principles, but the wires and screw are placed percutaneously often aided by stab wound incisions with a no. 11 blade. The radial styloidectomy and decortication of the opposing scaphoid and lunate articular surfaces are performed arthroscopically with mechanical burs. Rather than direct observation, scapholunate and lunocapitate reductions are observed fluoroscopically. Time should be taken at the beginning of the procedure to ensure adequate fluoroscopic visualization. We teach that several open RASL procedures should be done before arthroscopic RASL is attempted.

Results

A good outcome was achieved in 20 of 24 (83%) patients who underwent an open RASL procedure for chronic scapholunate injury (22 static and 2 dynamic tears an average of 16 months postinjury) with mean follow-up time of 62 months. The postoperative average visual analog score for pain was 1, and the average Disabilities of the Arm, Shoulder, and Hand (DASH) score was 23. Mean grip strength of the affected hand was 79% compared with the unaffected hand. Mean range of motion in flexion and extension was 103 degrees. Postoperative radiographs showed significant improvement of scapholunate diastasis (5.1 to 1.6 mm) and the scapholunate angle (81 to 53 degrees), and no significant change in carpal height ratio. Three patients needed reoperation because of chronic instability and pain and required intercarpal fusion or proximal row carpectomy. Two patients required screw removal at an average of 49 months after surgery because of screw head prominence. One patient is asymptomatic after screw removal, and the second patient has persistent instability and progressive arthritis.

Conclusion

Scapholunate ligament injuries are common, but they are often difficult to diagnose with many overlapping and confounding conditions. Inadequate treatment can lead to progressive instability because of changes in associated intrinsic and extrinsic ligaments. Arthroscopy plays a major role in staging the degree of chondral and ligamentous injuries and indicating treatment. Various arthroscopic procedures can be performed alone or in combination based on radiographic instability, location, and extent of the ligament injuries. These arthroscopic techniques include débridement, thermal capsuloligamentous shrinkage, transarticular wire placement, styloidectomy, and the RASL procedure. Increasingly severe static deformity resistant to reduction via the arthroscope should be repaired with an open procedure. Advanced arthritis should be treated with accepted salvage procedures.

REFERENCES

1. Morley J, Bidwell J, Bransby-Zachary M: A comparison of the findings of wrist arthroscopy and magnetic resonance imaging in the investigation of wrist pain. J Hand Surg [Br]. 2001; 26:544-546.

2. Haims AH, Schweitzer ME, Morrison WB, et al: Internal derangement of the wrist: indirect MR arthrography versus unenhanced MR imaging. Radiology. 2003; 227: 701-707.

3. Schmitt R, Christopoulos G, Meier R, et al: Direct MR arthrography of the wrist in comparison with arthroscopy: a prospective study on 125 patients. ROFO. 2003; 175: 911-919.

4. Rettig ME, Amadio PC: Wrist arthroscopy: indications and clinical applications. J Hand Surg [Br]. 1994; 19:774-777.

5. Ruch DS, Poehling GG: Arthroscopic management of partial scapholunate and lunotriquetral injuries of the wrist. J Hand Surg [Am]. 1996; 21:412-417.

6. Dautel G, Goudot B, Merle M: Arthroscopic diagnosis of scapho-lunate instability in the absence of x-ray abnormalities. J Hand Surg [Br]. 1993; 18:213-218.

7. Westkaemper JG, Mitsionis G, Giannakopoulos PN, et al: Wrist arthroscopy for the treatment of ligament and triangular fibrocartilage complex injuries. Arthroscopy. 1998; 14:479-483.

8. Sennwald G: Diagnostic arthroscopy: indications and interpretation of findings. J Hand Surg [Br]. 2001; 26:241-246.

9. Watson HK, Ballet FL: The SLAC wrist: scapholunate advanced collapse pattern of degenerative arthritis. J Hand Surg [Am]. 1984; 9:358-365.

10. Watson HK, Weinzweig J, Zeppieri J: The natural progression of scaphoid instability. Hand Clin. 1997; 13:39-49.

11. Taleisnik J: Current concepts review: carpal instability. J Bone Joint Surg Am. 1988; 70:1262-1268.

12. Berger RA: The anatomy of the ligaments of the wrist and distal radioulnar joints. Clin Orthop. 2001; 383:32-40.

13. Geissler WB, Freeland AE, Savoie FH, et al: Intracarpal soft-tissue lesions associated with an intra-articular fracture of the distal end of the radius. J Bone Joint Surg [Am]. 1996; 78: 357-365.

14. Berger RA: The gross and histologic anatomy of the scapholunate interosseous ligament. J Hand Surg [Am]. 1996; 21:170-178.

15. Berger RA, Imeada T, Berglund L, et al: Constraint and material properties of the subregions of the scapholunate interosseous ligament. J Hand Surg [Am]. 1999; 24:953-962.

16. Short WH, Werner FW, Green JK, et al: Biomechanical evaluation of ligamentous stabilizers of the scaphoid and lunate. J Hand Surg [Am]. 2002; 27:991-1002.

17. Burgess RC: The effect of rotatory subluxation of the scaphoid on radio-scaphoid contact. J Hand Surg [Am]. 1987; 12:771-774.

18. Ruch DS, Smith BP: Arthroscopic and open management of dynamic scaphoid instability. Orthop Clin North Am. 2001; 32:233-240.

19. Short WH, Werner FW, Green JK, et al: The effect of sectioning the dorsal radiocarpal ligament and insertion of a pressure sensor into the radiocarpal joint on scaphoid and lunate kinematics. J Hand Surg [Am]. 2002; 27:68-76.

20. Meade TD, Schneider LH, Cherry K: Radiographic analysis of selective ligament sectioning at the carpal scaphoid: a cadaver study. J Hand Surg [Am]. 1990; 15:855-862.

21. Blevens AD, Light TR, Jablonsky WS, et al: Radiocarpal articular contact characteristics with scaphoid instability. J Hand Surg [Am]. 1989; 14:781-790.

22. Berger RA, Blair WF, Crowninshield RD, et al: The scapholunate ligament. J Hand Surg [Am]. 1982; 7:87-91.

23. Ruby LK, An KN, Linscheid RL, et al: The effect of scapholunate ligament section on scapholunate motion. J Hand Surg [Am]. 1987; 12:767-771.

24. Boabighi A, Kuhlmann JN, Kenesi C: The distal ligamentous complex of the scaphoid and the scapho-lunate ligament: an anatomic, histological and biomechanical study. J Hand Surg [Br]. 1993; 18:65-69.

25. Mitsuyasu H, Patterson RM, Shah MA, et al: The role of the dorsal intercarpal ligament in dynamic and static scapholunate instability. J Hand Surg [Am]. 2004; 29:279-288.

26. Szabo RM, Slater RR Jr, Palumbo CF, et al: Dorsal intercarpal ligament capsulodesis for chronic, static scapholunate dissociation: clinical results. J Hand Surg [Am]. 2002; 27: 978-984.

27. Wintman BI, Gelberman RH, Katz JN: Dynamic scapholunate instability: results of operative treatment with dorsal capsulodesis. J Hand Surg [Am]. 1995; 20:971-979.

28. Lavernia CJ, Cohen MS, Taleisnik J: Treatment of scapholunate dissociation by ligamentous repair and capsulodesis. J Hand Surg [Am]. 1992; 17:354-359.

29. Weiss AP, Sachar K, Glowacki KA: Arthroscopic debridement alone for intercarpal ligament tears. J Hand Surg [Am]. 1997; 22:344-349.

30. Hirsh L, Sodha S, Bozentka D, et al: Arthroscopic electrothermal collagen shrinkage for symptomatic laxity of the scapholunate interosseous ligament. J Hand Surg [Br]. 2005; 30: 643-647.

31. Darlis NA, Weiser RW, Sotereanos DG: Partial scapholunate ligament injuries treated with arthroscopic debridement and thermal shrinkage. J Hand Surg [Am]. 2005; 30:908-914.

32. Steinberg BD, Plancher KD, Idler RS: Percutaneous Kirschner wire fixation through the snuff box: an anatomic study. J Hand Surg [Am]. 1995; 20:57-62.

33. Whipple TL: The role of arthroscopy in the treatment of scapholunate instability. Hand Clin. 1995; 11:37-40.

34. Peicha G, Seibert F, Fellinger M, et al: Midterm results of arthroscopic treatment of scapholunate ligament lesions associated with intra-articular distal radius fractures. Knee Surg Sports Traumatol Arthrosc. 1999; 7:327-333.

35. Wyrick JD, Youse BD, Kiefhaber TR: Scapholunate ligament repair and capsulodesis for the treatment of static scapholunate dissociation. J Hand Surg [Br]. 1998; 23:776-780.

36. Muermans S, De Smet L, Van Ransbeeck H: Blatt dorsal capsulodesis for scapholunate instability. Acta Orthop Belg. 1999; 65:434-439.

37. Yao J, Osterman AL: Arthroscopic techniques for wrist arthritis (radial styloidectomy and proximal pole hamate excisions). Hand Clin. 2005; 21:519-526.

38. Lipton CB, Ugwonali OF, Sarwahi V, et al: Reduction and association of the scaphoid and lunate for scapholunate ligament injuries (RASL). Atlas Hand Clin. 2003; 8:249-260.

39. Rosenwasser MP, Miyasaka KC, Strauch RJ: The RASL procedure: reduction and association of the scaphoid and lunate using the Herbert screw. Tech Hand Upper Extrem Surg. 1997; 1:263-272.

40. Lipton C, Ugwonali O, Sarwahi V, et al: The treatment of chronic scapholunate dissociation with reduction and association of the scaphoid and lunate (RASL). Atlas Hand Clin. 2003; 8:95-105.

41. Amin F, Gardner TR, Ko BH, et al: The RASL procedure (reduction and association of the scaphoid and lunate using the Herbert screw): an evaluation of inter-carpal kinematics in cadaveric wrists. Presented at the American Association for Hand Surgery Meeting, Tucson, AZ, January 2006.

Dorsal Capsulodesis

48

Robert M. Szabo, MD, MPH

Rationale and Basic Science Pertinent to the Procedure

Scapholunate dissociation is the most frequently diagnosed pattern of carpal instability.[1] If left untreated, it leads to scapholunate advanced collapse and progressive painful arthritis of the wrist.[2] Treatment for scapholunate dissociation remains controversial and has varied from limited wrist arthrodeses[3-6] to soft tissue procedures, including dorsal capsulodesis[7-11] and scapholunate interosseous ligament reconstruction using tendon graft.[12-14]

Soft tissue reconstructions have several theoretical advantages that make them attractive alternatives to other procedures. In contrast to arthrodeses, soft tissue reconstructions preserve more intercarpal motion, including scaphoid flexion and extension with radial and ulnar wrist deviation. Arthrodeses limit motion. The scaphotrapeziotrapezoid limited arthrodesis results in a loss of 16% to 45% of wrist flexion, 25% of wrist extension, and 45% of radial deviation.[3-6] Scaphocapitate arthrodesis, also advocated for scapholunate dissociations, has been shown to produce similar reductions in wrist range of motion and in relative intercarpal motion to scaphotrapeziotrapezoid arthrodesis.[15] There has been a renewed interest in tendon reconstructions[12,14]; however, historically early results, although promising, have not stood the test of time.[13]

With a dorsal capsulodesis procedure, which is a soft tissue procedure rather than an arthrodesis, greater intercarpal motion is preserved, including scaphoid flexion and extension with radial and ulnar wrist deviation. Blatt[7] popularized the capsulodesis using a radius-based flap of wrist capsule inserted into the distal pole of the scaphoid. That procedure has been reported to result in a significant decrease in wrist flexion by some investigators, however, including Blatt, who reported a mean loss of 20 degrees of flexion.[7,16] Although it corrects the flexed posture of the scaphoid by crossing the radiocarpal joint and tethering the scaphoid, it nevertheless fails to correct the diastasis between the scaphoid and lunate seen radiographically.

Seeking to address these problems, we developed the dorsal intercarpal ligament capsulodesis (DILC) for the treatment of scapholunate dissociation based on the dorsal intercarpal ligament of the wrist. In a cadaver model, we tested our hypothesis that the DILC can restore the scapholunate relationship with improved wrist range of motion and function.[17] In our model, the scapholunate interosseous ligament was sectioned, and the results of the DILC were compared with the results of a Blatt capsulodesis.[17] To perform the capsulodesis using the dorsal intercarpal ligament, a 5-mm strip of the portion of the ligament that inserts onto the trapezoid was dissected free. The dorsal intercarpal ligament has some fibers that insert onto the dorsal ridge of the scaphoid, but none that insert onto the distal pole of the scaphoid; the remainder of the ligament inserts onto the trapezoid. The scaphoid and lunate were reduced anatomically. The prepared dorsal intercarpal ligament was rotated proximally on its origin from the triquetrum, stretched as tightly as possible, and held in position with a forceps. The ligament was secured to the distal pole of the scaphoid with a suture anchor (**Figs. 48-1 and 48-2**).

DILC restored the normal scapholunate relationship more completely than did a Blatt capsulodesis. After a Blatt capsulodesis, the scapholunate diastasis remained significantly increased ($P < .05$) compared with the intact specimens when the wrist was placed in radial deviation, ulnar deviation, and the clenched fist position. In contrast, there were no significant differences in scapholunate gap between the intact specimens and DILC in any wrist position. In addition to the differences seen when comparing the intact group with each reconstructed group, there were significant differences between the two reconstructed groups. In the clenched fist position, in which the repair is stressed maximally, there was a significant increase in the scapholunate diastasis measured after a Blatt capsulodesis compared with DILC (5.8 ± 1.07 mm versus 3.1 ± 1.03 mm; $P < .05$). Similar significant differences were noted between reconstruction methods when the wrist was in extension and radial deviation. Both reconstruction techniques reduced the scapholunate angle. The scapholunate angle decreased more after DILC than after Blatt capsulodesis in all conditions except flexion, in which they were equal; however, the differences were not statistically significant owing to lack of power of the study.

Indications

DILC has a role in the treatment of dynamic scapholunate instability and flexible chronic static scapholunate dissociation in the absence of arthritic changes. The procedure also is useful as an augmentation for patients with an acute perilunate dislocation undergoing open reduction and repair of the scapholunate interosseous ligament.

With regards to age range, the procedure has no limitations. It is our preferred choice in skeletally immature individuals with scapholunate instability because growth should not be disturbed. DILC can be done in the acute setting because raising the dorsal intercarpal ligament based ulnarly provides a good exposure to repair the scapholunate interosseous ligament if needed. DILC can be done anytime in the chronic setting. There are no time limits for the procedure.

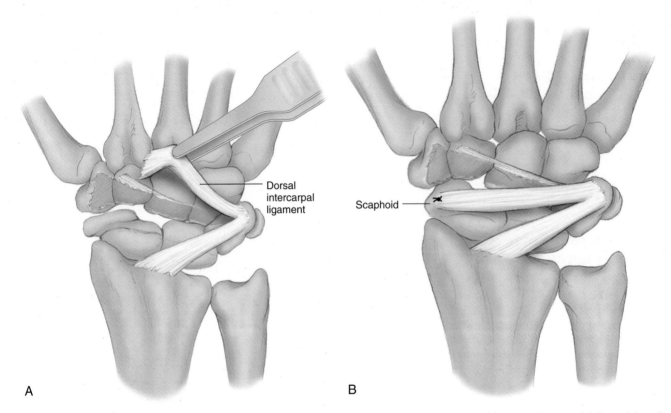

A   B

FIGURE 48-1 A and **B,** Dorsal intercarpal ligament capsulodesis from a dorsal perspective. The dorsal intercarpal ligament is elevated from its insertion on the trapezium and trapezoid (**A**), rotated proximally, and secured to a previously prepared bony trough in the distal pole of the scaphoid (**B**) using a suture anchor and additional nonabsorbable sutures as needed. *(From Szabo RM, Slater RR Jr, Palumbo CF, et al: Dorsal intercarpal ligament capsulodesis for chronic, static scapholunate dissociation: clinical results. J Hand Surg [Am]. 2002; 27:978-984.)*

Contraindications

DILC is absolutely contraindicated in patients with irreducible (inflexible) chronic static scapholunate dissociation and in patients with any arthritic changes indicative of a scapholunate advanced collapse wrist. This procedure is not indicated for patients with chronic, static scapholunate gaps of 1 cm or greater.

The procedure may be relatively contraindicated in patients who require high demand of wrist strength as judged by the physician and patient. These patients may be best served by a scaphocapitate or scaphotrapeziotrapezoid arthrodesis, although those procedures also have not provided a predictable solution to this problem.[3,4]

Web Video
48-1

Surgical Technique

A longitudinal skin incision is made dorsally over the patient's wrist, centered over Lister's tubercle. The superficial soft tissues are dissected off the extensor retinaculum, being careful to avoid injuring the cutaneous branches of the ulnar and radial nerves. The extensor pollicis longus is unroofed by incising the retinaculum over the third extensor compartment in a step-cut fashion to facilitate subsequent closure, and the tendon is retracted radially. A surgical sponge is used to wipe the dorsal ligamentous and capsular structures clean so that the interval between the dorsal radiocarpal and the dorsal intercarpal ligament can be identified in line with the long finger. An umbilical tape is passed around the dorsal intercarpal ligament, which is dissected out as it traverses the operative field (**Fig. 48-3**). It is then divided off its insertion on the trapezoid and trapezium (**Fig. 48-4**). A 5-mm-wide strip of the ligament is harvested and reflected ulnarly,

exposing the scaphocapitate and scaphotrapeziotrapezoid joints (**Fig. 48-5**).

Care is taken not to injure the vascular pedicle entering the scaphoid at its dorsal ridge. Next, the dorsal wrist capsule is incised longitudinally over the joint, and the dissection is continued proximally and subperiosteally beneath the second and fourth extensor compartments as necessary to allow adequate exposure.

To facilitate the actual reduction of the scaphoid and lunate, two 0.045-inch Kirschner wires (K-wires) are drilled in the posteroanterior direction to use as controlling joysticks—one in the scaphoid proximal pole and one in the lunate. The bones are reduced into normal anatomical alignment by extending the scaphoid and flexing the lunate and compressing them in the radial-ulnar direction. While maintaining the reduction, one or two parallel 0.045-inch K-wires are drilled percutaneously through the scaphoid into the lunate, and an additional 0.045-inch K-wire is drilled across the distal pole of the scaphoid into the capitate.

Appropriate reduction and wire placement are confirmed by direct inspection and intraoperative fluoroscopy. Particular attention is paid to the scapholunate gap on the anteroposterior view, the scapholunate angle on the lateral view, and the alignment of the distal scaphoid and the trapezium on the lateral view (**Fig. 48-6**). The remnant of the scapholunate interosseous ligament is reattached when possible using 4-0 nonabsorbable sutures via drill holes in a roughened spot in the dorsal proximal pole of the scaphoid, or alternatively via a small suture anchor.

A bony trough is prepared on the dorsal surface of the distal pole of the scaphoid adjacent to the scaphotrapezial joint, well

A

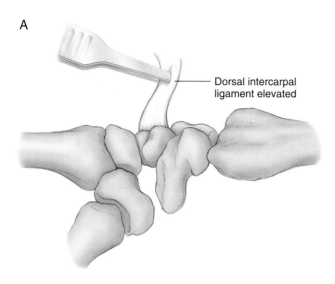

B

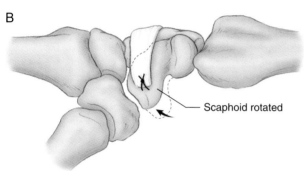

Scaphoid rotated

Dorsal intercarpal ligament elevated

FIGURE 48-2 A and **B,** Dorsal intercarpal ligament capsulodesis from a lateral perspective. **A,** After the dorsal intercarpal ligament is elevated, the scaphoid is rotated back into normal alignment with the trapezium. **B,** The completed ligament transfer is shown. The soft tissue reconstruction is reinforced with Kirschner wires for the first 8 weeks after surgery. *(From Szabo RM, Slater RR Jr, Palumbo CF, et al: Dorsal intercarpal ligament capsulodesis for chronic, static scapholunate dissociation: clinical results. J Hand Surg [Am]. 2002; 27:978-984.)*

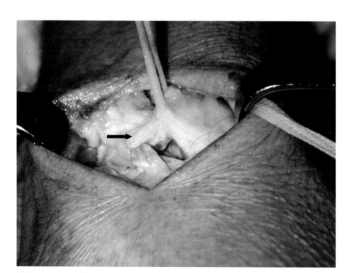

FIGURE 48-3 The dorsal intercarpal ligament is dissected and tagged with an umbilical tape. This ligament is a stout structure to be differentiated from capsular tissue. *Arrow* points to origin on the triquetrum.

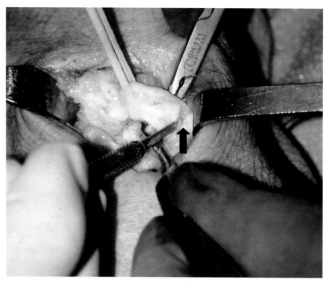

FIGURE 48-4 A hemostat is beneath the dorsal intercarpal ligament, which is being released from its insertion on the trapezium and trapezoid (*arrow*).

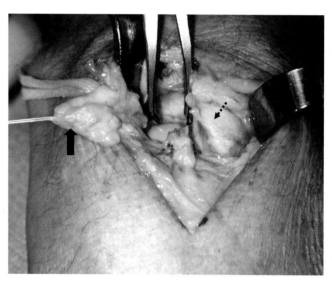

FIGURE 48-5 The dorsal intercarpal ligament is reflected ulnarly (*thick arrow*).The scapholunate diastasis is being shown with a laminar spreader. The scaphoid (*dashed arrow*) is flexed almost 90 degrees.

distal to the scaphoid's axis of rotation. A mini-Statack suture anchor (Zimmer, Inc., Warsaw, IN) attached to a 2-0 braided polyester suture is drilled into place at the base of the trough. One end of the suture anchor is passed through the end of the dorsal intercarpal ligament and then brought back out creating a Krackow stitch,[18] which is tied securely to bring the ligament firmly and snugly down into the trough on the scaphoid. Additional 4-0 nonabsorbable sutures are used to secure further the transferred ligament to its new insertion. The capsule is closed over the scapholunate interval, the extensor pollicis longus is replaced in its compartment, and the retinaculum is closed over the extensor tendons. The skin is closed in routine fashion.

Postoperatively, the extremity is immobilized in a bulky thumb spica dressing that extends above the elbow, reinforced with plaster splints. After 8 to 10 days, the sutures are removed, and the dressing is changed to a thumb spica cast extending above the

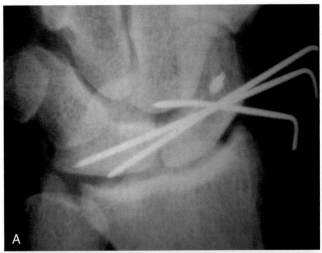

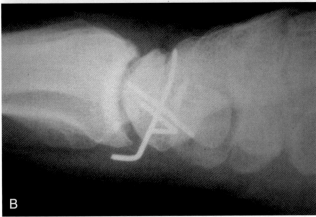

FIGURE 48-6 A and **B,** Postreduction x-rays illustrating the position of the suture anchor in the distal pole of the scaphoid, two Kirschner wires across the scapholunate joint, and one Kirschner wire across the scaphocapitate joint. **A,** Anteroposterior view. **B,** Lateral view. Restoration of the scapholunate angle must be confirmed on this view.

elbow for 3 weeks followed by a below-elbow thumb spica cast for an additional 4 weeks. The K-wires are removed 8 weeks after surgery, at which time gentle range of motion exercises under supervision are begun; a removable protective splint is worn between exercise sessions. Immobilization is discontinued 3 months after surgery. Patients are instructed to avoid forceful axial loading of the wrist, particularly in extension, such as with weightlifting or pushups, for 6 months after surgery.

Practical Tips

It is important to identify clearly the dorsal intercarpal ligament from surrounding capsular tissue. Rubbing the dorsal structures from medial to lateral with gauze helps with this visualization. It also is acceptable to leave some of the fibers of the dorsal intercarpal ligament that are attached to the scaphoid and just use the distal portion to advance.

Potential Pitfalls

Failure to reduce the scapholunate gap and correct the scapholunate angle would lead to carpal collapse. Using this procedure on patients with established arthritis would lead to continued pain. It is a good idea to inspect the radiocarpal joint at the time of surgery and have an alternative plan if arthritis is found. Care should be taken to ensure that suture anchors are secure and

placed completely subchondral so that they do not erode cartilage.

Controversies

Although we were encouraged from biomechanical studies and early clinical follow-up of the DILC, we noted that many other soft tissue capsulodesis techniques were reportedly successful at 1- or 2-year follow-up. Moran and associates[11] reviewed their intermediate-term results (average 54 months) after Blatt or Mayo capsulodesis, and noted that the results of their capsulodesis did not hold up over time. Although dorsal capsulodesis provided pain relief for patients with dynamic and static scapholunate instability, it did not provide maintenance of radiographic carpal alignment in cases of chronic scapholunate dissociation.[11] It remains controversial whether soft tissue procedures or limited arthrodesis is better. Zarkadas and colleagues[19] performed a study to evaluate the practice pattern of specialized hand surgeons in the management of acute and chronic scapholunate instability. They mailed a survey to the 1628 members of the American and Canadian Societies for Surgery of the Hand and received 468 responses from hand surgeons. The study showed that the management of chronic scapholunate instability varied greatly among the respondents. Favored management of chronic scapholunate dissociation included the Blatt capsulodesis alone, capsulodesis combined with a scapholunate ligament repair, or scaphotrapeziotrapezoid arthrodesis.[19] Treatment of chronic scapholunate dissociation remains an unsolved problem.

Complications

Complications are related to the K-wires used for fixation in this procedure. Some patients have irritation of the soft tissue surrounding the pins. Occasionally, patients present with pain and erythema around the pins and are treated with oral antibiotics prophylactically. With early pin loosening, there can be a loss of reduction.

Results

Previous studies have reported good clinical results using a dorsal capsulodesis to treat static scapholunate instability. Blatt[7] reported good results in 12 patients and a mean recovery of 80% of grip strength. Lavernia and colleagues[8] reported good results in 17 of 21 patients treated with scapholunate interosseous ligament repair combined with a dorsal capsulodesis procedure. Wintman and coworkers[16] showed that dorsal capsulodesis also can be used effectively to treat dynamic scapholunate instability. In a series of 20 procedures in 19 patients, subjective and objective evaluations improved substantially after surgery. After surgery, the symptoms of pain and clunking decreased significantly. Functional status was improved, most strikingly in the tasks of opening jars, sweeping, shoveling, and throwing. The investigators noted a meaningful improvement in wrist stability determined by the scaphoid shift maneuver.

One problem with these previously described procedures is that they limit wrist motion, particularly flexion, because the transferred capsule tethers the distal pole of the scaphoid to the distal radius. In Blatt's series,[7] loss of wrist flexion averaged 20 degrees. In the series reported by Lavernia and coworkers,[8] mean loss of flexion was 17 degrees. Wintman and colleagues[16] reported a mean loss of 12 degrees of flexion. In addition, none of the described procedures were successful at decreasing the scapholunate gap directly.

DILC conceptually has certain advantages over other soft tissue techniques. Because it links the triquetrum to the distal pole of the scaphoid directly, DILC seems to keep the proximal carpal row linked together to function as a unit. Our cadaver study confirmed that DILC decreased the scapholunate diastasis better than a Blatt capsulodesis, even when maximally loaded in the clenched fist position. We believe that the direction of the soft tissue tether in DILC may partly or entirely account for the observed decreased diastasis. We also believe that with DILC, the reduction of the scapholunate angle is accomplished in part because the transferred dorsal intercarpal ligament rests over the proximal pole of the capitate, which acts as a pulley to support the ligament and prevent the distal pole of the scaphoid from flexing excessively. DILC links the proximal carpal row together to decrease the scapholunate diastasis that develops after scapholunate interosseous ligament disruption. It decreases the diastasis better than a Blatt capsulodesis, and it corrects the scapholunate angle equally well. Neither DILC nor the Blatt capsulodesis restores normal wrist mechanics completely. The finding that DILC was strong enough to restore scapholunate gap and angle to near-normal conditions, even with loads applied across the wrist, was encouraging enough for us to start offering this procedure to patients.

We reported the results of a prospective study of 21 patients (22 wrists), 16 to 62 years old, followed 1 to 4 years.[10] For this study, all patients returned to complete a questionnaire and have a physical examination performed by physicians and therapists independent of the treating surgeons, and to obtain standardized radiographs of the wrists. Patient demographics, mechanism of injury, range of motion, and grip strength were recorded. Patients completed the Mayo wrist, Short-Form-12, and Disabilities of the Arm, Shoulder, and Hand (DASH) questionnaires. The scapholunate angle improved significantly ($P < .01$) from a mean preoperative value of 65 degrees to 54 degrees immediately postoperatively and remained at 50 degrees at final follow-up ($P < .01$). The scapholunate gap improved significantly from a mean preoperative value of 4.5 mm to 2.6 mm immediately postoperatively and remained at 2.7 mm at final follow-up ($P < .01$). There was no significant change in grip strength. Wrist flexion decreased by 10% postoperatively compared with a 15% decrease in wrist extension. Radial deviation decreased by 20%, whereas ulnar deviation decreased by 11% postoperatively.

Patients were satisfied with the outcomes. The mean DASH score for this group of patients was 17 (SD 17, range 1 to 69). The mean SF-12 score was 83 (SD 21, range 14 to 100). Two patients scored below the national mean of 50. The mean Mayo wrist score was 77 (SD 15, range 50 to 95). There were five excellent, seven good, five fair, and five poor results according to Mayo wrist scores. The DASH and the SF-12 score did not correlate with the Mayo wrist score, postoperative grip strength, or postoperative range of motion.

Our results confirmed that our hypothesis shown in vitro actually occurred in vivo. The scapholunate angle and diastasis were reduced and maintained over the duration of follow-up in this study. Longer follow-up is warranted, however, to see if this outcome is permanent. We are starting to see patients after 5 years show radiographic deterioration, although clinically they appear better than their x-rays. We continue to monitor our patients for longer term follow-up.

REFERENCES

1. Gelberman RH, Cooney WP 3rd, Szabo RM: Carpal instability. Instr Course Lect. 2001; 50:123-134.

2. Watson HK, Ballet FL: The SLAC wrist: scapholunate advanced collapse pattern of degenerative arthritis. J Hand Surg [Am]. 1984; 9:358-365.

3. Kleinman WB: Long-term study of chronic scapho-lunate instability treated by scapho-trapezio-trapezoid arthrodesis. J Hand Surg [Am]. 1989; 14:429-445.

4. Kleinman WB, Carroll CT: Scapho-trapezio-trapezoid arthrodesis for treatment of chronic static and dynamic scapho-lunate instability: a 10-year perspective on pitfalls and complications. J Hand Surg [Am]. 1990; 15:408-414.

5. Watson H, Hempton R: Limited wrist arthrodesis, I: the triscaphoid joint. J Hand Surg [Am]. 1980; 5:320-327.

6. Watson HK, Belniak R, Garcia-Elias M: Treatment of scapholunate dissociation: preferred treatment—STT fusion vs other methods. Orthopedics. 1991; 14:365-368; discussion 368-370.

7. Blatt G: Capsulodesis in reconstructive hand surgery: dorsal capsulodesis for the unstable scaphoid and volar capsulodesis following excision of the distal ulna. Hand Clin. 1987; 3:81-102.

8. Lavernia CJ, Cohen MS, Taleisnik J: Treatment of scapholunate dissociation by ligamentous repair and capsulodesis. J Hand Surg [Am]. 1992; 17:354-359.

9. Wyrick JD, Youse BD, Kiefhaber TR: Scapholunate ligament repair and capsulodesis for the treatment of static scapholunate dissociation. J Hand Surg [Br]. 1998; 23:776-780.

10. Szabo RM, Slater RR Jr, Palumbo CF, et al: Dorsal intercarpal ligament capsulodesis for chronic, static scapholunate dissociation: clinical results. J Hand Surg [Am]. 2002; 27:978-984.

11. Moran SL, Cooney WP, Berger RA, et al: Capsulodesis for the treatment of chronic scapholunate instability. J Hand Surg [Am]. 2005; 30:16-23.

12. Garcia-Elias M, Lluch AL, Stanley JK: Three-ligament tenodesis for the treatment of scapholunate dissociation: indications and surgical technique. J Hand Surg [Am]. 2006; 31:125-134.

13. Glickel SZ, Millender LH: Ligamentous reconstruction for chronic intercarpal instability. J Hand Surg [Am]. 1984; 9:514-527.

14. Brunelli GA, Brunelli GR: A new technique to correct carpal instability with scaphoid rotary subluxation: a preliminary report. J Hand Surg [Am]. 1995; 20:S82-S85.

15. Garcia-Elias M, Cooney WP, An KN, et al: Wrist kinematics after limited intercarpal arthrodesis. J Hand Surg [Am]. 1989; 14:791-799.

16. Wintman BI, Gelberman RH, Katz JN: Dynamic scapholunate instability: results of operative treatment with dorsal capsulodesis. J Hand Surg [Am]. 1995; 20:971-979.

17. Slater RR Jr, Szabo RM, Bay BK, et al: Dorsal intercarpal ligament capsulodesis for scapholunate dissociation: biomechanical analysis in a cadaver model. J Hand Surg [Am]. 1999; 24:232-239.

18. Krackow KA, Thomas SC, Jones LC: A new stitch for ligament-tendon fixation: brief note. J Bone Joint Surg [Am]. 1986; 68:764-766.

19. Zarkadas PC, Gropper PT, White NJ, et al: A survey of the surgical management of acute and chronic scapholunate instability. J Hand Surg [Am]. 2004; 29:848-857.

Modified Brunelli Tenodesis for the Treatment of Scapholunate Instability

49

Lisa A. Whitty, MD and Steven L. Moran, MD

Rationale and Basic Science Pertinent to the Procedure

Scapholunate instability is the most common form of carpal instability. Injury to the scapholunate interosseous ligament leads to alterations in the kinematic loads passing through the radiocarpal joint and a progressive degeneration of the secondary stabilizers of the carpus.[1] Eventual deterioration of these secondary stabilizers leads to fixed changes within the lunate and midcarpal joint leading to radiocarpal and midcarpal arthritis. Early within this process of scapholunate instability, pain is present over the dorsum of the wrist as overload to the remaining scapholunate ligament results in scaphoid subluxation, synovitis, and internal ligamentous strain.[2,3]

Despite its frequency, a standardized treatment protocol for scapholunate instability has not been established. Several surgical procedures have been recommended for the treatment of this disease process, including scaphotrapeziotrapezoidal and scaphocapitate fusion, capsulodesis alone, ligament repair in conjunction with dorsal capsulodesis, tenodesis, and bone-ligament-bone reconstruction.[1,4-12]

Tenodesis, in particular, attempts to re-establish the scapholunate relationship and scapholunate interosseous ligament through the use of various tendon weaves. Palmer and colleagues[13] described the use of the extensor carpi radialis longus tendon, which is routed through the tuberosity of the scaphoid, brought out dorsally through the lunotriquetral ligament, and then buried into a hole in the capitate. Taleisnik[14] used a strip of the flexor carpi radialis passed from palmar to dorsal through the lunate and into the scaphoid to recreate the dorsal scapholunate ligament. The graft is then introduced into a drill hole in the radius to create a deep radioscapholunate ligament. Many clinical series using similar tenodesis techniques have reported good results; however, because of the technical demands of these procedures and the complication associated with multiple bone tunnels, many of these procedures were abandoned in favor of scaphotrapeziotrapezoidal fusion or dorsal capsulodesis.[13-15] Inherently, any tenodesis procedure has attendant difficulties in tensioning the carpal bones because the elastic modulus of tendon is much larger than that of ligament. A reconstructed ligament that is snug enough to restore the scapholunate relationship would often result in a significant restriction in wrist motion that may approximate that following a partial wrist fusion.

In 1995, Brunelli and Brunelli[7] described a tenodesis technique using a slip of the flexor carpi radialis tendon that is tunneled through the distal portion of the scaphoid and attached to the distal radius to correct the abnormal scaphoid flexion deformity and to stabilize the scapholunate interval. Brunelli's original assumption was that rotary subluxation of the scaphoid is best corrected by stabilization of the scaphotrapeziotrapezoid ligament, rather than by reinforcing the scapholunate interosseous ligament.[7,16] Although this theory itself is still controversial, Brunelli's results were encouraging. In addition, the procedure itself required less bone tunneling with minimal destruction of the volar carpal ligaments. The initial results with the Brunelli repair have been comparable to the results reported for dorsal capsulodesis.[7,17,18]

Modifications of Brunelli's original procedure have been described by Van Den Abbeele and colleagues and Garcia-Elias and colleagues.[3,18,19] This modified technique involves tunneling the flexor carpi radialis tendon through the scaphoid from the distal pole to the dorsal tuberosity, in contrast to Brunelli's original description, in which the flexor carpi radialis is passed parallel to the scaphotrapeziotrapezoidal joint surface. The tendon is passed through the dorsal radiocarpal ligament, which also has been referred to as the dorsal radiolunotriquetral ligament. The distal end of the tendon is flipped back and secured to itself and the underlying lunate. This also is in contrast to Brunelli's original description, in which the flexor carpi radialis graft was originally anchored to the dorsal distal radius. This modified technique (now termed the "three-ligament tenodesis" because the weave is believed to stabilize the scaphotrapeziotrapezoidal, scapholunate interosseous, and dorsal radiocarpal ligaments) has yielded encouraging medium-term results for chronic scapholunate instability.[3,19]

Pertinent Anatomy

Adequate execution of the tenodesis procedure is predicated on a thorough understanding of wrist anatomy, including the secondary ligamentous constraints of scaphoid motion and the dorsal and volar wrist capsule. The ligaments of the wrist can be divided into two general categories. The first category includes the interosseous ligaments, which run between carpal bones and include the scapholunate and lunotriquetral interosseous ligaments (**Fig. 49-1A**). These two ligaments are the major stabilizers of the proximal carpal row and carpus.[20,21] The scaphotrapeziotrapezoidal ligament, also an interosseous ligament, connects the scaphoid with the trapezium and trapezoid (**Fig. 49-1B**).[22,23] Garcia-Elias and others[24-26] characterized the distal ligament connections of the scaphoid further into two separated complexes—the mediolateral scaphotrapeziotrapezoidal ligament and the anteromedial scaphocapitate ligament; both ligaments provide distal support to the scaphoid.

The second group of ligaments comprises the extrinsic wrist ligaments, which connect the forearm bones to the carpal bones. There are palmar and dorsal extrinsic wrist ligaments. These tend

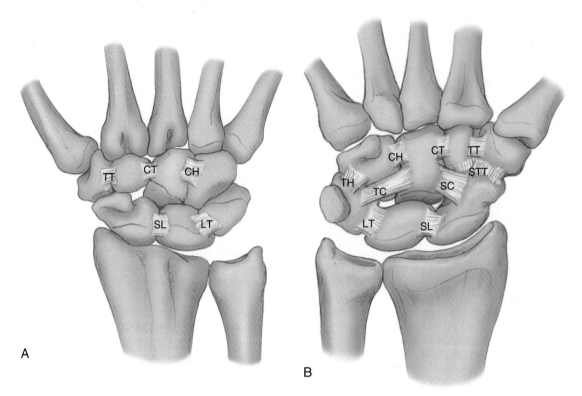

FIGURE 49-1 Intrinsic ligaments of the wrist are ligaments that originate and insert among the carpal bones. **A,** Dorsal view of the wrist shows the scapholunate (SL), lunotriquetral (LT), trapeziotrapezoid (TT), capitotrapezoid (CT), and capito-hamate (CH) intrinsic ligaments. **B,** Volar view of the wrist illustrates the volar aspect of the same ligaments in addition to the scaphotrapeziotrapezoid (STT), scaphocapitate (SC), triquetrocapitate (TC), and triquetrohamate (TH) ligaments. *(Copyright Mayo Clinic; reproduced with permission of the Mayo Foundation.)*

to serve as secondary stabilizers of carpal motion. The palmar extrinsic ligaments form a configuration of two "V"-shaped bands with a space between the bands. This space or gap, which has minimal ligamentous support and is an inherent point of weakness, is known as the space of Poirier (**Fig. 49-2A**). The dorsal carpal ligaments include the dorsal intercarpal and dorsal radiocarpal ligaments. These extrinsic ligaments are thinner and weaker than their palmar counterparts, but also provide structural support to the carpus (**Fig. 49-2B**).

The volar extrinsic ligaments, which act as major secondary constraints of scaphoid motion, include the radioscaphocapitate ligament, long radiolunate ligament, scaphotrapezial ligament, and scaphocapitate ligament (see Fig. 49-2A). The radioscaphocapitate ligament originates from the radial palmar rim of the radius and passes beneath the scaphoid waist to attach to the capitate. During its course, it gives off attachments to the lunate.[27] These fibers interdigitate with fibers from the ulnocapitate ligament to form the so-called arcuate ligament of the wrist.[28] The long radiolunate ligament lies ulnar to the radioscaphocapitate ligament and may also support the scapholunate relationship through its direct connections to the palmar component of the scapholunate interosseous ligament (see Fig. 49-2A).[29,30] Short and coworkers[31,32] showed that after disruption of the scapholunate interosseous ligament, division of the scaphotrapezial and radioscaphocapitate ligaments results in additional instability in scapholunate motion.

Important secondary dorsal stabilizers of the scapholunate joint include the dorsal intercarpal and dorsal radiocarpal ligaments. The dorsal intercarpal ligament originates from the dorsal ridge of the triquetrum and attaches to the dorsal distal aspect of the lunate and into the dorsal rim of the scaphoid. The ligament gives attachments to the scapholunate interosseous ligament and lunotriquetral interosseous ligament during its course.[32] The dorsal radiocarpal ligament, or the dorsal radiolunotriquetral ligament, originates from the dorsal margin of the distal radius just ulnar and distal to Lister's tubercle. The ligament extends obliquely with fibers inserting into the lunate, inserting into the lunotriquetral interosseous ligament, and finally inserting into the dorsal ridge of the triquetrum.[32] The dorsal intercarpal and dorsal radiocarpal ligaments create a "V" shape over the dorsal wrist capsule and contribute to the stability of the scaphoid and lunate (see Fig. 49-2B). Viegas and others[33,34] have noted that the dorsal portion of the scapholunate interosseous ligament is intertwined with portions of the dorsal capsule. Short and colleagues[32] and Ruch and Smith[35] have shown that injury to the dorsal intercarpal ligament can change carpal kinematics.

Finally, the flexor carpi radialis runs through a fibro-osseous canal at the scaphoid tuberosity and trapezial groove before inserting into the trapezial crest directly and then proceeding to the base of the second metacarpal.[36] Its course may be easily palpated subcutaneously beneath the skin in the radial aspect of the forearm.

Indications

The primary goals of the treatment of scapholunate instability include pain relief, re-establishment of carpal alignment, and maintenance of wrist mobility. The use of the modified Brunelli procedure is reserved for patients with a history of wrist pain

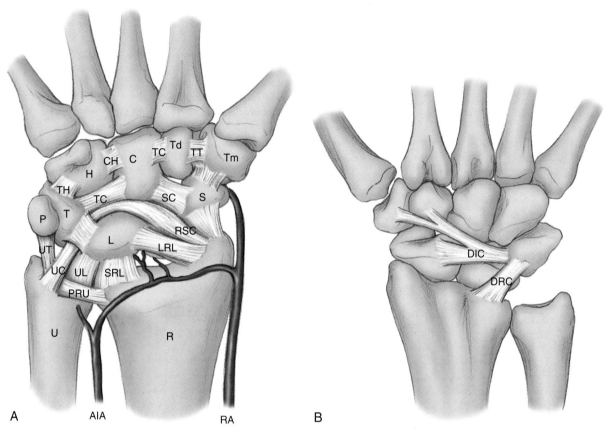

FIGURE 49-2 Extrinsic ligaments of the wrist include ligaments that originate outside the carpal bones and insert onto the carpal bones. **A,** From a volar view, the proximal ligaments from radial to ulnar include the radioscaphocapitate (RSC), long radiolunate (LRL), short radiolunate (SRL), ulnolunate (UL), ulnocapitate (UC), and ulnotriquetral (UT). AIA, anterior interosseous artery; C, capitate; H, hamate; P, pisiform; PRU, palmar radioulnar ligament; R, radius; RA, radial artery; S, scaphoid; T, triquetrum; Td, trapezoid; Tm, trapezium; U, ulna. **B,** From a dorsal view, there is only one true extrinsic ligament, the radiotriquetral or dorsal radiocarpal (DRC) ligament. The scaphotriquetral or dorsal intercarpal (DIC) ligament is by definition an intrinsic ligament, but is easier to illustrate here. *(Copyright Mayo Clinic; reproduced with permission of the Mayo Foundation.)*

lasting longer than 2 to 3 months. Patients with scapholunate instability seen within 6 to 8 weeks of injury usually are treated with attempted primary open or arthroscopic repair.

Dynamic and static instability can be treated with this procedure. Dynamic and static instability refer to the radiographic appearance of the patient's wrist at the time of presentation. Patients with static scapholunate instability present with a scapholunate diastasis greater than 3 mm and a scapholunate angle greater than 60 degrees. Patients also may present with radiographic signs of a dorsal intercalated segment instability pattern, which is manifested as an increased scapholunate angle greater than 60 degrees and an increased radiolunate and capitolunate angle. Patients with dynamic instability have normal static radiographs, but may show an increased scapholunate with stress radiographs (clenched fist view). The diagnosis of a dynamic scapholunate injury in these patients is often suspected on physical examination, but the definitive diagnosis is made at the time of arthroscopy. Patients presenting with wrist pain, normal radiographs, and only mild scapholunate instability, such as a Geissler grade 1 or 2[37] seen at the time of arthroscopy, may be better treated with an arthroscopic scapholunate interosseous ligament shrinkage or pinning versus an open repair combined with a dorsal capsulodesis, rather than a tenodesis procedure.[9]

The ideal patient for tenodesis is a patient with chronic scapholunate instability who has an easily reducible scaphoid and

lunate, without evidence of chondrolysis in the radioscaphoid fossa or midcarpal joint.[19] Concomitant ligamentous injuries, such as lunotriquetral injuries or triangular fibrocartilage complex injuries, can be repaired at the same time as the tenodesis procedure and are not a contraindication for this surgery.

Contraindications

Absolute contraindications to a tenodesis include radiographic evidence of advanced degenerative arthritis or significant cartilage loss that is visualized at the time of arthrotomy. Patients with degenerative arthritis confined to the radial styloid (grade 1 scapholunate advanced collapse) may be considered for a tenodesis in conjunction with a radial styloidectomy.

At the time of surgery, Kirschner wires (K-wires) are placed into the dorsal aspect of the scaphoid and the lunate. These joysticks are used to correct the increased scaphoid flexion and dorsal angulation of the lunate. If it is difficult to restore the normal alignment of the scaphoid and lunate with the use of K-wires, long-term success with the tenodesis procedure is unlikely. Patients with an irreducible lunate or scaphoid are better treated with some form of salvage procedure. A percentage of irreducible scaphoids can be converted to reducible scaphoids by resection of the fibrous tissue that develops along the medial corner of the scaphoid tuberosity and the proximal edge of the lunate.[3,7] If the scaphoid and lunate are easily reducible after resection of the fibrosis, one can proceed with the tenodesis procedure. Finally, if there is a repairable dorsal scapholunate interosseous ligament or an avulsed scapholunate interosseous ligament, one should attempt a primary repair before considering a tenodesis procedure.

Surgical Technique

Web Video

49-1 and 49-2

The modified Brunelli tenodesis technique is performed as described by Van Den Abbeele and colleagues[18] and Talwalkar and associates[19] using dorsal and volar approaches. A standard dorsal wrist incision is made, and the wrist capsule is opened using a ligament-sparing capsulotomy as described by Berger and Bishop[38] (**Fig. 49-3A**). The radiocarpal and midcarpal joints are inspected for signs of degenerative arthritis. Any scar tissue within the joint is excised. At this point, the surgeon confirms that the scaphoid and lunate are easily reducible; if not, the procedure is abandoned, and an alternative procedure is chosen.

Volarly, an incision is made over the flexor carpi radialis, and dissection proceeds distally to the scaphoid tuberosity (**Fig. 49-3B**). A strip of the flexor carpi radialis tendon (about one third of its width) is cut proximally, preserving its distal attachment to the base of the second metacarpal. A K-wire is drilled dorsal to volar from the bare area of the scaphoid dorsally to the scaphoid tubercle palmarly. Fluoroscopy is used to verify the position of the wire (**Fig. 49-4A and B**). A 3.5-mm cannulated drill is passed over the K-wire to create a channel for the tendon slip. The slip of tendon is passed from volar to dorsal through the bone tunnel made in the scaphoid (**Fig. 49-4C**). Placing the tendon slip on tension reduces the scaphoid, although K-wire joysticks also may be used to aid in reduction. The reduced scaphoid is held with one to two K-wires (**Fig. 49-5**). A small trough is created in the dorsal portion of the scaphoid and lunate within which the tendon will lie (**Fig. 49-6A**). The flexor carpi radialis is secured onto the scaphoid and the lunate using one or two suture anchors (**Fig. 49-6B and C**).

The dorsal radiocarpal ligament is identified as it passes over the triquetrum at the ulnar margin of the capsular flap. An opening is made in the dorsal radiocarpal ligament with a tendon passer. The tail of the flexor carpi radialis is weaved through the proximal margin of the dorsal radiocarpal ligament and then sewn back to itself. The tendon is secured with 3-0 nonabsorbable suture attached to the suture anchors. The capsular flap is repaired with an absorbable 3-0 suture. The suture tails attached to the

suture anchors are left long and are used to reef the wrist capsule to the tendon. Additional absorbable sutures may be placed between the tendon and the capsular flap as necessary. Finally, the extensor retinaculum is closed with an absorbable suture, and the skin is closed with nylon after release of the tourniquet and meticulous hemostasis.

An additional wire is placed between the scaphoid and capitate to stabilize the midcarpal joint (**Fig. 49-7**). A long arm cast is worn for 2 weeks followed by a short arm cast until wire removal. Wires are left for 6 to 8 weeks, at which time gentle range of motion exercises are permitted. A splint is worn for an additional 6 weeks. Unrestricted activity is allowed at 5 to 6 months.

Results

Overall results of the tenodesis procedure are encouraging, but most patients can expect some reduction in wrist flexion, and 30% to 40% of patients may continue to have wrist pain with heavy exertion. Brunelli and Brunelli's original report[7] of 13 patients noted a reduction in wrist motion ranging from 30% to 60% of the contralateral wrist. Grip strength improved 50% over preoperative values, and all patients in this study were able to return to work during the follow-up period. In the study by Talwalkar and associates[19] of 162 patients performed over 7 years, 62% of patients had no to mild pain at an average follow-up of 4 years. Range of motion was reduced by 26% compared with the contralateral side, and grip strength was 80% of the nonoperated side. Of patients, 79% were satisfied with the results of surgery, and 88% thought they would have had the same operation again.[19] There was no significant difference in outcomes for patients presenting with dynamic or static instability. These results were comparable to earlier published results from the same institution.[18]

More recently, Garcia-Elias and colleagues[3] have reported their 46-month results in 38 patients. In this group, 74% of patients noted pain relief at rest, and 76% were able to return to their normal vocational activities. Grip strength averaged 65% of the normal side, and postoperative wrist flexion and extension were approximately 75% of the contralateral side. None of these patients have required secondary surgery during the follow-up period.

Finally, Moran and colleagues[17] reported on a retrospective comparison of 15 patients undergoing the modified Brunelli procedure and 14 patients undergoing dorsal capsulodesis for

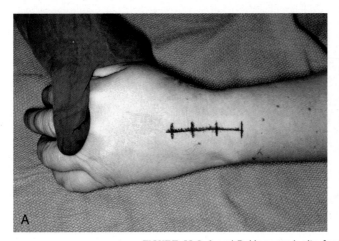

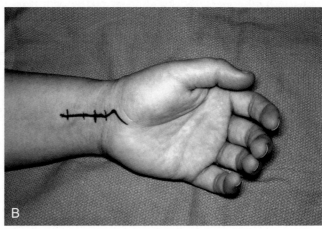

FIGURE 49-3 **A** and **B,** Lines mark site for typical dorsal (**A**) and palmar (**B**) incisions.

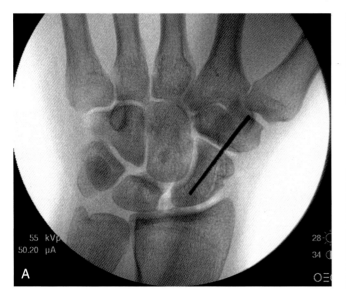

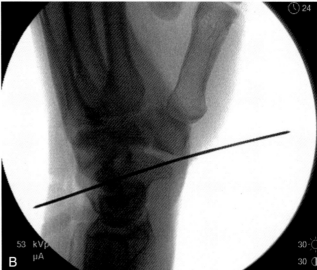

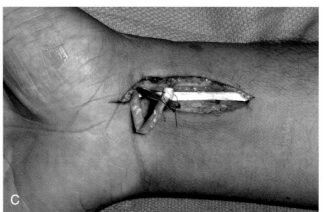

FIGURE 49-4 The initial guidewire is placed from a dorsal to palmar direction from the dorsal ridge or bare area of the scaphoid to the distal volar tuberosity. **A** and **B,** Intraoperative radiographs showing the ideal position of the guidewire in the anteroposterior (**A**) and lateral (**B**) planes. This wire is then used as the guide for a 3.5-mm cannulated drill, which creates the bone tunnel for the flexor carpi radialis. When the tunnel is created, a cannulated awl is passed from dorsal to proximal into the palmar incision. **C,** The flexor carpi radialis tendon slip is tied to the cannulated awl and withdrawn into the dorsal incision.

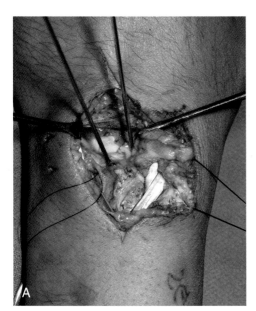

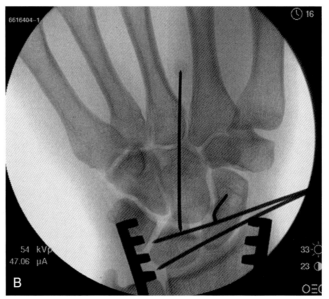

FIGURE 49-5 Before tensioning the flexor carpi radialis tendon slip, the scapholunate relationship is re-established with the aid of Kirschner wires placed dorsally into the scaphoid and lunate. These Kirschner wires are used as joysticks to correct rotatory subluxation of the scaphoid and dorsal angulation of the lunate. When the anatomical relationship has been re-established, the scaphoid and lunate are pinned with one or two Kirschner wires. **A,** Standard dorsal approach to carpus with Kirschner wires in scaphoid and lunate. **B,** Intraoperative radiograph shows position of the Kirschner wires within the scaphoid and lunate after restoration of scapholunate relationship.

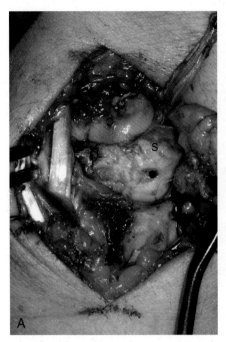 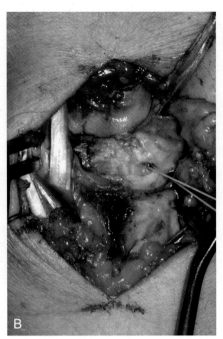 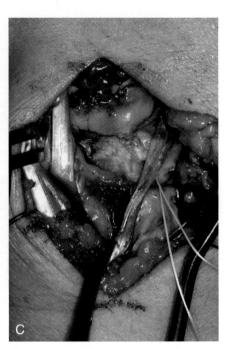

FIGURE 49-6 A, After pinning the scapholunate joint, a bone trough is cut into the scaphoid and lunate with the use of a small rongeur. **B,** A bone anchor is placed at the base of the trough in the scaphoid, and a separate bone anchor is placed into the lunate. **C,** The flexor carpi radialis tendon is tensioned and secured to the floor of the trough using the sutures from the bone anchors. The tail of the flexor carpi radialis is based through the dorsal radiocarpal and then sutured back to itself. C, capitate; L, lunate; S, scaphoid.

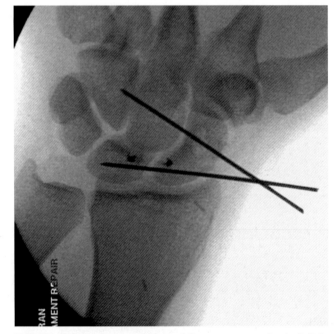

FIGURE 49-7 At the completion of the case, one wire is left to stabilize the scapholunate relationship, and an additional wire is placed across the scaphocapitate joint to minimize stresses on the scaphoid during the early postoperative course.

the treatment of chronic scapholunate instability with an average 3-year follow-up (**Fig. 49-8**). Final wrist range of motion was 63% to 64% of the normal side in both groups. The postoperative grip strength remained unchanged in both groups, measuring 91% of normal side in the capsulodesis group and 86.5% of normal side in the tenodesis group. There was one failure requiring wrist fusion in the tenodesis group. Motion decreased from 89% of the contralateral side preoperatively to 63% postoperatively. The preoperative scapholunate angle averaged 63 degrees (range 45 to 95 degrees) and was corrected to 54 degrees (range 35 to 95 degrees) on final follow-up.[17] There was a statistical long-term improvement in the scapholunate angle in the tenodesis group that was not seen in the capsulodesis group, suggesting that the modified Brunelli procedure may provide a benefit over capsulodesis in controlling scaphoid flexion and preserving carpal dynamics; however, further prospective trials are required to determine the ideal long-term treatment for this difficult problem.

Summary

The modified Brunelli tenodesis procedure provides pain relief, restores carpal height, reduces the scaphoid to its anatomical position, and allows reconstruction of the volar scaphotrapezio-trapezoidal ligament. The procedure is appropriate for patients with either static or dynamic scapholunate instability. It is contraindicated in patients with evidence of radiocarpal arthritis and patients with an irreducible scaphoid and lunate. Early results have shown that this technique provides better radiographic restoration of the scapholunate relationship compared with capsulodesis procedures.

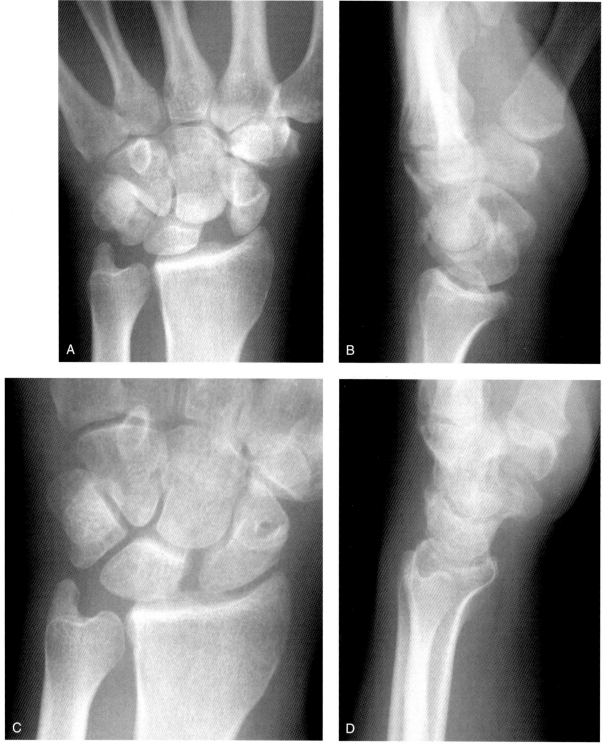

FIGURE 49-8 **A** and **B,** Preoperative anteroposterior (**A**) and lateral (**B**) radiographs of a patient with a chronic scapholunate dissociation and significant dorsal intercalated segment instability. **C** and **D,** The patient was treated with a tenodesis procedure with good restoration of the scapholunate gap (**C**) and scapholunate angle (**D**) at 2-year follow-up. *(From Moran SL, Ford KS, Wolfe CA, et al: Outcomes of dorsal capsulodesis and tenodesis for treatment of scapholunate instability. J Hand Surg. 2006; 31:1436-1438.)*

REFERENCES

1. Gelberman RH, Cooney WP, Szabo RM: Carpal instability. Instr Course Lect. 2000; 82A:578-594.

2. Linscheid RL, Dobyns JH, Beabout JW, et al: Traumatic instability of the wrist: diagnosis, classification and pathomechanics. J Bone Joint Surg Am. 1972; 54:1612-1632.

3. Garcia-Elias M, Lluch AL, Stanley JK: Three-ligament tenodesis for the treatment of scapholunate dissociation: indications and surgical technique. J Hand Surg [Am]. 2006; 31:125-134.

4. Watson HK, Hempton RF: Limited wrist arthrodeses, I: the triscaphoid joint. J Hand Surg [Am]. 1980; 5:320-327.

5. Kleinman WB, Carroll C: Scapho-trapezio-trapezoid arthrodesis for treatment of chronic static and dynamic scapho-lunate instability: a 10-year perspective on pitfalls and complications. J Hand Surg [Am]. 1990; 15:408-414.

6. Davis CA, Culp RW, Hume EL, et al: Reconstruction of the scapholunate ligament in a cadaver model using a bone-ligament-bone autograft from the foot. J Hand Surg [Am]. 1998; 23:884-892.

7. Brunelli GA, Brunelli GR: A new technique to correct carpal instability with scaphoid rotary subluxation: a preliminary report. J Hand Surg [Am]. 1995; 20(3 Pt 2):S82-S85.

8. Blatt G: Capsulodesis in reconstructive hand surgery: dorsal capsulodesis for the unstable scaphoid and volar capsulodesis following excision of the distal ulna. Hand Clin. 1987; 3:81-102.

9. Lavernia CJ, Cohen MS, Taleisnik J: Treatment of scapholunate dissociation by ligamentous repair and capsulodesis. J Hand Surg [Am]. 1992; 17:354-359.

10. Wolf JM, Weiss AP: Bone-retinaculum-bone reconstruction of scapholunate ligament injuries. Orthop Clin North Am. 2001; 32:241-246.

11. Wyrick JD, Youse BD, Kiefhaber TR: Scapholunate ligament repair and capsulodesis for the treatment of static scapholunate dissociation. J Hand Surg [Br]. 1998; 23:776-780.

12. Wintman BI, Gelberman RH, Katz JN: Dynamic scapholunate instability: results of operative treatment with dorsal capsulodesis. J Hand Surg [Am]. 1995; 20:971-979.

13. Palmer AK, Dobyns JH, Linscheid RL: Management of post-traumatic instability of the wrist secondary to ligament rupture. J Hand Surg [Am]. 1978; 3:507-532.

14. Taleisnik J: Wrist: anatomy, function, injury. Instr Course Lect. 1978; 27:61-68.

15. Almquist EE, Bach AW, Sack JT, et al: Four corner ligament reconstruction for treatment of chronic complete scapholunate separation. J Hand Surg. 1991; 16:322-327.

16. Brunelli GA, Brunelli GR: Rotary subluxation of the scaphoid: correction using the flexor carpi radialis. In Watson HK, Weinzweig J, eds: The Wrist. Philadelphia: Lippincott Williams & Wilkins, 2001.

17. Moran SL, Ford KS, Wolfe CA, et al: Outcomes of dorsal capsulodesis and tenodesis for treatment of scapholunate instability. J Hand Surg. 2006; 31:1436-1438.

18. Van Den Abbeele KL, Loh YC, Stanley JK, et al: Early results of a modified Brunelli procedure for scapholunate instability. J Hand Surg [Br]. 1998; 23:258-261.

19. Talwalkar SC, Edwards AT, Hayton MJ, et al: Results of tri-ligament tenodesis: a modified Brunelli procedure in the management of scapholunate instability. J Hand Surg [Br]. 2006; 31:110-117.

20. Berger RA, Blair WF, Crowinshield RD, et al: The scapholunate ligament. J Hand Surg [Am]. 1982; 7:87-91.

21. Landsmeer JM: Studies in the anatomy of the carpus and its bearing on some surgical problem. Acta Morphol Neederlando-Scand. 1960; 3:304-321.

22. Drewniany JJ, Palmer AK, Flatt AE: The scaphotrapezial ligament complex: an anatomic and biomechanical study. J Hand Surg. 1985; 10:492-498.

23. Moritomo H, Viegas SF, Nakamura K, et al: The scaphotrapezio-trapezoidal joint, part I: an anatomic and radiographic study. J Hand Surg. 2000; 25:899-910.

24. Garcia-Elias M: Kinetic analysis of carpal stability during grip. Hand Clin. 1997; 13:151-158.

25. Masquelet AC, Strube F, Nordin JY: The isolated scapho-trapezio-trapezoid ligament injury: diagnosis and surgical treatment in four cases. J Hand Surg [Br]. 1993; 18:730-735.

26. Garcia-Elias M, Geissler WB: Carpal instability. In Green DP, Hotchkiss RN, Pederson WC, et al, eds: Green's Operative Hand Surgery. Philadelphia: Elsevier Churchill Livingstone, 2005.

27. Berger RA, Landsmeer JM: The palmar radiocarpal ligaments: a study of adult and fetal human wrist joints. J Hand Surg [Am]. 1990; 15:847-854.

28. Patterson R, Moritomo H, Yamaguchi S, et al: Scaphoid anatomy and mechanics: update and review. Atlas Hand Clin. 2004; 9:129-140.

29. Berger RA: The anatomy of the ligaments of the wrist and distal radioulnar joints. Clin Orthop. 2001; 383:32-40.

30. Berger RA: The gross and histologic anatomy of the scapholunate interosseous ligament. J Hand Surg [Am]. 1996; 21:170-178.

31. Short WH, Werner FW, Green JK, et al: Biomechanical evaluation of the ligamentous stabilizers of the scaphoid and lunate, part II. J Hand Surg. 2005; 30:24-34.

32. Short WH, Werner FW, Green JK, et al: The effects of sectioning the dorsal radiocarpal ligament and insertion of a pressor sensor into the radiocarpal joint on scaphoid and lunate kinematics. J Hand Surg. 2002; 27:68.

33. Viegas SF, Yamaguchi S, Boyd NL, et al: The dorsal ligaments of the wrist: anatomy, mechanical properties, and function. J Hand Surg. 1999; 24:456.

34. Mizuseki T, Ikuta Y: The dorsal carpal ligaments: their anatomy and function. J Hand Surg [Br]. 1989; 14:91.

35. Ruch DS, Smith BP: Arthroscopic and open management of dynamic scaphoid instability. Orthop Clin North Am. 2001; 32:233.

36. Bishop AT, Gabel G, Carmichael SW: Flexor carpi radialis tendinitis, part I: operative anatomy. J Bone Joint Surg Am. 1994; 76:1009-1014.

37. Geissler WB, Freeland A, Savoie FH III, et al: Intraarticular soft-tissue lesions associated with an intraarticular fracture of the distal end of the radius. J Bone Joint Surg Am. 1996; 78:357-365.

38. Berger RA, Bishop AT: A fiber-splitting capsulotomy technique for dorsal exposure of the wrist. Tech Hand Upper Extrem Surg. 1997; 1:2-10.

Bone-Ligament-Bone Reconstruction

50

Greg Merrell, MD and Arnold-Peter C. Weiss, MD

Rationale and Basic Science

Scapholunate dissociation is a vexing problem facing hand surgeons. It is the most common form of carpal instability.[1-4] Untreated scapholunate interosseous ligament (SLIL) disruption leads to significant degenerative changes of the carpus.[4-8] A multitude of treatment options are described, which suggests that an optimal strategy has yet to be discovered.[5,9-41] Partial wrist fusion, although a durable solution, trades off improvements in pain with decreased range of motion and strength.[38]

The great strides made in anatomical anterior cruciate ligament reconstruction over the past 30 years have led some hand surgeons to consider a similar model for SLIL reconstruction. Biomechanical studies show that the dorsal portion of the ligament is strongest and most important functionally.[8,42-47] The yield strength of the dorsal region was 260N, more than twice that of the palmar region.[42] Reconstruction of the dorsal ligament also is appealing given the ease of exposure through a standard dorsal approach. Various composite grafts have been investigated, including bone-retinaculum-bone from the distal radius,[30] navicular-cuneiform autograft,[27,41] SLIL allograft,[5,12] metacarpal-carpal composite,[48] and capitohamate ligament,[42] in an attempt to match the strength, stiffness, and functionality of the native SLIL (Fig. 50-1).

Indications and Contraindications

The ideal candidate is a patient with an acute or chronic rupture of the SLIL and only dynamic instability. Patients with a history consistent with an SLIL tear, pain over the scapholunate interval, or stress views showing widening at the scapholunate interval were considered for operative intervention. The definitive diagnosis of dynamic instability was made by direct arthroscopic examination in all patients. The reconstruction is rarely necessary in Geissler grade 1, but is commonly performed for grades 2 through 4. Patients with static scapholunate widening generally have not done well with bone-tendon-bone reconstruction, which is a relative contraindication. Sclerosis of the lunate (sometimes seen in cases of perilunate or lunate dislocation) also is a relative contraindication because of the risk of graft pullout. Degenerative changes of the carpus would be an absolute contraindication. An inability to reduce anatomically the scapholunate gap and rotation would be another absolute contraindication. Low-demand patients and elderly patients may be better served with a definitive procedure, such as a proximal row carpectomy.

Navicular-Cuneiform Autografts

Davis and colleagues[41] reported on the use of the dorsomedial portion of the navicular–first cuneiform ligament. Although weaker than the SLIL, its minimal donor morbidity made it an acceptable clinical choice. The graft is harvested through a medial incision with posterior retraction of the tibialis anterior. Each bone plug measures $10 \times 5 \times 5$ mm and is secured with small screws. The same group of investigators reported several cases of tissue elongation without loss of angulation.[49] Commentary on donor site morbidity has not been published at this point. Svoboda and associates[27] reported on the biomechanics of several other bone-tendon-bone complexes in the foot (e.g., tarsometatarsal ligament); however, none of these have been reported in clinical use.

Metacarpal-Carpal Autografts

Metacarpal-carpal grafts have several appealing features. The articulation at the base of the second or third metacarpal is relatively immobile and perhaps expendable. It can be harvested through the same dorsal incision as the reconstruction. These grafts more closely approximate the strength and stiffness of the SLIL than distal radius retinaculum grafts.[48] Early results from a small case series are encouraging.[50] The two main complications—graft pullout and graft stretching—are similar to reports with other types of bone-tendon-bone grafts. Graft stretching typically occurs after several months, perhaps during the revascularization phase of healing. There is loss of a tight SLIL interval, but the scapholunate angle is usually maintained. Graft pullout is seen more often in cases with poor lunate bone quality. A vascularized third metacarpal-carpal bone graft may have some benefit in these cases.[49]

Capitohamate Autografts

Berger's group[51] pioneered the use of the capitohamate graft for SLIL reconstruction. There are three capitohamate interosseous ligaments—dorsal, deep, and palmar. The dorsal ligament has a load to failure of 133N. The dorsal ligament is clinically feasible to harvest, and preservation of the deep and palmar ligaments is likely to maintain the capitohamate orientation. Berger supplements the repair with a capsulodesis and pins. Protected motion is started at 4 weeks, and pins are removed at 8 weeks. There are no clinical results published yet on this technique. Berger has commented that he does not perform this reconstruction if the lunate is translated ulnarly more than 50% out of the fossa.[49]

Authors' Preferred Technique (Distal Radius Retinaculum Graft)

A standard dorsal midline approach is made. The extensor pollicis longus is released on the ulnar side and transposed radially. Using a small osteotome, a single $20 \times 8 \times 8$ mm bone block with the overlying periosteum and retinaculum is harvested from the distal

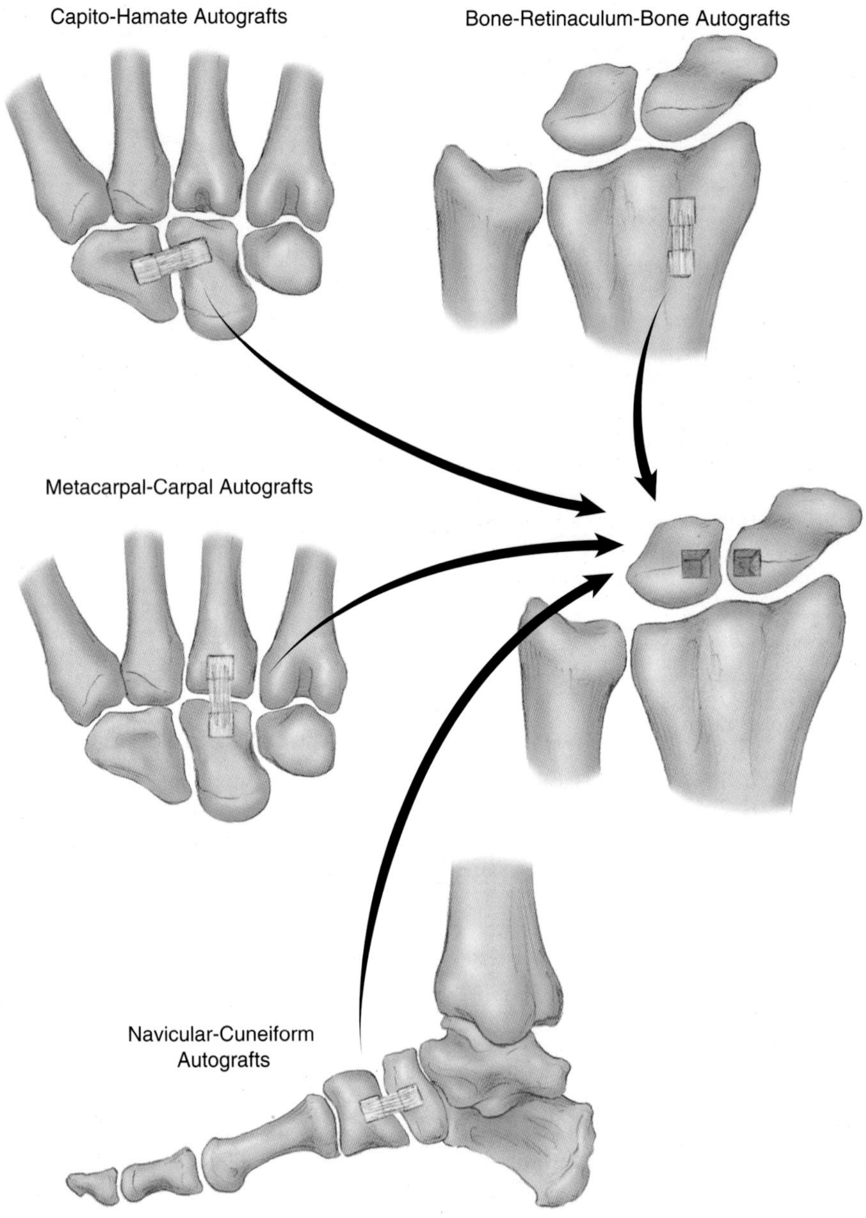

Capito-Hamate Autografts

Bone-Retinaculum-Bone Autografts

Metacarpal-Carpal Autografts

Navicular-Cuneiform
Autografts

FIGURE 50-1 Schematic diagram of the various sources of autograft used in scapholunate ligament reconstruction. All of the techniques have the same method of inset into the scapholunate interval as described by Weiss.[30,31]

radius near Lister's tubercle between the second and third compartments (**Fig. 50-2**). A 2- to 3-mm segment of cancellous and cortical bone is removed from the midportion of the bone block with a fine rongeur. Care is taken not to disrupt the overlying periosteum and retinaculum.

The capsule between the second and fourth compartment is incised longitudinally or via a ligament-sparing incision to expose the scapholunate interval. The wrist is flexed to improve visibility of the joint, and Kirschner wires (K-wires) are placed into the scaphoid and lunate for use as joysticks (**Fig. 50-3**). After reduction is confirmed on fluoroscopy, two 0.045-inch K-wires are drilled from the scaphoid into the lunate to capture the reduction. The joystick K-wires are removed. With a small osteotome, troughs are cut in the scaphoid and lunate adjacent to the joint, matching the size of the harvested graft (**Fig. 50-4**). The graft is digitally impacted into the scaphoid and lunate. A 1.3-mm screw is placed into each graft, securing them to the

scaphoid and lunate (**Fig. 50-5**). Intraoperative fluoroscopy is used to check the alignment and placing of the screws and K-wires (**Fig. 50-6**). The capsule is repaired with imbrication as needed. Short arm spica immobilization in wrist extension is used for 6 weeks.

Harvey and colleagues[49] reported on 20 patients with a distal radius bone-retinaculum-bone reconstruction augmented with a Herbert screw, placed percutaneously from the radial side. The screw is removed at 9 to 12 months. One patient had screw pullout with gapping of the scapholunate interval, and another had a fixed dorsal intercalated segment instability deformity. Eighty percent of their first 20 patients returned to their previous occupations.

Results

In 1998, Weiss[31] first reported on 19 patients treated with distal radius bone-retinaculum-bone fixation of the SLIL. Three of the

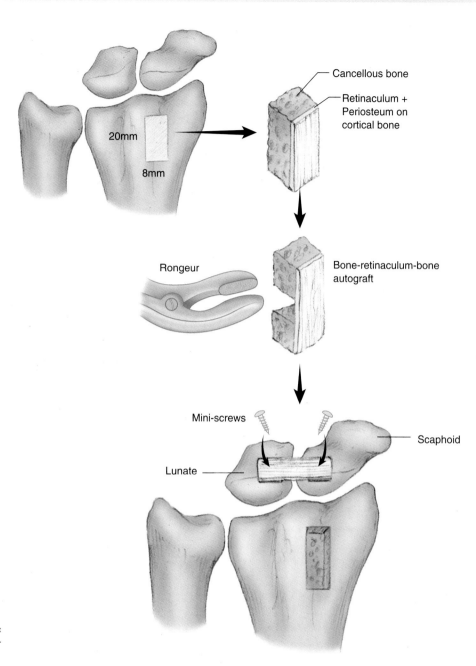

FIGURE 50-2 Overall diagram of the basic method for implanting a bone-retinaculum-bone autograft.

five patients in this group with a static deformity went on to further surgery (proximal row carpectomy, radioscapholunate fusion, wrist arthrodesis). In a longer term examination of the 14 patients (15 wrists) with dynamic instability, we report the following results. Five could not be located. Of the remaining nine, three had subsequent surgery (one had proximal row carpectomy, and two had wrist arthrodesis). The reason for failure of these three is unknown. It could be that the ligament reconstruction tears through the soft tissue substance. We have not seen evidence that the bone plugs displace. For the other six, follow-up averaged 8.5 years. Average grip strength was 119 lb. Wrist flexion averaged 49 degrees, and wrist extension averaged 58 degrees (**Fig. 50-7**). Three patients had no pain, and three had mild pain with activity. All returned to work at their previous occupation. Mayo wrist scores were three excellent, two good, and one fair. The graft does

not seem to stretch out over time. The natural history postoperatively is that if the graft remains intact for 6 to 12 months, it will stay so. We have noticed minor degenerative changes (usually around the junction of the scaphoid and lunate with slight spurring), but no loss of height of the radiolunate or radioscaphoid joints.

Over the follow-up period there have been few modifications to the procedure. If the quality of the soft tissue is robust, we use only the bone-retinaculum-bone graft with a single mini-screw fixation in each plug. In one case, the soft tissue quality was suspect, so we augmented the repair with a dorsal capsulodesis. In one case, not included in this series of pure bone-retinaculum-bone reconstructions, we found the tissue of such poor quality that we placed a headless screw across the scapholunate joint for additional temporary fixation.

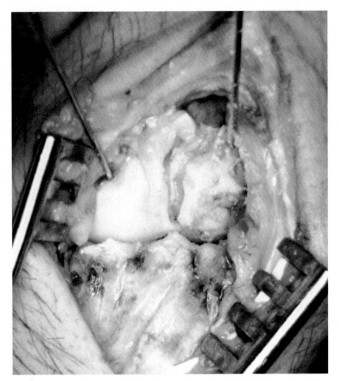

FIGURE 50-3 The use of Kirschner wires as joysticks to reduce the scapholunate interval before transfixing with Kirschner wires is essential.

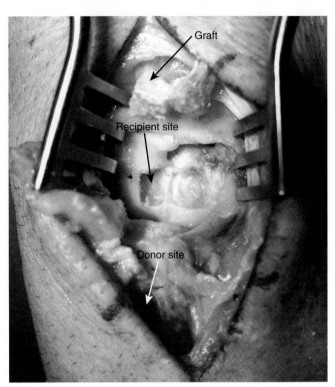

FIGURE 50-4 From the bone block removed with its retinaculum and periosteum intact, a 2- to 3-mm segment of cancellous and cortical bone is removed from the midportion of the bone block with a fine rongeur resulting in the bone-retinaculum-bone autograft. Care is taken not to disrupt the overlying periosteum and retinaculum. Recipient troughs are fashioned in the scaphoid and lunate of a similar size to accept the bone-retinaculum-bone graft.

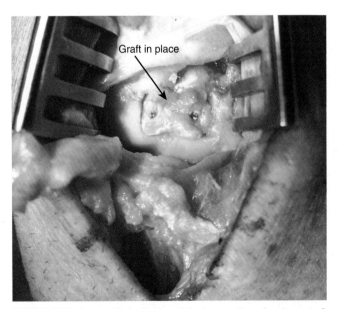

FIGURE 50-5 A press-fit application of the bone-retinaculum-bone graft into the troughs is performed followed by fixation with mini-screws.

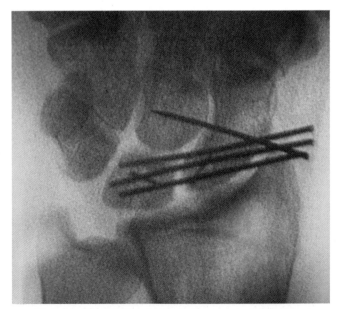

FIGURE 50-6 Intraoperative fluoroscopy is used to check for appropriate placement of all hardware.

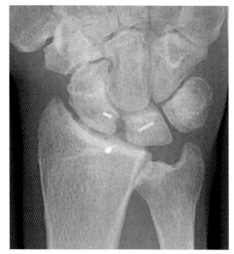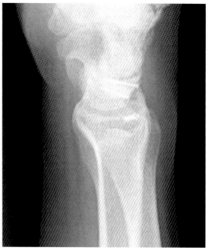

FIGURE 50-7 A 3-year follow-up examination revealed excellent maintenance of the scapholunate gap and little degenerative changes on posteroanterior and lateral radiographs. The patient has excellent function without pain even with strenuous exercise.

REFERENCES

1. Dobyns J, Linscheid F, Chao E, et al: Traumatic instability of the wrist. Instr Course Lect. 1975; 24:182-199.
2. Linscheid R: Scapholunate instabilities (dissociations, subdissociations, distraction). Ann Chir Main. 1984; 3:323-330.
3. Mayfield J: Wrist ligamentous anatomy and pathogenesis of carpal instability. Orthop Clin. 1984; 15:209-216.
4. Watson HK, Weinzweig J, Zeppieri J: The natural progression of scaphoid instability. Hand Clin. 1997; 13:39-49.
5. Ashmead D, Watson H, Damon C, et al: Scapholunate advanced collapse wrist salvage. J Hand Surg [Am]. 1994; 19:741-750.
6. Krakauer J, Bishop A, Cooney WP: Surgical treatment of scapholunate advanced collapse. J Hand Surg [Am]. 1994; 19:751-759.
7. Linscheid RL: Scapholunate ligamentous instabilities (dissociations, subdislocations, dislocations). Ann Chir Main. 1984; 3:323-330.
8. Viegas SF: The dorsal ligaments of the wrist. Hand Clin. 2001; 17:65-75.
9. Augsberger S, Necking L, Horton J, et al: A comparison of scaphoid-trapezium-trapezoid fusion and four bone tendon weave for scapholunate dissociation. J Hand Surg [Am]. 1992; 17:360-369.
10. Beredjiklian PK, Dugas J, Gerwin M: Primary repair of the scapholunate ligament. Tech Hand Upper Extrem Surg. 1998; 2:269-273.
11. Bickert B, Sauerbier M, Germann G: Scapholunate ligament repair using the Mitek bone anchor. J Hand Surg [Br]. 2000; 25:188-192.
12. Coe M, Spitellie P, Trumble T, et al: The scapholunate allograft: A biomechanical feasibility study. J Hand Surg [Am]. 1995; 20:590-596.
13. Cohen MS, Taleisnik J: Direct ligamentous repair of scapholunate dissociation with capsulodesis augmentation. Tech Hand Upper Extrem Surg. 1998; 2:18-24.
14. Harvey EJ: Hand based autograft replacement of the scapholunate ligament: early clinical outcome. American Society for Surgery of the Hand Annual Meeting, Seattle, WA, 2000.
15. Lavernia CJ, Cohen MS, Taleisnik J: Treatment of scapholunate dissociation by ligamentous repair and capsulodesis. J Hand Surg [Am]. 1992; 17:354-359.
16. Linscheid RL, Dobyns JH: Treatment of scapholunate dissociation: Rotatory subluxation of the scaphoid. Hand Clin. 1992; 8:645-652.
17. Lutz M, Haid C, Steinlechner M, et al: Scapholunate ligament reconstruction using a periosteal flap of the iliac crest: A biomechanical study. Arch Orthop Trauma Surg. 2004; 124:262-266.
18. Minami A, Kaneda K: Repair and/or reconstruction of scapholunate interosseous ligament in lunate and perilunate dislocations. J Hand Surg [Am]. 1993; 18:1099-1106.
19. Minami A, Kato H, Iwasaki N: Treatment of scapholunate dissociation: ligamentous repair associated with modified dorsal capsulodesis. Hand Surg. 2003; 8:1-6.
20. Misra A, Hales P: Blatt's capsulodesis for chronic scapholunate instability. Acta Orthop Belg. 2003; 69:233-238.
21. Muermans S, De Smet L, Van Ransbeeck H: Blatt dorsal capsulodesis for scapholunate instability. Acta Orthop Belg. 1999; 65:434-439.
22. Palmer A, Dobyns J, Linscheid F: Management of post-traumatic instability of the wrist secondary to ligament rupture. J Hand Surg. 1978; 3:507-532.
23. Saffar P, Sokolow C, Duclos L: Soft tissue stabilization in the management of chronic scapholunate instability without osteoarthritis: a 15-year series. Acta Orthop Belg. 1999; 65:424-433.
24. Schweizer A, Steiger R: Long-term results after repair and augmentation ligamentoplasty of rotatory subluxation of the scaphoid. J Hand Surg [Am]. 2002; 27:674-684.
25. Shin SS, Moore DC, McGovern RD, et al: Scapholunate ligament reconstruction using a bone-retinaculum-bone autograft: A biomechanic and histologic study. J Hand Surg [Am]. 1998; 23:216-221.
26. Slater RR Jr, Szabo RM, Bay BK, et al: Dorsal intercarpal ligament capsulodesis for scapholunate dissociation: biome-

chanical analysis in a cadaver model. J Hand Surg [Am]. 1999; 24:232-239.

27. Svoboda S, Eglseder W, Belkoff S: Autografts from the foot for reconstruction of the scapholunate interosseous ligament. J Hand Surg [Am]. 1995; 20:980-985.

28. Viegas SF, Dasilva MF: Surgical repair for scapholunate dissociation. Tech Hand Upper Extrem Surg. 2000; 4:148-153.

29. Watson H, Hempton R: Limited wrist arthrodesis, I: the triscaphe joint. J Hand Surg. 1980; 5:320-327.

30. Weiss AP: Scapholunate ligament reconstruction using a bone-retinaculum-bone autograft: a new technique. AAOS Trans. 1996; 213:169.

31. Weiss AP: Scapholunate ligament reconstruction using a bone-retinaculum-bone autograft. J Hand Surg [Am]. 1998; 23:205-215.

32. Weiss AP, Sachar K, Glowacki KA: Arthroscopic debridement alone for intercarpal ligament tears. J Hand Surg [Am]. 1997; 22:344-349.

33. Wintman B, Gelberman R, Katz J: Dynamic scapholunate instability: results of treatment with dorsal capsulodesis. J Hand Surg [Am]. 1995; 20:971-979.

34. Wolf JM, Weiss AP: Bone-retinaculum-bone reconstruction of scapholunate ligament injuries. Orthop Clin North Am. 2001; 32:241-246.

35. Wyrick JD, Youse BD, Kiefhaber TR: Scapholunate ligament repair and capsulodesis for the treatment of static scapholunate dissociation. J Hand Surg [Br]. 1998; 23:776-780.

36. Zarkadas PC, Gropper PT, White NJ, et al: A survey of the surgical management of acute and chronic scapholunate instability. J Hand Surg [Am]. 2004; 29:848-857.

37. Blatt G: Capsulodesis in reconstructive hand surgery: dorsal capsulodesis for the unstable scaphoid and volar capsulodesis following excision of the distal ulna. Hand Clin. 1987; 3:81-102.

38. Kleinman W, Carrol C: Scapho-trapezio-trapezoid arthrodesis for treatment of static and dynamic scapholunate instability: a ten year prospective on pitfalls and complications. J Hand Surg [Am]. 1990; 15:408-414.

39. Brunelli F, Spalvieri C, Bremner-Smith A, et al: [Dynamic correction of static scapholunate instability using an active

tendon transfer of extensor brevi carpi radialis: preliminary report]. Chir Main. 2004; 23:249-253.

40. Brunelli GA, Brunelli GR: A new technique to correct carpal instability with scaphoid rotary subluxation: a preliminary report. J Hand Surg [Am]. 1995; 20(3 Pt 2):S82-S85.

41. Davis CA, Culp RW, Hume EL, et al: Reconstruction of the scapholunate ligament in a cadaver model using a bone-ligament-bone autograft from the foot. J Hand Surg [Am]. 1998; 23:884-892.

42. Berger RA, Imeada T, Berglund L, et al: Constraint and material properties of the subregions of the scapholunate interosseous ligament. J Hand Surg [Am]. 1999; 24:953-962.

43. Kauer J: Functional anatomy of the wrist. Clin Orthop. 1980; 149:9-20.

44. Short W, Werner F, Fortino M, et al: A dynamic biomechanical study of scapholunate ligament sectioning. J Hand Surg [Am]. 1995; 20:986-999.

45. Short WH, Werner FW, Green JK, et al: Biomechanical evaluation of the ligamentous stabilizers of the scaphoid and lunate: part II. J Hand Surg [Am]. 2005; 30:24-34.

46. Tang JB, Ryu J, Omokawa S, et al: Wrist kinetics after scapholunate dissociation: the effect of scapholunate interosseous ligament injury and persistent scapholunate gaps. J Orthop Res. 2002; 20:215-221.

47. Viegas SF, Yamaguchi S, Boyd NL, et al: The dorsal ligaments of the wrist: anatomy, mechanical properties, and function. J Hand Surg [Am]. 1999; 24:456-468.

48. Harvey E, Hanel D: Autograft replacements for the scapholunate ligament: a biomechanical comparison of hand based autografts. J Hand Surg [Am]. 1999; 24:963-967.

49. Harvey EJ, Berger RA, Osterman AL, et al: Bone-tissue-bone repairs for scapholunate dissociation. J Hand Surg [Am]. 2007; 32:256-264.

50. Harvey E, Hanel D: What is the ideal replacement for the scapholunate ligament in a chronic dissociation? Can J Plast Surg. 2000; 8:143-146.

51. Ritt MJ, Berger RA, Kauer JM: The gross and histologic anatomy of the ligaments of the capitohamate joint. J Hand Surg [Am]. 1996; 21:1022-1028.

Dorsal Radiocarpal Ligament Tears

51

David J. Slutsky, MD

Various authors have cast light on the importance of the dorsal radiocarpal ligament (DRCL) in maintaining carpal stability.[1-4] Tears of the DRCL have been linked to the development of volar and dorsal intercalated segmental instabilities and may be implicated in the development of midcarpal instability.[5-7] Despite this growing body of evidence, there is still a paucity of literature on the incidence of DRCL tears. An isolated tear of the DRCL also can be a source of chronic wrist pain.[8] The existence of a DRCL tear when combined with a tear of a primary wrist stabilizer indicates a chronic lesion, which may negatively affect the prognosis after treatment.[9,10]

In most series, the DRCL is overlooked during the typical arthroscopic examination of the wrist. It is hard to visualize a DRCL tear through the standard dorsal wrist arthroscopy portals because the torn edge of the DRCL tends to float up against the arthroscope while viewing through the 3,4 and 4,5 portals, which makes identification and repair of the DRCL tear cumbersome. It can be seen obliquely through the 1,2 and 6U portals, but visualization of the DRCL across the radiocarpal joint may be laborious in a tight or small wrist, especially if synovitis is present. Wrist arthroscopy through a volar radial portal (VR) is the ideal way to assess the DRCL because of the straight line of sight.[11-13]

Clinical Relevance

Elsaidi and colleagues[14] showed the importance of the DRCL on scaphoid kinematics through a series of sectioning studies. They sequentially divided the radioscaphocapitate, long radiolunate, radioscapholunate, and short radiolunate ligaments. They next divided the central and proximal scapholunate interosseous ligament (SLIL), then the dorsal SLIL, and finally the dorsal capsule insertion on the scaphoid. There was no appreciable change in the radiographic appearance of this wrist. When the DRCL was divided, a dorsal intercalated segmental instability deformity occurred.

In another series of biomechanical studies on ligament sectioning using 24 cadaver arms, Short and coworkers[15] determined that the SLIL is the primary stabilizer of the scapholunate articulation, and that the DRCL, the dorsal intercarpal ligament, the scaphotrapezial ligament, and the radioscaphocapitate ligament are secondary stabilizers. They found that dividing the dorsal intercarpal or scaphotrapezial ligament alone followed by 1000 cycles of wrist flexion-extension and radial-ulnar deviation had no effect on scaphoid and lunate kinematics. Dividing the DRCL alone did cause increased lunate radial deviation when the wrist was in maximum flexion. Dividing the SLIL after any of the ligaments tested produced increased scaphoid flexion and ulnar deviation while the lunate extended. Short and coworkers[15] also

hypothesized that cyclic motion seems to cause further deterioration in carpal kinematics owing to plastic deformation in the remaining structures that stabilize the scapholunate.

These data provide a rationale for repairing the DRCL. The data also suggest that consideration should be given to augmenting the stability of the scaphotrapezial ligaments concomitant with treatment of the SLIL instability. Similar studies have established that the triangular fibrocartilage complex (TFCC) and the dorsal and volar radioulnar ligaments are primary stabilizers of the ulnocarpal joint.[16] DRCL tears that are found during the arthroscopic treatment of ulnar-sided lesions are handled in a similar fashion.

Indications

Geissler and colleagues[17] proposed an arthroscopic grading scale of interosseous ligament instability that has gained wide acceptance. In Geissler grade 1 and 2 lesions, there is no to minimal instability owing to ligament attenuation, but no tearing; these are synonymous with a dynamic instability. Grade 3 and 4 lesions represent partial and complete tears with greater degrees of carpal instability. This classification quantifies the resultant instability, and not the actual size of the tear. Based on this grading scale, an arthroscopic classification of DRCL tears is proposed in **Table 51-1**.

The treatment of DRCL tears is summarized in **Table 51-2**. An arthroscopic repair is indicated for isolated DRCL tears, which often leads to resolution of the wrist pain.[8,10] DRCL tears are commonly associated with SLIL tears or instability or both. Geissler grade 1 and 2 SLIL injuries are still amenable to arthroscopic treatment. In these situations, an arthroscopic repair of any associated DRCL tears is indicated because it may augment the coronal stability of the SLIL repair.[8-10] In open SLIL repairs, sagittal plane stability is often supplemented by adding a dorsal capsulodesis or using a tendon weave, such as the modified Brunelli procedure. Arthroscopic thermal shrinkage of the scaphotrapezial ligaments also theoretically may enhance the sagittal plane stability of the scapholunate joint. This is currently under investigation, but no data are available to recommend this procedure as yet.

Geissler grade 3 SLIL injuries represent a relative gray area for arthroscopic treatment methods alone. Investigators have shown, however, that this type of ligament injury can be treated successfully with thermal shrinkage and pinning. In the author's view, any associated DRCL tears should be repaired arthroscopically at the same time. Tears or instability of the lunotriquetral interosseous ligament are treated in similar fashion to the SLIL. DRCL repairs are indicated for Geissler grade 1 and 2 lunotriquetral interosseous ligament injuries and can be combined with

TABLE 51-1 Classification of Dorsal Radiocarpal Ligament Tears*

Stage 1	Isolated DRCL tear
Stage 2	DRCL tear with associated SLIL or LTIL instability (Geissler grade 1/2) and/or TFCC tear
Stage 3A	DRCL tear with associated SLIL or LTIL tear (Geissler grade 3) and/or TFCC tear
Stage 3B	DRCL tear with associated SLIL or LTIL tear (Geissler grade 4) and/or TFCC tear
Stage 4	Chondromalacia with widespread carpal pathology

*The ligament with the highest Geissler grade determines the stage.
DRCL, dorsal radiocarpal ligament; LTIL, lunotriquetral interosseous ligament; SLIL, scapholunate interosseous ligament; TFCC, triangular fibrocartilage complex.

TABLE 51-2 Treatment of Dorsal Radiocarpal Ligament Tears

Stage 1	Arthroscopic DRCL repair
Stage 2	Arthroscopic DRCL repair, SLIL or LTIL débridement ± shrinkage, TFCC repair/débridement ± wafer
Stage 3A	Arthroscopic DRCL repair, SLIL or LTIL shrinkage + pinning, TFCC repair/débridement ± wafer (consider scaphotrapezial ligament shrinkage)
Stage 3B	Open SLIL repair/reconstruction ± capsulodesis, LTIL repair/reconstruction, TFCC repair/débridement ± wafer/ulnar shortening
Stage 4	Partial carpal fusion versus PRC

DRCL, dorsal radiocarpal ligament; LTIL, lunotriquetral interosseous ligament; PRC, proximal row carpectomy; SLIL, scapholunate interosseous ligament; TFCC, triangular fibrocartilage complex.

lunotriquetral interosseous ligament shrinkage and débridement with or without pinning. Because there is a marked association of DRCL tears in the presence of long-standing TFCC tears, in my view DRCL repairs should be performed concomitantly with débridement or repair of the TFCC tear.

Contraindications

In cases in which the treatment of an SLIL tear or dynamic scapholunate instability includes some type of dorsal capsulodesis, the dorsal incision followed by the creation of a dorsal capsular checkrein to restrain palmar flexion of the scaphoid renders any separate treatment of the DRCL tear unfeasible. When the DRCL tear is seen in association with palmar midcarpal instability, a soft tissue repair of the dorsal ligaments would not by itself correct the midcarpal instability.[18] The results of a DRCL repair in association with two or more other intracarpal lesions are often inconsistent, and open repair methods should be considered, especially if they include a Geissler grade 3 ligament injury.[9] Geissler grade 4 ligament injuries are beyond the realm of arthroscopic treatment and require open repair or reconstruction (see Table 51-2).

Equipment and Implants

Generally, a 2.7-mm, 30-degree angled arthroscope with a camera attachment is necessary. A fiberoptic light source, video monitor, and printer also are standard equipment. Newer digital systems provide superior video quality compared with analog cameras and allow direct writing to a CD. A 3-mm hook probe is needed for palpation of intracarpal structures. Some method of overhead traction is useful. This may include traction from the overhead lights or a shoulder holder along with 5- to 10-lb sandbags attached to an arm sling. A traction tower, such as the Linvatec tower (Conmed-Linvatec Corp, Largo, FL) or the ARC wrist traction tower (Arc Surgical LLC, Hillsboro, OR), greatly facilitates instrumentation. A motorized shaver and suction punch forceps are useful for débridement. Some type of diathermy unit, such as the Oratec radiofrequency probe (Smith & Nephew, New York, NY), is needed in cases where augmentation of the repair with capsular shrinkage is desired. Various curved and straight 18-gauge spinal needles are used for passage of an absorbable 2-0 suture for the outside-in repair. A suture lasso or grasper is needed to retrieve the suture ends.

Optional Equipment

Various suture repair kits, including the Linvatec TFCC repair kit (Conmed-Linvatec Corp, Largo, FL) and the Arthrex TFCC repair kit (Arthrex, Inc, Naples, FL), are commercially available.

Surgical Technique

An inside-out arthroscopic repair technique of the DRCL was performed earlier An outside-in repair is technically easier and has been used more recently. The VR portal is established by making a 2-cm longitudinal incision in the proximal wrist crease, exposing the flexor carpi radialis tendon sheath. The sheath is divided, and the flexor carpi radialis tendon is retracted ulnarly. The radiocarpal joint space is identified with a 22-gauge needle, and the joint is inflated with saline. A blunt trochar and cannula are introduced through the floor of the flexor carpi radialis sheath, which overlies the interligamentous sulcus between the radioscaphocapitate ligament and the long radiolunate ligament.

A 2.7-mm, 30-degree arthroscope is inserted through the cannula. The repair is performed by spearing the radial side of the DRCL tear with a curved 21-gauge spinal needle placed through the 3,4 portal while viewing through the arthroscope in the VR portal. A 2-0 absorbable suture is threaded through the spinal needle and retrieved with a grasper or suture snare inserted through the 4,5 portal (Fig. 51-1A-F). A curved hemostat is used to pull either end of the suture underneath the extensor tendons, and the knot is tied either at the 3,4 portal or at the 4,5 portal. The repair is augmented with thermal shrinkage if the torn edge of the DRCL is voluminous and still protrudes into the joint after the sutures are tied (Fig. 51-1H).

Rehabilitation

After the repair, the patient is placed in a below-elbow splint with the wrist in neutral rotation. Finger motion and edema control are instituted immediately. At the first postoperative visit, the sutures are removed, and the patient is placed in a below-elbow cast for 6 weeks, followed by wrist mobilization.

Clinical Studies

A retrospective chart review of 21 patients who underwent a DRCL repair was published in 2005. None of the wrists showed

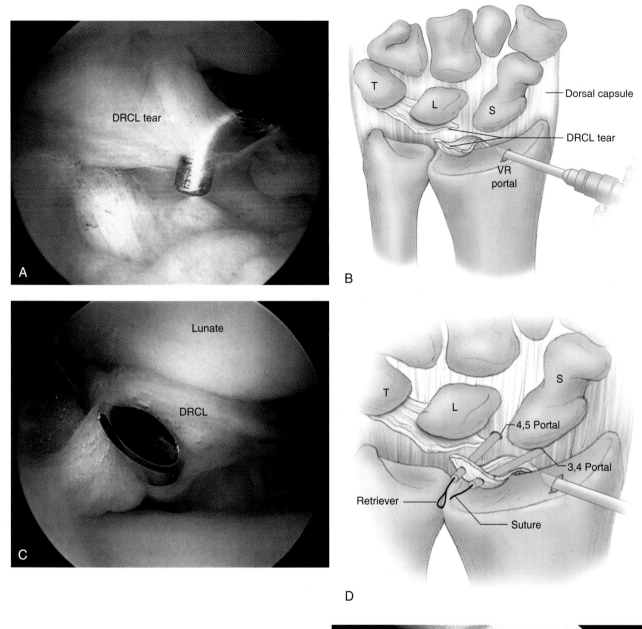

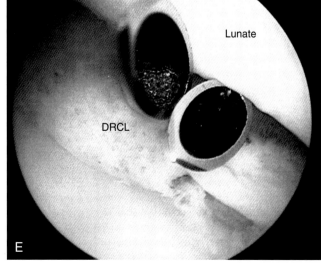

FIGURE 51-1 Outside-in dorsal radiocarpal ligament (DRCL) repair technique. A, Arthroscopic view of DRCL tear from the VR portal. **B,** Drawing of DRCL tear. **C,** Insertion of curved spinal needle through edge of DRCL tear. **D,** Drawing of outside-in technique using two spinal needles and a suture retriever. **E,** Insertion of second spinal needle.

Continued

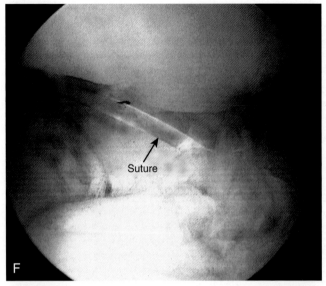

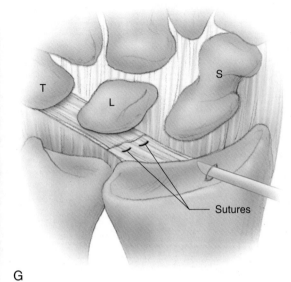

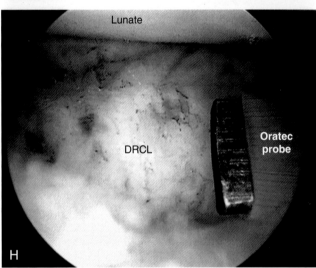

FIGURE 51-1, cont'd   **F,** Arthroscopic view of suture loop before tying. **G,** Drawing of completed repair. **H,** Repair augmented with thermal shrinkage after suture has been tied. *(A, C, E, F, and H from Slutsky DJ: Clinical applications of volar portals in wrist arthroscopy. Tech Hand Upper Extrem Surg. 2004; 8:229-238; B, D, and G from Slutsky DJ: Arthroscopic repair of dorsal radiocarpal ligament tears. J Arthrosc Related Surg. 2005; 21:1486e1-1486e8.)*

a static carpal instability pattern on x-ray. Preoperative magnetic resonance imaging (MRI) was performed by the referring physician in six patients. Preoperative arthrograms were performed as a part of the diagnostic workup for wrist pain in 20 patients. None of the DRCL tears in this series were identified with preoperative arthrography or MRI. Preoperative MRI in one patient with a DRCL tear was misinterpreted as representing a dorsal wrist ganglion. There were 6 men and 16 women. The average patient age was 40 years (range 25 to 62 years). All patients failed a trial of conservative treatment with wrist immobilization, cortisone injections, and work restrictions. The average length of conservative treatment was 7 months. The time interval between injury and surgical intervention averaged 25 months (range 8 to 53 months).

At the time of arthroscopy, four patients were found to have an isolated DRCL tear that was solely responsible for their wrist pain. The remaining 17 patients had additional ligamentous pathology. A dorsal capsulodesis was done in seven patients as the primary treatment for the SLIL instability or tear. Thirteen of the 21 patients underwent an arthroscopic DRCL ligament repair with or without thermal shrinkage as described earlier (repair in

5, repair + shrinkage in 6, shrinkage in 2). Ten of these patients underwent ancillary procedures for treatment of the coexisting wrist pathology. Lunotriquetral ligament tears were treated with débridement with or without pinning. Triangular fibrocartilage tears were débrided or repaired. Scapholunate ligament tears or instability were treated with capsulodesis with or without open repair. One patient had generalized arthrofibrosis, which precluded a DRCL repair. Concomitant nerve entrapment was a common finding, which was treated at the same time.

The average duration of follow-up was 16 months (range 7 to 41 months); one patient was lost to follow-up at 4 weeks. Pain was graded as none, mild, moderate, and severe. Wrist extension, wrist flexion, radial deviation, ulnar deviation, and grip strength were assessed. Wrist range of motion was compared with presurgical values. Grip strength was compared with the contralateral side at follow-up evaluation.

The four patients who underwent an isolated DRCL repair were satisfied with the outcome of surgery and would repeat the surgery again because it improved their symptoms. All four patients graded their pain as none or mild. None of these patients were taking pain medications. All returned to their previous occupations without restriction. Their wrist motion was unchanged compared with the preoperative status. Grip strengths were 90% to 130% of the opposite side.

A dorsal capsulodesis was performed as the primary treatment for an SLIL tear or a dynamic scapholunate instability in seven patients instead of a DRCL repair. The capsulodesis was ineffective in controlling pain in the remaining four patients, three of whom had additional wrist pathology. This is consistent with other studies, which have shown that although pain is improved, it does not resolve completely after a dorsal capsulodesis in most cases.[19] Cadaver studies suggest that dynamic scaphoid instability results from an isolated injury to the SLIL without damage to the dorsal intercarpal and DRCL ligaments.[4] I found the corollary to hold true in that four of seven patients with dynamic scapholunate instability had a DRCL tear, but an intact scapholunate ligament.

The remaining 10 patients had a DRCL tear in combination with ulnar-sided pathology. One patient was lost to follow-up. Of the nine patients, six had chronic residual pain, with three of these patients having arthroscopic evidence of osteoarthritis. Soft tissue procedures alone were ineffective in controlling their symptoms. There was a trend toward a worse outcome when there was coexisting ulnar-sided carpal pathology, which may reflect more severe or longer standing carpal instability. This trend was not invariable, however, because two of nine patients in this group had only occasional, mild pain after treatment. The final patient in this subgroup had an associated palmar midcarpal instability with laxity of the lunotriquetral joint. Although a DRCL repair and lunotriquetral joint pinning improved his symptoms, it did not correct the midcarpal instability, which remained mildly symptomatic.

Current Experience

Sixty-four patients have now undergone arthroscopy for the investigation and treatment of refractory wrist pain. Thirty-five patients were found to have DRCL tears, for an overall incidence of 55%. Five patients had an isolated DRCL tear. Thirteen patients in this series had an SLIL instability or tear or both; 7 of 13 (54%) also had a DRCL tear. Of this subgroup, four patients had a Geissler grade 1 or 2 instability, and three had a Geissler grade 3 or 4 tear. Seven patients had a lunotriquetral interosseous ligament instability or tear or both; two of seven (28%) also had a DRCL tear. Of this subgroup, one patient had a Geissler grade 2 instability, and one had a Geissler grade 3 or 4 tear. Two patients had a capitohamate ligament tear; one of these patients also had a DRCL tear. Seven patients had a solitary TFCC tear; six of seven (86%) were in association with a DRCL tear. One patient had a chronic ulnar styloid nonunion and a DRCL tear. There was TFCC fraying, but no tear or detachment. Two or more lesions were present in 23 patients; DRCL tears were present in 12 patients (52%). Sixty-two percent of the combined lesions that were associated with a DRCL tear also included a TFCC tear.

Summary

DRCL tears are found in approximately 50% of cases when there is a chronic intracarpal derangement. It is prudent that the arthroscopist is diligent in recognizing and treating this condition. Ongoing research into the ideal method of treatment of these combined injuries is still needed.

REFERENCES

1. Short WH, Werner FW, Green JK, et al: The effect of sectioning the dorsal radiocarpal ligament and insertion of a pressure sensor into the radiocarpal joint on scaphoid and lunate kinematics. J Hand Surg [Am]. 2002; 27:68-76.
2. Mitsuyasu H, Patterson RM, Shah MA, et al: The role of the dorsal intercarpal ligament in dynamic and static scapholunate instability. J Hand Surg [Am]. 2004: 29:279-288.
3. Viegas SF, Yamaguchi S, Boyd NL, et al: The dorsal ligaments of the wrist: anatomy, mechanical properties, and function. J Hand Surg [Am]. 1999; 24:456-468.
4. Ruch DS, Smith BP: Arthroscopic and open management of dynamic scaphoid instability. Orthop Clin North Am. 2001; 32:233-240.
5. Viegas SF, Patterson RM, Peterson PD, et al: Ulnar-sided perilunate instability: an anatomic and biomechanic study. J Hand Surg [Am]. 1990; 15:268-278.
6. Moritomo H, Viegas SF, Elder KW, et al: Scaphoid nonunions: a 3-dimensional analysis of patterns of deformity. J Hand Surg [Am]. 2000; 25:520-528.
7. Horii E, Garcia-Elias M, An KN, et al: A kinematic study of luno-triquetral dissociations. J Hand Surg [Am]. 1991; 16:355-362.
8. Slutsky DJ: Arthroscopic repair of dorsal radiocarpal ligament tears. Arthroscopy. 2002; 18:E49.
9. Slutsky D: Arthroscopic repair of dorsoradiocarpal ligament tears. J Arthrosc Related Surg. 2005; 21:1486e1-1486e8.
10. Slutsky DJ: Management of dorsoradiocarpal ligament repairs. J Am Soc Surg Hand. 2005; 5:167-174.
11. Slutsky DJ: Wrist arthroscopy through a volar radial portal. Arthroscopy. 2002; 18:624-630.
12. Slutsky DJ: Volar portals in wrist arthroscopy. J Am Soc Surg Hand. 2002; 2:225-232.
13. Slutsky DJ: Clinical applications of volar portals in wrist arthroscopy. Tech Hand Upper Extrem Surg. 2004; 8:229-238.
14. Elsaidi GA, Ruch DS, Kuzma GR, et al: Dorsal wrist ligament insertions stabilize the scapholunate interval: cadaver study. Clin Orthop. 2004; 425:152-157.
15. Short WH, Werner FW, Green JK, et al: Biomechanical evaluation of the ligamentous stabilizers of the scaphoid and lunate: part III. J Hand Surg [Am]. 2007; 32:297-309.
16. Palmer AK, Werner FW: The triangular fibrocartilage complex of the wrist—anatomy and function. J Hand Surg [Am]. 1981; 6:153-162.
17. Geissler WB, Freeland AE, Savoie FH, et al: Intracarpal soft-tissue lesions associated with an intra-articular fracture of the distal end of the radius. J Bone Joint Surg Am. 1996; 78:357-365.
18. Goldfarb CA, Stern PJ, Kiefhaber TR: Palmar midcarpal instability: the results of treatment with 4-corner arthrodesis. J Hand Surg [Am]. 2004; 29:258-263.
19. Moran SL, Cooney WP, Berger RA, et al: Capsulodesis for the treatment of chronic scapholunate instability. J Hand Surg [Am]. 2005; 30:16-23.

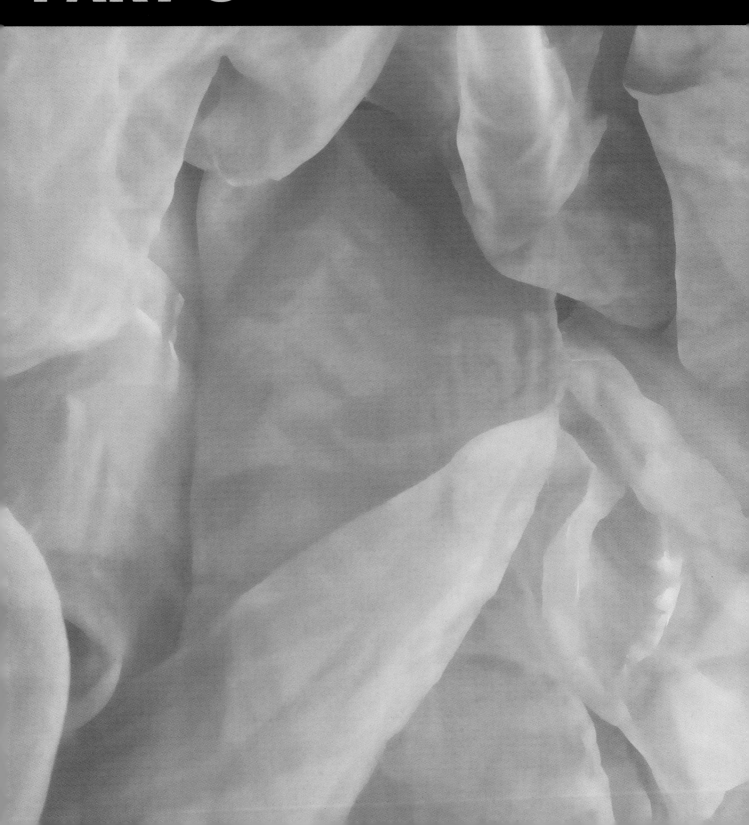

PART 8 TREATMENT OF COMPLICATIONS

Arthroscopic Release of Wrist Contracture

52

Joseph Bergman, MD and Gregory Bain, MBBS

Rationale and Basic Science Pertinent to the Procedure

Wrist contracture is a difficult problem with significant clinical implications. It has a variety of causes with trauma to the distal radius and carpus being the most common. The authors recommend that the wrist contracture be classified as extra-articular, capsular, or intra-articular. Extra-articular causes include heterotopic bone and changes in joint orientation, as might be seen after an extra-articular distal radius fracture; intra-articular causes include intra-articular distal radius or carpal fractures and carpal instability. Extra-articular and intra-articular pathology should be dealt with to address these sources of wrist stiffness.

Causes of capsular stiffness include fractures, surgery, arthritis, and immobilization to the wrist. In cases of capsular stiffness, initial treatment should include physiotherapy directed at stretching and splinting. In most cases, this regimen yields satisfactory results.

In refractory cases, surgical intervention may be warranted given the effectiveness of the technique when used with other joints.[1-5] Open and arthroscopic techniques have been described for the wrist, although there is a paucity of literature regarding clinical outcomes. Nonetheless, for cases where conservative management is inadequate, there seems to be a role for surgical management. In cases in which the source of the restriction in motion is the capsule, release or resection of the capsule would provide an increased range of motion, much as it does in other cases of arthrofibrosis.

Anatomy

Numerous nerves and blood vessels traverse the wrist joint. Their proximity is important in choosing arthroscopic portals and during release of contractures. The ulnar and median nerves and the radial artery are most at risk during this procedure, and their proximity to the capsule is relevant to the safety of the release (**Fig. 52-1**).

Ulnar Nerve

The ulnar nerve is at risk in many of its branches for portal selection and in its proximity to the ulnar volar joint capsule. It courses from beneath the flexor carpi ulnaris to the radial side of the tendon, and passes radial to the pisiform at an average distance of 6 mm (range 4 to 12 mm). Because the ulnar carpal ligaments are left untouched in this procedure, the ulnar nerve is principally of issue with respect to portal placement.

The ulnar nerve has two significant superficial branches, which originate approximately 10 cm proximal to the wrist joint—the dorsal cutaneous branch, and the volar cutaneous branches of the ulnar nerve. Placement of the 6R portal should be done using blunt dissection to avoid injury to the dorsal superficial ulnar cutaneous nerve. The portal should be placed in the proximal fifth (19%) of an imaginary line drawn from the ulnar styloid to the fourth web space.[6]

Median Nerve

The median nerve's course on the central volar aspect of the wrist within the carpal tunnel places it away from the joint capsule. It is the most superficial structure within the carpal tunnel and sits 13 mm underneath the skin surface.[7] It passes an average of 6.9 mm volar to the volar wrist capsule and at closest, 4 mm.[8] The median nerve passes radially within the carpal tunnel and is, on average, 18 mm radial to the pisiform and 8 mm ulnar to the scaphoid tubercle. It is protected by the mass of the finger flexors during capsular excision.

Radial Artery

The radial artery is located radially to the flexor carpi radialis tendon and sheath. It is at least 3 mm away from the volar radial capsule (average >5 mm). During capsular release, the radial artery is the structure most at risk, but careful division of the radioscaphocapitate ligament and the long radiolunate ligaments avoids the artery.

Indications

An arthrofibrotic wrist in which stiffness is the principal presenting complaint is most appropriate for arthroscopic release of the wrist capsule. Patients for whom stiffness is not the dominant symptom are not ideal.

Ideal Candidate

The ideal candidate for arthroscopic capsular release is a patient with functional loss of range of motion and for whom conservative therapy, including splinting, has failed. There is no upper limit to timing, but the joint should have stabilized in terms of pathology and range of motion before initiating any surgical release. In practice, this should be at least 6 months from the time of injury.

Capsular contracture should be diagnosed as the origin of the stiffness, and bony architecture should be ruled out as a reason for limitation of motion. There should be normal articular cartilage with a normal anatomical joint surface. Stiffness should be the sole reason for the contracture, with a painless but limited range of motion. Lastly, there should not be a generalized arthropathy likely to lead to recurrence of stiffness.

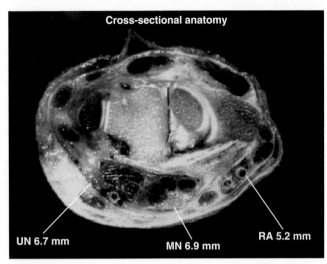

Cross-sectional anatomy

UN 6.7 mm   MN 6.9 mm   RA 5.2 mm

FIGURE 52-1 Cadaver cross section showing the relative locations of the major neurovascular structures of concern, including the ulnar nerve (UN), the median nerve (MN), and the radial artery (RA). *Used with permission from The Journal of Arthroscopic and Related Surgery, Vol 16, No. 1 (Jan-Feb), 2000.*

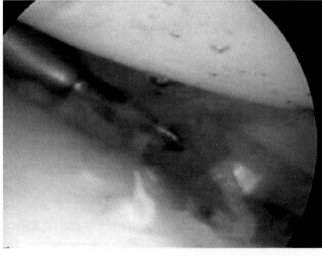

FIGURE 52-2 Video frame showing division of the volar extrinsic ligaments with the use of electrocautery. Note the pericapsular fat seen adjacent to the divided ligaments.

Contraindications

Absolute Contraindications

There is a risk to vital neurovascular structures during portal placement and capsular release. The volar portals and capsular release procedures should be considered advanced techniques that should be performed only by trained and experienced surgeons. Training on cadaver specimens is recommended before performing these procedures.

Significant prior soft tissue–distorting trauma or surgery that would preclude a safe procedure would be a contraindication. Previous compound fractures may have distorted anatomy. Global contraindications include active infection, compromised or lacerated skin overlying the wrist, and general contraindications to anesthesia.

Relative Contraindications

As described previously, in any situation in which the joint stiffness is due to multiple factors, capsular release alone is unlikely to provide significantly improved range of motion and is likely to recur. A painful joint or one where the joint architecture or articular surface is compromised is a relative contraindication. Complex intra-articular fractures with carpal instability are unlikely to improve with a capsular release.

Web Video ## Surgical Technique

52-1

A standard arthroscopic setup is used.[9] The patient is supine, with a tourniquet and finger traps. A 5-kg weight to distract the joint is used to assist in visualization. A 2.7-mm arthroscope is used in most cases, although a 1.9-mm arthroscope can be used in a smaller or more restricted joint. Using the 3,4 and 6R working portals, diagnostic arthroscopy and débridement are performed.

Volar Capsular Release

There is often synovitis on the volar capsule that should be débrided to improve visualization and make subsequent capsular release easier. To perform the capsular release, a hooked electro-

TABLE 52-1 Distance from the Radiocarpal Joint Capsule: Results from Magnetic Resonance Imaging Scans and Cadaver Sections

Structure	Average (mm)	Range (mm)
Median nerve	6.9	4-9
Ulnar nerve	6.7	4-9
Radial artery	5.2	3-7

cautery probe is introduced through the 6R portal and advanced in a radial direction as far as possible. Cautery is used to divide the volar capsule and volar carpal ligaments as shown in **Figure 52-2**. The long and short radiolunate ligaments, the radiocapitate ligament, and part of the radioscapholunate ligament are divided. Figure 52-2 also shows the division of the volar capsule down to periarticular fat. Based on the work of Viegas and colleagues,[10] the authors believe that leaving part of the radioscaphocapitate ligament intact is important to prevent the potential complication of ulnar translocation of the carpus. We have not seen this complication, but predict that it could occur, and that it would be extremely difficult to treat.

The triangular fibrocartilaginous complex is left intact, including the ulnotriquetral and ulnolunate ligaments. Division of the radial side of the volar capsule should continue until the flexor carpi radialis tendon is seen, and extracapsular fat is exposed. The surgeon must not delve into this volar periarticular fat because this may lead to significant neurovascular injury. Distances to important anatomical structures are shown in **Table 52-1**. Although the median and ulnar nerves are at least 4 mm away from the capsule, the radial artery can lie as close as 3 mm to the radial volar capsule.

After release of the volar capsule, the joint is taken through a range of motion to assess whether a satisfactory range has been obtained. In most cases, a volar release is all that is required. If marked contracture still exists, however, a dorsal capsular release can be performed.

Dorsal Capsular Release

In our opinion, the dorsal capsular release is more technically difficult than the volar release because of the proximity of the extensor tendons. The extensor tendons lie directly adjacent to the dorsal capsule so that there is no safety margin between the capsule to be released and the tendon to be preserved. In contrast to the volar release, in which there is a distinct layer of periarticular fat that acts as a buffer for the volar neurovascular structures, no such protection exists for the extensor tendons.

Our preferred technique for dorsal capsular release is to use a volar radial portal as a viewing portal as described by Slutsky, Ashwood, and Abe and their colleagues,[11-13] and the 3,4 dorsal portal as a working portal. Blunt dissection using a hemostat is used to pass a nylon tape through the 3,4 portal, down to the level of the tendon-capsule interface and across to the 6R portal. By applying tension to the nylon tape, it can be used as a retractor to protect the tendons from injury during release of the dorsal capsule. The nylon tape is positioned between the capsule and extensor tendons.

The capsule is excised using basket forceps with one jaw visualized intra-articularly and the other jaw placed between the capsule and the nylon tape retracting the tendons as shown in **Figure 52-3**. The capsulectomy proceeds from the 3,4 portal, ulnarly to the point of the 6R portal. The use of the basket forceps to release the dorsal capsule down to the level of the tendon-capsule interface, at which the retracting nylon tape is seen.

Figure 52-4 shows a summary of the ligaments to be divided during either a volar or a dorsal procedure. Following either procedure, a gentle closed manipulation is performed.

Complications

Our series of arthroscopic contracture release is small, and no complications were observed. With a volar release, major neurovascular complications can occur. The surgeon should not advance into the periarticular fat volarly. Ulnar translocation of the carpus also can occur, and this complication should be avoided by maintaining half of the radioscaphocapitate ligament.

With a dorsal release, injury to the extensor tendons can occur. This complication can be avoided through retraction and protection of the extensor tendons with a nylon tape. Using the volar viewing portal ensures that the surgeon is directly visualizing the capsule and extensor tendons. Other potential complications include those common to any surgical procedure, such as deep infection, wound problems, and hematoma.

Results

Wrist contracture is an uncommon problem, and cases that are refractory to conservative management make up an even smaller cohort. There are only two case series in the literature that describe any form of arthroscopic release of the wrist. The first is an article that describes the technique as presented here. Patients with a range of motion less than the functional range described by Palmer and colleagues[14] were treated with the capsular release as described previously. The range of motion increased from 20% to 70% of the contralateral side, and the grip strength increased from one third to more than two thirds of the contralateral side.[8] This improvement in grip strength is due to better wrist extension, which facilitates grip function.

A second article describes arthroscopic release of a scapholunate sagittally oriented curtain of tissue found between the scapholunate interval and the midradial ridge.[15] Although we did not see this feature in our series, if such a structure is found, it should be débrided. Hattori and associates[15] found that after débridement

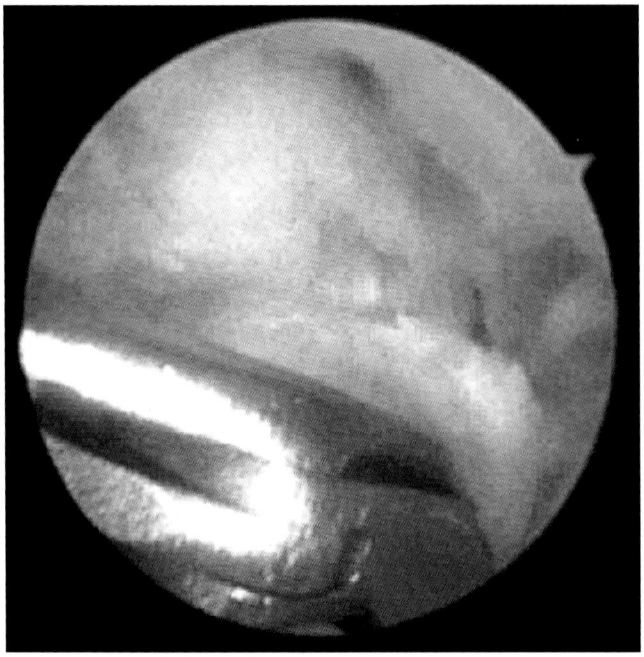

FIGURE 52-3 Video frame showing the use of the basket forceps to divide the dorsal capsule. Note the nylon tape seen immediately adjacent to the forceps and the vertically oriented extensor tendons just past the nylon tape.

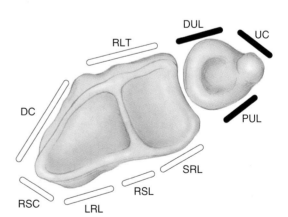

FIGURE 52-4 Schematic of wrist ligaments. Ligaments shaded black including the dorsal ulnar ligament (DUL), the ulnar carpal ligament (UC), and the palmar ulnar ligament (PUL) are not resected. Volar and dorsal ligaments shaded white are resected with the exception of the radioscaphocapitate ligament (RSC), which is partially resected, preserving at least 50%. Volar ligaments including short and long radiolunate ligaments (SRL, LRL), and the radioscapholunate ligament (RSL) are resected for a volar release, whereas the dorsal capitate ligament (DC) and the radiolunotriquetral ligament (RLT), also known as the dorsal radiocarpal ligament, are resected for a dorsal release. *Used with permission from The Journal of Arthroscopic and Related Surgery, Vol 16, No. 1 (Jan-Feb), 2000.*

of this band of tissue, improvements in range of motion were seen.

Arthroscopic capsular release allows for improved motion in patients with a localized capsular contracture. It is performed with minimal collateral damage to the wrist. It is not a technically demanding technique, although it is most suitable for an experienced surgeon. A familiarity with the anatomy of the volar and dorsal wrist and training or familiarization with a cadaver model are recommended.

REFERENCES

1. Richmond JC, Gladstone J, MacGillivray J: Continuous passive motion after arthroscopically assisted anterior cruciate ligament reconstruction: comparison of short- versus long-term use. Arthroscopy. 1991; 7:39-44.

2. Jones GS, Savoie FH 3rd: Arthroscopic capsular release of flexion contractures (arthrofibrosis) of the elbow. Arthroscopy. 1993; 9:277-283.

3. Vaquero J, Vidal C, Medina E, et al: Arthroscopic lysis in knee arthrofibrosis. Arthroscopy. 1993; 9:691-694.

4. Ogilvie-Harris DJ, Biggs DJ, Fitsialos DP, et al: The resistant frozen shoulder: manipulation versus arthroscopic release. Clin Orthop. 1995; 319:238-248.

5. Utsugi K, Sakai H, Hiraoka H, et al: Intra-articular fibrous tissue formation following ankle fracture: the significance of arthroscopic debridement of fibrous tissue. Arthroscopy. 2007; 23:89-93.

6. Tindall A, Patel M, Frost A, et al: The anatomy of the dorsal cutaneous branch of the ulnar nerve—a safe zone for positioning of the 6R portal in wrist arthroscopy. J Hand Surg [Br]. 2006; 31:203-205.

7. Sora MC, Genser-Strobl B: The sectional anatomy of the carpal tunnel and its related neurovascular structures studied by using plastination. Eur J Neurol. 2005; 12:380-384.

8. Verhellen R, Bain GI: Arthroscopic capsular release for contracture of the wrist: a new technique. Arthroscopy. 2000; 16:106-110.

9. Bain GI, Richards RS, Roth JH: Wrist arthroscopy. In Lichtman DM, Alexander AH, eds: The Wrist and Its Disorders. 2nd ed. Philadelphia, W.B. Saunders, 1997.

10. Viegas SF, Patterson RM, Ward K: Extrinsic wrist ligaments in the pathomechanics of ulnar translation instability. J Hand Surg [Am]. 1995; 20:312-318.

11. Slutsky DJ: Wrist arthroscopy through a volar radial portal. Arthroscopy. 2002; 18:624-630.

12. Ashwood N, Bain GI: Arthroscopically assisted treatment of intraosseous ganglions of the lunate: a new technique. J Hand Surg [Am]. 2003; 28:62-68.

13. Abe Y, Doi K, Hattori Y, et al: Arthroscopic assessment of the volar region of the scapholunate interosseous ligament through a volar portal. J Hand Surg [Am]. 2003; 28:69-73.

14. Palmer AK, Werner FW, Murphy D, et al: Functional wrist motion: A biochemical study. J Hand Surg [Am]. 1985; 10:39-46.

15. Hattori T, Tsunoda K, Watanabe K, et al: Arthroscopic mobilization for contracture of the wrist. Arthroscopy. 2006; 22:850-854.

Management of Lost Pronosupination

53

Marc Garcia-Elias, MD, PhD

Pronosupination is important in most activities of daily living. A loss of forearm rotation may be compensated by internally or externally rotating the humerus with the elbow semiextended, but this implies a high risk of developing degeneration of the rotator cuff. Without pronosupination, numerous common tasks, such as pouring water from a pitcher into a glass, or fastening a brassiere, are extremely difficult. A forearm with limited pronosupination is a substantial handicap, almost as serious as an unstable distal radioulnar joint (DRUJ).

For a full forearm rotation, not only do proximal and distal radioulnar joints need to be well aligned, with matching lengths and congruent cartilages, but also the soft tissue stabilizing structures must function properly.[1-3] Pronosupination is a multifactorial phenomenon that can be affected in many different ways, the more common being distal radius misalignment, radioulnar length discrepancy, joint incongruity, and soft tissue (capsule or muscle or both) contracture.[4]

As in any other complex problem, treatment of DRUJ stiffness is based on a thorough clinical examination and adequate radiographic investigation of the cause of the problem. Properly obtained lateral radiographs and axial tomograms are helpful in assessing the spatial relationship of the bones involved. Arthroscopy is an excellent tool to evaluate the status of all intracapsular soft tissues involved in pronosupination, whereas magnetic resonance imaging provides information on the extracapsular DRUJ stabilizers.

Frequently, the loss of supination is secondary to a dorsally malunited distal radial fracture. In such instances, if the triangular fibrocartilage complex (TFCC) has been stretched out or avulsed off the basistyloid fovea, the ulnar head is forced into a dorsally subluxed position relative to the sigmoid notch. Such joint incongruity prevents the normal combination of joint spinning and gliding necessary for a full forearm rotation. Treatment in these cases consists of a radial corrective osteotomy.[5]

In other circumstances, the ulna may be excessively long as a result of trauma (shortened distal radial fracture) or a congenital defect, and may impinge the lunate during supination and wrist extension, producing pain. Such an abutment may explain a reduced range of forearm rotation. In these cases, any form of ulnar length reduction (i.e., ulnar shortening osteotomy or wafer procedure) is mandatory.[6]

If the lack of rotation is due to joint incongruity secondary to trauma or cartilage degeneration, many different options exist[2]: (1) total ulnar head resection,[7] (2) "matched ulna" resection,[8] (3) hemiresection and fibrous interposition,[9] (4) DRUJ fusion plus creation of a metaphyseal pseudarthrosis,[10] (5) ulnar head implants,[11,12] and (6) total DRUJ prosthesis.[13] All of these options are discussed elsewhere in this book, so they are not covered here.

This chapter concentrates on the loss of forearm rotation secondary to soft tissue (capsular or muscle or both) contracture.

Pathomechanics

To understand the consequences of specific DRUJ soft tissue contractures, it is important to analyze how the radius is prevented to rotate around the ulna beyond its normal limits.

Supination Constraints

As the radius rotates from neutral toward supination, very few changes in ligament tension appear in either the palmar or the dorsal radioulnar ligaments. The horizontal portion of the TFCC, consisting of the articular disc (central zone) and the two peripheral radioulnar ligaments, moves as a unit (**Fig. 53-1A and B**).[3,14] Tension in the palmar radioulnar ligament does not increase until a certain degree of supination is reached (**Fig. 53-1C**). At this point, the distance between the two ends of the ligament (fovea and palmar corner of the radius) starts increasing until the palmar radioulnar ligament is fully taut, at about 70 degrees of supination.[14] If the palmar capsule was not elastic, that would be the limit of supination. The capsule is very lax, however,[15] and allows some degree of dorsal subluxation of the radius, with the ulnar head displacing palmarward, decreasing tension in the anterior radioulnar ligament (**Fig. 53-1D**). This decrease in tension allows further supination up to about 80 degrees, until the dorsal radioulnar ligament becomes fully taut.[1]

An important dynamic control of the final stages of supination is the pronator quadratus, which in supination becomes stretched and promotes coaptation of the joint, avoiding its subluxation (**Fig. 53-2**).[3,16,17] The palmar radioulnar ligament can be thought of as the primary stabilizer of the early stages of supination,[1] whereas the dorsal radioulnar ligament,[14] the palmar capsule,[15] and the pronator quadratus muscle[16,17] are secondary stabilizers avoiding dorsal dislocation of the radius relative to the ulna.

Pronation Constraints

A similar phenomenon occurs during pronation: No substantial changes in tension develop in the two radioulnar ligaments until a certain degree of pronation is achieved (**Fig. 53-3A, B**). At about 60 degrees of pronation, the dorsal ligament becomes maximally taut (**Fig. 53-3C**).[14] This would stop pronation if it were not for the elastic dorsal capsule, which allows some palmar subluxation of the radius relative to the ulna. As the ulna glides dorsally, there is increasing tensioning of the anterior radioulnar ligament and the dorsal capsule, the two ultimate constraints of pronation (**Fig. 53-3D**).[1]

The extensor carpi ulnaris muscle has a similar role to that of the pronator quadratus in that it is an effective dynamic stabilizer

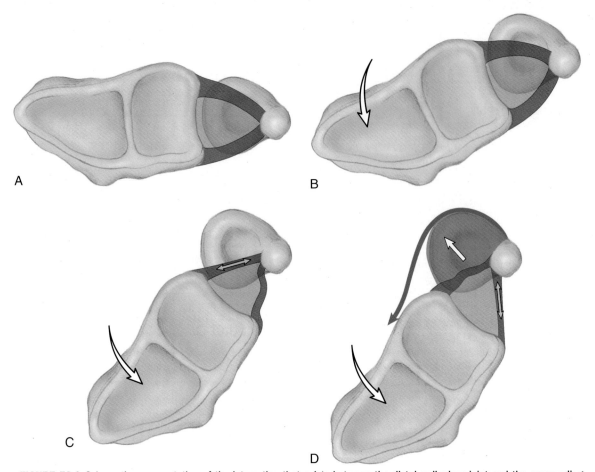

FIGURE 53-1 Schematic representation of the interaction that exists between the distal radioulnar joint and the surrounding soft tissues during supination. **A** and **B,** As the radius initiates a rotation around the ulna, very few changes in tension of the palmar and dorsal radioulnar ligaments appear. **C,** Tension in the palmar radioulnar ligament does not increase significantly until a certain degree of supination is reached (*yellow arrow*). This tension generates a palmar translation vector to the ulnar head. **D,** As the ulna subluxes palmarly (*white arrow*), the dorsal radioulnar ligament becomes taut (*yellow arrow*), preventing further displacement. The palmar radioulnar capsule (*in pink*) helps in stabilizing the joint at the extreme of supination and the pronator quadratus muscle (*in green*).

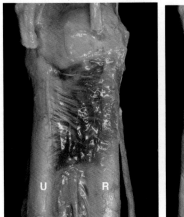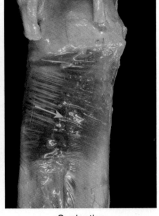

Pronation   Supination

FIGURE 53-2 The pronator quadratus muscle is fully stretched during supination, increasing its mechanical advantage as distal radioulnar joint dynamic stabilizer. If this muscle sustains a disruption, it is most likely to occur during supination. In pronation the muscle belly of the pronator quadratus does not offer resistance to a palmar displacement of the ulnar head.

of the DRUJ during pronation. As emphasized by Spinner and Kaplan,[18] the extensor carpi ulnaris tendon is maintained in a close relationship with the head of the ulna by a fibrous tunnel, independent from the rest of the extensor retinaculum. Because of this, at full pronation, the extensor carpi ulnaris tendon lies medial to the ulnar head and promotes coaptation of this bone against the dorsal rim of the sigmoid cavity, maximizing stability (**Fig. 53-4**).[3,18] The dorsal radioulnar ligament can be thought of as the primary stabilizer of the early stages of pronation,[14] whereas the palmar radioulnar ligament,[1] the dorsal capsule,[15] and the extensor carpi ulnaris muscle[18] are secondary stabilizers avoiding palmar dislocation of the radius relative to the ulna.

Clinical Forms of Soft Tissue Contractures around the Distal Radioulnar Joint

Contractures around the DRUJ may cause three forms of forearm limitation: (1) loss of pronation, (2) loss of supination, and (3) combined pronation and supination loss. The third form of forearm limitation, combining pronation and supination losses, usually falls into the category of intra-articular stiffness (arthrofibrosis), and often results from complex trauma or inflammatory

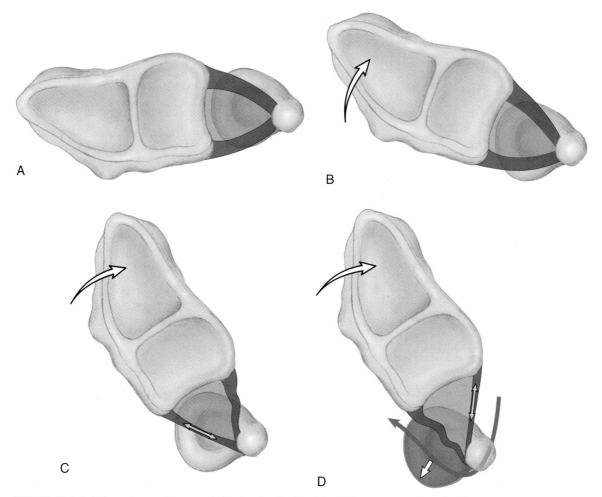

FIGURE 53-3 **Soft tissue interaction around the distal radioulnar joint during pronation. A** and **B**, Rotation around the neutral position does not imply significant changes in tension of the radioulnar ligaments. **C**, The dorsal radioulnar ligament becomes taut (*yellow arrow*) before reaching the extreme of pronation. With this, the ulna is forced toward the dorsum. **D**, As the ulna subluxes dorsally, the palmar radioulnar ligament becomes taut preventing further displacement. The dorsal radioulnar capsule (*in pink*) and the extensor carpi ulnaris tendon (*in green*) stabilize the joint at the extreme of pronation.

disease generating intra-articular cartilage destruction and invasion by scarring fibrotic tissue.[2] This is a difficult condition to treat effectively and most often requires a salvage intervention.[4] It is rarely seen after a common distal radial fracture. If releasing an arthrofibrotic joint is believed to be necessary, however, a double palmar and dorsal approach following the guidelines proposed by Kleinman and Graham[15] is recommended (see later).

Loss of Pronation

Of the four structures the scarring or contracture of which may theoretically affect pronation (see Fig. 53-3D), only the dorsal capsule is shown to be directly involved in the rare cases where there is truly an isolated lack of pronation owing to soft tissue contracture.[15] The dorsal capsule may disrupt, lose its elasticity, and become thick in several ways; most often, this occurs as the consequence of an extra-articular, palmarly angulated distal radial fracture (Smith type), or in Galeazzi's fracture-dislocation.[4] If the fracture is not properly reduced and stabilized, and particularly if the forearm is immobilized in an above-elbow cast for too long, these injuries may induce a deficit of pronation. Plate fixation and early mobilization of these types of fractures is common practice because the need for a secondary dorsal capsular release is almost anecdotic.

Permanent scar retraction of a partial injury to the radioulnar ligaments producing limitation of forearm rotation is very rare. When they fail, these ligaments tend to avulse or disrupt creating instability, but seldom stiffness.[19] Detaching the radioulnar ligaments to achieve increased pronosupination should be considered only exceptionally.

Extensor carpi ulnaris tendinitis may result in muscle contracture and slight limitation of pronation.[20] Reduction of forearm rotation is not static, but most often the result of pain produced by the synovitic tendon when stretched during pronation. Proper treatment of the condition (e.g., splinting, glucocorticoid injections, eventually a synovectomy) is all that is needed to recover full pronosupination.

Loss of Supination

Post-traumatic palmar capsular thickening inducing a supination deficit is common.[15] Distal radial fractures with mild dorsal displacement are particularly prone to create DRUJ capsular defects in the palm, which may eventually cause this problem. The reason for it is as follows.

The hyperextended carpus pulls the ulnar head anteriorly by means of the strong ulnocarpal ligaments (**Fig. 53-5**).[3] As the distal radius displaces dorsally, a shear stress in the DRUJ is

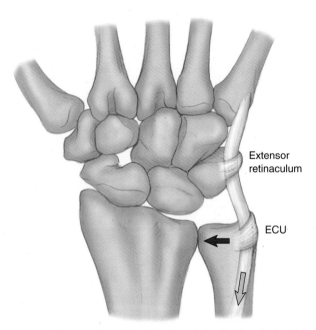

FIGURE 53-4 **Mechanism of stabilization of the distal radioulnar joint by the extensor carpi ulnaris tendon.** The extensor carpi ulnaris has its own compartment over the groove on the dorsum of the ulnar head. The sheath that covers the tendon is independent from the extensor retinaculum. In pronation, that compartment is located on the medial aspect of the bone. The tendon in that position has an S-shaped configuration. Contracture of the extensor carpi ulnaris muscle produces a radial directed force that compresses the joint and helps prevent a dorsal subluxation of the ulna relative to the radius.

created. If the TFCC, including the ulnocarpal ligaments, does not fail, the ulnar head promotes tearing of the palmar capsule in its attempt to sublux palmarly relative to the dorsally angulated distal radius. If, in addition, there is a supination moment involved in the injury, the fully stretched pronator quadratus muscle may be unable to resist the palmar push of the ulna, and may sustain substantial elongation. Such muscle injury would not have major consequences, however, if not for the fact that this muscle is contained in its own small compartment,[21,22] which the fracture fills with abundant hematoma, creating the conditions for a localized compartment syndrome.[23,24] Increased pressure on the muscle may seriously affect its contractability, inducing its later fibrotic retraction and subsequent limitation of supination.

As stated earlier, supination contractures usually appear after poorly displaced distal radial fractures. This can be easily understood by considering the pathomechanism of injury. The deep fascia usually is disrupted in badly displaced fractures. This disruption eliminates the possibility of a pronator quadratus compartment syndrome and later pronator quadratus muscle retraction. If the fracture is grossly displaced, the TFCC is most often pulled off the ulna. With this, the antepulsion vector created by the ulnocarpal ligaments onto the ulna no longer appears. As a consequence, the ulnar head does not cause any substantial volar capsular disruption, eliminating the chances for later scar retraction and lack of supination.

Management of Distal Radioulnar Joint Soft Tissue Contracture

The management of a patient with reduced pronosupination depends on the chronicity of the problem and the location of the

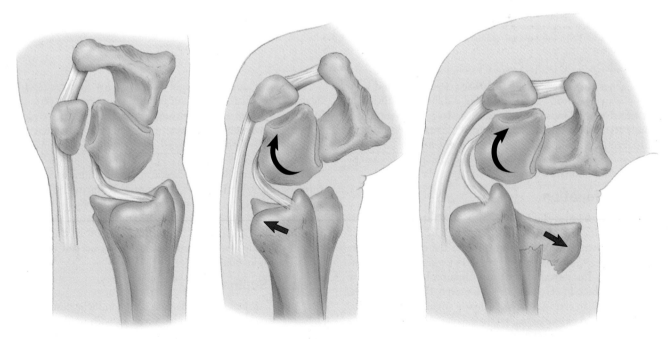

FIGURE 53-5 Most palmar capsular derangements, eventually resulting in a deficit of supination, are the result of distal fractures without detachment of the triangular fibrocartilage complex (TFCC). If the ulnocarpal ligaments maintain the normal origin of the TFCC into the fovea, wrist extension promotes a palmar translation of the ulna relative to the radius. If there is a concomitant dorsal displacement of the radius, the ulnar head protrudes further palmarly and may disrupt the palmar capsule. By contrast, if there is avulsion of the TFCC, including the ulnocarpal ligaments, there is no palmar translation force to the ulna, and the chances for a palmar capsular derangement are minimal.

structures involved. As stated earlier, if there is bone deformity or joint incongruity, this needs to be resolved first. No soft tissue release would ever correct a bone-related stiffness problem. If this problem has been ruled out, an aggressive supervised therapy program is always recommended. The aim is to recover progressively the elasticity of all retracted structures through deep massage, gentle passive mobilization, and application of passive splints with progressive rotation angles. Dynamic splinting also may be considered. Failing this, surgery is indicated.

Distal Radioulnar Joint Capsular Release

A volar approach to the DRUJ capsule is usually performed through a 5-cm longitudinal or zigzag incision along the medial border of the flexor carpi ulnaris tendon. Alternatively, the joint may be approached through a longitudinal incision along the interval between the ulnar neurovascular bundle and the flexor digitorum tendons (see **Fig. 53-6D**). In the first case, a careful dissection and protection of the dorsal branch of the ulnar nerve is mandatory. Gentle retraction of the neurovascular bundle allows exposure of the deep fascia that covers the pronator quadratus muscle. Complete fasciectomy of the area covering the DRUJ is recommended. Excision of the volar capsule is accomplished, as described by Kleinman and Graham,[15] by first incising its insertion on the radius. A second transverse incision paralleling the proximal margin of the palmar edge of the TFCC is then made. The proximal border of the capsule is cut, circumscribing the area of the ulna covered by cartilage. With this, a volar "silhouette" resection of the DRUJ capsule is excised, while protecting the articular surfaces of the distal ulna and sigmoid notch of the radius (see **Fig. 53-6F**).[15] At this point, if the only problem is capsular thickening, full passive supination should be obtained. If there is still a lack of supination, the procedure needs to address the associated pronator quadratus muscle problem.

When there is a true pronator quadratus muscle contracture owing to muscle disruption, its distal and ulnar fibers usually appear whitish and fibrotic (see **Fig. 53-6E**). By contrast, when contracture is the consequence of a localized compartment syndrome, the entire muscle looks fibrotic and does not contract when stimulated with the scalpel.[23,24] In the first instance, the superficial belly of the muscle is detached off the ulna, and its fibrotic portion is excised. In the second case, the entire muscle needs to be released and extracted.

Aside from capsular and muscle contracture, the joint may have developed arthrofibrosis (intra-articular adhesions) requiring further arthrolysis (see **Fig. 53-6G**). A blunt Freer elevator is used to unblock the joint until full passive supination is achieved, and the ulnar head can be passively displaced back and forth on the sigmoid notch. Detachment of the foveal insertion of the TFCC is seldom indicated. If liberation of all intra-articular adhesions does not allow full forearm rotation, a dorsal approach is preferred.

The dorsal DRUJ capsule is approached by retracting the extensor digiti quinti from the fifth extensor compartment.[25] An ulnar retinacular flap is elevated from the underlying dorsal capsule. The thickened and adhesive capsule is excised following the "silhouette" method of capsulectomy described for the palmar side.[15] After passive intraoperative assessment of forearm rotation and translation of the ulnar head within physiological limits, the dorsal retinaculum is repaired, and all wounds are closed. A bulky compression dressing with an above-elbow supination splint is placed for 1 week, after which patients are encouraged to pursue active hand therapy. Night splints in full supination may be used eventually.

Results

We have recently reviewed six patients (five women and one man, average 36 years old [range 20 to 51 years old]) who had undergone a DRUJ capsular release for a loss of forearm rotation. Three of the six patients had sustained mildly displaced fractures of the distal radius, all having been treated nonoperatively in a cast. One had had a radial head fracture treated with internal plate fixation, one had a direct blow to the palmar surface of his wrist, just proximal to the palmar crease, and the last one had an episode of intense wrist pain after a racket ball game. All patients with a radial fracture had acceptable radial length and congruent articular surfaces at the DRUJ (see **Fig. 53-6B**).

Careful clinical and radiographic examination excluded any other bone pathology that could affect pronosupination. All patients except one had marked limitation of supination (average 15 degrees [range 0 to 35 degrees]) and an almost normal pronation (average 72 degrees). The patient who had a proximal radial head fracture had supination and pronation limited to less than 20 degrees. All patients had a volar capsular excision, plus detachment of the pronator quadratus muscle. The patient with the radial head fracture required further dorsal capsulectomy to increase pronation. One patient required extensive arthrolysis to remove fibrotic tissue obliterating the empty spaces of a chronic dorsally subluxed DRUJ.

The average interval between injury and surgery was 16 months (range 4 to 30 months). At an average follow-up of 15 months (range 7 to 52 months), patients were evaluated for pain relief, range of motion, and grip strength. Pain relief at rest was obtained in all patients, with two complaining of mild discomfort during strenuous activity. All patients resumed their normal activities except one who had to downgrade the strength level of her job. Average ranges of forearm rotation at follow-up were for supination 68 degrees (84% of contralateral) and pronation 80 degrees (95%). Average grip strength relative to the contralateral normal side improved from 45% to 65%. A case example of the technique and the results obtained is shown in **Figure 53-6**.

Our results are similar to the results published by Kleinman and Graham in 1998.[15] In their series, six patients with recalcitrant limited forearm rotation required a palmar capsulectomy, whereas three had a combined palmar and dorsal capsulectomy. Their range of forearm rotation improved from an average 54 to 21 degrees of pronation-supination to 82 to 72 degrees at follow-up.

Summary

The most common causes of loss of pronosupination after wrist injury are an alteration of the normal length, alignment, or congruency of the radius, the ulna, or both. Frequently, there is a concomitant soft tissue contracture that should not be underestimated. Capsular thickening may result from a tear caused by DRUJ subluxation, whereas pronator quadratus muscle contracture may result from a localized compartment syndrome. In all cases, when the rotation deficit does not resolve with adequate hand therapy, a surgical release of the DRUJ capsule plus pronator quadratus muscle detachment from the ulna may have acceptable results.

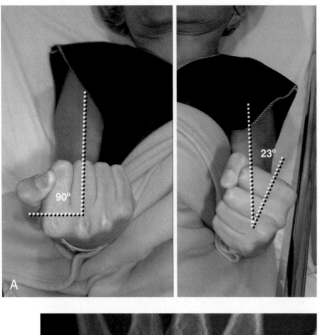

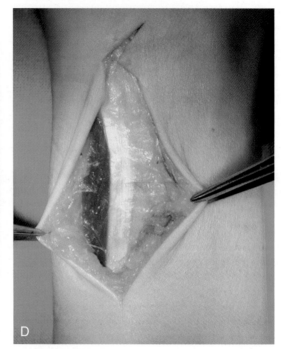

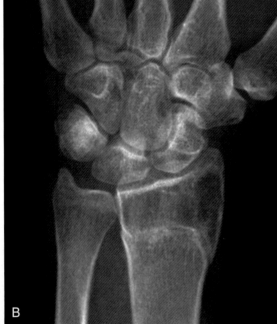

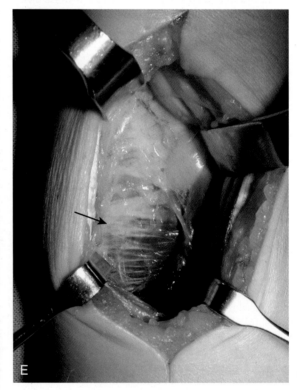

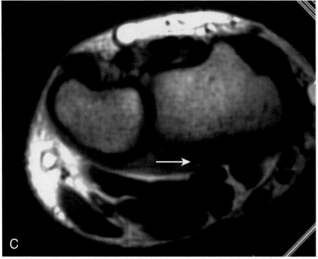

FIGURE 53-6 Illustrative case of a 52-year-old woman who presented with lack of supination 6 months after a mildly displaced distal radius fracture treated conservatively. The patient recalled having had intense pain at the palmar aspect of the wrist after the fracture (possibly pronator quadratus compartment syndrome). **A,** Clinical photographs of the maximum range of active supination that was present before surgery. Passive motion was identically reduced. **B,** Neither joint incongruity nor length discrepancy could be blamed for the lack of rotation. **C,** Transverse magnetic resonance imaging showed retraction of the pronator quadratus muscle. **D,** The joint was approached palmarly along the lateral border of the flexor carpi ulnaris tendon, taking care to protect the ulnar neurovascular bundle that courses behind the tendon. **E,** Appearance of the pronator quadratus muscle, with a whitish distal medial corner (*arrow*) as a result of fibrosis.

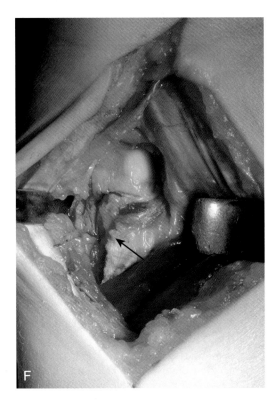

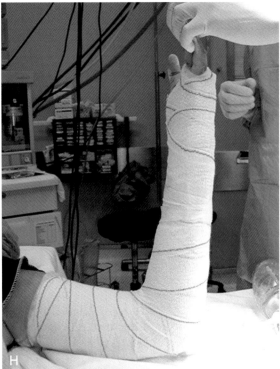

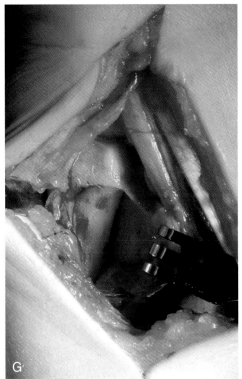

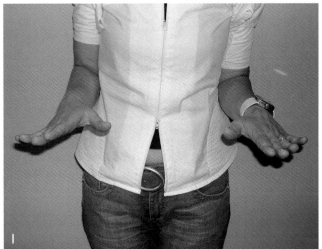

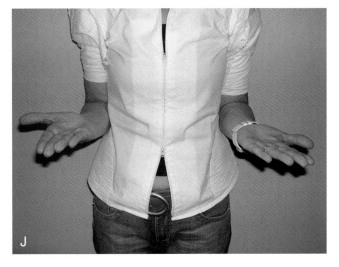

FIGURE 53-6, cont'd **F,** Despite excision of the volar distal radioulnar joint capsule and detachment of the pronator quadratus muscle (*arrow*), supination was still blocked. **G,** Elevation of the pronator quadratus muscle disclosed the existence of fibrotic bands within the joint, excision of which allowed recovery of full supination. **H,** The arm was immobilized in an above-elbow supination splint for 1 week followed by an active program of supervised physiotherapy. In this case, it took 5 months to obtain full active pronosupination. **I** and **J,** At 1 year, the range of forearm rotation was still normal and painless.

REFERENCES

1. Hagert CG: The distal radioulnar joint in relation to the whole forearm. Clin Orthop. 1992; 275:56-64.

2. Lichtman DM, Ganocy TK, Kim DC: The indications for and techniques and outcomes of ablative procedures of the distal ulna. Hand Clin. 1998; 14:265-277.

3. Garcia-Elias M: Soft-tissue anatomy and relationships about the distal ulna. Hand Clin. 1998; 14:165-176.

4. Bowers WH: Instability of the distal radioulnar articulation. Hand Clin. 1991; 7:311-327.

5. Prommersberger KJ, Van Schoonhoven J, Lanz UB: Outcome after corrective osteotomy for malunited fractures of the distal end of the radius. J Hand Surg. 2002; 27:55-60.

6. Chun S, Palmer AK: The ulnar impaction syndrome: Follow-up of ulnar shortening osteotomy. J Hand Surg [Am]. 1993; 18:46-53.

7. Darrach W: Forward dislocation at the inferior radio-ulnar joint, with fracture of the lower third of the shaft of the radius. Ann Surg. 1912; 56:801-802.

8. Watson HK, Gabuzda GM: Matched distal ulnar resection for posttraumatic disorders of the distal radioulnar joint. J Hand Surg. 1992; 17:724-730.

9. Bowers WH: Distal radioulnar joint arthroplasty: the hemiresection-interposition technique. J Hand Surg. 1985; 10:169-178.

10. Kapandji IA: The Kapandji-Sauvé operation: its techniques and indications in non-rheumatoid diseases. Ann Chir Main. 1986; 5:181-193.

11. van Schoonhoven J, Fernandez DL, Bowers WH, et al: Salvage of failed resection arthroplasties of the distal radio-ulnar joint using a new ulnar head prosthesis. J Hand Surg [Am]. 2000; 25:438-446.

12. Berger RA, Cooney WP: Use of an ulnar head endoprosthesis for treatment of an unstable distal ulnar resection: review of mechanics, indications, and surgical technique. Hand Clin. 2005; 21:603-620.

13. Scheker LR, Babb BA, Killion PE: Distal ulnar prosthetic replacement. Orthop Clin North Am. 2001; 30:365-376.

14. Schuind F, An KN, Berglund L, et al: The distal radioulnar ligaments: a biomechanical study. J Hand Surg [Am]. 1991; 16:1106-1114.

15. Kleinman WB, Graham TJ: The distal radioulnar joint capsule: clinical anatomy and role in posttraumatic limitation of forearm rotation. J Hand Surg [Am]. 1998; 23:588-599.

16. Johnson RK: Stabilization of the distal ulna by transfer of the pronator quadratus origin. Clin Orthop. 1992; 275: 130-132.

17. Stuart PR: Pronator quadratus revisited. J Hand Surg [Br]. 1996; 21:714-722.

18. Spinner M, Kaplan EB: Extensor carpi ulnaris: its relationship to the stability of the distal radioulnar joint. Clin Orthop. 1970; 68:124-129.

19. Szabo RM: Distal radioulnar joint instability. J Bone Joint Surg. 2006; 88:884-894.

20. Allende C, Le Viet D: Extensor carpi ulnaris problems at the wrist—classification, surgical treatment and results. J Hand Surg. 2005; 30:265-272.

21. Sotereanos DG, McCarthy DM, Towers JD, et al: The pronator quadratus: a distinct forearm space? J Hand Surg [Am]. 1995; 20:496-499.

22. Gerber A, Masquelet AC: Anatomy and intracompartmental pressure measurement technique of the pronator quadratus compartment. J Hand Surg [Am]. 2001; 26:1129-1134.

23. Summerfield SL, Folberg CR, Weiss APC: Compartment syndrome of the pronator quadratus: a case report. J Hand Surg [Am]. 1997; 22:266-268.

24. Schumer ED: Isolated compartment syndrome of the pronator quadratus compartment: a case report. J Hand Surg [Am]. 2004; 29:299-301.

25. Garcia-Elias M, Smith DE, Llusá M: Surgical approach to the triangular fibrocartilage complex. Tech Hand Upper Extrem Surg. 2003; 7:134-140.

Treatment of Ununited Fractures of the Distal Radius 54

David C. Ring, MD, PhD

Rationale

Nonunion of the distal radius—long considered to be extremely rare[1,2]—has been noted more frequently in recent years.[3-7] Although some authors have speculated that the advent of external fixation and other techniques for maintaining the length of the radius has created bony defects that can lead to nonunion,[7] nonunion also is seen after internal fixation or nonoperative treatment (**Figs. 54-1 through 54-3**).[3-7] There seems to be an association with concomitant fracture or dislocation of the distal ulna (see Fig. 54-2).[4,5]

Although the cause and incidence of nonunion of the distal radius are uncertain, the need for operative treatment is clear. Most nonunions are synovial.[4-7] The wrist is usually deformed, unstable, and painful. Some patients have a severe radial deviation deformity reminiscent of congenital clubhand, which has been referred to as acquired or post-traumatic clubhand (**Fig. 54-4**).[8,9]

Operative treatment can improve upper limb function in patients with nonunion of the distal radius by either fusing the wrist or healing the fracture. Improved implants and operative techniques have improved healing of the fracture, preserving some wrist motion.[5,6] Even small amounts of wrist motion can enhance upper limb function.[10]

Indications

Unstable ununited fractures are disabling and warrant operative treatment in all but the most severely infirm patients. A fracture of the distal radius that remains ununited in a distracted position (e.g., with external fixation) may heal after the fracture has been allowed to settle. Any fracture that remains unstable greater than 6 weeks after injury is likely to have healing problems and should be considered for operative treatment.

Contraindications

Concomitant infection should be treated with serial débridement and organism-specific parenteral antibiotics. Definitive treatment is delayed until the infection is eradicated. Very infirm, debilitated, or severely demented patients can be managed with a brace.

Operative Techniques
Treatment Options

The most common treatment of ununited fractures of the distal radius has been wrist arthrodesis,[4,7] probably because attempts at internal fixation of the small, metaphyseal distal radius fragment seem risky. The appeal of retaining some wrist motion along with the development of better implants and techniques for the fixa-

tion of small articular fractures has influenced us to offer our patients an attempt to heal the fracture with internal fixation and autogenous cancellous bone grafting.[5,6]

Two principles have proved useful. First, the concept of applying two plates in orthogonal planes—as practiced at other anatomical sites, such as the distal humerus,[11] and as supported by mechanical principles—is particularly useful in the distal radius, where the distal fragment can be very small.[5] A second, orthogonal plate provides a greater number of fixation points in the distal fragment. Second, the use of fixed-angle devices instead of standard screws for osteoporotic bone—also used in the humerus[12]—can provide more secure fixation of bone in which preexisting osteoporosis has often been exacerbated by disuse of the limb.[13]

Wrist arthrodesis may be optimal in infirm patients and patients with limited functional demands in whom pain relief is the primary goal, and as a salvage of failed attempts to gain union. Some nonunions, in particular complex articular nonunions, are not amenable to operative fixation, and wrist fusion is the only option (see Fig. 54-3). Some authors have suggested that when there is less than 6 mm of bone between the lunate facet of the distal radius articular surface and the fracture site, there is insufficient bone to support internal fixation.[7] I believe that although this increases the challenge of internal fixation, there is usually a larger amount of bone in the radial styloid portion of the distal fragment that can accept internal fixation (see Fig. 54-2).

Wrist Arthrodesis

Standard wrist arthrodesis techniques using specific wrist fusion plates[14] have proved adequate for ununited fractures of the distal radius.[4,7] In this situation, the nonunion represents another "articulation," which must be débrided, bone grafted, and stabilized with the plate. Bone graft can be obtained from the resected ulna when a concomitant Darrach procedure is performed, from the radial styloid, or from the iliac crest (see Fig. 54-2).

Open Reduction and Internal Fixation

A volar Henry[15] exposure provides access to the volar and radial aspects of the distal radius. The fracture site is identified, and fibrous or synovial tissues are removed. The sclerotic fracture ends are opened with rongeurs and curets and drilled repeatedly with a small bit to open the intramedullary canal. Opening of the sclerotic fracture ends and intramedullary canal facilitates the ingress of a vascular supply providing cells, nutrients, and growth factors to support healing.

To facilitate and stabilize reduction, a small skeletal distractor or other external fixator can be applied between two 2.5-mm Schantz screws, one placed in the distal fragment and one in the proximal fragment. The Schantz screws are placed so that distrac-

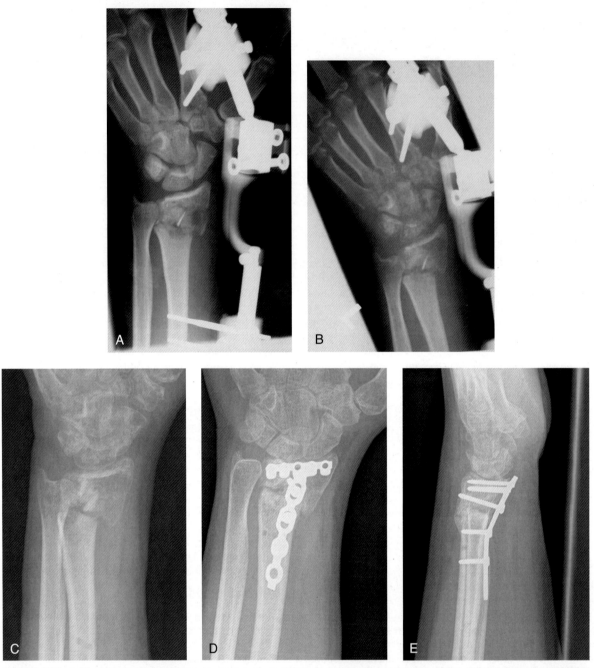

FIGURE 54-1 A 42-year-old man was injured in a race car accident. **A,** A comminuted fracture of the distal radius was stabilized and distracted with an external fixator. **B,** The fracture failed to heal, his hand became stiff, and there was osteopenia related to disuse. **C,** After removing the external fixator and rehabilitating the hand, the fracture remained ununited. **D,** Débridement of the nonunion, autogenous cancellous bone grafting, and internal fixation achieved union. **E,** The use of a plate with fixed-angle metaphyseal screws enhanced the security of the fixation.

tion between them realigns the fragments, but the screws themselves do not interfere with internal fixation devices. In patients with a severe radial deviation deformity, consideration is given to releasing or Z-lengthening the brachioradialis and flexor carpi radialis tendons to facilitate realignment of the distal radius, but this is rarely necessary if the decision has been made to accept the shortening of the radius and resect the distal ulna.

Many patients benefit from Darrach resection of the distal ulna. This procedure is preferable in patients with substantial deformity of the distal radius in whom length and alignment cannot be restored without creating a large bony defect. In

addition, attempts to realign the distal radioulnar joint often risk painful arthrosis if either the realignment is inadequate or the joint has degenerated during the period of nonunion and deformity. The distal ulna usually provides sufficient bone graft so that obtaining additional bone from the iliac crest is usually unnecessary.

With the skeletal distractor holding the fragments reduced—sometimes with an ancillary Kirschner wire transfixing the fragments—the plates and screws are applied. A variety of volar plates with fixed-angle (locked) screws are now available. The fixed-angle screws or pins are better suited to fixation of the metaphy-

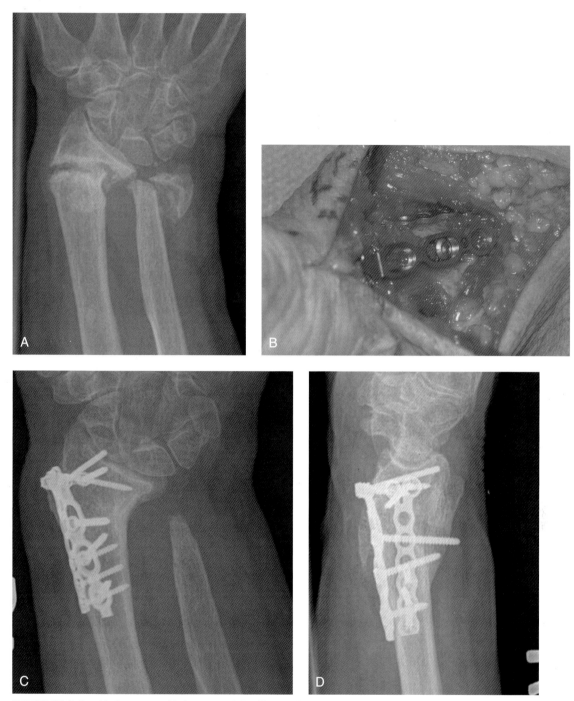

FIGURE 54-2 An elderly woman with fractures of the distal radius and ulna was treated in a cast. **A,** Synovial nonunions of both fractures with an ulnar deviation deformity ensued. **B,** Through a volar exposure, orthogonal plates (one volar, one direct radial) were applied. **C,** Good fixation of the radial styloid was achieved. **D,** The use of locking screws enhanced the security of fixation in the osteoporotic metaphyseal bone. *(Case Courtesy of J.B. Jupiter MD.)*

seal bone of the distal radius, which is often osteopenic. In some patients with very small distal fragments, it can be useful to enhance the fixation in the more substantial radial styloid portion of the distal fragment by applying a second plate, orthogonal to the volar plate on the direct radial surface of the distal radius. Several implants are designed for placement on this part of the bone, many with locking screws. Autogenous cancellous bone graft is applied to the defect, and the wound is closed.

Rehabilitation

Active-assisted motion of the hand and forearm is encouraged the morning after surgery. A removable plastic wrist splint is used to help support the wrist for 4 to 6 weeks after surgery. Approximately 6 weeks after the surgery, the splint is discarded, and active-assisted wrist motion is allowed. Strengthening exercises are restricted until radiographic healing is established.

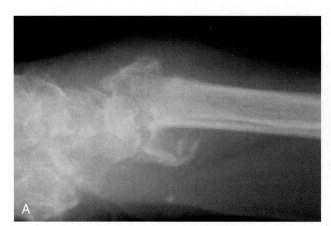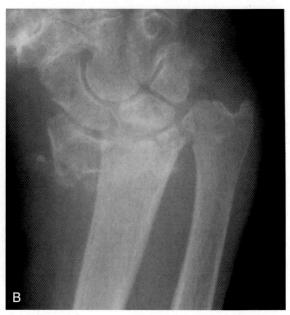

FIGURE 54-3 A 75-year-old woman injured her wrist and believed that it was just a sprain. **A,** On presentation 6 weeks later, she had an unstable complex ununited fracture of the distal radius. **B,** This nonunion with associated complex articular injury was thought not to be amenable to attempts at repair and was salvaged with a wrist arthrodesis.

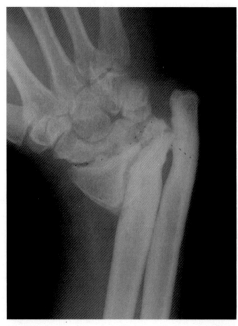

FIGURE 54-4 Some nonunions of the distal radius are associated with a marked radial deviation deformity—the so-called post-traumatic radial clubhand.

Complications

We have not encountered infection, wound problems, or nerve injury.[5,6] If the fracture fails to heal, the implants eventually loosen or break, and the decision to undertake further attempts to heal the fracture or to salvage the situation with wrist arthrodesis is based on the specific circumstances and the desires of the patient. Wrist motion is never returned to normal, and some patients regain very little wrist motion. Progressive arthrosis also can compromise the result and may require subsequent wrist arthrodesis

in rare cases. The implants often irritate the overlying tendons and can lead to tendon rupture. I have a low threshold for recommending implant removal when implants are associated with pain, swelling, or crepitance of the tendons over the plate.

Results

Segalman and Clark[7] reported on 12 nonunions of the distal radius treated over a 24-year period at the Curtis Hand Center. This report is testament to the relative rarity of the problem. Also, the findings should be interpreted in the context of the older treatment methods available at the time many of the patients were managed. Segalman and Clark[7] divided the nonunions into two groups:

1. Nine nonunions with less than 5 mm of bone at the lunate facet (six treated with wrist arthrodesis and three without further surgery)
2. Three nonunions with 5 mm or greater bone at the lunate facet that had operative attempts to gain union

The authors recommended that nonunions with less than 5 mm of bone at the lunate facet be treated with wrist arthrodesis.

In contrast, Prommersberger and colleagues[6] supported attempts at gaining fracture healing in all patients in their report of a multicenter retrospective series of 23 patients, including 13 patients with an ununited fracture of the distal radius in whom the distal fragment had more than 5 mm of subchondral bone supporting the articular surface distal to the site of the nonunion and 10 patients with an ununited fracture of the distal radius with a smaller distal fragment. Bony union was achieved in 22 of 23 patients, an average of greater than 80 degrees of wrist flexion arc was maintained, and grip strength averaged greater than 59% of the opposite arm. One patient in the large fragment group failed to heal the fracture and had wrist arthrodesis. There were no significant differences in the radiological and clinical outcome between the two groups. These findings may reflect what is possible with newer implants and techniques.

REFERENCES

1. Watson-Jones R: Fractures and Other Bone and Joint Injuries. 2nd ed. Edinburgh: Livingstone, 1942.
2. Bacorn RW, Kurtzke JF: A study of two thousand cases from the New York State Workmen's Compensation Board. J Bone Joint Surg Am. 1953; 38:643-658.
3. Harper WM, Jones JM: Non-union of Colles' fracture: report of two cases. J Hand Surg [Br]. 1990; 15:121-123.
4. McKee MD, Waddell JP, Yoo D, et al: Nonunion of distal radial fractures associated with distal ulnar shaft fractures: a report of four cases. J Orthop Trauma. 1997; 11:49-53.
5. Fernandez DL, Ring D, Jupiter JB: Surgical management of delayed union and nonunion of distal radius fractures. J Hand Surg [Am]. 2001; 26:201-209.
6. Prommersberger KJ, Fernandez DL, Ring D, et al: Open reduction and internal fixation of un-united fractures of the distal radius: does the size of the distal fragment affect the result? Chir Main. 2002; 21:113-123.
7. Segalman KA, Clark GL: Un-united fractures of the distal radius: a report of 12 cases. J Hand Surg [Am]. 1998; 23:914-919.
8. Netrawichien P: Radial clubhand-like deformity resulting from osteomyelitis of the distal radius. J Pediatr Orthop. 1995; 15:157-160.
9. Ono CM, Albertson KS, Reinker KA, et al: Acquired radial clubhand deformity due to osteomyelitis. J Pediatr Orthop. 1995; 15:161-168.
10. Adams BD, Grosland NM, Murphy DM, et al: Impact of impaired wrist motion on hand and upper-extremity performance. J Hand Surg [Am]. 2003; 28:898-903.
11. Helfet DL, Hotchkiss RN: Internal fixation of the distal humerus: a biomechanical comparison of methods. J Orthop Trauma. 1990; 4:260-264.
12. Ring D, Perey B, Jupiter JB: The functional outcome of the operative treatment of ununited fractures of the humeral diaphysis in elderly patients. J Bone Joint Surg Am. 1999; 81:177-189.
13. Perren SM: Evolution of the internal fixation of long bone fractures: the scientific basis of biological internal fixation: choosing a new balance between stability and biology. J Bone Joint Surg Br. 2002; 84:1093-1110.
14. Hastings H, Weiss AP, Quenzer D, et al: Arthrodesis of the wrist for post-traumatic disorders. J Bone Joint Surg Am. 1996; 78:897-902.
15. Henry AK: Extensile Exposure. 2nd ed. Edinburgh: Churchill Livingstone, 1973.

Scaphoid Hemiresection and Arthrodesis of the Radiocarpal Joint

55

Soheil Payvandi, DO and William H. Seitz, Jr., MD

Indications and Contraindications

The underlying pathology of radiocarpal arthritis frequently is due to trauma or degenerative changes or both. The leading causes are malunited or nonunited fractures of the radius or scaphoid, radiocarpal or intercarpal dislocations or dissociations, or forms of primary osteoarthritis or inflammatory arthritis. Management has focused on reducing pain to increase function, while, when possible, preserving some degree of motion, with total wrist arthrodesis being the ultimate salvage procedure.[1,2] Surgical approaches that attempt to preserve some motion have included proximal row carpectomy, four-corner fusion with and without scaphoid excision, radiolunate arthrodesis, radioscapholunate arthrodesis, and lunocapitate arthrodesis.[2-7]

Motion-sparing surgical procedures require healthy articular cartilage at the site of preserved motion. For proximal row carpectomy, a healthy capitate head and lunate fossa are required; for a four-corner fusion, the lunate and its fossa of the radius must have a healthy articular surface. Radiolunate and radioscapholunate arthrodesis require a healthy midcarpal joint and can provide stability, but result in a significantly limited arc of motion and a moderately high failure rate because the scaphoid acts as a strut between the proximal and distal carpal rows.[2,8]

Biomechanical studies have shown the effect of preserving versus osteotomizing the scaphoid on midcarpal joint motion, with osteotomy significantly increasing the degree of allowable motion through the midcarpal joint.[5,8] When the lunate and the scaphoid fossae are arthritic, but the midcarpal articulation of the capitate in its lunate and scaphoid fossae remains healthy, it is logical to attempt to preserve and use the midcarpal joint to retain motion, while eliminating pain through an arthrodesis of the arthritic radiocarpal surfaces.[2,9]

This chapter describes a step-by-step technique of using a tensioned, flexible plating system (Small Bone Innovations, Morrisville, PA) to perform a scaphoid hemiresection and recessed arthrodesis of the radiocarpal joint (the SHARC procedure). This procedure allows the capitate to move within its midcarpal joint as a "universal" joint.[8] The ideal candidate is a patient with radiocarpal arthritis and a healthy midcarpal articulation. Contraindications to performing the procedure are active local infection, systemic disease, midcarpal arthrosis, and unwillingness of the patient to comply with postoperative instructions and rehabilitation protocols.

Preoperative Planning

Patients with radiocarpal arthritis should have a thorough history, physical examination, and radiographic assessment. Patients usually have an extended history of wrist-related complaints with or without previous wrist trauma. These complaints may include pain, loss of strength, and considerable restriction of motion. Radiographic analysis (including computed tomography scans if needed) should show a smooth, regular contour of the capitate with maintenance of healthy articular cartilage of the midcarpal joint. The hamate and proximal pole of the scaphoid should have structural viability (no evidence of a vascular necrosis or collapse). ·

Surgery

For this outpatient procedure, patients are positioned supine, and standard preparing and draping techniques are applied. After appropriate preoperative antibiotics have been administered, an upper arm tourniquet is generally inflated to 250 mm Hg. The surgeries are performed under either regional axillary block anesthesia or general anesthesia. The patient's arm is placed on the hand table in a fully pronated position. The surgeon is seated on the axilla side of the table with an assistant facing across.

Technique

55-1

A dorsal midline incision is used in all cases. The extensor retinaculum is step-cut and reflected, and the extensor tendons from the first through the fifth compartment are mobilized and retracted (**Fig. 55-1**). As an adjunct for postoperative pain relief, a posterior interosseous sensory neurectomy is performed (**Fig. 55-2**).[10] The radiocarpal joint capsule is incised longitudinally and elevated medially and laterally exposing the entire distal radius, scaphoid, lunate, and midcarpal joint. The radiocarpal articulation should be assessed at this point, confirming the preoperative diagnosis of arthritic degeneration of the radioscaphoid and radiolunate articular surfaces with preservation of a healthy articulation at the capitolunate joint (**Fig. 55-3**).

Residual degenerative articular surface of the proximal lunate and scaphoid is removed with a curet, rongeur, or high-speed bur (**Fig. 55-4**), and a bur is used to create a complementary recessed "cup" in the distal radial metaphysis (**Fig. 55-5**). The scaphoid is next osteotomized at its waist, and the distal half of the scaphoid is morcellated and sharply excised (**Fig. 55-6**). The proximal scaphoid and lunate, with exposed raw cancellous bone along their entire proximal surfaces, are recessed into the hollowed-out distal radius in a neutral position (**Fig. 55-7**). From the Wrist-Fit fixation set (Small Bone Innovations, Morrisville, PA), 0.045-inch Kirschner wires (K-wires) are inserted from dorsal distal to palmar proximal in an oblique fashion, placing at least three K-wires between the scaphoid and the lunate into the radius (**Fig. 55-8**).

Alternatively, the pin plates from the distal radius fixation system (Tri-Med, Valencia, CA) may be used. In most cases, two K-wires are placed in the scaphoid longitudinally, and two are

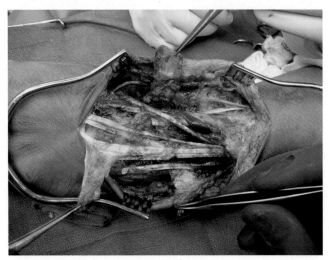

FIGURE 55-1 Extensor retinaculum is step-cut and reflected with extensor tendons from the first through the fifth compartment mobilized.

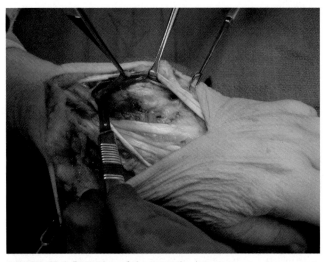

FIGURE 55-2 Resection of the posterior interosseous sensory nerve for postoperative pain relief.

placed in the lunate transversely. Three flexible conforming plates are slid over the K-wires (**Fig. 55-9**), held in place while the screw holes are predrilled, measured, and secured down with cortical screws, "tension-locking" the pin plate constructs into place. The depth of the K-wires is measured, and the K-wires are replaced with high angle screws from the set (**Fig. 55-10**). X-ray confirmation ensures satisfactory alignment of the recessed scapholunate arthrodesis and maintenance of the capitate within the scapholunate midcarpal fossa, now functioning as a "universal joint" (**Fig. 55-11**).

When secure fixation is achieved, the capsule is reapproximated and closed anatomically; a slip of the step-cut extensor retinaculum is sometimes placed beneath the extensor tendons over the distal portion of the pin plates, while the more proximal portion of the retinaculum is reapproximated holding the extensor tendons in place (**Fig. 55-12**). The overlying subcutaneous tissue is approximated with interrupted inverted absorbable sutures, and the skin is closed with a running absorbable subcuticular 6-0 suture.

Postoperative Management

After closure, a bulky soft dressing with a volar resting splint is applied for 7 to 10 days, after which a removable thermoplastic splint is used, and the patient is started on range of motion exercises. At 6 weeks, the splint is discontinued. The patient begins progressively more aggressive stretching, strengthening, and endurance exercises over the next 4 to 12 months and is allowed to begin to resume normal activities when radiographic evidence of healing of the arthrodesis is noted, and motion, strength, and levels of comfort permit.

Results

The senior author (W.H.S.) has now successfully used this technique in more than 30 cases. In an initial review presented at the 59th American Society for Surgery of the Hand (ASSH) annual meeting (2004, New York City) and submitted for publication, 12 patients with radiocarpal arthritis were managed with the SHARC procedure. The authors used a tension plating system (Small Bone Innovations, Morrisville, PA, or Tri-Med, Valencia, CA) designed and contoured for distal radius fractures. There

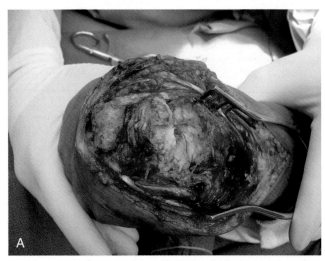

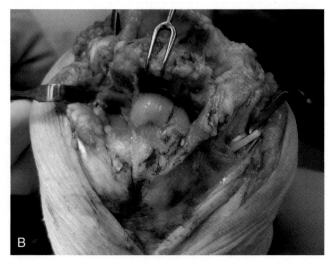

FIGURE 55-3 **A** and **B,** Inspection of the radiocarpal articulation showing arthritic degeneration of the radioscaphoid and the radiolunate articular surfaces with preservation of a healthy articulation at the capitolunate joint.

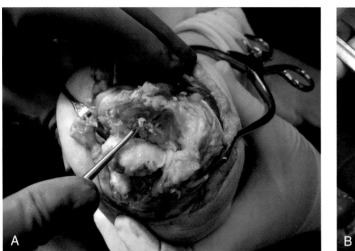 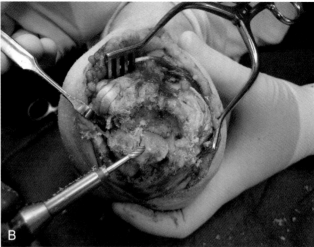

FIGURE 55-4 **A** and **B,** Cartilage remnants are removed with a curet, and the residual degenerative articular surface of the proximal lunate and scaphoid is removed with a high-speed bur, exposing a cancellous surface.

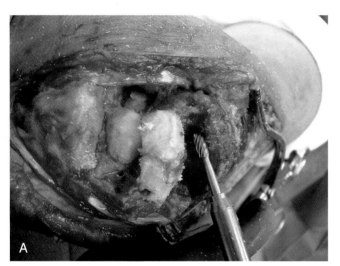 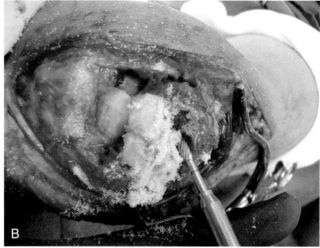

FIGURE 55-5 **A** and **B,** A bur is used to create a complementary recessed "cup" in the distal radial metaphysis.

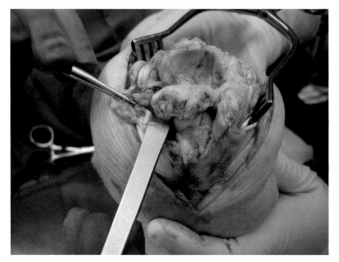 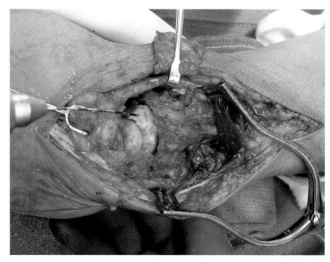

FIGURE 55-6 The scaphoid is osteotomized at its waist, and the distal half of the scaphoid is morcellated and sharply excised.

FIGURE 55-7 The proximal scaphoid and lunate are recessed into the hollowed-out distal radius in a neutral position.

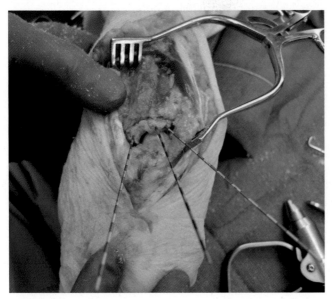

FIGURE 55-8 Kirschner wires from the Wrist-Fit fixation set (Small Bone Innovations, Morrisville, PA) are inserted from dorsal distal to palmar proximal in an oblique fashion.

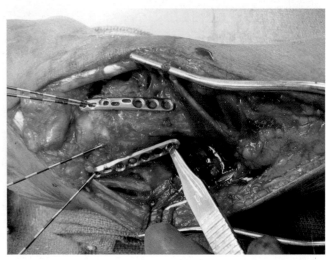

FIGURE 55-9 Flexible conforming pin plates are slid over the Kirschner wires.

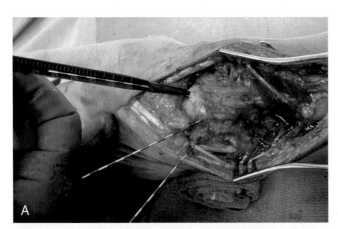

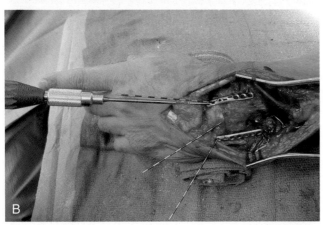

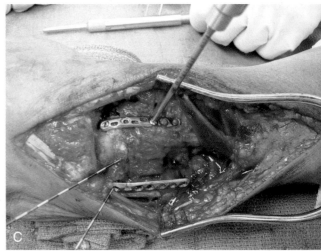

FIGURE 55-10 A to C, The pin plate construct is "tension-locked" into place by insertion of 2.7-mm cortical screws. The Kirschner wires are used to make screw length measurements and replaced with high angle screws from the set.

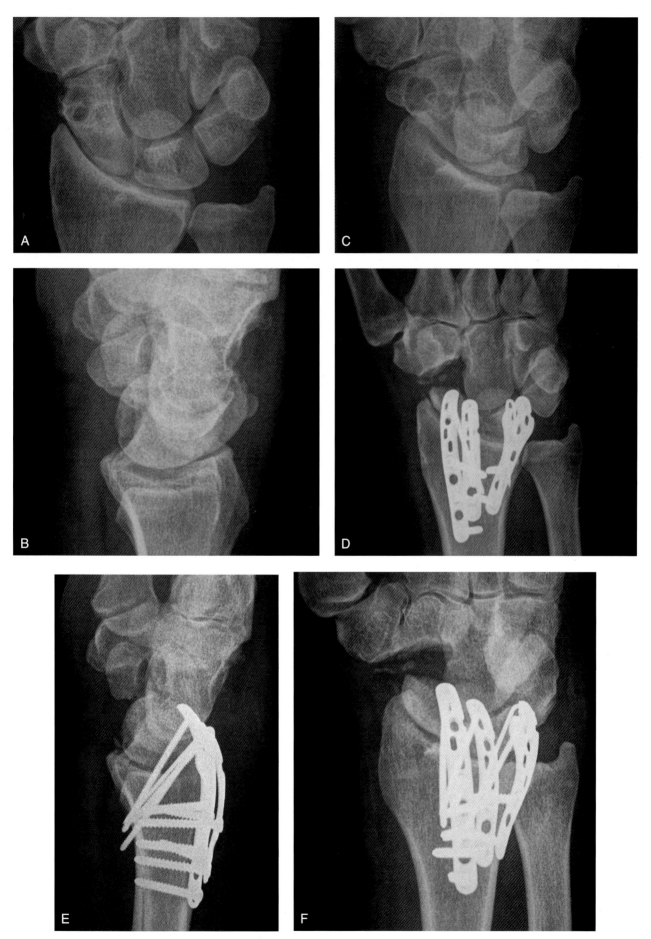

FIGURE 55-11 **A** to **F,** Preoperative and postoperative x-rays of a sample case.

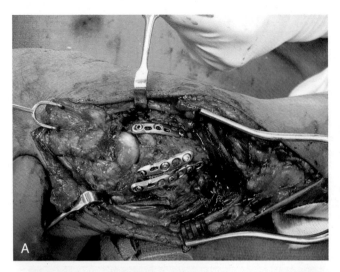

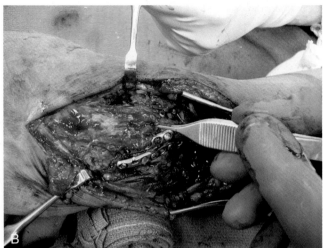

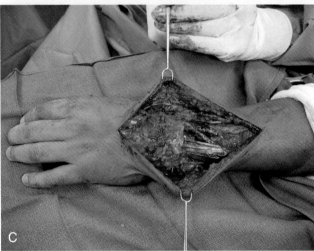

FIGURE 55-12 **A** to **C**, The capsule is reapproximated and closed anatomically, and the more proximal portion of the retinaculum is reapproximated holding the extensor tendons in place.

were 11 men and 1 woman an average age of 57.1 years (age range
28 to 79 years). Diagnoses included post-traumatic arthritis following malunited distal radius fracture (three patients), fracture-
dislocation of the wrist (four patients), scapholunate dissociation
with advanced collapse (four patients), and scaphoid nonunion
with advanced collapse (one patient).

Since we started performing this specific technique, we have
carefully followed 12 patients postoperatively for 2 to 5 years with
an average follow-up of 2.8 years. Five patients were gainfully
employed previously, and all five returned to their prior level of
employment. The other seven patients all were retired at the time
of their treatment, and all returned to activities of daily living
and recreational activities without limitations. Postoperatively,
flexion-extension arc of motion increased to 85.8 degrees with a
range of 65 to 120 degrees, whereas radioulnar deviation range
of motion arc increased to an average of 15 degrees with a range
of 10 to 20 degrees. Grip strength increased postoperatively to
an average of 81.3% of the contralateral side with a range of 70%
to 90%. The level of pain the patients have perceived at follow-up
on a visual analog scale of 0 to 10 averaged 1.1 (range 0 to 2).
All patients acknowledged a significant decrease in pain and
increase in motion, strength, and function. All 12 patients believed
they had significantly improved, and all 12 stated they would have
the surgical procedure again because it provided a significant

improvement in their overall symptoms from the preoperative
state.

Since that initial series, an additional 20 patients have undergone the SHARC procedure. Of the cohort of 32 patients, 2 have
required revision surgery (one total wrist arthrodesis and one
total wrist arthroplasty). The remaining patients have exhibited a
high level of function, range of motion, and pain relief.

Discussion

Radiocarpal arthritis of various etiologies frequently involves the
radioscaphoid articulation, but sometimes spares the radiolunate
joint. When the proximal lunate articular surface and its fossa
within the radius are well preserved, proximal row carpectomy
and four-corner fusion have been shown to be effective, motion-
preserving reconstructive procedures, relieving the pain of arthritis.[3,5-7] Similarly, midcarpal arthritis is well treated with four-corner
fusion.[3-5]

When the scaphoid and the lunate fossae of the radius are
degenerated with reciprocal scaphoid and lunate articular wear,
attempting to maintain radiocarpal motion at the lunate facet
with either the lunate itself or the capitate is not an option.
Radioscapholunate arthrodesis alone has been attempted with
only modest success.

Because the scaphoid represents a stable strut between the proximal and distal rows, its integrity precludes significant midcarpal motion. When it remains intact after radioscapholunate arthrodesis, there is a much longer lever arm acting to create motion at the attempted arthrodesis site, which can lead to nonunion. Conversely, if union is obtained, stresses may now be transmitted to the scaphotrapezial joint, creating painful arthrosis at this location. The biomechanical effect of this stable strut between the proximal and distal rows also explains why excision can enhance motion even when four-corner fusion is performed.[4,5,8]

Recessing the scaphoid and lunate into the hollowed-out metaphysis of the distal radius maximizes contact for healing and provides enhanced room for secure capsular closure without the need to overtighten the capsule. This allows ample motion through the midcarpal joint when combined with the excision of the distal half of the scaphoid. The capitate now sits as a "ball" within the "socket" formed by the lunate and proximal half of the scaphoid, functionally converting the midcarpal joint into a "universal joint."

Limited, "anatomy-specific" fixation using tensioned K-wires or screws with flexible contoured plates and cortical screws has been shown to provide an extremely secure fixation around the distal radius.[11] Application of this technique uses a minimal amount of hardware to provide secure fixation of the lunate and proximal half of the scaphoid into the concavity of the distal radius, while allowing early controlled motion through the new midcarpal "universal" joint.

In the authors' experience, total wrist arthrodesis or possibly total wrist arthroplasty are the alternative procedures, and in our estimation should be reserved as salvage procedures. In the face of advanced diffuse radioscapholunate arthritis with evidence of a healthy midcarpal joint, the SHARC procedure is an effective reconstructive procedure, providing stability, relieving pain, and preserving functional mobility. Results of the SHARC procedure are comparable to the results of other successful motion-sparing procedures, providing an alternative when the entire radial articular surface is degenerative.[2,3,5-7] It provides a functional alternative to wrist arthrodesis and enhanced motion compared with radioscapholunate arthrodesis alone, with more functional outcomes and fewer complications.[1,2] This procedure does not preclude salvage with total wrist arthrodesis or arthroplasty.

REFERENCES

1. De Smet L, Truyen J: Arthrodesis of the wrist for osteoarthritis: outcome with a minimum follow-up of 4 years. J Hand Surg. 2003; 28B:575-577.
2. Nagy L, Büchler U: Long-term results of radioscapholunate fusion following fractures of the distal radius. J Hand Surg. 1997; 22B:705-710.
3. Krakauer JD, Bishop AT, Cooney WP: Surgical treatment of scapholunate advanced collapse. J Hand Surg. 1994; 19A:751-759.
4. Kobza PE, Budoff JE, Yeh ML, et al: Management of the scaphoid during four-corner fusion—a cadaveric study. J Hand Surg. 2003; 28A:904-909.
5. Tomaino MM, Miller RJ, Cole I, et al: Scapholunate advanced collapse wrist: proximal row carpectomy or limited wrist arthrodesis with scaphoid excision? J Hand Surg. 1994; 19A:134-142.
6. Tomaino MM, Delsignore J, Burton RI: Long-term results following proximal row carpectomy. J Hand Surg. 1994; 19A:694-703.
7. Wyrick JD: Proximal row carpectomy and intercarpal arthrodesis for the management of wrist arthritis. J Am Acad Orthop Surg. 2003; 11:277-281.
8. McCombe D, Ireland DCR, McNab I: Distal scaphoid excision after radioscaphoid arthrodesis. J Hand Surg. 2001; 26A:877-882.
9. Garcia-Elias M, Lluch A, Ferreres A, et al: Treatment of radiocarpal degenerative osteoarthritis by radioscapholunate arthrodesis and distal scaphoidectomy. J Hand Surg. 2005; 30A:8-12.
10. Berger RA: Partial denervation of the wrist: a new approach. Tech Hand Upper Extrem Surg. 1998; 2:25-35.
11. Dodds SD, Cornelissen S, Jossan S, et al: A biomechanical comparison of fragment-specific fixation and augmented external fixation for intra-articular distal radius fractures. J Hand Surg. 2002; 27A:953-964.

Osteotomy for Extra-articular Malunion of the Distal Radius

56

Diego L. Fernandez, MD

Distal radius fractures, first described in the 18th century by Petit[1] and Pouteau[2] commonly account for 10% of all fractures[3] and 72% of all forearm fractures.[4] For most authors, the most common complication of distal radius fractures is malunion, with a prevalence that ranges from 5% to 70% of all distal radius fractures, depending on the articles reviewed.[5-12]

Etiology and Pathophysiology

Approximately 25% of distal radius fractures treated by closed means heal with deformities that exceed general parameters of acceptance (dorsal tilt of 20 degrees in the sagittal plane and 10 degrees in the coronal plane, <10 degrees of rotation, <2 mm radial shortening, and <2 mm intra-articular step-off).[8,9,11,13-16] When these fractures are treated by surgical means, however, regardless of the stabilization method employed, the incidence rate of malunion decreases to 10% or less.[16,17] As a result, almost 80% of corrective osteotomies for malunion of the distal radius are done after failed closed treatment, and the remaining 20% are done after failed osteosynthesis, usually procedures done with minimally invasive techniques, such as external fixators or percutaneous Kirschner wires (K-wires).[5,8,9,11,14,15,18-21]

Distal radius malunion may be (1) extra-articular, characterized by metaphyseal angulation and radial shortening; (2) intra-articular, involving distortion of the radiocarpal or distal radioulnar joints, or both; or (3) a combination of the two (intra-articular and extra-articular). Distal radioulnar joint (DRUJ) disorders associated with malunited distal radius fractures can be grouped into one of three basic conditions: (1) incongruency, (2) impaction (abutment), and (3) instability. Other, less frequent DRUJ problems associated with malunions are painful nonunions of the ulnar styloid, capsular contractures, and radioulnar impingement after distal ulnar resections. This chapter addresses the indications and surgical tactics for corrective osteotomies, compares newer trends in management with the available literature, evaluates outcome after deformity correction, and discusses associated complications.

Diagnosis, Indications, and Timing

The need for surgical correction is multifactorial. Wrist deformity after fracture, even when exceeding the previously mentioned parameters of acceptance, may or may not produce symptoms. Differentiating symptomatic from asymptomatic malunion is paramount to decide whether treatment is necessary. Adequate, painless wrist function can be expected despite radiographic evidence of deformity, shortening, and degenerative changes. By necessity, the surgical decision is based on limitation of joint motion, grip strength, level of pain, and degree of cosmetic deformity. The intensity of these symptoms and their relative impact on activities of daily living, as correlated with radiocarpal radio-graphic findings, help define deformity tolerance and indications for corrective surgery.[5,7,8,16,22]

Pain

A malunited radius fracture may be a source of pain for various and often overlapping reasons, each of which must be assessed carefully because each sheds relevance in the selection of treatment. Intra-articular incongruence, be it at the radiocarpal joint or DRUJ, can produce early and often incapacitating pain.[7,23,24] Loss of radial length can result in ulnocarpal abutment and may be a source of ulnar-sided wrist pain. Depending on the integrity of the distal radioulnar ligaments (volar and dorsal) of the triangular fibrocartilage complex, the abutment pain may be associated with limited forearm rotation (ligaments intact) or an unstable DRUJ (ligaments disrupted).[25-27] A significant dorsal deformity (>20 to 30 degrees in the sagittal plane) displaces the proximal carpal row dorsally and overloads the articular cartilage in this reduced surface area (Fig. 56-1). Not only is this a common source of pain, but it also has been considered a prearthritic condition.[28,29]

Capsular contractures and synovitis that result from positional abnormalities within the carpal rows are responsible for painful limitation of wrist flexion. At the midcarpal articulation, a dorsally malunited fracture can result in several distinct problems and compensatory deformities: (1) an adaptive (type I) dorsal intercalated segment instability (DISI), in which the midcarpal flexion is lax and fully correctable by radial osteotomy (Fig. 56-2A-D)[30,31]; (2) a fixed (type II) DISI malalignment, which does not improve after radial osteotomy and may represent a chronic stage of scapholunate instability, not diagnosed at the time of injury, or the stiffening with time of a previously lax deformity (Fig. 56-2E)[9,30,32]; and (3) the already mentioned dorsal subluxation of the entire carpus.[25] Differentiating DISI types I and II can be done with a lateral x-ray of the wrist taken in the same amount of extension as the dorsal angulation of the malunited distal radius (see Fig. 56-2).[30,32]

Grip Strength

Another important parameter when deciding whether a corrective osteotomy is indicated is the loss of grip strength. Grip strength, when compared with the uninjured side or with cohorts of the healthy general population, often represents the degree of deformity and the associated functional impairment.[33] Although there is no generally established quantity of weakness to warrant an osteotomy, it is thought that a grip of at least 30 kg is needed for most activities of daily living.[34] In addition to the loss of strength secondary to pain, the spatial angulations that result from malunion alter the flexor and extensor tendinous vectors of traction.[7] The change in position of the wrist's center of rotation results in diminished efficiency of the tendon lever arms.

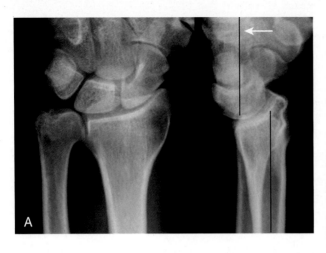

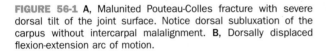

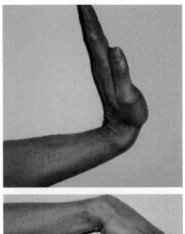

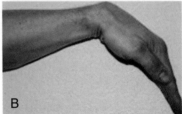

FIGURE 56-1 **A,** Malunited Pouteau-Colles fracture with severe dorsal tilt of the joint surface. Notice dorsal subluxation of the carpus without intercarpal malalignment. **B,** Dorsally displaced flexion-extension arc of motion.

Range of Motion

The third evaluation criterion for corrective osteotomy is limitation of joint motion. Malunions with intra-articular incongruity greater than 2 mm have considerable limitations in range of motion.[23,24] It is common to have less than 40 degrees in extension or supination or both in a Smith fracture and flexion of only 30 degrees in a Colles' fracture.[32] Limited motion may be severe enough to indicate a corrective osteotomy alone, despite adequate grip strength and absence of pain. When combined with pain and weakness, decreased function significantly limits activities of daily living.

Cosmetic Appearance

For certain patients, malunion deformity may be so obvious that esthetic considerations may incline the surgeon toward correction despite nonsuggestive functional and radiographic parameters. An isolated deformity does not justify corrective osteotomy.[7,16,22] Regardless, it is rare for such deformities to occur in the absence of symptoms.

Radiographic Findings

My colleagues and I do not believe in the use of fixed radiographic angles for determining if correction is needed. Certain parameters that are associated with rapid degenerative changes, such as an articular incongruence greater than 2 mm or the prearthritic deformity of a dorsal defect greater than 20 to 30 degrees, are considered formal surgical indications, independent of patient symptoms, especially in a young patient. Lanz and Kron[35] suggest comparisons of the affected wrist with statistical radiographic standards to quantify amount of deformity.[3,15,22,36] In contrast, a comparison tailored to the patient's particular anatomy can be obtained with radiographs of the uninjured wrist, as suggested in an earlier work.[7]

Timing

Although correction of extra-articular deformity can be safely delayed until the soft tissues offer an ideal surgical environment,

and maximal residual function of the wrist has been regained, intra-articular deformity should be dealt with as soon as possible, before irreversible articular damage occurs. Jupiter and Ring[37] compared the results of early and late osteotomies in two similar cohorts and concluded that early correction provided easier radial and DRUJ realignment because of the absence of soft tissue and capsular contractures. The need for structural iliac crest bone graft is diminished because the local nascent callus material can be used to fill defects. Jupiter and Ring[37] concluded that although functional results are similar in both groups, early surgery resulted in considerably less total disability and earlier return to work.

Surgical Correction of Extra-articular Dorsal Deformity: Management Options
Dorsal Opening Wedge Osteotomies

Because radial shortening is a constant component of the dorsal deformity, an opening wedge osteotomy that is transverse in the frontal plane and oblique (parallel to the joint surface) in the sagittal plane, to provide lengthening, is recommended. The osteotomy should accomplish a reorientation of the radiocarpal joint surface to improve load distribution, re-establish the mechanical balance of the midcarpal joint, and restore the anatomical relationships of the DRUJ. Variations in technique for creating a dorsal opening wedge osteotomy have been described. All allow radial lengthening of 10 to 12 mm, and permit correction of the volar tilt in the sagittal plane, radial inclination in the frontal plane, and rotational deformity in the coronal plane.

Dorsal Approach
Preoperative Planning

A careful preoperative plan incorporating K-wires that mark the angles of correction is characteristic of this technique (**Fig. 56-3**). These angles are mandatory to simplify the procedure, guarantee

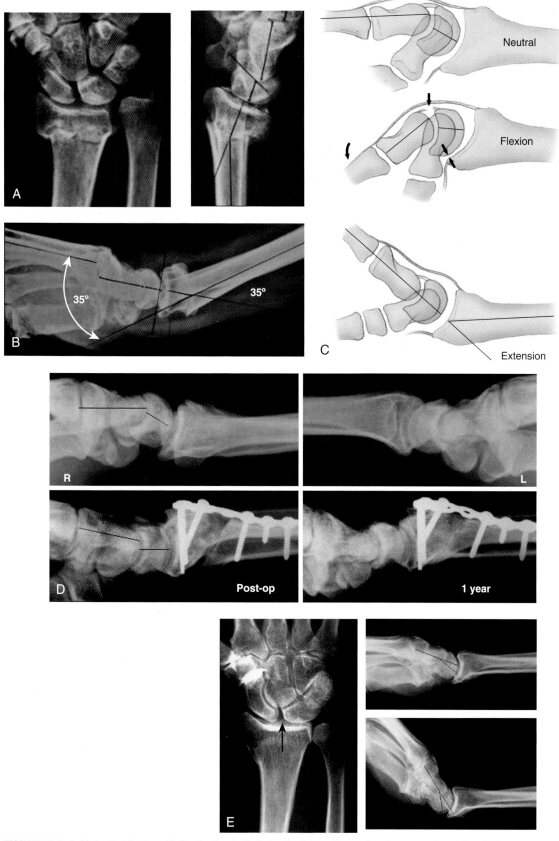

FIGURE 56-2 A, Malunited Pouteau-Colles fracture with "adaptive" dorsal intercalated segment instability (DISI) malalignment. **B,** The carpus is realigned in a lateral x-ray taken in the same amount of dorsiflexion as the dorsally displaced distal fragment (35 degrees in this patient). **C,** Schematic representation of the type I "lax" adaptive DISI in dorsally angulated malunions. **D,** *Top,* Comparative lateral radiographs of a patient with a malunited right Colles' fracture with type I adaptive DISI. *Bottom,* Restoration of normal carpal alignment after osteotomy. **E,** Type II fixed DISI malalignment. Notice that carpal alignment does not improve with wrist extension. Slight widening of the scapholunate interval (*arrow*) suggests a chronic stage of scapholunate instability.

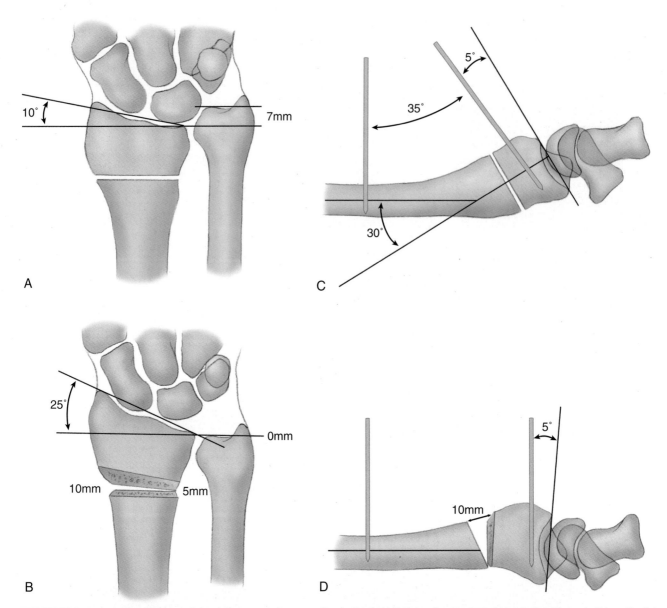

FIGURE 56-3 Preoperative planning of the osteotomy. A, For correction in the frontal plane, the amount of shortening (7 mm in this patient) is measured between the head of the ulna and the ulnar corner of the radius on the anteroposterior radiograph. The lines for the measurement are perpendicular to the long axis of the radius. The ulnar tilt is reduced to 10 degrees in this patient. **B,** To restore the ulnar tilt to normal (average 25 degrees), the osteotomy is opened more on the dorsoradial than on the dorsoulnar side. **C,** For correction in the sagittal plane, the dorsal tilt (30 degrees in this patient) is measured between the perpendicular to the joint surface and the long axis of the radius on the lateral radiograph. The Kirschner wires are introduced so that they subtend the angle that corresponds to the dorsal tilt plus 5 degrees of volar tilt (30 degrees + 5 degrees = 35 degrees in this patient). **D,** After opening the osteotomy by the correct amount, the Kirschner wires lie parallel to each other.

an accurate angular correction, and diminish the need for intraoperative image control. Prerequisites for this planning process are standard radiographs of the injured and uninjured side. When superimposed, these images allow localization of the osteotomy site and measurement of angular deformity in the two orthogonal projections: the lateral view (sagittal plane) and the anteroposterior view (frontal plane).

Rotational deformity is more accurately measured by superimposing tracings of symmetrical computed tomograms of both forearms. The proximal cuts of the scan should include the bicipital tuberosity, and the distal cuts should be at the level of Lister's tubercle. The "radial torsion angle" is defined as the angle between the proximal and distal reference axes.[38] The difference between the radial torsion angles for the injured and contralateral side represents the true bony rotational malalignment.

The osteotomy entails a wedge opening on the dorsal and radial side, with a volar and ulnar hinge. Two K-wires are planned for intraoperative monitoring and inserted precisely in the sagittal plane, converging at the intended angle of correction. The osteotomized distal fragment is outlined and tilted around the respective hinge at the predetermined correction angles. The resulting length is evaluated and checked with respect to the distal ulna and adjusted if necessary. For a true hinge or wedge (unicortical osteotomy), its height at the ulnopalmar corner is zero and at the ulnodorsal corner equals the dorsal gap from the lateral projection. The radiopalmar corner is taken from the plan converting the arc of correction in millimeters. The radiodorsal height is the sum of the two aforementioned measurements. For a trapezoidal-shaped defect (bicortical osteotomy), the dimensions are calculated in the same manner, in addition to its depth, which is given by the sagittal and frontal diameter of the radius at the level of the cut.

Technique

The incision begins at a point 2 cm distal to Lister's tubercle and extends 5 cm proximally in the forearm. The extensor retinaculum is incised longitudinally between the third and fourth dorsal compartments. Next, the extensor pollicis longus tendon is dissected out of its groove and retracted. The distal part of the radius is exposed ulnarly by separating the extensor tendons of the fourth and fifth compartments with their fibrosynovial sheaths. Raising these structures close to bone protects the posterior interosseous nerve as it is displaced ulnarward. Radially, a periosteal elevator is passed under the wrist extensor tendons. The tendons

are separated from bone, placing two small Hohmann retractors on both sides of the future osteotomy site.

To ensure proper orientation and location of the osteotomy, a fine K-wire is inserted through the dorsal capsule into the radiocarpal joint along the articular surface of the radius, indicating the sagittal plane of the joint. If a single angular correction is planned, the osteotomy cut has to be exactly parallel to the joint surface in the sagittal plane. If correction of radial inclination and malrotation is needed, the cut has to be aligned perpendicular to the distal fragment in both planes (i.e., in the anteroposterior view as well). Otherwise, rotation along a nonorthogonal interface results in secondary angular malpositioning. According to the operative plan, two threaded 2.5-mm K-wires are inserted subtending the angle of correction on both sides of the future osteotomy (**Fig. 56-4**). These K-wires not only serve to guide intraoperative correction, but also to manipulate and maintain the distal fragment in the correct position. A small external fixator may be used temporarily to maintain correction, if needed.

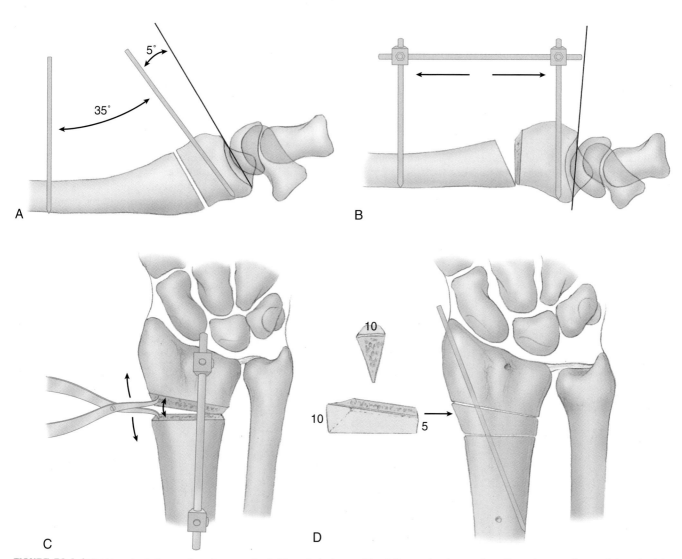

FIGURE 56-4 Osteotomy technique—dorsal approach. A, Threaded wires subtend the angle of correction. The osteotomy is parallel to the joint surface in the sagittal plane. Note the fine Kirschner wire introduced into the radiocarpal joint. **B** and **C,** The osteotomy is opened dorsally and radially with a small spreader clamp. A fixator bar maintains the correction. **D,** An iliac graft shaped to conform to the defect is inserted, and one oblique Kirschner wire is driven through the radial styloid and graft into the radial metaphysis. The fixator is removed, and definitive plate fixation is carried out.

Protecting the volar soft tissues, the osteotomy is performed with the oscillating saw parallel to the distal K-wire, taking care not to osteotomize completely the volar cortex. The osteotomy is opened dorsally and radially by manipulating the wrist into flexion and with the assistance of a small laminar spreader. The osteotomy is opened until both K-wires are parallel in the sagittal plane. Complete tenotomy of the brachioradialis or Z-lengthening is recommended to facilitate radial lengthening. Next, a corticocancellous strut graft is harvested from the iliac crest, shaped according to the resulting osteotomy defect, incorporated with the cortical portion oriented dorsally, and temporarily fixed with K-wires. If rotational correction is needed, one or two K-wires are inserted through the graft into the proximal fragment to secure the correct axial alignment. Then the distal fragment can be rotated (usually pronated) on the graft to the desired position. The amount of rotational correction is monitored with the two K-wires in the sagittal plane.

Various methods of stable fixation are available. In our practice, a 2.7-mm condylar plate or the use of two 2.4-mm locking plates are preferred for the following reasons: (1) The 2.7-mm condylar plate can be completely covered by the fourth compartment and does not interfere with the extensor pollicis longus or the wrist extensors, diminishing the risk of attrition tendinitis; (2) its fixed-angle component minimizes loss of correction by fragment settling; (3) by virtue of the low profile of the plate, extensor tendon irritation is uncommon, and removal of hardware is seldom necessary; and (4) stability of the construct can be augmented by inserting a separate oblique lag screw across the osteotomy. If the 2.4-mm distal radius plates are used, one is applied on the radial border between the wrist extensors and the first dorsal compartment, and the other is applied dorsoulnarly under the fourth compartment (**Fig. 56-5**).

If fixed-angle devices are used, morcellized cancellous grafts may be used because the chances of loss of correction are minimized, especially if the distal locking screws are placed in the subchondral area of the epiphysis.[20] With increasing stability of the construct, an earlier return of unrestricted active wrist motion can be offered. During wound closure, the extensor pollicis longus is protected from the plate by the interposition of an extensor retinacular flap or returned to its groove, if Lister's tubercle has been preserved. Deep suction drainage of the wound is recommended for 24 hours postoperatively.

Postsurgical Care

Generally, we prefer to immobilize the wrist in a volar plaster splint for 10 to 14 days to permit the surrounding soft tissues to heal. When the sutures have been removed, gentle active wrist motion is permitted in cases in which stable internal fixation was accomplished in the presence of good bone quality. A removable wrist splint to perform such exercises is recommended. For cases in which K-wire fixation was used, a below-elbow cast is worn for about 4 weeks. Strenuous activities are not allowed until there is radiographic evidence of bony healing, which usually takes at least 8 to 12 weeks after osteotomy. Dorsal plates usually are removed 3 to 6 months after surgery to prevent attrition tendinitis of the extensor pollicis longus tendon. Volar plates may be left in place.

Volar Approach

The volar approach, originally described by Lanz and colleagues,[35,39] consists of performing the dorsal correction through a volar approach, and internally fixing the distal radius with an anatomically congruent, fixed-angle volar plate. This method, although technically challenging, has the undeniable advantage of an automatic correction of deformity by the correct placement of an anatomically congruent volar plate to the distal fragment (**Fig. 56-6**). There is no risk of extensor tendinitis, provided that screws do not protrude through the dorsal cortex,[34] and the approach permits an "en-bloc" manipulation of the osteotomized fragment.

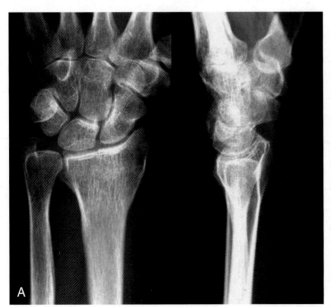
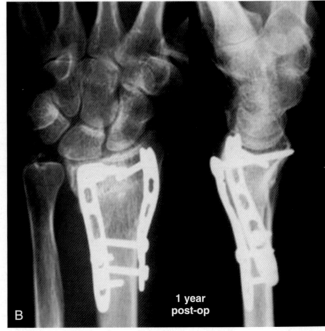

FIGURE 56-5 A, A malunited Pouteau-Colles fracture with 30 degrees of dorsal tilt and slight shortening. B, Radiographs 1 year after osteotomy.

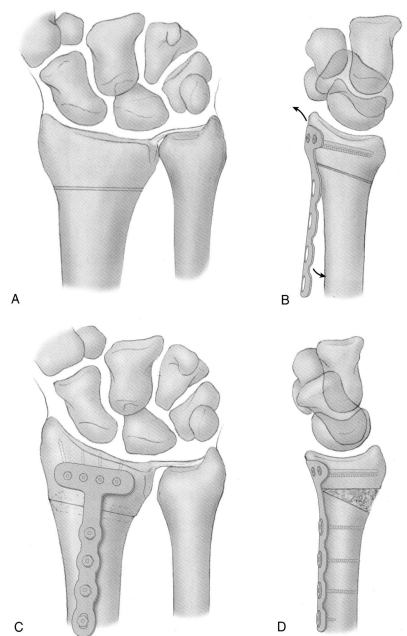

A

B

C

D

FIGURE 56-6 Schematic representation of a dorsal opening wedge osteotomy performed through a volar approach with a fixed-angle distal radius plate.

Technique

The distal part of the Henry approach between the flexor carpi radialis and radial artery is used (**Fig. 56-7**). After detachment of the pronator quadratus, the lateral border of the radius is exposed. This exposure is facilitated with detachment or a Z-tenotomy of the brachioradialis and by opening the floor of the first dorsal compartment.[40] At this point, a flat Hohmann retractor should be carefully placed under the extensor tendons (see **Fig. 56-7B**). Two 2-mm K-wires subtending the correction angle are driven into the shaft and distal fragment. The distal K-wire should be parallel to the joint surface in the sagittal plane (see **Fig. 56-7C**). Before the osteotomy cut, the distal component of the plate is fixed temporarily to the distal radius (see **Fig. 56-7D**).

The drill holes for the most ulnar and radial fixed-angle pegs of the proximal row of holes in the DVR plate are prepared at this point. The plate is removed, and the osteotomy cut is per-

formed at the old fracture site from volar dorsal parallel to the distal K-wire (see **Fig. 56-7E**). As described for the dorsal approach, the same principles for preoperative planning, and making the osteotomy cut perpendicular to the axis of the radius in the anteroposterior plane and parallel to the joint surface in the sagittal plane, apply. After completion of the osteotomy, the distal fragment is supinated and extended while the shaft is maintained pronated. This maneuver facilitates dorsal exposure to visualize and resect the dorsal callus and periosteum, diminishing the danger of damaging the extensor tendons. A dorsal release also is imperative to permit ease of correction and restoration of radial length. Next the plate is fixed with subchondral fixed-angle pegs and screws to the distal fragment (see **Fig. 56-7F-H**).

Correction in all three planes occurs simultaneously as the proximal part of the plate is progressively reduced to the radial shaft with a bone clamp. A laminar spreader may be used

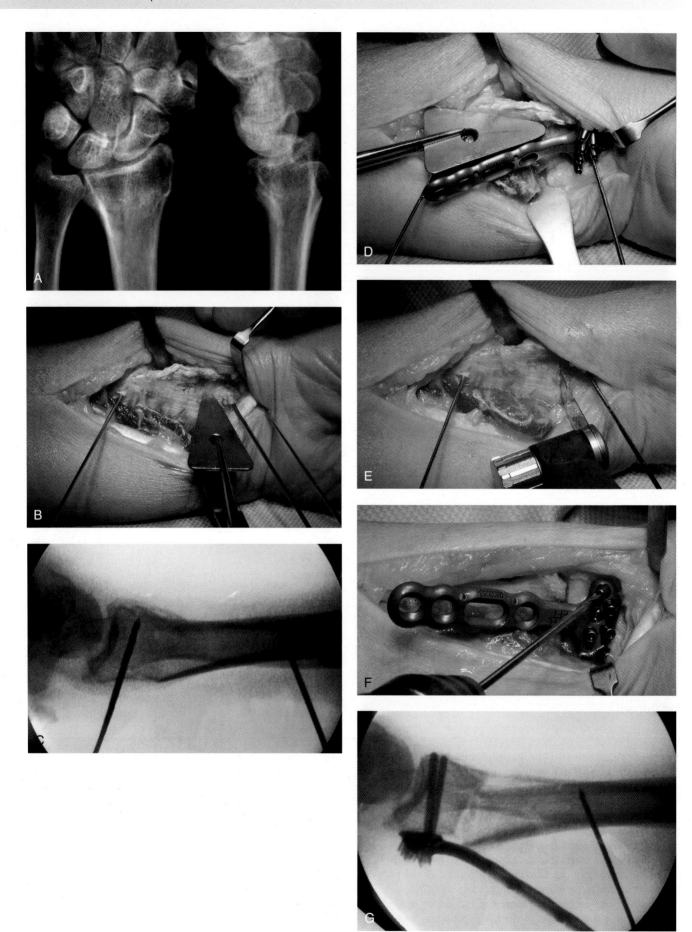

FIGURE 56-7 Osteotomy technique—volar approach. A, Radiographs of a distal radius malunion with 30 degrees of dorsal angulation. Correction through a volar approach and fixation with a fixed-angle plate was planned. **B,** Malunion exposed through volar flexor carpi radialis extended approach. Kirschner wires subtend the correction angle of 30 degrees. The distal Kirschner wire is parallel to the one inserted in the radiocarpal joint. **C,** Fluoroscopic view showing the position of the Kirschner wires. The distal Kirschner wire is parallel to the joint surface in the sagittal plane. **D,** The DVR plate has been temporarily fixed to the distal radius with one Kirschner wire. The angle between the plate and radial shaft equals the correction angle of 30 degrees. **E,** The osteotomy is performed with the oscillating saw blade parallel to the distal Kirschner wire. Notice soft tissue protection with a Hohmann retractor placed dorsally under the extensor tendons. **F,** The plate is fixed to the distal fragment with subchondral fixed-angle pegs and screws. **G to I,** Fluoroscopic control of plate position in the lateral and anteroposterior planes. Notice subchondral placement of half-threaded pegs. **J and K,** Intraoperative fluoroscopy views showing anatomical realignment of the distal fragment and DRUJ congruency. **L and M,** Radiographs 1 year after surgery. Notice complete bone remodeling at the osteotomy site and no loss of initial correction.

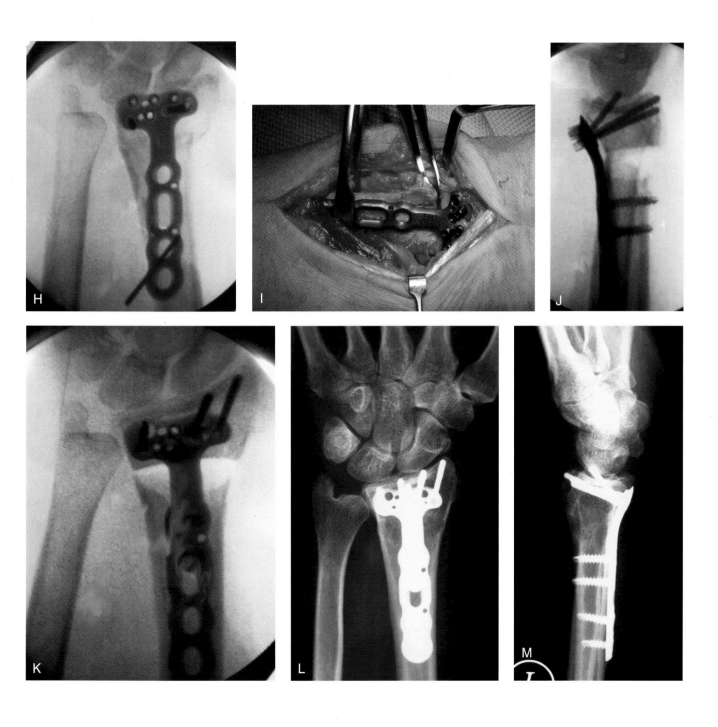

simultaneously to open the dorsal wedge and help in restoring length and performing frontal plane corrections (see **Fig. 56-7I**). After fluoroscopic verification of correction, the plate is fixed to the radial shaft (see **Fig. 56-7J and K**).

The intrinsic stability of these fixed-angle devices, especially when distal pegs are placed subchondrally, guarantees the maintenance of length. These devices have become the implant of choice for fixation of osteoporotic bone and have allowed us to extend the indications of radial osteotomy in elderly patients. For the same reasons, there is no need of structural corticocancellous bone grafts, and the gap may be filled with morcellized autologous grafts or even with bone substitutes. At 1 year, complete radio-graphic bone remodeling of the bone defect may be observed (see **Fig. 56-7L and M**).

Volar Closing Wedge Osteotomies

Because most of the failures of reconstructive surgery after distal radius fracture are due to persistent symptoms arising from the DRUJ, some authors have advocated distal ulnar resection at the time of the corrective radial osteotomy. Posner and Ambrose[41] described a closing wedge osteotomy associated with a Darrach procedure, fixed with K-wires and protected with plaster immobilization. This approach has clear advantages for malunions in

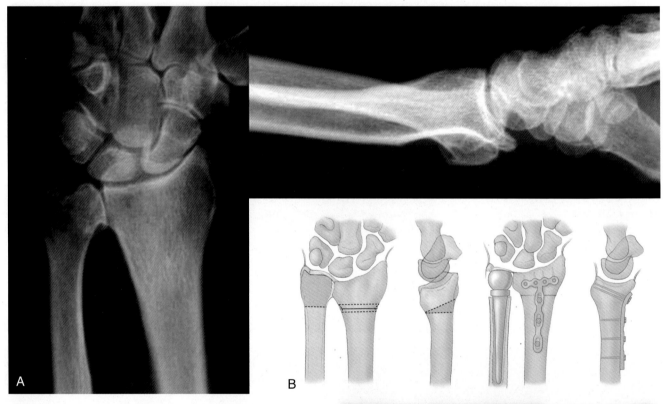

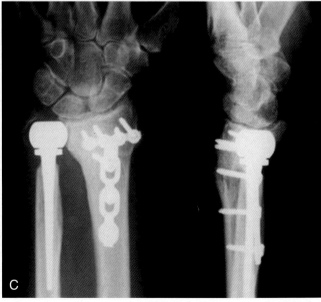

FIGURE 56-8 **A,** Malunion of the distal radius with severe degenerative changes of the distal radioulnar joint. **B,** A palmar closing wedge osteotomy and DRUJ prosthetic replacement was planned. **C,** Radiographs 5 years after osteotomy. The prosthesis is stable, and the patient was free of symptoms.

elderly patients with osteoporotic bone and degenerative changes of the DRUJ or associated intra-articular sigmoid notch involvement in the radius malunion. A similar technique was proposed by Viso and colleagues,[42] whereas other authors[11,12] recommend an ulnar shortening osteotomy, if the DRUJ shows no degenerative changes. If degenerative changes of the DRUJ are present, I prefer a closing wedge palmar osteotomy and primary prosthetic ulnar head replacement with restoration of a 0-mm ulnar variance.[43,44] I no longer resect the distal ulna (Bowers or Darrach) in these situations in an effort to maintain the integrity of the DRUJ, the load transmission of the ulnar side of the carpus, and the kinematics of forearm rotation (**Fig. 56-8**).

Surgical Correction of Metaphyseal Volar Deformity (Malunited Smith-Goyrand Fractures)

The classic symptoms of malunion following volarly displaced fractures include decreased wrist extension, ulnar deviation, and supination. Because of the tendency for Smith's fractures to heal with a pronation deformity of the distal radius, the lack of supination may be especially troublesome for the patient. Volarly angulated malunions following Smith's fractures require a palmar open wedge osteotomy. A straight volar incision between the flexor carpi radialis tendon and the radial artery is performed. The pronator quadratus muscle is detached radially, and the flexor pollicis longus muscle is mobilized from the radial shaft. The malunion is approached subperiosteally by dissecting the pronator quadratus muscle to the ulnar side, and the soft tissues are protected with Hohmann retractors. The palmar opening wedge osteotomy, grafting, and plating are done in a "reversed" fashion—as in Colles' deformity, but from the volar side (**Fig. 56-9**).

Care must be taken not to overcorrect the physiological palmar tilt of 10 degrees when manipulating the distal fragment into dorsiflexion. The application of a volar buttressing T-plate auto-matically derotates the pronated distal fragment by virtue of the flat surface of the plate.[3,21,45,46] Plate fixation is strongly recommended on the volar side because practically all malunited Smith's fractures have a pronation deformity of the distal fragment and an apparent dorsal subluxation of the distal ulna. Most available volar radial plates have been procontoured to fit the anatomical concavity of the distal radial volar surface, so that now overcorrection into a dorsal tilt is a rare complication. Care has to be taken with the screw length; attrition tendinitis and tendon ruptures may occur with the screw protruding dorsally. Dorsiflexion of the distal fragment and derotation and lengthening reorient the sigmoid notch of the radius with respect to the head of the ulna, restoring articular congruity of the radioulnar joint.

Discussion

In a meta-analysis of the results of almost 600 corrective osteotomies published in the French and English literature, Gonzalez del Pino and associates[34] noted that overall results depended fundamentally on the quality and exactness of the correction obtained. Approximately 40% of the cases require a second or third surgical procedure for implant extraction (most cases), treatment of complications, or correction of residual deformity or to address problems in the DRUJ. Obtaining an adequate correction is not always possible. Good and excellent results were obtained in 72% of the cases, fair results were obtained in 15% to 20%, and poor results were obtained in the remaining 10% to 15%. Given the multiple techniques employed, and the variation in deformity, patient selection, and methods of outcome evaluation, these figures serve as rough estimates of a general trend.

Despite the fact that corrective osteotomy for a malunited distal radius has become a standardized surgical procedure, and that advances in diagnosis, instrumentation, and surgical technique continue to evolve, it remains obvious that the best treatment is prevention (immediate surgical fracture stabilization). Major advances include the use of fixed-angle plates that allow

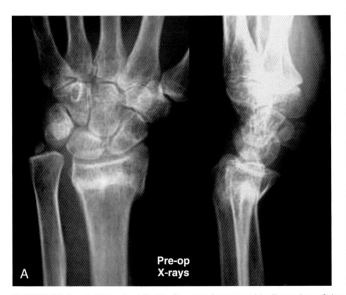
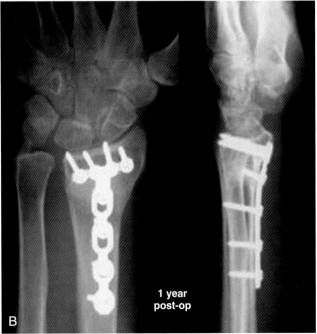

FIGURE 56-9   A, Malunited Smith-Goyrand fracture with disruption of the distal radioulnar joint. **B,** At late follow-up, x-rays show adequate angular correction. The patient had a painless forearm rotation despite residual slight widening of the distal radioulnar joint.

rigid fixation of the osteotomy even in osteoporotic bone, obviating the need for structural bone grafting. Prosthetic replacement of the ulnar head provides a sound alternative to DRUJ salvage and rescue of postresection radioulnar impingement.

Conclusion

Surgical reconstruction of post-traumatic wrist deformity is not a problem with a simple solution, and these malunions are in most instances significantly disabling. In my experience, the keys to a good result are directly related to careful patient selection, accurate angular correction, and recognition and simultaneous treatment of the associated distal radioulnar pathology.

REFERENCES

1. Petit J: L'Art de Guerir les Maladies de l'Os. Paris: d'Houry, 1705.
2. Pouteau C: Oeuvres posthumes de M Pouteau: Memoire, contenant quelques reflexions sur quelques fractures de l'avant-bras sur les luxations incomplètes du poignet et sur le diastasis. Paris: Pierres, 1783.
3. Prommersberger KJ, Van Schoonhoven J, Laubach S, et al: Corrective osteotomy for malunited, palmarly displaced fractures of the distal radius. Eur J Trauma. 2001; 27:16-24.
4. Alffram P, Bauer G: Epidemiology of fractures of the forearm: A biomechanical investigation of bone strength. J Bone Joint Surg Am. 1962; 44:105-114.
5. Brown JN, Bell MJ: Distal radial osteotomy for malunion of wrist fractures in young patients. J Hand Surg [Br]. 1994; 19:589-593.
6. Hunt TR, Hasting H 2nd, Graham TJ: A systematic approach to handling the distal radio-ulnar joint in cases of malunited distal radius fractures. Hand Clin. 1998; 14:239-249.
7. Jupiter JB, Fernandez DL: Complications following distal radial fractures. J Bone Joint Surg Am. 2001; 83:1244-1265.
8. Ladd AL, Huene DS: Reconstructive osteotomy for malunion of the distal radius. Clin Orthop. 1996; 327: 158-171.
9. McGrory BJ, Amadio PC: Malunion of the distal radius. In Cooney WP, Linscheid RL, Dobyns JH, eds. The Wrist: Diagnosis and Operative Treatment. St. Louis: Mosby, 1998.
10. McKay SD, MacDermid JC, Roth JH, et al: Assessment of complications of distal radius fractures and development of a complications checklist. J Hand Surg [Am]. 2001; 26: 916-922.
11. Sennwald G, Fischer W, Stahelin A: Le cal vicieux du radius distal et son traitement: a propos de 122 radii. Int Orthop. 1992; 16:45-51.
12. Voche P, Merle M, Dautel G: Les cals vicieux extra-articulaires du radius distal: evaluation et techniques de correction. Rev Chir Orthop Reparatrice Appar Mot. 2001; 87:263-275.
13. Fourrier P, Bardy A, Roche G, et al: Approche d'une definition du cal vicieux du poignet. Int Orthop. 1981; 4:299-305.
14. Hove LM, Mölster AO: Surgery for posttraumatic wrist deformity: Radial osteotomy and/or ulnar shortening in 16 Colles' fractures. Acta Orthop Scand. 1884; 65:434-438.

15. Prommersberger KJ, van Schoonhoven J, Lanz UB: Outcome after corrective osteotomy for malunited fractures of the distal end of the radius. J Hand Surg [Br]. 2002; 27:55-60.
16. Wright T: Osteotomy for distal radius malunion. Tech Hand Upper Extrem Surg. 2000; 4:222-235.
17. Saffar P, Cooney WP, eds: Treatment of distal intra-articular malunions. In: Fractures of the Distal Radius. London: Martin Dunitz, 1995.
18. Linder L, Stattin J: Malunited fractures of the distal radius with volar angulation: corrective osteotomy in 6 cases using the volar approach. Acta Orthop Scand. 1996; 67:179-181.
19. Oskam J, Bongers KM, Karthaus AJ, et al: Corrective osteotomy for malunion of the distal radius: the effect of concomitant ulnar shortening osteotomy. Arch Orthop Trauma Surg. 1996; 115:219-222.
20. Ring D, Roberge C, Morgan T, et al: Osteotomy for malunited fractures of the distal radius: a comparison of structural and non-structural autogenous bone grafts. J Hand Surg [Am]. 2002; 27:216-222.
21. Shea K, Fernandez DL, Jupiter JB, et al: Corrective osteotomy for malunited, volarly displaced fractures of the distal end of the radius. J Bone Joint Surg [Am]. 1997; 79: 1816-1826.
22. Prommersberger KJ, Lanz UB: Corrective osteotomy for malunited Colles' fractures. Orthop Traumatol. 1998; 6: 75-87.
23. Knirk JL, Jupiter JB: Intra-articular fractures of the distal end of the radius in young adults. J Bone Joint Surg Am. 1986; 68:647-659.
24. Marx RG, Axelrod TS: Intraarticular osteotomy of distal radius malunions. Clin Orthop. 1996; 327:152-157.
25. Adams BD: Effects of radial deformity on distal radioulnar joint mechanics. J Hand Surg [Am]. 1993; 18:492-498.
26. Bronstein AJ, Trumble TE, Tencer AF: The effects of distal radius fracture malalignment on forearm rotation: a cadaveric study. J Hand Surg [Am]. 1997; 22:258-262.
27. Kihara H, Palmer AK, Werner FW, et al: The effect of dorsally angulated distal radius fractures on distal radioulnar joint congruency and forearm rotation. J Hand Surg [Am]. 1996; 21:40-47.
28. Pogue DJ, Viegas SF, Patterson RM, et al: Effects of distal radius fracture malunion on wrist joint mechanics. J Hand Surg [Am]. 1990; 15:721-727.
29. Short WH, Palmer AK, Werner FW, et al: A biomechanical study of distal radial fractures. J Hand Surg [Am]. 1987; 12:529-534.
30. Fernandez DL: Reconstructive procedures for malunions and traumatic arthritis. Orthop Clin North Am. 1993; 24(2): 341-364.
31. Psychoyios VN, Ring D, Roberge C, et al: Carpal alignment after corrective osteotomy for malunited fractures of the distal radius. J Hand Surg [Br]. 2000; 25:38.
32. Park MJ, Cooney WP 3rd, Hahn ME, et al: The effects of dorsally angulated distal radius fractures on carpal kinematics. J Hand Surg [Am]. 2002; 27:223-232.
33. Torres M, Gonzalez del Pino J, Yánez J, et al: Estudio dinamometrico de la mano y el pulgar. Rev Ortop Traumatol. 1999; 43:321-326.

34. Gonzalez del Pino J, Bartolomé del Valle E, Lopez Graña G, et al: Consolidaciones viciosas tras fracturas del extremo distal del radio: patogenia, indicaciones y técnicas quirúrgicas. Rev Ortop Traumatol. 2003; 47(Suppl 1):55-69.

35. Lanz U, Kron W: Neue Technik zur Korrektur in Fehlstellung verheilter Radiusfrakturen. Hand Chir Mikrochir Plast Chir. 1976; 8:203-206.

36. Kwasny O, Fuchs M, Schabus R: Opening wedge osteotomy for malunion of the distal radius with neuropathy: 13 cases followed for 6 (1-11) years. Acta Orthop Scand. 1994; 65:207-208.

37. Jupiter JB, Ring D: A comparison of early and late reconstruction of malunited fractures of the distal end of the radius. J Bone Joint Surg Am. 1996; 78:739-748.

38. Bindra RR, Cole RJ, Yamaguchi K, et al: Quantification of the radial torsion angle with computerized tomography in cadaver specimens. J Bone Joint Surg Am. 1997; 79:833-837.

39. Prommersberger KJ, Moossavi S, Lanz U: Ergebnisse der Korrekturosteotomie fehlverheilter Extensionsfrakturen der Speiche an typischer Stelle. Handchir Mikrochir Plast Chir. 1999; 31:234-240.

40. Orbay J, Indriago I, Badia A, et al: Corrective osteotomy of dorsally malunited fractures of the distal radius via the extended FCR approach. J Hand Surg [Br]. 2003; 28(Suppl 1):2-3.

41. Posner MA, Ambrose L: Malunited Colles' fractures: correction with a biplanar closing wedge osteotomy. J Hand Surg [Am]. 1991; 16:1017-1026.

42. Viso R, Wegener EE, Freeland AE: Use of a closing wedge osteotomy to correct malunion of dorsally displaced extra-articular distal radius fractures. Orthopedics. 2000; 23:721-724.

43. van Schoonhoven J, Fernandez DL, Bowers WH, et al: Salvage of failed resection arthroplasties of the distal radio-ulnar joint using a new ulnar head prosthesis. J Hand Surg [Am]. 2000; 25:438-446.

44. Fernandez DL: Management of acute and chronic derangement of the distal radioulnar joint following radius fractures. In Jakob RP, Fulford P, Horan F, eds: EFORT Instructional Course Lectures. J Bone Joint Surg Br. 1999; 41-53.

45. Fernandez DL: Correction of post-traumatic wrist deformity in adults by osteotomy, bone-grafting, and internal fixation. J Bone Joint Surg Am. 1982; 64:1164-1178.

46. Fernandez DL, Jupiter JB: Fractures of the Distal Radius: A Practical Approach to Management. 2nd ed. New York: Springer, 2002.

Arthroscopic-Assisted Osteotomy for Intra-articular Malunion of the Distal Radius

57

Francisco del Piñal, MD

Rationale and Basic Science Pertinent to the Procedure

Classically, management of a young patient with a step-off in the distal radius has been panarthrodesis. Several pioneer surgeons, such as Saffar,[1] Fernandez,[2] and others,[3-8] opened the door to the possibility of cutting again the displaced fragments and reducing them in anatomical position. The gold standard for the most common sagittal step (anteroposterior) is to do the osteotomy through a dorsal route partly under fluoroscopy guidance.[4,5,7,8] For volar shearing type malunions, the joint is approached volarly, the external callus is removed, and with an osteotome directed toward the joint, the fragment is slowly cut away, with the hope that the osteotome follows the original fracture line.[5,6,8] All these procedures and others can be grouped under "outside-in osteotomy techniques."

Good results have been reported with outside-in osteotomy techniques, but fears of devascularization and inaccurate reduction exist. Fernandez[2] considered the technique appropriate only for single line fractures, although Gonzalez del Pino and Ring[4,5] used it for the more complex four-part fractures.

In my experience with outside-in osteotomy techniques, the main problem I had encountered was the difficulty having visual control of the step-off before the osteotomy, which became an "impossible" feat when the fragment was "reduced" as the joint space closed. One then had to rely on fluoroscopy (an unreliable method),[9] and on palpation with a Freer elevator. Another problem was that sometimes the step-offs did not have a linear trace amenable to a simple cut, but rather a complex irregular shape (**Fig. 57-1**). To obtain better visual control, a very aggressive capsular release is necessary. This aggressive capsular release may increase the risk of avascular necrosis of the ostetomized fragments, virtually contraindicating outside-in techniques.

Bearing in mind these limitations, we sought a method for assessing the status of the articular cartilage in the area of malunion, which at the same time allowed us to identify the fracture line accurately. This chapter outlines our present experience with a method to perform the osteotomy under arthroscopic guidance from "inside-out."[10]

Indications

Any candidate for an outside-in osteotomy correction[1-7] can be eligible for an arthroscopic-guided osteotomy. Absolute indications are a malunion in the coronal plane (shearing-type fractures) causing secondary carpal subluxation and any fracture with a step-off of 2 mm or more, whether or not the patient is symptomatic. Some authors[11] believe that step-offs of just 1 mm also can be symptomatic, and it seems sensible in young patients with

an intrafacetary step-off to go ahead with the operation. Low-demand patients or silent areas (e.g., the interfacetal sulcus) are better served by a conservative approach.

Timing is important, and delaying the operation would have a negative impact on the outcome in two ways. First, healthy areas of cartilage would wear out, particularly in intrafacetary step-offs.[2,12] Second, the operation would be technically more difficult, and the reduction obtained would be less accurate; this is because the gap would be filled with mature bone (rather than scarred bone and granulating tissue), making it more difficult to achieve reduction and to close the gap. Additionally, overzealous resection of tissue in the gap may cause narrowing of the radius in the frontal plane (see **Fig. W9-5** online) causing ulnar translocation of the carpus.

Although my experience is limited to malunions less than 3.5 months old, I cannot see any contraindication in older malunions, provided that the cartilage is preserved. Surgical tactics vary slightly for older malunions (see later). Delaying the operation in the hope that some cases may not be symptomatic does not seem reasonable because midterm osteoarthritis has been shown to occur in most intra-articular malunions in young individuals.[13,14]

Contraindications

Apart from the customary contraindications to any wrist arthroscopy (mainly active infection locally), I cannot see any reason for not trying to correct a malunited fragment or fragments if local conditions are met. Wearing out of the cartilage on the opposing carpal bone is a contraindication for the procedure because restoration of the joint congruency would not prevent osteoarthrosis in the short term. As discussed previously, intrafacetary malunions are probably tolerated worse than interfacetary malunions, but to contraindicate the procedure on timing alone is unwise. A patient with a huge step-off who has not moved the wrist much would wear the cartilage out less than a patient who has a small step-off but has undergone intensive physiotherapy. Another contraindication for this procedure is when an area of multifragmentation with scarring is found on the distal radius. In these cases, the patient would be better served with other options.

Surgical Technique

Web Video

The surgical technique is more cumbersome and complicated than the average wrist arthroscopy.[10] First, it requires an open exposure of the distal radius for plate fixation of the fragments in addition to the arthroscopic-aided osteotomy. Second, it requires alternating the hand from a suspended position to flat on the operating table. We use a custom-made system that allows easy fastening and release of the hand to and from the bow

57-1

543

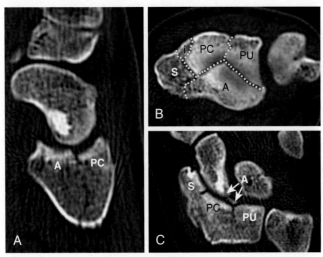

FIGURE 57-1 Preoperative computed tomography scan of a C3.1 fracture. **A**, A 3.5-mm step-off on the scaphoid fossa. A, anterior fragment; PC, posterior central fragment. **B**, Corresponding axial view of the same case, showing a multipiece fracture. The styloid (S), posterior central (PC) fragment, and small (i) intermiddle fragment are depressed, in relation to the anterior fragment (A) and the posteroulnar fragment (PU) (see **C**). **C**, Coronal computed tomography scan showing the depression of the styloid (S) and posterior central (PC) fragment in relation to the posteroulnar (PU) and anterior (A) fragments. Only the former fragments require correction. *(From del Piñal F, Garcia-Bernal FJ, Delgado J, et al: Correction of malunited intra-articular distal radius fractures with an inside-out osteotomy technique. J Hand Surg [Am]. 2006; 31:1029-1034; with permission from the American Society for Surgery of the Hand.)*

(**Fig. 57-2**).[10] Third, fluoroscopy is used periodically during the procedure, which is facilitated by placing the hand flat. The osteotomes and probes that are used need to be sturdier than the average arthroscopic instruments (**Fig. 57-3**). Finally, the assistance of another experienced surgeon is integral to the procedure (**Fig. 57-4**). It is important that everyone on the surgical team is prepared and familiar with their assigned role to diminish the operative time because the whole procedure needs to be done in less than tourniquet time. It is helpful for the surgeon to preplan the osteotomies beforehand based on a review of the preoperative x-rays and, if possible, the original fracture films. I have found a good-quality preoperative computed tomography scan to be invaluable because the intraoperative view of the joint disruption can be quite misleading (see Fig. 57-1).

The key of the whole operation is to perform the arthroscopy without infusion water, which we have called "dry arthroscopy."[15] This dry technique prevents the constant vision losses owing to water escaping through the portals that we experienced with the classic (wet) technique and that made us abandon our initial attempts to perform the osteotomy. The dry technique has two additional advantages: There is no risk of massive fluid extravasation causing compartment syndrome, and the open part of the operation is done without the tissues being infiltrated with water. Not infusing water engenders a new set of difficulties secondary to vision loss owing to splashes and blood staining. Numerous tricks are available to deal with these hindrances, and these are discussed separately later in this chapter.

Osteotomy

The arm is exsanguinated and stabilized to the table with a strap at the arm. In early malunions, the procedure is started by preparing the proposed site of plate fixation with the arm lying on the

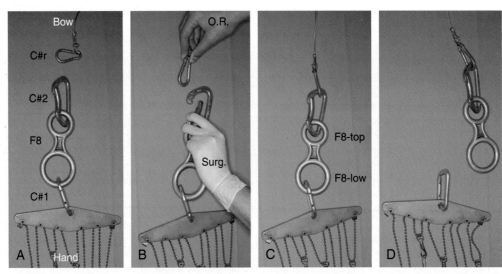

FIGURE 57-2 Method for maintaining sterility when changing from a vertical traction position, suitable for arthroscopy, to a standard surgical position, with the hand flat on the table. **A**, The hand, held with Chinese traps, hangs from "carabiner 1" (C#1), a figure-of-eight descender (F8), "carabiner 2" (C#2), and the "bow's rope carabiner" (C#R). (Carabiners and figure-of-eight descenders can be purchased at any climbing shop.) **B**, The surgeon, under sterile conditions, connects C#2 to C#R, which is held by the operating room personnel. **C**, During arthroscopy, only the lower hole of F8 is considered sterile (F8-low) because the other hole (F8-top) comes into indirect contact with C#R. **D**, To transfer the hand to a horizontal position, the surgeon unfastens C#1. To put the hand into traction again, the surgeon needs only to fasten C#1 to F8-low, which maintains sterility at all times. All but C#R are sterile. *(From del Piñal F, Garcia-Bernal FJ, Delgado J, et al: Correction of malunited intra-articular distal radius fractures with an inside-out osteotomy technique. J Hand Surg [Am]. 2006; 31:1029-1034; with permission from the American Society for Surgery of the Hand.)*

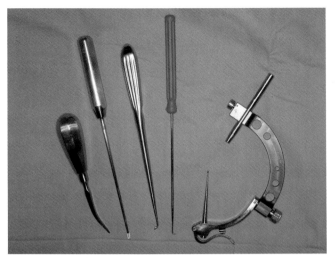

FIGURE 57-3 Instrumentation required for the procedure *(from left to right)*: impactor, osteotome, strong angled curet, shoulder probe, small joint arthroscopic guide. *(From del Piñal F, Garcia-Bernal FJ, Delgado J, et al: Correction of malunited intra-articular distal radius fractures with an inside-out osteotomy technique. J Hand Surg [Am]. 2006; 31:1029-1034; with permission from the American Society for Surgery of the Hand.)*

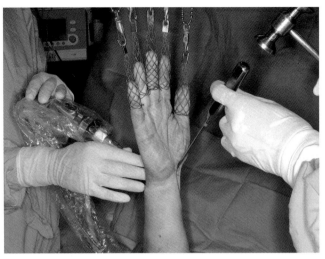

FIGURE 57-5 The osteotomy is being done through the volar-radial portal, while the assistant is holding the camera. Often at the same time, the second surgeon is directing the osteotomy through a dorsal 3,4 portal. *(From del Piñal F: Correction of mal-united intraarticular distal radius fractures with an inside-out osteotomy technique. In Slutsky D, Nagle D, eds: Techniques in Wrist and Hand Arthoscopy. Elsevier, 2007.)*

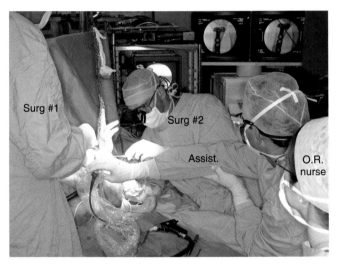

FIGURE 57-4 **The setup.** The first surgeon is controlling the reduction, while the second surgeon is stabilizing the reduction by introducing the distal pegs on the plate. A resident is holding the camera (Ass#1). The first surgeon has in front the arthroscopic tower and the fluoroscopy display. *(From del Piñal F: Correction of mal-united intraarticular distal radius fractures with an inside-out osteotomy technique. In Slutsky D, Nagle D, eds: Techniques in Wrist and Hand Arthoscopy. Elsevier, 2007.)*

hand table. A limited volar-ulnar incision is used for a volar shearing type of intra-articular malunion. A limited Henry approach is used in cases of a malunited radial styloid fragment or multifragmented malunion. A plate is preplaced and held in position with a single screw through its stem. Then the arthroscopic part begins.

The surgical tactics for late-presenting malunions (>3 months) or for cases in which a high suspicion of carpal ligament injury exists are reversed. In these cases, an exploratory arthroscopy, to assess the quality of the cartilage articular surface or the integrity of the ligaments, is recommended first. If local conditions are met, the hand is released from traction, and with the hand lying flat, the appropriate incision and plate are placed. In both instances,

when the plate is preplaced, the hand is then placed in traction with the fingers pointing upward. In most cases, we use 7 kg (15.5 lb) of traction applied to all fingers.

The standard 3,4 and 6R portals are developed. Transverse 1-cm skin incisions are preferred on the dorsum of the wrist because they heal with a minimal scar. To avoid lacerating any nerve or tendon, a superficial skin incision is made with a no. 15 blade. A hemostat is used to widen the portal to permit the smooth entrance of the osteotomes and other necessary instruments. Apart from dorsal portals, a volar radial (VR) portal is always used. If a Henry type of incision is planned, the portal is developed as recommended by Levy and Glickel[16]; otherwise, we follow the techniques of Doi and coworkers[11] or Slutsky[17] (**Fig. 57-5**). The quality of the articular cartilage over the adjacent scaphoid and lunate is assessed along with exploration of the midcarpal joint if there is any doubt about the integrity of the interosseous ligaments.

Initially, a 2.7-mm scope is introduced through the 3,4 portal, and the joint is palpated (for this we prefer the stronger shoulder probe). The consistency of the cartilage and the presence and location of steps are assessed. A shaver can be helpful to remove the synovitis and fibrin, which are always present and obscure the view (2.9-mm incisor blade; 2.9-mm barrel abrader; Dyonics, Smith & Nephew Inc., Andover, MA). Air should flow freely into the joint when the suction of the synoviotome or bur is working; otherwise, the suction sucks the capsule in, obscuring the view. Sufficient air enters through the side tube of the arthroscope's sheath. The surgeon should keep the valve open throughout the procedure.

When major cartilage destruction has been ruled out, and the fragments to be mobilized are defined, the scope is moved to the 6R portal, and the 3,4 and VR portals are used for instrumentation. For cutting the fragments, we use periosteal elevators that are commercially available for shoulder surgery (Artrex AR-1342-30° and AR-1342-15°; Artrex, Naples, FL). These elevators have a width of 4 mm and are strong enough to cut the fragments by gently tapping with a hammer. More recently, we have incorporated straight and curved osteotomes (Artrex AR-1770 and AR-

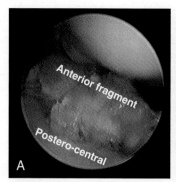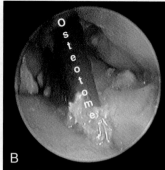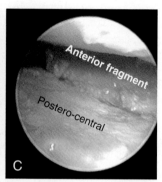

FIGURE 57-6 Correction of a step-off in the same patient as shown in Figure 57-1. Right wrist, the arthroscope is in 6R; at the very far upper left corner is the styloid. **A,** Step-off on the scaphoid fossa. **B,** The osteotome (entering the joint through the volar-radial portal) is separating the malunited fragments. **C,** Corresponding view after reduction. *(From del Piñal F, Garcia-Bernal FJ, Delgado J, et al: Correction of malunited intra-articular distal radius fractures with an inside-out osteotomy technique. J Hand Surg [Am]. 2006; 31:1029-1034; with permission from the American Society for Surgery of the Hand.)*

1771), which can be helpful because their different shapes are ideally suited to following the irregular shape of the fracture lines. To avoid the risk of lacerating extensor tendons when introducing the "osteotomes" through the 3,4 portal, the blade of the osteotome should be introduced parallel to the tendon under direct visual control and then rotated while inside the joint. Gentle maneuvers are necessary when hammering from dorsal to volar because there is a risk of cutting flexor tendons if plunging volarly or extensor tendons when doing the reverse maneuver.

I have found that it is easier when there is an established metaphyseal callus to start by removing this callus and doing the osteotomy in this area. The osteotome blade is directed perpendicular to the shaft of the radius, precutting the malunited fragment. Then, during the arthroscopy, the surgeon would have to cut only the cartilaginous malunion, and the fragment would be free without undue maneuvers that may damage the cartilage.

The displaced fragments are fully mobilized by carefully prying them apart with the osteotome. In most cases, the fragments are disimpacted and easily elevated by hooking them with a strong shoulder probe and pulling upward. On one occasion, we had to resort to elevation of a fragment from the outside with the use of a Steinmann pin that was introduced into the exact spot and advanced through a small arthroscopic guide (Ref 4291; Dyonics, Smith &Nephew Inc., Andover, MA).

Often scar and new bone formation between the fragments impede reduction. This early granulation tissue should be resected with the help of small curets or burs introduced through the portals. When the reduction is acceptable (**Fig. 57-6**), one surgeon maintains the position of the fragments, while the assistant inserts the distal locking pegs in the plate. This step may be difficult because the flexor carpi radialis and digital flexors are under tension (owing to the traction) and impede insertion of any ulnar screws in the plate. This step is facilitated by backing off the wrist traction sufficiently to allow tendon retraction by insertion of a Farabeuf type of retractor. A compromise must be made to prevent a complete collapse of the radiocarpal space.

When the articular fragments have been secured under arthroscopic control, the hand is laid flat on the operating table, and the rest of the screws are inserted in the plate. The type of fixation depends on the configuration of the malunion. In one case, we used a single screw to secure the volar-ulnar fragment. In

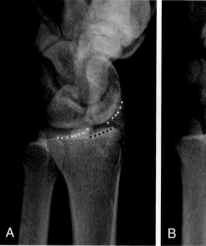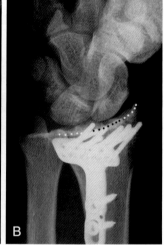

FIGURE 57-7 **A,** Preoperative x-ray of the same patient in Figures 57-1, 57-6, and 57-8 (depressed fragments highlighted by *black dots*). **B,** Restoration of the articular line (6 weeks). *(From del Piñal F, Garcia-Bernal FJ, Delgado J, et al: Correction of malunited intra-articular distal radius fractures with an inside-out osteotomy technique. J Hand Surg [Am]. 2006; 31:1029-1034; with permission from the American Society for Surgery of the Hand.)*

another, a 2.7-mm buttress plate was used to stabilize a styloid fragment. In the most common situation in which there are four or more fragments, a plate with locking distal pegs is preferred (DVR; Hand Innovations, Miami, FL) (**Fig. 57-7**).

The hand is suspended again under traction for a final inspection of the articular surface. The joint is irrigated with 10 to 30 mL of saline introduced through the scope's side tube, and a shaver is used to remove all the debris. Fluoroscopy can be used repeatedly throughout the procedure by releasing the hand from the traction bow (see Fig. 57-2). Some authors find it easier to perform wrist arthroscopy with the hand lying flat on the table, but we have no experience with this technique.[18]

The portals are closed with paper tape or a single stitch, and the wrist is placed in a removable splint. In all our cases, the fixation was sufficiently stable to start protected range of motion on the first postoperative visit (48 hours) (**Fig. 57-8**).

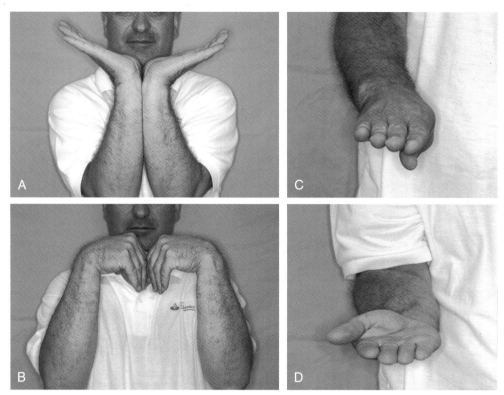

FIGURE 57-8 Results of the same patient as in Figure 57-7 after 18 months (right wrist).

Modifications to Improve Vision When Using the Dry Technique

The dry technique introduces a new set of difficulties derived from vision loss secondary to splashes of blood or soft tissue debris that may stick to the scope tip. Removing the scope and wiping off the lens with a wet sponge is efficacious but time-consuming. Poor vision quality or being immersed in a "red sea" may make the surgeon abandon this technique, which has a lot to offer. Based on our experience with more than 100 dry wrist arthroscopies, we have found the following technical tips helpful[15]:

+ First, avoid getting too close with the tip of the scope when working with burs or osteotomes to avoid splashes that might block your vision. It is preferable first to inspect the area of interest and then slightly pull the scope back before inserting your working instrument. For the same reason, avoid touching the tip of the scope with your instruments (e.g., probe, synoviotomes).

+ If you get a minor splash at the tip of your scope, you can remove it by gently rubbing the tip of the scope on the local soft tissue (e.g., capsule, fat). This maneuver clears the view sufficiently.

+ If there is blood or blood clots (as after a fracture), you can clear any debris by injecting with 10 to 20 mL of saline through the side valve of the scope and then aspirating with the synoviotome. This should provide a sufficiently dry field.

+ It is ideal to have an absolute dry field, and for this we use small (13 × 13 mm) or medium (25 × 25 mm) surgical patties (Ref 800-04000, size ½ inch × ½ inch; Ref 800-04003, size 1 inch × 1 inch [25 × 25 mm]; Neuray; Xomed, Jacksonville, FL). The small patty can be rolled and directly introduced into the joint by a grasper. The large patties have to be slightly modified by cutting them into the shape of a triangle, which facilitates removal from the joint. If the patties become entangled, they can be removed by pulling on the tail or by retrieving with a grasper (**Fig. 57-9**).

+ The synoviotome, bur, or any other instruments connected to a suction machine can clog because the aspirated debris dries out. Frequent clearing is required by injecting saline through the tubing. This clogging can be minimized by periodic saline aspiration from an external basin.

+ If the arthroscopy is done immediately after elevating the tourniquet, vision can be poor, improving as the operation proceeds. We realized the vision impairment was caused by condensation at the tip of the scope as a consequence of the different temperatures (the joint still was warm and the scope at room temperature). As time passes, vision improves as the hand cools down. This is easily overcome by immersing the tip of the scope tip in warm saline for a few minutes before beginning surgery.

+ Finally, most times the vision is not completely clear, but still sufficient to accomplish the goals of the procedure safely. Having a completely clear field except for specific times during the procedure is unnecessary and wastes valuable time.

Results

The technique presented here is drawn from experience in five patients with nascent intra-articular malunions of short duration (5 weeks to 3.5 months) with a follow-up of 6 months to 2.5 years. Two patients had a single fragment mobilized (one antero-medial fragment, one styloid fragment) with severe functional limitation (**Fig. 57-10**). The other three patients had two or more

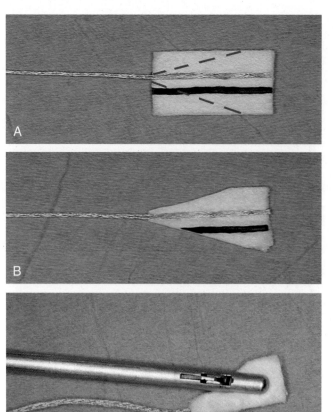

FIGURE 57-9 **A** and **B**, To dry out the surgical field, the neurosurgical patties have been modified (**A**), and the squared tail part has been cut to facilitate its removal (**B**). **C**, The patty is rolled and introduced into the joint with a grasper. To prevent the patty from entangling or breaking inside the joint, the grasper (not the tail) is used to retrieve it. Breakage is not much of a problem because the remaining segment can be retrieved easily with the grasper. *(From del Piñal F, Garcia-Bernal FJ, Regalado J, et al: Dry arthroscopy: surgical technique. J Hand Surg [Am]. 2007; 32:119-123, with permission from the American Society for Surgery of the Hand.)*

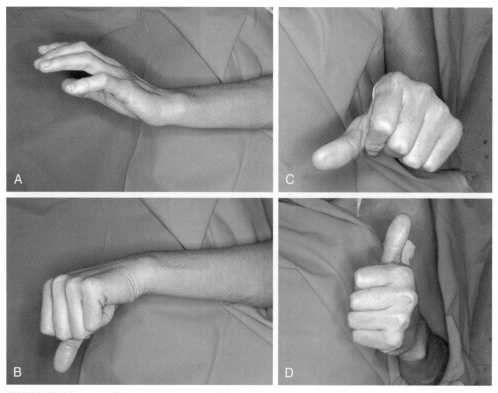

FIGURE 57-10 **A** to **D**, This patient was seen 3.5 months after sustaining a distal radius fracture treated with an external fixator and Kirschner wires. Notice total blockage of supination.

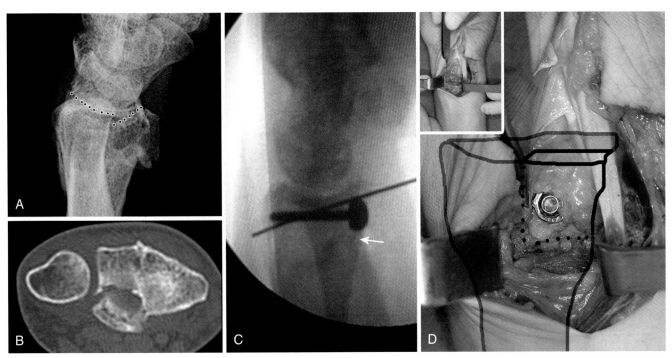

FIGURE 57-11 **A** and **B**, A displaced volar-ulnar fragment involving the radiocarpal and the distal radioulnar joint was evident. This single fragment was responsible for minimal range of motion and loss of supination. **C**, The malunited fragment was reduced provisionally with a Kirschner wire, and then, with the hand lying on the table, a 2.7-mm screw with a washer was used for fixation. (Fluoroscopic control; *arrow* points to the reduced volar cortex). **D**, Notice minimal disturbance of the soft tissue attachments around the fragment at the end of the operation.

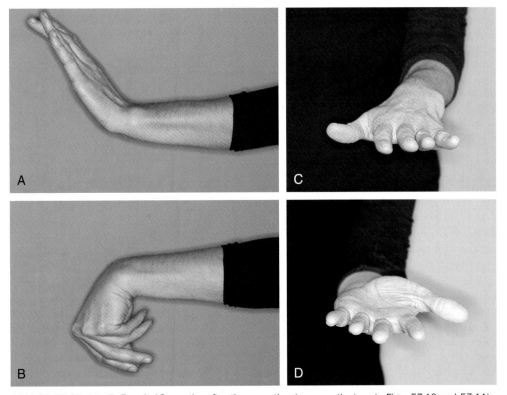

FIGURE 57-12 **A** to **D**, Result 18 months after the operation (same patient as in Figs. 57-10 and 57-11).

fragments mobilized (all had C31 fractures of the AO classification). Gaps of less than 1 mm were unavoidable after the operation because of a preexisting loss of cartilage and early granulation tissue, but intra-articular steps were reduced to 0 mm (from a maximum of 5 mm).

It may be argued that fragments may be more easily defined early on by simply breaking the external callus. Based on the experience of our group and others, however, impacted cartilage containing fracture fragments is soundly healed by 3 to 4 weeks and needs to be redefined with the use of an osteotome.[3,19] Piecemeal fragmentation can occur if the mobilization is not done carefully. Herein lies the main advantage of the procedure: The arthroscope allows us to follow the exact line of chondral fracture under magnification and to restore the anatomy of the cartilaginous surface. Additionally, the risk of avascular necrosis of the mobilized fragments is minimized as nominal interference with the soft tissue connections of the fragments occurs. Finally, the capsular ligaments are not violated (**Fig. 57-11**). All these facts together with rigid fixation allow rapid healing and permit immediate mobilization (**Fig. 57-12**).

The inside-out technique is a minimally invasive procedure that allows full assessment of the articular deformity, a more precise osteotomy, and mobilization of the displaced fracture fragments. Irregular fragments, not amenable to other techniques, can be dealt with by this procedure. Correction of step-offs was achieved in every case with an accuracy of 0 mm. Residual gaps of about 1 mm were common owing to cartilage loss, interposition of newly formed bone, and presumably cartilage destruction from the original injury. Understanding of the intricacies of the dry technique is needed to perform the procedure in a safe, efficient manner. An accomplished arthroscopist would not have any undue difficulty incorporating the dry technique. As for any change from a familiar technique to one less so, some patience is needed at the beginning to overcome the initial frustrations secondary to vision losses. A giant leap is made when the surgeon understands and accepts that a perfect view is not needed except for some steps of the operation. The procedure can be incorporated easily by any surgeon familiar with wrist arthroscopy (see Video 57-1).

REFERENCES

1. Saffar P: Treatment of distal radial intra-articular malunions. In Saffar PH, Cooney WP III, eds: Fractures of the Distal Radius. London: Martin Dunitz, 1995.

2. Fernandez DL: Reconstructive procedures for malunion and traumatic arthritis. Orthop Clin North Am. 1993; 24: 341-363.

3. Marx RG, Axelrod TS: Intraarticular osteotomy of distal radius malunions. Clin Orthop. 1996; 327:152-157.

4. Gonzalez del Pino J, Nagy L, Gonzalez Hernandez E, et al: Osteotomías intraarticulares complejas del radio por fractura. Indicaciones y técnica quirúrgica. Rev Ortop Traumatol. 2000; 44:406-417.

5. Ring D, Prommersberger KJ, Gonzalez del Pino J, et al: Corrective osteotomy for malunited articular fractures of the distal radius. J Bone Joint Surg Am. 2005; 87:1503-1509.

6. Thivaios GC, McKee MD: Sliding osteotomy for deformity correction following malunion of volarly displaced distal radial fractures. J Orthop Trauma. 2003; 17:326-333.

7. Apergis E: Proceedings of the 9th Congress of the International Federation of Societies for Surgery of the Hand, Budapest, Hungary, June 13-17, 2004.

8. Prommersberger KJ, Ring D, Del Pino JG, et al: Corrective osteotomy for intra-articular malunion of the distal part of the radius: surgical technique. J Bone Joint Surg Am. 2006; 88(Suppl 1, Pt 2):202-211.

9. Edwards CC 2nd, Haraszti CJ, McGillivary GR, et al: Intra-articular distal radius fractures: arthroscopic assessment of radiographically assisted reduction. J Hand Surg [Am]. 2001; 26:1036-1041.

10. del Piñal F, Garcia-Bernal FJ, Delgado J, et al: Correction of malunited intra-articular distal radius fractures with an inside-out osteotomy technique. J Hand Surg [Am]. 2006; 31:1029-1034.

11. Doi K, Hattori Y, Otsuka K, et al: Intra-articular fractures of the distal aspect of the radius: arthroscopically assisted reduction compared with open reduction and internal fixation. J Bone Joint Surg Am. 1999; 81:1093-1110.

12. Wagner WF Jr, Tencer AF, Kiser P, et al: Effects of intra-articular distal radius depression on wrist joint contact characteristics. J Hand Surg [Am]. 1996; 21:554-660.

13. Knirk JL, Jupiter JB: Intra-articular fractures of the distal end of the radius in young adults. J Bone Joint Surg Am. 1986; 68:647-659.

14. Trumble TE, Schmitt SR, Vedder NB: Factors affecting functional outcome of displaced intra-articular distal radius fractures. J Hand Surg [Am]. 1994; 19:325-340.

15. del Piñal F, Garcia-Bernal FJ, Regalado J, et al: Dry arthroscopy: surgical technique. J Hand Surg [Am]. 2007; 32:119-123.

16. Levy HJ, Glickel SZ: Arthroscopic assisted internal fixation of volar intraarticular wrist fractures. Arthroscopy. 1993; 9:122-124.

17. Slutsky DJ: Clinical applications of volar portals in wrist arthroscopy. Tech Hand Upper Extrem Surg. 2004; 8:229-238.

18. Huracek J, Troeger H: Wrist arthroscopy without distraction: a technique to visualise instability of the wrist after a ligamentous tear. J Bone Joint Surg Br. 2000; 82:1011-1012.

19. del Piñal F, Garcia-Bernal FJ, Delgado J, et al: Results of osteotomy, open reduction, and internal fixation for late-presenting malunited intra-articular fractures of the base of the middle phalanx. J Hand Surg [Am]. 2005; 30:1039-1050.

Index

Note: Page numbers followed by *f* and *t* indicate figures and tables, respectively. Page numbers followed by *b* indicate boxed material.